W9-COD-961

What People Are Saying About This Book . . .

This is a much needed book. There is no other publication like it. David has done a marvelous job in presenting the chemistry of essential oils in a clear, readable, and enjoyable way for everyone. A good scientific work. Lots of good data. I recommend this book to everyone who uses therapeutic oils and wants to understand how and why they work.

Terry Shepherd Friedmann, M.D., A.B.H.M.
Cofounder, American Board of Holistic Medicine
Author of *Freedom Through Health* and other books

Dr. Stewart has created another masterpiece! With a kiss of the Divine with nature, he has brilliantly woven his artistry to bring the Spiritually etheric oils into the Scientific realm for our understanding of nature's physicality and purpose. In this informative, practical and down-to-earth book, Dr. Stewart takes the reader on a chemical journey from the infinitesimally small structure of a molecule to the Infinite Cosmos revealing God's signature in all of creation. God's love has also manifested through Dr. Stewart's dedication in his written words. This is a magnificent must read book for anyone using essential oils.

Sabina M. DeVita, Ed.D., D.N.M.
Author of *Saving Face* and other books
President, Institute for Energy Wellness Studies
Brampton, Ontario, Canada

He's done it again! Dr. Stewart's new book proves once again that nature is truly a testimony to God—even at the scale of atoms and electrons. Even a child can see why chemistry makes sense when described in terms of the Creator. If chemistry could have been this clear when I went to school, it would actually have been fun. The awesome order of God's creation on a molecular level helps me appreciate His providence more than ever before. A treasury of scientific detail in common language that gives expanded meaning to God's provisions for his children. This book fills an important need not met by any other publication.

Rev. Dennis Peterson
Author of *Unlocking the Mysteries of Creation*
Director of the Creation Resource Foundation
Eldorado, California

This book is fabulous. In fact, it's brilliant. An invaluable resource to any student studying essential oils. Dr. Stewart's knowledge and very honest views of the use of essential oils are excellent, tactfully described, and yet humorous to read. The information is really superb. I am adding this to my list of recommended books for my students as an absolute must.

> *Susan Duerden Neary, Certified Educator*
> Salon Owner and Aromatherapy Lecturer
> Clitheroe, Lancashire, Great Britain

A beautiful book. A chemistry book, yes. But it flows like music. A symphony in words.

> *Marriane W. Morse*
> *Aromatherapist and Raindrop Facilitator*
> *Marlborough, New Hampshire*

A truly inspired work of art. A blending of the spiritual and scientific wonders of the gift of essential oils on this planet. This book opens up a whole new world of intrigue with fascinating presentations that lead to an understanding of how and why oils work in sync with our physical, emotional, and spiritual bodies. Dr. Stewart creatively weaves in stories which are so valuable for insight, clarification, and making this a wonderfully flowing story of God's blessings. This book also has the best and clearest explanations I have ever found of pH, allergies, and other health-related topics. This is definitely the chemistry of essential oils made simple . . . as well as profound!

> *Connie Adams, C.M.T., F.C.C.I.*
> Certified Aromatherapy Instructor and Massage Therapist
> Fairfield, California

Your chemistry book is fabulous and will be a best-seller. I love the humor, simplicity, depth of knowledge, and the way you have brought science and religion together, as it should be. This is a book I definitely want to carry here at my center. It will help the lay person, as well as the scientist, to understand the profound healing effects of essential oils within the human body and how to use that information to both select oils and to prayerfully decide a course of action to facilitate healing. Thanks so much for taking the time to write this book!

> *Vicki Opfer*
> Diamond Distributor, Young Living Essential Oils
> Aromatherapy Educator and National Trainer
> Denver, Colorado

In his book, on *The Chemistry of Essential Oils*, Dr. David Stewart has, to my knowledge, gone where no author has ever gone before. He explains the complex organic chemistries, as well as some practical uses, of these natural plant-distilled oils so that anyone with a high-school education can comprehend them. And he has presented the material in a wonderfully engaging way, undergirded by a devout Scriptural perspective as well!

Readers will find in this volume a fresh, challenging, and complementary alternative point of view for the practice of medicine and the healing arts, which no doubt will stimulate some beneficial and much needed debate. I believe Dr. Stewart is on the "cutting edge" of a gentle revolution in American healthcare.

Robert W. Miner, M.D.
Christian Psychiatrist
Grand Rapids, Michigan

In this information-packed book, Dr. Stewart, a truly gifted writer and teacher takes us step-by-step from the basic building blocks of the physical universe to an understanding of how essential oils fit into the Divine Plan. This wonderful new book transcends the compartmentalism of modern science and religion, lifting us into a refreshing space where reality becomes a reverent understanding of God's magnificent creation.

Edward R. Close, Ph.D.
Author of several books, including *Transcendental Physics, Reality Begins with Conciousness,* and *Nature's Mold Rx*
Jackson, Missouri

This is the most beautiful love story in the guise of chemistry. It empowers me to say things in my church I was never able to say before. Yes, it is a chemistry book, but the way you explain the love of God in terms of chemistry, it make me cry every time I read it. It is like a book of devotions. Thank you. Thank you.

Nancy Day
Maggie Valley, North Carolina

I have just finished reading your chemistry book twice!!! I love it! You are amazing! I am wowed, enriched, and pleasantly surprised at the humor, love and simplicity of Chemistry explained by your Divine teaching. Thank you for sharing your precious gift with us!!!

Katrina Harrison
Essential Oils Teacher and Raindrop Facilitator
Cochrane, Alberta, Canada

It is often said the best way to make a contribution to society is to discover a need and fill it. Dr. David Stewart has done just that by offering technical, scientific, and what could have been very challenging information in a simplified, interesting, easy-to-understand manner. For thousands of us who use, work with, and educate about therapeutic-grade essential oils, this is the piece we have needed to better understand how to choose our oils wisely for the most effective results. It affords us the opportunity to become more professional in our craft.

Dr. Stewart is a rare individual who possesses the skill to combine his left-brain knowledge and expertise with a compassionate heart and a desire to bring his vast storehouse of information to the lay person in clear, understandable terms.

This book is an amazing blend of the factual and the spiritual, woven together with David's magical touch, which has produced a brilliant piece of work. This is an invaluable resource, and will take a prominent place in my library.

> *Joy Linsley*
> Ambassador Master Star
> Young Living Essential Oils
> Naperville, Illinois

This book was so enlightening to me. I thought your classes were great, but your book has really given me a deeper and fuller understanding in a way that is both useful in my practice and also for all people searching for answers to how these oils work and why they work so well. Your book is easy reading and the content perfect for myself as I have no background in chemistry. I will keep it with the rest of my most important reference books.

> *Barbara Newton, C.C.I.*
> Aromatologist and Raindrop Instructor
> Jerome, Michigan

Phenomenal! This book hardly deserves to be deemed a dry category of chemistry! Dr. Stewart makes, what is for many people a boring subject, something alive and full of interest. For the first time, I understand how chemistry and vibrational frequency relate. He has done a great service for those of us in healing work and in the art of aromatherapy. The book is truly a treasure for those with or without a scientific background.

> *Linda L. Smith R.N., M.S.*
> Author of *Healing Oils, Healing Hands,* and other books.
> President, Healing Touch Spiritual Ministry, Inc.
> Arvada, Colorado

We are delighted to recommend this book. It is the first to address positively the dilemma over supposedly toxic oils as well as the undoubtedly beneficial use of certain oils neat for certain conditions. It is refreshing to find someone else who feels our wonderful essential oils are unnecessarily maligned when all that is needed is more knowledge on the chemistry, which this book provides. The book also rightly explains how tests done on animals with single components or perfume quality oils cannot be related to the use of genuine essential oils on people.

Shirley and Len Price, Aromatherapy Instructors
Authors of *Aromatherapy for Health Professionals*
and *Understanding Hydrolats*
Hinckley, Great Britain

What a wonderful reference!! A must read for any one wanting to understand the chemistry of therapeutic essential oils and how they can be of value to mankind. A great source for both the layman and the professional alike. David has made the science and chemistry of essential oils easy to understand. This is one book I want in my library.

Joanne Schwarm, L.P.N .
Raindrop Practitioner,
Burlington, Iowa

As a nurse for almost 30 years, Dr. Stewart's book has finally given me "scientific permission" to follow the "whispers of God" in my heart. I've always felt led in the care of the patients God has brought to me, but I often yielded to what medicine mandates instead of honoring God's leadings. Dr. Stewart reminds each of us to listen and be inspired by God's handiwork. This is a historical work! I congratulate you and thank you, Dr. Stewart.

Fran Norton, R.N., S.C.C.I.
Aromatherapy Instructor
Certified Childbirth Educator (AHCC)
Wentzville, Missouri

I love reading your chemistry book. Your introduction even made me cry. Your heart is so pure and wonderful, it so shines in your book. It is so evident that you love what you are writing about. It makes reading the book so much fun!

Larkin Busby
Practicing Aromatherapist, Raindrop Facilitator, and Teacher
St. James, Missouri

A monumental work whose significance is surmounted only by its depth, breadth, heart, and soulful explanations of God's love manifest in even the tiniest quanta of his creation. For those who have ears, let them hear. Those who have eyes, let them see. For those who wish to know of God's love and those who want to love God in an ever greater or deeper way, this book must be read.

The power and love of God for every infinitesmal particle of creation is magnified, made clear, and visible for anyone to see in this book. Read it. It will change your life forever for the better. If there were only one book you could buy and read this year, you couldn't do better than this one. It rekindles a childlike awe for the wonder of God's love.

Jacqui Close, R.A.
Registered Aromatherapist
Aromatherapy Instructor, Southeast Missouri State University
Cape Girardeau, Missouri

Although I had made numerous attempts to study the chemistry of essential oils over the years, it wasn't until I read *The Chemistry Essential Oils Made Simple*, by Dr. David Stewart, that I was able to achieve breakthroughs in my understanding with such ease. "To get understanding is to be chosen above silver." (Proverbs 16:16) As you read this book, I encourage you to gaze in childlike delight while David gently lays his hand on your shoulder and focuses the lens as you read. Take a closer look, and learn more of our Creator, His love and care for you, through the intricate design He has placed in these precious, treasured gifts of essential oils.

Kathy Spohn, F.C.C.I.
Certified Instructor in Raindrop, Vitaflex, Oils of Scripture,
Essential Oil Chemistry, and Emotional Release
Wyoming, Michigan

I am so impresseed with your book. It is so well laid out and I just love the way you elucidate the facts of the matter and then apply the theory onto the oils and how they work. It really is brilliant. When I first saw a stack of the books at your workshop and read the title, "The Chemistry of Essential Oils Made Simple," I was thinking, "If it really is so simple, why is the book two inches thick?" But now I eat humble pie. You really have made it simple. It truly is an excellent work. I recommend it over and over again for the valuable insights you provide. Thank you.

Neena Love. Q.M.T., R.T.P.
Yandina, Queensland, Australia

THE
CHEMISTRY
OF ESSENTIAL OILS
MADE SIMPLE

*God's Love
Manifest in Molecules*

by

David Stewart, Ph.D., D.N.M.
Integrated Aromatic Science Practitioner

Care Publications
Fourth Printing
2013

ISBN 0-934426-99-6
LCCN 2004091768

1st printing 3,300 copies (2005) • 2nd printing 5,500 copies (2006)
3rd printing 5,500 copies (2010) • 4th printing 11,000 copies (2013)

Care Publications
RR 4, Box 646, Marble Hill, MO 63764
(800) 758-8629 • careclasses@raindroptraining.com
www.RaindropTraining.com or www.CarePublications.net

Price: $49.95 USD

IMPORTANT NOTICE

The information in this book is intended for education purposes only. It is not provided in order to diagnose, prescribe, or treat any disease, illness, or injured condition of the body. The author, publisher, and printer accept no responsibility for such use. Anyone suffering from any disease, illness, or injury should consult with a physician or other appropriate licensed health care professional.

Publisher's Cataloging–in–Publication
(Provided by Quality Books, Inc.)

Stewart, David, 1937 –
     The chemistry of essential oils made simple: God's love manifest in molecules / by David Stewart. -- 1st ed.
     p.cm.
     Includes bibliographical references and index.
     LCCN 20040911768
     ISBN 0-934426-99-6

     1. Aromatherapy. 2. Essences and essential oils--
Therapeutic use--Testing. 3. Bible--Criticism, interpretation, etc. I Title.

RM666.A68S84 2004   615'.321
                                                    QB104-800037

13 14 15 16 17 18 19 20

DEDICATION
TO MY WIFE, LEE,

who knows all my faults, has to live with them, and loves me any-how. She has been my life partner and best friend for more than fifty years and a constant source of insight and inspiration. Many of the thoughts and ideas in this book, and in most of my other publications, have come to me through her. This book, and the many other works that I do and have done, would not have been possible without her selfless support and endless hard work, which are largely unseen, unsung, and unknown to the public. She is my counselor, my lover, the mother of my children, a true mirror in which I can better see myself, a clear window through which I perceive the Divine, and a channel through which I daily receive His Blessings and His Grace.

ACKNOWLEDGMENTS

I wish to thank many people for their assistance in producing this book, including Connie Adams, CCI (Fairfield, CA), Fran Anderssen (Leopold, MO), Margaret Ann Brock (Perryville, MO), Karen Hanna (Lethbridge, AB), Mindy Kirby, CCI (Rutherfordton, NC), Lois Loyek (Battleford, SK), Neena Love, QMT (Australia), Barbara Newton, CCI (Jerome, MI), Fran Norton, RN, FCCI (Wentzville, MO), Anthony Stewart (Marble Hill, MO), Barbara Vissers (Jenison, MI), and others for their excellent proofing of this book, as well as Edward R. Close, Ph.D. (Jackson, MO), Rev. Dennis Peterson (El Dorado, CA), Rev. Jacqueline R. Heitmann (Paoli, PA), and Linda Smith, RN (Arvada, CO) for pointing me in directions I would not have otherwise been aware, and also B. Ray Knox, PhD (Bella Vista, AR), Robert W. Miner, MD (Grand Rapids, MI), Sheila Hay (Tok, AK), Maralyn A. Renner (Ferndale, CA), and Kathy Spohn, FCCI, for their scientific and spiritual insights, to Jacqui Close, RA, CCI (Jackson, MO) and Gloria Miller (Rolla, MO), for their thorough editing and many helpful suggestions. I also want to thank the hundreds of inquiring students who have taken my Chemistry courses over the years whose questions and interest have been the principal stimulus, inspiration, and springboard from which this work came to be written.

Cover Art Caption is on the next page . . .

COVER ART

• Galactic Storms and Aromatic Rings •

Seen here is a photo* of tornado-like structures of the Lagoon Nebula located in the Sagittarius constellation. The dusty brown gas of the Nebula is being continuously ionized by radiation from nearby, hot stars including 0 Herschel 36 (bright red, left center). This is causing a blue mist to evaporate from the Nebula's surface. The temperature difference between the hot surface and cool interior of the Nebula, combined with the radiation from the stars, produces strong shearing forces that twist the clouds into tornados.

This particular picture was chosen as an example of Psalm 19:1, "The heavens are telling the glory of God; and the firmament proclaims His handiwork."

Psalm 19 leads us to recall Romans 1:20, "God's eternal power and divine nature, invisible though they are, have been understood and seen through the things He has made." From this we see that "Invisible though they are, the atoms are also telling the glory of God and the molecules proclaim His handiwork."

The back cover features a resonance energy model of an aromatic (benzene) ring showing a colored spectrum of frequencies. The aromatic ring is a functional group of six carbon atoms with attached hydrogen atoms from which millions of different molecules are fashioned. Vibrational rings of carbon come in countless combinations and are active healing agents in every essential oil.

This is a book about the nature of God revealed through the chemistry of essential oils.

* (Photo by NASA through the Hubble Space Telescope. Images and text © 2003 Photo Researchers, Inc., New York, NY. Reproduced with permission. The aromatic spectral ring model was adapted from an illustration in *Organic Chemistry*, 4th ed., by Francis Cary.)

TABLE OF CONTENTS
Introduction

PART ONE
A SHORT COURSE IN CHEMISTRY
Chapter One

Chapter Two

♥ What Oils Do in Living Plants 51

Chapter Three

Chapter Five

Chapter Six

Chapter Seven

Chapter Eight

♥ Chemotypes and Environmental Factors 234

Chapter Nine

♥ Isoprenes, Terpenes, and PMS 255

Chapter Ten

Chapter Eleven

Chapter Twelve

❤ Practical Answers to Frequently Asked Questions 430

PART TWO
CATALOGS of Compounds
in Essential Oils

PART THREE
BEYOND CHEMISTRY

Preamble

Article One

Article Two

Article Three

Article Four

PART FOUR
APPENDICES & RESOURCES

The heavens are telling the glory of God; and the firmament proclaims his handiwork . . . There is no speech, nor are there words; their voice is not heard; yet their voice goes out through all the earth and their words to the end of the world.   *Psalm 19:1, 3-4*

Ask the plants; speak to the earth, and they will teach you.
                                    Job 12:8

God's eternal power and divine nature, invisible though they are, have been seen and understood through the things he has made.
                                    Romans 1:20

And God said, Let there be light: and there was light. And God saw the light, that it was good.
                                    Genesis 1:3-4

Pray without ceasing. Give thanks in all circumstances: . . .Prove all things. Hold fast to that which is good.   *I Thessalonians 5:17-18, 21*

Every plant yielding seed that is upon the face of all the earth, and every tree with seed in its fruit, I have given you . . .And God saw everything that he had made, and indeed, it was very good.
                                    Genesis 1:29, 31

God is love, and those who abide in love abide in God, and God abides in them.
                                    I John 4:16

♥ Introduction
A LETTER FROM ME TO YOU

Dear Readers,

The purpose of this book is not to make you a chemist. It is to inspire you to see God's hand in the creation of the molecules of essential oils. It is to help you appreciate, through a basic understanding of chemistry, that God loved us before he ever made us and that he was thinking of your well-being and mine when he crafted the molecules of essential oils.

According to Psalm 19, "The heavens are telling the glory of God; and the firmament proclaims his handiwork." The psalmist speaks of the power and nature of God as evidenced in the grandeur of the galaxies, the great dome of the sky, and the infinite scale of the cosmos. The scripture goes on to say that even though inanimate creation does not speak in words, it still has a voice resounding everywhere, to be heard and understood by the spiritually attuned.

While God's presence is visibly manifest in his grand and infinite forms, he can also be experienced in the infinitesimally small. Invisible though they are, the atoms are also telling the glory of God; and the molecules proclaim his handiwork. God is both mightily and minutely active in his creation. I see God's hand written all over the chemistry of essential oils.

This is a book on chemistry, but chemistry with a heart and soul. To you who have little or no background in chemistry, yet desire a basic understanding of the science of essential oils—this book was written for you.

To you who may even fear chemistry and avoided it in school—fear no more. This book was especially written for you.

And to you who may have degrees in chemistry—even advanced degrees—this book is for you, too, because the unique composition and character of essential oils is not found in college textbooks nor is it yet a part of the curriculum of most university regimens. And, as you will discover, the properties of essential oils that bring healing and maintain health cannot be explained solely by materialistic science as we know it. The power of the oils is more than chemistry.

My Life as a Chemist

I have always loved chemistry. My dad was a chemist. He was teaching high school science when I was born back in 1937. He later became a chemist for a local plate glass factory in Crystal City, Missouri. While other boys may have talked fishing and football with their fathers—my dad and I talked chemistry.

My dad loved nature, too, and so did I. We camped a lot as a family and my dad, who loved to teach, was always showing me interesting things about the plants and animals we found. He taught me to listen and learn directly from the forests, the flowers, the rocks, and the trees themselves. So I grew up in an environment that nurtured my hunger for an understanding of the nature of life and the universe and what made everything tick. While I often bombarded my dad with scientific questions on why this or why that, much of my free time as a child was spent alone exploring the woods and streams and caves around our small town. It was then that I learned to gain information and knowledge directly from Nature, herself, beyond what can be found in books or what could be conveyed by spoken words.

As a boy I always wanted a chemistry set. It took several years of asking before my parents fulfilled that dream. It was a Christmas present. I was soon entertaining my family (mom, dad, two sisters, and a brother) with displays of homemade fireworks.

Thus, I learned at an early age that one could get sparkling red colors from strontium nitrate, lavender from potassium, green from boron, orange from carbon, yellow from sodium, and a blinding white from burning magnesium. These were my first lessons in qualitative analysis.

But as a budding boy chemist, fireworks were not quite enough for me. My real desire was to make a bomb. Isn't that what most boys want with a chemistry set? I was eleven at the time.

Recipe for a Bomb

The instruction book that came with my chemistry set did not mention bomb making. Yet, somehow, I found a recipe. It was for making ammonium iodide—a compound that is stable under water, but which explodes on the slightest touch when dry. I had to visit our local pharmacy to purchase some pure iodine crystals. There weren't any in the chemistry set.

That evening after supper I quietly went to our basement where my "lab" was set up. Following the directions of my recipe, I concocted a small batch of ammonium iodide as a precipitate which I then carefully captured as a layer of brown particles onto a piece of filter paper. Gently laying the wet crystal-covered disk of paper on my work bench, away from the rest of my chemicals and apparatus, I then went upstairs to bed. "I'll come back tomorrow morning and set it off when it's dry," I thought to myself. I had not mentioned my plans or what I had done to anyone.

Later that night when I was asleep upstairs, my mom and dad started hearing popping noises coming from the basement. What was happening was that as the wet filter paper began to dry around the edges, some of the unstable crystals started to spontaneously go off one at a time.

Going down to the basement to investigate, my parents began looking around to find the source of the snap, crackle, and pop which was now occurring every few minutes. "Sounds like it's coming from David's table over there," my dad said to my mom, "but all I see is a piece of paper."

He then picked it up, shook it, and held it up to his ear. That's when it exploded. "I saw fire come out and go into his ear!" my mother reported. As for my dad, he had a ringing in his ear and couldn't hear very well for a long time after that.

But they were very nice. I was not punished. They recognized that their son was probably going to be a scientist someday and they didn't want to discourage him. All they said was, "Next time, please let us know what you are doing." They actually laughed about it. The experience provided a story my father would tell many times in the years to follow.

Of course, I was disappointed not to see my bomb go off, but glad there were no serious consequences—neither to my dad nor to myself. I never made another bomb. My boyhood desire had been satisfied.

But my enthusiasm for chemistry was undampened. A year or so later, when I was in the seventh grade, I ran across a copy of the table of the natural elements with their scientific names and symbols. I was so excited that I memorized the whole list just for fun—all 92 of them.

A couple of years later, during my freshman year in high school, I took my first upper level English class. The teacher gave us all an assignment for the semester. It was to write a report on any book of our choosing. I chose a chemistry book. It was entitled "*The Romance of Chemistry.*" When my teacher received the report, he couldn't believe it and asked, "Why?"

"Well," I replied, "you said <u>any</u> book we wanted."

I took every science and math course my high school offered, which wasn't much: one semester each of biology, chemistry, physics, algebra, geometry, and trigonometry. I was kicked out of chem lab one day when I dropped a nickel into some nitric acid to show my lab partner what would happen. The billowing smoky blue fumes in the back of the room gave us away.

Between high school graduation and college, I worked full time for the summer in the Missouri State Highway Department chemistry lab. Our job was to test and analyze all of the materials used to build roads, bridges, highway signs, and guard rails, etc., to make sure everything measured up to standards. This included all of the paints, asphalts, concretes, metals, and other materials. It was fun to see applied chemistry in action.

Introduction xxxiii

Science Meets Religion

My keen interest in the sciences from early childhood has never waned and was always there. But so was my interest in God and religion. My mother regularly read us Bible stories at bedtime and we never missed church on Sunday—morning or evening. My siblings and I were also active in the church youth fellowship and youth choir. Starting my sophomore year in high school, I also played the organ for Sunday morning services. We were Methodists.

When I was ten or twelve years old my Sunday school teacher taught us how to use a concordance to find Bible verses. Every week he would give us an unidentified verse to locate. If, by the next Sunday, we were successful in finding its source in the Bible, he'd give us a quarter. I never missed getting that quarter. Back in the 1940s, that was a lot of money, especially to a young boy.

My love for the Bible, nurtured by my mother's Bible stories and by the encouragement of that Sunday school teacher, has only grown greater throughout the years.

In 1955, when I chose my majors at Central Methodist College in Fayette, Missouri, it was to be in religion, philosophy, and English—not science. At that time I was planning to be a Methodist minister.

After three years of pre-theological training, I had a change of heart. I quit college. I had been the college photographer during my last year at Central. For the next four years, I became a professional photographer in Los Angeles, California. I did everything from camera to darkroom. I especially loved the chemistry of it.

In 1962, I returned to Missouri and married my wife, Lee. I loved her chemistry, too, and still do. It was then that I went back to college.

I first majored in history and social sciences, then biology and chemistry, and eventually math and physics. I finally received my Bachelor of Science degree with a double major in physics and mathematics from the University of Missouri at Rolla. That was in 1965. It had taken me six years of classes to complete my first college degree. My wife, who had already completed her degree before we were married, earned hers in just three years, majoring in business and music education.

My first job after college was as a hydraulic engineer and groundwater hydrologist with the United States Geological Survey in Southern California. I specialized in the chemistry of natural waters. While in their employ I completed a two year study to identify the sources of groundwater pollution in San Bernardino County.

In 1967 I returned to Rolla, Missouri, earning an MS degree in 1969 and a Ph.D. in 1971—specializing in continuum mechanics, the mathematics of vibratory energy, and spectral frequency analysis of wave phenomena. My doctoral dissertation contained hundreds of equations in tensor calculus for which I was awarded a degree in geophysics in theoretical seismology. This training has become invaluable in my study of vibratory medicine.

In 1973 I spent a semester in medical school, not for credit, but for first-hand information and experience. This was to prepare me for a writing/teaching career in the alternative health field—an area in which I was to be engaged for most of the next thirty years to the present.

After twelve years of college teaching in the earth sciences (seven years at University of North Carolina, Chapel Hill, and five years at Southeast Missouri State University, Cape Girardeau) I went to pastor's school. For three years, during the late 1990s, I served as a local United Methodist minister. I loved being a pastor. But my calling was to another ministry and this book is part of it.

Why Do You Need to Know Chemistry?

People who use essential oils, including some who enroll in my chemistry class, often ask, "Why do I need to know chemistry?"

My answer is this: "You don't have to know chemistry to use essential oils successfully and experience many benefits, but . . . if you can gain a little understanding of how and why essential oils work, you can apply and use them better and more effectively.

"And since your belief has something to do with how well oils perform, perhaps a little science will strengthen the level of your faith, which is another benefit you might gain from a chemistry seminar or a book such as this.

"And if you want to teach others how to use oils, they will ask questions and many of the questions can be answered only if you know some chemistry.

"You will also encounter professionals with a technical or medical background who want to know if there is any science to the practice of aromatherapy. To respond satisfactorily to such sincere inquiries, you need to know a little appropriate chemistry—or at least have a familiarity with the resources to which you can direct them for their answers."

However, the three reasons just stated are not the most important ones for studying chemistry. Healing with essential oils is intuitive and spiritual, a gift acquired by one's receptivity to the Divine. Intellectual study with a secular attitude, unappreciative of the source of all things, will block intuition. Such study is spiritually harmful. Such study will reduce and limit your finer sensitivities and right brain capabilities. This is the kind of study that dominates our schools and universities today. There is a better way.

Your left brain (reasoning) and right brain (intuition) are connected. To develop one to the neglect or suppression of the other is not good for either. Balance is the key. Intellectual study with a devotional attitude in recognition of God as the source of all knowledge will increase your intuitive gifts without limit. Applying and inhaling essential oils during your learning and creative activities helps to optimize all the gifts that God has given to you.

This is a chemistry book written in devotion and guided through prayer. You will find that the more you familiarize yourself with its contents, the more in tune you will become with the oils and their healing applications. Eventually, you may be able to discern the intimate chemistry of essential oils directly without a book because you will see God in them and he will speak to you and answer all of your questions. (John 16:13)

Introduction

What This Book Has for You

Part One of this book is the material I present in a five-hour seminar on the basic chemistry of essential oils. It is the course taught for credit by authorized instructors who teach for CARE International—The Center for Aromatherapy Research and Education. This is the teaching text as well as the text required of all students taking the course. This book is also the text for a chemistry course taught in the Institute for Energy Wellness (IEWS), Brampton, Ontario, Canada, which offers diplomas in aromatic science. For more on CARE and IEWS, see the Resource Section (pp. 842-845) at the end of this book.

Part Two includes a tabulation of representative chemical compositions of the major and minor compounds in 113 of the most common essential oils. Part Two also contains more than thirty tables of cross-indexes of every imaginable commutation and permutation of the compounds of essential oils, as well as their plant origins, plant families, and common names. This is the first time such a pragmatic and practical set of tables has ever been compiled for the constituents of essential oils.

Part Three, entitled "Beyond Chemistry," outlines the limits of science in exploring truth and reality and clarifies the relationship between God, science, religion, and ourselves as human beings. If one is to subscribe to science as a basis for information and understanding, he or she needs to comprehend its limits and how it relates (or does not relate) to personal living. In this section we will learn how the properties of essential oils lead into quantum and wave mechanics, relativity, and consciousness theory. Part Three is an optional section not taught in CARE classes, but demonstrates the fact that healing powers of oils are more than chemistry and that they offer more than can be explained by science as we know it.

Part Four includes a course outline, a glossary, an annotated bibliography, various resources, and an index.

Self-learning DVDs and audiotapes for chemistry are also available from CARE featuring the author. These audiovisual aids correspond to the chemistry course presented in Part One and outlined in Part Four. Periodically check the website, www.RaindropTraining.com, for the availability of these items, as well as classes available on the chemistry of essential oils taught from this book.

Vertical Education vs. Horizontal

Science and mathematics are vertical areas of study. You have to establish certain foundations and reach certain levels of understanding before you can go on to more advanced levels of comprehension. You can't grasp calculus until you have achieved some facility with algebra and trigonometry. In science and math, concepts are stacked one upon another in a vertical fashion like a tall building, with the stipulation that a solid base has to be established on each floor before you construct another one above it.

History and literature, on the other hand, are horizontal areas of study. You don't have to master American history in order to comprehend European, African, or Asian history. Neither do you have to master Shakespeare in order to appreciate writers of the nineteenth and twentieth centuries. In history and literature concepts can be acquired side by side in a horizontal fashion, like adding new wings to a one-story building complex.

Chemistry is a science, but acquiring a comprehension of it lies somewhere in between vertical and horizontal. Thus, it is possible, to a point, to write a book employing the advanced concepts of chemistry necessary to discuss essential oil science without having to construct a towering vertical structure to get there.

The best way to comprehend this book would be, of course, to start at the beginning and master each chapter in order as you go. That would be vertical education. However, if you prefer horizontal education, try skipping around wherever your curiosity leads you. The book is written and organized in a way that will allow that. Let the Table of Contents stimulate your appetite, like a menu. Then plunge in and go where it leads you. You can choose all the desserts first, if you wish, saving the items more difficult to chew and digest for later. Doing it that way, you may find chemistry more fun than you ever expected.

Introduction

How Science and Religion Got Separated

In cultures throughout the world, the healing arts of antiquity were closely allied with religion. The same is true for the beginnings of science as an approach to discover truth. Early scientists did not function in an atheistic vacuum. In their research, their relationship with God was never far from their consciousness.

When asked what motivated his life-long devotion to science and mathematics, Albert Einstein replied, "I want to know God's thoughts." Hippocrates, Pythagoras, Copernicus, Galileo, Da Vinci, Newton, Boyle, Pascal, Pasteur, Kepler, Carver, Burbank, Bose, Maxwell, Plank, Schroedinger, Bohr. . . the list goes on and on of spiritual men with great minds who pioneered the precepts that form the foundations of modern science—great minds that also recognized an eternal, omnipresent God whose thoughts are the objects of scientific research.

In a 1930 issue of the *New York Times Magazine*, Einstein stated, "I maintain that a cosmic religious feeling is the strongest and noblest motive for scientific research... In this materialistic age of ours, serious scientific workers are among the only profoundly religious people."

Einstein was not talking here about scientists whose motivation for research is principally for practical or commercial results. According to Einstein, pragmatic science, which is necessary to bring theory into practice to the benefit of humankind, can also lead to a "completely false notion" of reality and what true science is really all about. To Einstein and the other great scientists of history, true scientific endeavor must lead one to a greater understanding of and reverence for God. True science must always bring us closer to our creator.

When Einstein referred to true scientists as "profoundly religious people," he wasn't referring to religion as a formal sect or denomination or adherence to any dogma or particular set of scriptures. He was talking about a direct, personal relationship with God, independent of membership in any church, temple, synagogue, or mosque, or the social participation in organized religion of any kind. He was talking about the real thing, the common denominator of all religions—a one-on-one, ongoing relationship between a person and God, as a child relates to his or her earthly father.

True science and true religion should never be in conflict. They both seek the same end—the delineation of and the alliance with truth. There was a time in history when scientists seeking truth had to separate themselves from the institutions that controlled public religious practice. Centuries ago, when sincerely devout, God-loving men began, in their honesty, to discover aspects of the universe contrary to prevailing religious dogma, the ecclesiastical authorities who benefited from maintaining those dogmas declared them heretics.

Some early researchers, perceived to be in conflict with the church, were imprisoned. Others were tortured or killed in the name of God. Thus, to save their own lives, scientists who hungered for a more complete understanding of creation than was offered by formal religion had to seek means to develop science in a way that did not offend church leaders.

What developed was a philosophy of separation between church and science. So long as the church kept itself to "spiritual" matters only, and science kept strictly to "material" matters, then there would be no conflict. Religion was for the sanctuary and science was for the laboratory. The two were not to mix. As a result, today we have materialistic science and secular medicine, both of which claim no relationship to God in their practice. At the same time, we have religion that does not know how to incorporate science into its theology and has lost its healing ministry.

But the "separation" of science from religion is a false dichotomy. To deny God as the source of healing makes medicine impotent, ineffective, and incapable of true healing. To deny the spiritual as an integral part of the material makes science incapable of discerning the true nature of the universe. Both science and medicine have confined themselves inside a materialistic container where the ultimate answers they seek are all on the outside.

The separatist dogmas of formal religion have done the same as separatist science. Theologians have created boxes in which they restrict themselves to find God when, in truth, the complete revelation of God is to be found outside of their boxes, as well as inside. God's omnipresence includes the atoms and molecules of the material world, as well as those aspects we designate as spiritual.

No Boundaries

The truth is that things spiritual and things material are intimately interrelated. In fact they are inseparable. Without the spiritual world there would be no material world. Both are manifestations of the one God whose omnipresence and omniscience permeate everything from atoms to galaxies, from the tiniest creatures, to you and me.

Without the spiritual, the practice of medicine cannot heal. Without including the spiritual side of the universe, the endeavors of science can lead only to half-truths and dead ends.

A more detailed discussion of the relationship between the spiritual and the physical is given in Part Three of this book. There we will discuss the connection between mind and matter in terms of science in such a way that to believe in the laws of material science actually leads to the inevitable conclusion that there is a conscious, omnipresent, loving God and that we are created in his image. Any other conclusion would be illogical and incompatible with the laws of physics as we know them today. But we will leave that discussion for later. (also see pp. 741-42)

At the heart of it, this is a chemistry book focused on oils, but materialistic chemistry alone cannot completely account for the behavior of essential oils, or for the fact that they even exist. Neither this book, nor any other book on the science of essential oils, can be complete without stepping outside the materialistic paradigm.

Prayer: The Ultimate Tool of Science

D. Gary Young, N.D., is a noted authority on essential oils, a teacher, a healer, and author of several books on the subject. Dr. Young is my mentor and the one who first introduced me to the oils and to the science of their chemistry. That was in 1999.

Years before his books were published, Young engaged in a successful practice of naturopathic medicine. When he first encountered aromatherapy and began to incorporate that modality into his practice, there were no accessible references on the chemistry of therapeutic oils or on how they worked in the body and mind to bring about healing. "I studied the chemistry of oils through prayer," he said.

Dr. Young's "studies" have borne innumerable fruits through the years as countless people have been healed by the science he has developed "through prayer."

Let me suggest that in the end the science of prayer is always going to be your ultimate resource in studying and applying essential oils for therapeutic purposes. Neither this book nor any other will or can replace that direct contact with the source of all science, which is the conscious presence of a divine, guiding intelligence (God) permeating all creation. When you are faced with a healing crisis and don't know which way to go or what oils to apply, you can always ask God directly. He provides the ultimate textbook and is always near, waiting for you to ask.

"Ask the plants," as it says in Job 12:8, or "Speak to the earth," as in some translations, "and they will teach you." The great botanist George Washington Carver spoke to peanut plants and they told him how to make butter with their beans, plastics with their shells, and paint pigments with their oils. Likewise was the prayerful life of Luther Burbank, the horticultural genius whose communion with the plant kingdom led him to dozens of new fruits and vegetables, including Burbank plums, pears, and potatoes. Forty percent of the potatoes eaten today are Burbanks, including most potato chips. Luther even talked the thorns off of cacti with words of love and kindness, resulting in a spineless variety with altered DNA that willingly and gladly serve animals in the desert as food.

There is a book entitled, *The Secret Life of Plants* by Tompkins and Bird, mentioned in the bibliography. It tells of the lives of many inspired giants of science and their devotion to God as the source of their insights. Gary Young, and many scientists like these, have approached their work with an attitude of reverence and because of their receptivity to divine truth, God has been able to teach them and inspire them to share their findings and research to the benefit of all humankind.

Ask and It Will be Given

This source of infallible information, tapped by sincere devotional seekers of all times and places, is also available to you. "Ask and it will be given to you; search and you will find; knock and the door will be opened to you," says Matthew 7:7. However, James 4:3-4 gives us a qualifier: "You do not have, because you do not ask. You ask and do not receive, because you ask wrongly. . ."

In other words, while God wants to teach you and fill you with his truth, he cannot pour his truth into your vessel unless you ask with faith, trust, fearlessness, openness, a right attitude, a willingness to enlarge your vessel to receive his gift of wisdom, and a desire to share the knowledge and understanding you receive.

The great scientists have literally brought to the world direct revelations from God by their research. In so doing, at some level, they had to be reverent, patient, and humble—persisting until God answered them in his own time and in his own way. They gave God no deadlines by which to respond nor did they try to confine his word within a preconceived paradigm made by men. They were willing to set aside their thoughts and the prevailing ideas of their times in order to know God's thoughts and to articulate them as best they could to the good of us all.

It's Not Your I.Q.

In teaching the chemistry of essential oils to hundreds of students over the years, I have met many people who fear math and the sciences in general, and chemistry in particular. They say things like, "I just don't have the aptitude" or "the ability" or "the intelligence" to do well in chemistry. Let me offer you this word of encouragement. You do have the aptitude, ability, and intelligence. It's not a deficiency in your I.Q. It is an emotional block.

If you are one of those who find quantitative disciplines, such as math and science, too much of a challenge, let me suggest that you reflect back on your childhood. You will probably find that somewhere in your past there was a science or math teacher, a parent, or other authority figure who embarrassed, humiliated, ridiculed, intimidated, or otherwise abused you, perhaps repeatedly—thus creating an emotional block to your learning in science or math. Unfortunately, there are some verbally and emotionally abusive teachers in elementary and secondary schools who unknowingly produce mental blockages in their students—barriers that persist into adulthood and prevent them from learning certain subjects throughout their lives. Such barriers to learning do not have to be permanent.

If you have had difficulty in absorbing or understanding certain topics, you may have been a victim of such abuse and don't remember it. You can use essential oils to help you recall the trauma and overcome this obstacle to your learning. For example, you may inhale and anoint yourself with emotionally releasing oils such as cedarwood, lavender, frankincense, or myrrh. You can also apply the oil blend of Valor™—which clears fears and imbues one with a sense of confidence and courage.

Applying these principles, there are many students who thought they would never grasp nor understand chemistry, or any other science, who, upon dealing with certain forgotten memories and repressed emotions from the past, with the help of essential oils, suddenly found that learning chemistry was not so hard after all. In fact, it was fun. Some day, using essential oils as aids to learning will be routine in schools everywhere.

Mission and Conclusion

I have another book entitled, *Healing Oils of the Bible.* Its mission is to help bring God back into the health care system and to re-establish his presence as the foundation of the process of all true healing. This book, *The Chemistry of Essential Oils Made Simple*, has been written to help bring God back into the sciences and to re-establish his presence as the foundation of the process of true scientific research.

Religion and science can both be abused to promulgate untruth. This can happen when theologians neither understand nor accept true science and/or when scientists fail to recognize the divine source of all truth. By uniting the two in a proper way, the path to truth is certain. Religion makes science relevant. And science, in its proper role, makes religion honest. Neither is complete without the other. Together, they both lead to God. Separately they can both become false gods. As Paul admonished us in I Thessalonians 5:21, "Prove all things." That statement was meant for all our endeavors—both in science and in spirit.

Why did I write this book? I see God in the atoms and molecules of this world. I want everyone to be blessed with such vision. The message and mission of this book is to unite spiritual experience with material science and to bring science back to a closer walk with religion through the chemistry of essential oils.

Sincerely,

David Stewart, Ph.D., D.N.M., I.A.S.P.
December 25, 2004

♥ How This Book Came to Be

• More than four years in the making, this book is an outgrowth of the feedback from students in dozens of chemistry classes I taught during 2001-2004 throughout the United States and Canada. My research and data compilation on essential oils began in July 1999.

The first Essential Oil Chemistry Class I offered was on January 6, 2001, at St. James, Missouri. During the next few months, classes were taught throughout Missouri in Eldon, Webster Groves, Cape Girardeau, Jefferson City, O'Fallon, Jackson, and St. Louis. Between every class I revised and expanded the notes in response to the questions and feedback from the students in order to find all the the right topics and develop better ways to teach them simply and understandably.

My first chemistry class in another state was in Burlington, Iowa, October 26, 2001, as part of the very first CARE Intensive. The actual writing of this book began August 26, 2003, with a pencil on a yellow pad. I was in a cabin at Baker Creek, Alberta, Canada (near Lake Louise) during a break between chemistry classes taught in Calgary and Edmonton, Alberta.

The writing was completed in my home on a farm near Marble Hill, Missouri, on January 5, 2005. The glossary and index were accomplished during January and February 2005. The first edition was released on St. Valentine's Day—February 14, 2005, with a printing of 3,300 copies. The second printing was in August, 2006 with 5,500 copies. The third was in 2010 with another 5.500 copies.

It took me four years to assemble this book and commit it to paper, but it took me a lifetime to gather, absorb, and integrate the material contained here.

Throughout my writing career of more than a dozen books, it has always been most comfortable for me to write with pencil on a yellow pad. I did not realize the significance of this until after this book was completed. Until recently, lead pencils were always made of cedarwood which is the fragrance most associated with pencil writing. The smell of cedarwood oil, and the smell of wood in general, is very calming and grounding. It clears the mind and brain, thus improving one's focus and concentration. Meanwhile the color yellow works in the same direction, facilitating the making of decisions and wise choices, many of which are required in the process of writing.

It is interesting to note that King Solomon built his temple and palace of cedarwood, thus permeating his environment with a fragrance that would assist him in thinking clearly and making wise decisions on a daily basis. (I Kings 6:9-15) Maybe Solomon understood the properties of cedarwood and knew what he was doing, but as for me, I just followed my instincts.

PART ONE

A SHORT COURSE ON THE CHEMISTRY OF ESSENTIAL OILs

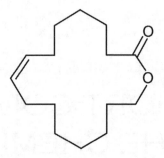

Structural Formula for
A Molecule of Ambrettolide
$C_{15}H_{26}O_2$

A musky smelling sesquiterpene lactone
with hormonal qualities found in

Hibiscus Seed Oil
(*Abelmoschus moschatus*)

♥ CHAPTER ONE
REVIEW & CRITIQUE OF RESOURCE LITERATURE

The purpose of this Chapter is to familiarize you with books that relate to essential oil chemistry without your having to spend the money and take the time to review all of them yourself. One could easily spend thousands of dollars on such references. By reading this section you won't need to do that. The following pages provide you with an overview of the literature of essential oil chemistry and related topics and will enable you to find what you need when you need it.

This chapter will also introduce you to the idea of becoming a Certified Aromatherapist (CA), a Registered Aromatherapist (RA), A Certified CARE Instructor (CCI), a Certified Clinical Aromatherapist (CCA) and/or an Integrated Aromatic Science Practitioner (IASP).

All of the books mentioned in this section are listed in the bibliography at the end of this book. Here, and in the bibliography, I have evaluated the references as I see them. You don't have to take my word for anything. My judgment could be faulty, and you may disagree with my evaluations. If you disagree, let me know. Your opinions may prompt me to change my commentary in future editions.

My purpose is to provide you with a broad exposure to the various texts and make recommendations that will prevent you from spending unnecessary funds for books you don't need, are redundant, or are incompatible with the healing principles of therapeutic aromatherapy, which we espouse in this book.

Most books on aromatherapy contain at least some information on the chemistry of essential oils. Some of them contain a lot while others only a little. All of them are generally good in their chemistry presentations, but not all such books are to be recommended. Upon completing this chapter you will be better equipped to know what books may be of benefit to you, which ones you may wish to acquire, and which ones you really don't need.

Before you can intelligently review an essential oil textbook, you need to understand three things: (1) The four ways oils are taken into the body; (2) The three schools of aromatherapy; and (3) The two basic kinds of oil.

Four Ways to Take Oils

There are four basic portals through which essential oils can enter the body: through the lungs, through the skin, through the digestive tract, and through the absorbent tissues of our body orifices.

By "digestive tract" we are referring to oils taken by mouth, and swallowed so that they are actually absorbed through the stomach and intestines by digestive processes.

By "body orifices" we are referring to oils applied by suppositories or a bulb syringe to be absorbed directly through the lining of the rectum or vagina and also to oils to be absorbed by the tissues of the oral cavity where they are not swallowed, but held in the mouth. Holding oils in the mouth allows them to be absorbed directly into the blood stream through the tissues under the tongue and through the inside lining of the cheeks (buccal cavity).

Swallowing the oils to be assimilated through the digestive tract results in a major portion being destroyed by the stomach acids. Hence, a greater quantity of oil is required when swallowed than when simply held in the mouth. However, some oils are too strong to be held in the mouth so that when internal administration is desired, swallowing them in capsules is an effective alternative. Another pleasant means of taking oils orally is by putting a drop or two in your food or drink. All pathways for oils to enter your body are effective.

Suggestion: For maximum retention and ease of comprehension as you read this book, try inhaling or diffusing peppermint, lemon, or cedarwood oil or anointing your head with Brain Power™ or 3 Wise Men™ as you read. If chemistry has been an intimidating topic for you, anoint yourself with Valor™ beforehand and put some cedarwood on your right thumb (right brain reflex point) to help release any emotional blockages you may have to learning a science.

Three Schools of Aromatherapy

The various modes of administration of essential oils have given rise to three schools of aromatherapy.

The German school emphasizes inhalation as the best way to receive the benefits of essential oils. Inhalation puts oil molecules directly into the blood stream through the alveoli of the lungs as well directly to the brain through the olfactory nerves which connect to the central brain.

The English emphasize massage with neutral carrier oils containing 2–5% essential oils as the best practice of aromatherapy. In the English school skin is the primary organ of absorption for essential oils applied diluted in low concentrations.

The French emphasize taking essential oils orally, but in practice they utilize all four methods of administration, including oils applied neat (undiluted) on the skin. In reality, all four ways are valid, each with their advantages and disadvantages. In rare cases, those of the French school may also administer essential oils directly into living tissues via hypodermic injections, as with certain cancerous tumors. However, this practice is reserved for licensed physicians only.

The best way to optimize the benefits of aromatic oils is to be open to administering them by any and all pathways—by nose, skin, mouth, intestines, rectum, and/or vagina—depending on the situation. This is what we recommend. This is what the leading aromatherapists of the world recommend—including authorities such as D. Gary Young, N.D. and Terry Friedman, M.D. of the United States, Kurt Schnaubelt, Ph.D. of Germany, and Daniel Penoel, M.D., of France.

Regarding aromatherapy in the United States and Canada, only the French and British schools predominate. If you are not deeply involved with American aromatherapy, or have been involved only a short time, you may not be aware of the competition between the British and the French schools around the world. To understand the nature of the conflict, some explaining is in order. This will help you to understand why there are some contradictions between books of different schools.

The British School Explained

The British School of Aromatherapy emphasizes massage with essential oils diluted in carrier oils in 2–5% concentrations and discourages the use of essential oils neat (undiluted) on the skin or taken orally. Aromatherapy came to Great Britain in 1950 when Madam Marguerite Maury, who was French, moved to England. She was a biochemist who had studied the oils in Paris, and was familiar with the medical applications of aromatherapy. However, as a non-physician, she felt that she should focus on non-medical usages and established a model of diluting oils for massage and beauty applications. Later, others in Great Britain, such as Robert Tisserand, who were associated with the massage and fragrance industries became proponents of the Maury model. It was in this way that the British came to emphasize "aroma" more than "therapy" because the leading early proponent, Madam Maury, was neither therapist nor health professional.

The British rely on scientific research on animals, using oils that are often perfume or food grade, and usually applying only certain compounds isolated from essential oils rather than the whole oil. This has led to a host of invalid applications of scientific data to the human use of oils.

The British School emphasizes that aromatherapy can be unsafe and states many cautions and contraindications for oils taken neat or orally. They forbid the use of many essential oils entirely. These warnings are probably valid when non-therapeutic grade oils are applied. The British school emphasizes that because essential oils have their hazards, aromatherapy is best practiced by trained, certified professionals—some even going so far as to promote government licensing and regulation.

Most formally trained aromatherapists in the U.S. are of the British school, relying on British sources or sources influenced by that philosophy. The British school does not condone certain beneficial American practices, such as raindrop technique, which apply essential oils neat (undiluted) to the skin. The National Association of Holistic Aromatherapists (NAHA) and the Aromatherapy Registration Council (ARC) are two American institutions that lean toward the British school and, with few exceptions, recognize only those educational programs that are of British philosophy.

The French School Explained

The French School of Aromatherapy emphasizes oral and neat applications of essential oils but also recommends oils by inhalation, massage in fatty oil bases, as well as rectal and vaginal applications. Modern aromatherapy started in France during the 1920s and was developed by medical doctors whose interest was in healing disease and maintaining health—including relaxation, massage, and the emotional aspects of wellness. Among those early medical pioneers was Jean Valnet, M.D., who was a contemporary of Madam Maury and who wrote the first modern book (in French) on the practice of aromatherapy as a healing art. During World War II, Dr. Valnet found essential oils to treat the wounded to be invaluable and dedicated his life to promoting aromatherapy among his medical colleagues. It was in this way that the French came to emphasize "therapy" more than on "aroma" because a leading early proponent, Jean Vanet, M.D., was a therapist and health professional.

The French rely on scientific research with people using whole oils of therapeutic grade quality and, to a great extent, the empirical and anecdotal experience of their practices.

Dr. Valnet's book was translated and published in English in 1980 with the assistance of Robert Tisserand who was the editor. The French school emphasizes that aromatherapy is safe and can be practiced, with common sense, by anyone whether trained in the healing arts or not. Jean Valnet, M.D., who pioneered and promoted aromatherapy in France in the mid-twentieth century, strongly advocated the practice of aromatherapy by anyone (with minimal training) as being safe and effective. In Dr. Valnet's view, applying essential oils was not a practice to be commandeered for the exclusive use of professionals. To his way of thinking, government licensing of aromatherapy would be completely inappropriate.

This has led to hundreds of thousands of ordinary, relatively untrained people using oils on themselves, friends, and relatives throughout the United States, Canada, and Europe, as well as the Middle East, Asia, and Australia. It has also led to a popular protocol of applying essential oils called "raindrop technique," where a variety of oils are applied undiluted to the back and feet with various techniques of massage, addressing the therapeutic needs of one's whole body, inside and out. This highly successful method can be learned by anyone and has been performed on hundreds of thousands with benefit and with none of the harms the British seem to fear. (See *Statistical Validation of Raindrop* listed in the bibliography.)

Differences of Opinion

There is a certain rivalry between the British and French schools in North America resulting in confrontations usually initiated by practicing aromatherapists of the British school toward those of the French school. Meanwhile those who apply essential oils after the fashion of the French model just want to be left alone to enjoy the benefits of their ways of applying aromatic oils.

We who use oils neat, take them orally, and do raindrop technique are following the methods of the French school. If you are new to American aromatherapy, you may not yet be aware this conflict of opinions, but if you read a variety of aromatherapy books and articles and meet a variety of people using essential oils, you are very likely to encounter it. This information is provided to give you insight, as well as answers for rebuttal, should a member of the anti-French group come into your life and attempt to attack the credibility, safety, and efficacy of what you are doing. (See *A Statistical Validation of Raindrop* and the books by Higley, Manwaring, Young, Franchomme, and Penoel mentioned later in this chapter for data on the benefits and safety of oils applied undiluted.)

Oils That Heal vs. Oils That Don't

Before exploring the literature on essential oil chemistry, it is important to understand the framework in which various authors write. As described earlier in this chapter, there are four pathways of administering aromatic oils to the body and three different schools of thought in aromatherapy. These factors are important to know when interpreting any book or article on aromatherapy.

There are also two general categories of essential oils—those that heal and those that do not (i.e. those that are therapeutic and those that are not). Authors of aromatherapy literature do not always identify which kind of oils they are addressing. When a writer issues warnings about the potential risks and toxicities of a certain essential oil and is not clear that they are referring only to non-therapeutic grades, a reader could be misled to believe that certain oils should always be avoided, not realizing that there may be therapeutic versions of that species which are safe and effective. Thus misinformed, readers could be led to deny themselves of the valid therapies such oils can afford.

Conversely, when non-therapeutic brands of oils are mistaken for therapeutic ones and are applied with an intent to heal, not only is healing unlikely, but actual harm can result.

Definition of a Therapeutic Grade Oil

A therapeutic grade essential oil is defined here as one that is specially distilled from plants that are cultivated organically or grown wild in a clean environment (not gathered along a busy highway). Plants should be from the proper botanical genus, species, and cultivar. No chemical fertilizers are added to the soil, and crop cultivation is free of herbicides and pesticides. Essential oils should be extracted by steam distillation at minimum temperatures and pressures, as was done in ancient times. No chemical solvents are to be used in the extraction process.

The essential oil must be distilled using low-pressure, low-temperature steam for the proper length of time to ensure that a complete essential oil is extracted, and that there is no significant loss or exclusion of lighter fractions (e.g. monoterpenes) or heavier fractions (e.g. diterpenes) from the oil. Moreover, distillation, condensation, and separation should be performed in vessels constructed of relatively inert materials, such as food-grade stainless steel or glass.

Finally, the chemical profile of the principal constituents in the oil must fall within the parameters of certain minimum standards such as those of AFNOR (*Association Francaise de Normalization*). AFNOR is a French agency that regulates the quality of thousands of French products, including essential oils. Their website is www.afnor.fr. The ISO (International Standardization Organization) in Geneva, Switzerland, has adopted the AFNOR standards for oils as the international standard. There are also European Commission (EC) standards, which also correspond to AFNOR.

As of this publication, there are no standards for therapeutic-grade essential oils set by any government agency in North America. The United States Pharmacopoeia Convention (USP), founded in 1830, used to publish standards for herbs and essential oils, and may do so again in the near future, but today its main focus is to publish the latest FDA-enforceable standards for manufacturing drugs and medicines, as well as some vitamins and nutritional supplements. (More on USP, pp. 39-40.) At this time, there is only one North American company that regularly sends samples to Europe to ascertain compliance with EC-AFNOR-ISO standards for essential oils. (See the Resources, pp. 843-845.)

Limitations of AFNOR Standards

As AFNOR authorities have pointed out, their standard is only for a minimum profile of compounds and concentrations that must be present in an oil before it can be labeled as such and such a species. Complete, natural oils are mixtures of hundreds of compounds, but the AFNOR-ISO standard focuses only on a few ingredients, usually less than six. As an example, for an oil to be called "Peppermint Oil (*Mentha piperita*)" by AFNOR standards, it must contain 35-45% menthol, 10-20% menthone, 4-9% methyl acetate, and 3-7% 1,8 cineole. But these are only four compounds of hundreds present in a complete, natural oil. An unethical company could synthesize these four compounds, mix them in these proportions with a suitable filler oil and it would pass the AFNOR test. Such an oil would have a fragrance and taste like peppermint, but not its healing capabilities.

Fulfilling the AFNOR-ISO standard is not sufficient to prove if an oil is of therapeutic value. The healing properties of an oil also have to do with the way it was grown, harvested, distilled, and packaged. These are factors not considered by AFNOR-ISO. For more, visit www.RaindropTraining.com and download the AFNOR article from the archives of the *Raindrop Messenger*, Vol. 3, No. 3.

Therapeutic-grade essential oil should be bottled as it comes from the still, with none of its natural constituents removed and with nothing added. The container and its lid, or seal, must be non-reactive, air tight, and a shield from light, such as bottles of brown, amber, or blue glass.

Thus derived, an essential oil will contain hundreds of constituents, most of them in trace amounts and measured in fractions of a percent. Yet every constituent is vital to the healing potential of the oil. It is the balance of these many constituents that forms the foundation of its therapeutic value. While salt is never a major ingredient in any recipe for fine food, trace amounts of it can make all the difference in the flavor and even the nutritional value. The same with our bodies. We need only traces of iodine, selenium, boron, chromium, cobalt, and many other elements, but when our bodies are devoid of even one trace element, malfunction, disease, and even death can result.

Thus it is with a therapeutic grade oil. Its delicate balance is the result of having been grown in a nurturing environment of love, gently coaxed from the plant, and packaged in a protective container guarded from light, heat, and air. Once delivered from the still, not one constituent is removed nor is anything synthetic added, lest the life of the oil be compromised and its ability to administer healing obliterated or reduced.

In general, with the exercise of moderation and common sense—whether inhaled, taken internally, or applied to the skin—therapeutic grade oils are safe and effective even when administered straight and concentrated (neat), without dilution in a fatty base. Therapeutic oils may also be called "healing oils." (For details on usages, see the books of Higley, Manwaring, or Young mentioned on p. 14 in this chapter.)

Food and Flavor Grade Oils

The vast majority of essential oils (over 95%) are produced for flavor and fragrance and do not fulfill therapeutic standards. Such oils are not considered suitable for use in healing applications. Out of the hundreds of constituents comprising a natural, therapeutic grade oil, the fragrance industry is interested only in the few components that contribute to aroma. The same goes for the flavor industry. All they care about are the components that contribute to taste. The spearmint, cinnamon, wintergreen, and peppermint oils used in trace amounts to make mints, mouthwash, toothpaste, and chewing gum need only have the compounds that comprise the flavor.

Thus, the hundreds of components that comprise a natural oil in balanced proportions. and which are responsible for its healing properties, are typically absent from an oil produced for fragrance or flavor. In fact, some perfume and food grade oils are entirely artificial, formulated in a laboratory by synthesizing and mixing the one, two, or three main compounds that dominate its natural odor or taste. In England, for example, natural wintergreen oil is virtually non-existent.

Instead, laboratory-produced methyl salicylate (the main ingredient in wintergreen) is bottled and labeled "oil of wintergreen" when, in fact, it was not derived from a wintergreen plant, *Gaultheria procumbens*, at all.

In addition to their focus only on the qualities of an oil that serve their purposes, the food and flavor industries are most concerned with economics. Their interest is in producing the necessary oils as inexpensively as possible to maximize profits. In contrast to therapeutic oils, which are grown organically, food and fragrance grade oils are normally distilled from plants cultivated with chemical fertilizers, herbicides, fungicides, and pesticides. Most of these are intrinsically toxic and inevitably end up as contaminants in the oils.

Consequences of Chemical Fertilizers

Chemical fertilizers reduce the quality of essential oils indirectly in that they destroy the very soils that plants need to grow strong and vigorous to produce therapeutically active oils. Proper, organically nourished soil is a living thing, teeming with millions of microbes, earthworms, and other burrowing creatures that till and transform the soil into a feast of nutrients and minerals upon which plants thrive. Many of the vital trace elements needed for healthy plant life are actually created in the soil by biodynamic processes that literally transform elements. (See Biotransmutation, p. 655.)

Inorganic fertilizers should be called "soilicides" or "terracides." They assassinate the soil and kill the earth. The myriad life forms that inhabit healthy soil and maintain its spectrum of minerals all die with the application of such chemicals. Dead soils cannot rejuvenate themselves. The elements plants need for health may still be in the soil, but they are no longer in forms easily utilized or absorbed. At the same time, many minerals, formerly present and bioilogically replenished, simply disappear. In the absence of vital elements, having killed nature's mechanisms for replacement, farmers and gardeners become dependent on using more and more chemical fertilizers, which is exactly what fertilizer manufacturers want.

Impoverished soils produce impoverished plants, which is why our fruits and vegetables no longer contain the nutrients they used to have. Plants grown in such soil become deficient, weak, and unhealthy. Because their immune systems have been compromised, they cannot ward off the attack of fungi, bacteria, and insects. Thus they require toxic fungicides and pesticides for protection, which further degrades their health and adds further damage to the soil.

Such plants may look good, but they are like a person who appears healthy on the outside, while being sick on the inside. Sick plants are not capable of producing top quality healing oils, but they can provide the basic components for flavor and/or fragrance. This is why you want to use only essential oils grown in a proper organic way.

Tricks of the Trade for Fragrance and Flavor

Therapeutic plant oils are extracted by steam distillation at minimum temperatures and pressures, over an extended period of time, as was done in ancient times, in order to preserve as many of the subtle constituents as possible. By contrast, oils for food or fragrance are extracted at maximum temperatures and pressures to minimize the distillation times in order to save on fuel and labor. By such processes, the desired taste and scent may have been preserved, but not the balance of the numerous constituents that provide therapy.

Chemical solvents are also used in the extraction process to squeeze every drop of useable oil from the plant mass, again for reasons of economy. Such solvents contribute additional contaminants to the oil. With food grade and fragrance grade oils, these processes are often performed in vessels of materials that interact with the oils, thus contaminating them with various metals and other substances which further compromise their potential for healing.

Finally, while the chemical profile of a therapeutic grade oil must fall naturally within the parameters of certain standards such as EC-AFNOR, when it comes to oils for foods and perfumes, all that matters is taste and smell. If these do not measure up to the artificial standards of the industry, various constituents are removed and/or synthetic compounds are added until the taste and smell are right. The result is a dead oil with little or no therapeutic value which may be toxic if applied neat or taken orally in its concentrated form.

Aromatherapy books about non-therapeutic grade oils are full of precautions and warnings. Such oils are safe only when diluted to less than 5% in a vegetable oil or used in minute proportions for flavorings. These oils are used in candles, bath oils, body lotions, shampoos, toothpaste, mouth washes, air fresheners, oil lamps, and potpourri. These are the oils usually sold in most retail outlets, including many health food stores. This is recreational aromatherapy, not therapeutic aromatherapy.

Deliberate Fraud

There are, as of yet, no standards for therapeutic-grade essential oils set by any government agency in North America. Hence, labeling fraud is rampant. Therefore, to be sure you are getting therapeutic grade oils, you need to know your grower, your distiller, your packager, and your distributor because anywhere along this chain of delivery, oils can be compromised.

There is nothing dishonest about producing food or perfume grade oils. The problem comes when such oils are bottled, labeled, and presented as if they were therapeutic when they are not. Such oils contain the flavor and aromatic components desired by their respective industries, but are usually missing the therapeutic compounds that do not contribute to taste or smell.

A common practice is to take a decent grade of essential oil and dilute it 90% to 95% with an odorless, colorless solvent (usually an inexpensive petrochemical) so that what was a pound of good oil becomes ten or twenty pounds of diluted oil to be sold as if it were the original substance, thus multiplying the profit. Such diluted oils often carry labels saying "Genuine" or "100% pure," which is allowed by the U.S. FDA. However, when you see a bottle of fluid labeled as "frankincense" for $10–$20 for a full ounce, you can be sure it has been diluted because you can't gather the resins from the Arabian and Somalian deserts, transport them to France or England to be distilled, and then import them to North America (or any other country) for that price and maintain quality and purity.

Mysteriously, for every pound of frankincense distilled in the world, more than a dozen pounds are eventually sold. Pure, unadulterated frankincense should cost around $140 per ounce. In Biblical times, a pound of frankincense oil was more precious than a pound of gold. In fact, in ancient times it was called "liquid gold." Today, a pound of gold is worth about

$4,800 while on the retail market a pound of pure frankincense is worth about $2,400, which is still pretty precious.

If you have smelled true frankincense, then you will know the difference immediately when given a sample of the diluted versions that are common on the market. I have tested several brands of anointing oils labeled as frankincense and/or myrrh sold in Christian bookstores and have not found a single one that is true. When only the common names (Frankincense and Myrrh) are used and the latin names (*Boswellia carteri* and *Commiphora myrrha*) are missing from the label, that is a clear warning that the contents are probably not genuine, and certainly not therapeutic.

Finding such oils for sale in a clear white glass bottle is another clue that the contents are not real essential oils, even though the label may say so. Essential oils exposed to light will polymerize and lose both their fragrance and their healing properties. Genuine essential oils must be stored in light proof containers or dark glass—like amber or blue.

Books With Essential Oil Chemistry Info

The foregoing discussions on modes of application, schools of thought, and types of oils are to prepare you to be a discriminating reader of essential oil books. Now we are ready to dive into the literature.

If one searches the library for books containing essential oil chemistry, they will find a variety of resources, most of them British publications. Even among those published in the United States, most seem to be written from the British point of view, which is considerably different than the French and German schools to which we subscribe.

In this section we shall review a number of books containing chemistry information and related areas. We will recommend those we think are the best and most complete and will caution you about those whose point of view is counterproductive to the benefits that can be realized through aromatic oils.

For the most part, unless you are intending to pursue an in-depth study of the science of essential oils, you won't need to purchase any of these books. We will make some recommendations. Depending on the intensity of your interest, you can take our suggestions or leave them.

The bibliography contains more than seventy publications

relevant to the science of essential oils in one way or another. Extensive commentary is given there to help you judge whether you would want to read or purchase such books. We will discuss only a few selected titles for this chapter.

Of the seventy plus books in the annotated bibliography, thirty-three are mentioned in this chapter. The first five are American texts, the next two are by a German author and eight are British, while the last one (#33) is French. In addition, we shall briefly review five general chemistry texts, four allopathic references (USP and the PDRs), and eight other books that pertain to essential oil science. The first three American texts are as follows:

1. **Reference Guide for Essential Oils**
   by Connie and Alan Higley

2. **Essential Oils Desk Reference**
   edited by Brian Manwaring

3. **Essential Oils Integrative Medical Guide**
   by D. Gary Young

These three books are all compatible with the point of view of this book, which is the French school of aromatherapy. They each contain considerable information on chemistry, expressed in lay terms, and give the main compounds comprising about 90 different oils. Their recommendations on the safe administration of oils is appropriate and consistent with common sense. Their suggested applications are comprehensive and excellent, covering a broad spectrum of diseases and conditions. All the oils, products, and blends of oils mentioned in the first two books ("Reference Guide" and "Desk Reference") are sold by Young Living Essential Oils, Inc., an American grower, distiller, and vendor of high quality therapeutic grade essential oils.

The third book, *Integrative Medical Guide*, refers to all the same oils, products, and blends as the first two, but in a generic way not associated with any particular brand or company. Formulas for many blends are given in this book.

The content of these three books overlap by about 70% so that if you purchased any one of them, you would have 70% of what is contained in the others. We highly recommend all three, but from a practical point of view, you really only need one of them.

4. Pharmacognosy and Pharmacobiotechnology
by James Robbers, Marilyn Speedie, & Varro Tyler

The preface of (4) *Pharmacognosy and Pharmacobiotechnology* states, "The goal of this textbook is to provide primary knowledge of natural product drugs to the pharmacy student." The book is about the chemistry of natural medicinal substances, including considerable information on essential oil compounds—both natural and synthetic.

There is a whole chapter on terpenoids and another on phenylpropanoids—two of the most important classes of compounds found in essential oils. These two types of compounds are responsible for some of the most dramatic healing properties possessed by natural botanical oils.

This book is a grandchild and descendant of older texts that date back to when pharmacists stocked herbs to compound into remedies. Pharmacobiotechnology is a new field of biological engineering where plants and bacteria are genetically manipulated with human genes to create hybrids that produce useful drugs. These include diagnostic proteins, antibiotics, and human growth hormone. Thus, mushrooms and *Escherichia coli* have been cultivated to produce human insulin while soybeans and yams have been manipulated to make cortisone and prednisone.

As to whether or not you need this book to learn about essential oil chemistry, I say "No, you don't need it." Most of the material in this book does not apply to essential oils and much of what does, you can find in more easy-to-understand terms elsewhere.

5. The Merck Index: An Encyclopedia of Chemicals, Drugs, and Biologicals edited by
Susan Budavari

The Merck Index: An Encyclopedia of Chemicals, Drugs, and Biologicals. This excellent reference was first published in 1899 and republished in its 13th edition in 2001. It is the most comprehensive reference on natural organic compounds available. More than 100 oils are discussed. The book is over 2,400 pages in length. In it more than 10,000 compounds are described in detail with all of their physical and chemical parameters, their toxicities and indications, their structural formulas, and lists of their isomers. Virtually every constituent found in essential oils is described in this massive volume along with many herbs and their attributes. For in-depth studies of the chemistry of essential oils, this book is a must reference. However, unless you are writing a book, doing research, or intend to work in the field of chemical analyses of natural substances, you don't need this exhaustive work. It is expensive. It costs around $100. If you really want to check it out, go to a library and use their copy.

6. Advanced Aromatherapy: The Science of Essential Oils
   by Kurt Schnaubelt

7. Medical Aromatherapy: Healing with Essential Oils
   by Kurt Schnaubelt

These two books are in English while both are German in origin and French in orientation. Dr. Schnaubelt (PhD) is a student of Dr. Daniel Penoel (MD), a Frenchman and leading practicing aromatherapist in Europe. These books are both from the French point of view. They are compatible with the safety and application recommendations of this book and those of the first three books mentioned earlier.

We highly recommend these two books for those who seek additional insights and a more in-depth understanding of essential oil chemistry. Dr. Schnaubelt presents a two-dimensional scheme for classifying oils according to their chemistry which is also found in Penoel's book (See p. 48).

Dr. Schnaubelt is Director of the Pacific Institute of Aromatherapy, San Rafael, California (415) 479-9121, which offers various classes on aromatherapy, including training in essential oil chemistry. Dr. Schnaubelt's Institute also offers a home study course. (See the Resources Section at the back of this book.)

Books from a British Point of View

To one extent or another, all of the books listed below are from the English point of view of aromatherapy. All but one of them (Sheppard-Hanger) are by British authors.

8. **Aromatherapy for Health Professionals**
   by Shirley and Len Price

9. **Chemistry of Essential Oils: Introduction for Aromatherapists, Beauticians, Retailers, & Students.**
   by David G. Williams

10. **Essential Chemistry for Safe Aromatherapy**
    by Sue Clarke

11. **Essential Oil Safety**
    by Robert Tisserand and Tony Balacs

12. **Aromatherapy Practitioner Reference Manual**
    by Sylla Sheppard-Hanger

13. **Natural Aromatic Materials - Odours & Origins**
    by Tony Burfield

14. **Clinical Aromatherapy for Pregnancy and Childbirth**
    by Denise Tiran

15. **Clinical Aromatherapy: Essential Oils in Practice**
    by Jane Buckle

British aromatherapy focuses on massage where essential oils comprise only a small percent (1–5%) in a neutral fatty base oil such as grape seed, sweet almond, olive, jojoba, etc. The British also do not look favorably on oral applications of essential oils.

The British are very concerned about what they perceive as risks and hazards of the neat (undiluted) application of essential oils to the skin. In fact, they are so concerned that within their scope of practice, neat applications of oils are almost totally prohibited, with the exceptions of tea tree oil (*Melaleuca alternifolia*) on the feet and some limited applications of lavender (*Lavandula angustifolia*). Lemon oil (*Citrus limon*) is considered safe to take orally by most British aromatherapy authorities, but this is an exception. Following British protocol would abolish most applications of essential oils as practiced by the French, and by most Canadians and Americans—including the highly beneficial and safe practice of raindrop technique, which applies eight essential oils undiluted directly to the skin.

Forbidden Oils

There are lists of oils that many British aromatherapists don't use at all, even diluted, because they consider them too dangerous to use for any human purpose. The various lists of forbidden oils by different British authors are not all the same, but almost all of them include wintergreen (*Gaultheria procumbens*), calamus (*Acorus calamus*), and tansy (*Tanacetum vulgare*) as taboo oils. In her book, *The Complete Book of Essential Oils*, British author, Valerie Worwood, says these three oils "should NOT be used under any circumstances."

Other oils on British black-lists include basil (*Ocimum basilicum*), oregano (*Origanum compactum or vulgare*), cassia (*Cinnamomum cassia*), cinnamon (*Cinnamomum verum*), clove (*Syzygium aromaticum*), savory (*Satureja montana*), fennel (*Foeniculum vulgare*), thuja (*Thuja plicata*), and two species of birch (*Betula lenta* and *Betula alleghaniensis*). The oils of marjoram (*Origanum marjorana*), rosemary (*Rosmarinus officinalis CT cineole*), sage (*Salvia officinalis*) and clary sage (*Salvia sclarea*) are prohibited in pregnancy by most British aromatherapists for fear of inducing a miscarriage. While the British concerns are probably right when referring to perfume grade oils, they do not apply when it comes to therapeutic grade oils.

For example, birch, basil, oregano, wintergreen, and marjoram are oils that are safely applied neat in raindrop technique, a procedure that has been experienced by tens of thousands of Americans and Canadians with great benefits. But the British, in general, do not acknowledge these benefits, and neither do the North American aromatherapists trained in the British way of thinking. (For data on the safety of raindrop technique, see, *A Statistical Validation of Raindrop*, in the bibliography.)

Regarding cassia, calamus, and cinnamon, they were all ingredients of the holy anointing oil decreed by God and used by Moses and Aaron in Biblical times (Exodus 30:22-31). This blend also contained myrrh (*Commiphora myrrha*) and olive oil (*Olea europea*). According to the formula given in the Bible, this blend was 82% essential oils and only

18% fatty oil of olive, which does not comply with the British requirement of keeping the essential components to less than 5%. This blend was safely used by the Israelites to anoint priests for more than twelve centuries. (For information on the Biblical use of these oils, see *Healing Oils of the Bible*, listed in the bibliography.)

As for clove, it has been safely used for thousands of years, from the days of ancient Egypt, and has been applied neat in the oral cavity as a local anesthetic by dentists for more than 500 years. In addition to its effectiveness in pain relief, clove has also demonstrated itself as an anti-inflammatory and as a blood thinner. Clove oil is also the most concentrated antioxidant known with an ORAC (Oxygen Radical Absorbance Capacity) value of over 1,000,000. By comparison the ORAC score is only 2,400 for blueberries, 1,260 for spinach, 750 for oranges, and 210 for carrots. Rather than eat a bushel of carrots every day, I personally swallow a capsule of clove oil on a regular basis with no ill effects, only benefits.

When it comes to the oils of marjoram, rosemary, sage, or clary sage posing a threat of miscarriage, there has never been a scientific study, or even a documented case of this happening. While marjoram does seem to have an affinity with the involuntary muscles (including the uterus), many expectant mothers have safely received raindrop technique, which employs marjoram oil neat. The sage oils can be hormonal in their properties, and thousands of women report achieving hormonal balance with the help of these oils. Rosemary oil has been used by women, even during pregnancy, for effective treatment of candida. We do recommend that one consult with a licensed health professional during pregnancy when considering ingesting or applying any substance that could cross the placental barrier. Thus far, no valid research has implicated essential oils in common sense applications as abortifacients.

When aromatherapists apply oils with fears and reservations, they do not see the healings and miracles so abundantly experienced by those who annoint with oils in faith.

The Toxicity of Tansy

As for the toxicity of wild (Idaho) tansy (*Tanacetum vulgare*), once when I was lecturing, there were some British oriented aromatherapists in the audience. They were being somewhat disruptive to my presentation when one of them raised her hand saying, "Isn't tansy poisonous and too dangerous to use in aromatherapy?"

I responded by saying, "That's a great question. Thank you for asking. It just happens that I have a bottle of tansy oil right here with me." I then opened it and poured a few drops directly in my mouth saying, "Let's just find out if it is poisonous or not. If I am still alive at the end of my talk, then we will know." With that, the hecklers ceased their interruptions and, of course, I was still alive at the end of the program.

One does need to be careful about ingesting oils if they are not of good quality and integrity. If you are looking for a source of pure, effective therapeutic essential oils that are safe to breathe into your system, take orally, and/or apply neat to the skin, check the resource section at the end of this book.

Commentary on Eight British Texts

(8) *Aromatherapy for Health Professionals* by Shirley and Len Price, stands out significantly from the other British books we have listed. It is mostly written from the French school. The authors trained in France and the foreword is by the famed French aromatherapist, Daniel Penoel, MD. In addition to many practical suggestions and applications, the book also tabulates some of the most detailed chemical analyses for essential oils available—including data for 66 different oils. Hence, I highly recommend this well organized book.

(9) *Chemistry of Essential Oils: Introduction for Aromatherapists, Beauticians, Retailers, and Students* by David G. Williams, is an excellent essential oil chemistry book. However, as Williams clearly points out, his book is addressed to the fragrance industry to whom he has been a consultant throughout his career. His book does not deal with therapeutic oils. Nevertheless, Williams' book is a

good reference for basic chemistry. It is well written and easy to understand. Williams' book is unique in that it features several pages of gas chromatograph analyses of specific oils along with scratch-and-sniff swatches by which you can experience the smell of the oil under discussion. Williams is clearly an excellent teacher. This book, published in England, is difficult to obtain in North America.

(10) *Essential Chemistry for Safe Aromatherapy* by Sue Clarke is actually one of the best books on essential oil chemistry easily available in the United States. It is definitely British in its overly conservative view with respect to oil safety. Clarke even goes so far as to caution one performing massage to work carefully around any cuts or breaks in the skin so as not to get oil directly in the lesion. Of course, those who use good grade oils know that putting an appropriate essential oil directly into an open wound not only protects it against infection, but facilitates rapid healing. For an excellent and thorough treatment of basic oil chemistry, I do recommend Clarke's well presented, well organized book. Just don't let her safety precautions deter you from using essential oils undiluted for healing purposes. Follow the guidance offered by the first three texts mentioned in this chapter and you will be fine. (i.e. Higley, Manwaring, and Young)

Animal and Single Compound Studies

The next publication in the list of eight is (11) *Essential Oil Safety* by Robert Tisserand and Tony Balacs. This book is not recommended for people who use good quality therapeutic grade oils because this book does not contain any information relevant to such oils. However, an unwary reader may not realize this if they don't study the preface carefully where the authors state "This text was largely an extrapolation of toxicological reports from the Research Institute for Fragrant Materials." In other words, this is a book on the toxicity of perfume grade oils.

Furthermore, as the authors also point out, in all of the studies they cite as indications of toxicity in oils, the data are for animals (not people) and/or the tests were not for a whole oil but for isolated compounds of an oil. These types of studies are not valid indicators of the behavior of oils in actual practice. Animals are generally more sensitive to essential oils. For example, the sense of smell of a dog is at least 10,000 times more sensitive than human smell. The skins of many animals are also more absorbent than human skin. In the animal studies often cited as indications of oil toxicity, massive overdoses were administered to determine lethal toxicity. It is not valid to translate such research into guidelines of aromatherapy practice for normal human usage.

Clinical aromatherapy is a wholistic modality, and the only valid research on an aromatic oil is with the whole oil, not just a fraction. Testing isolated single compounds of an oil would be like testing the toxicity of concentrated doses of pure sea salt (NaCl + trace minerals) separately from the foods in which it is used. Such a test could cause one to conclude that foods containing sea salt are potentially harmful and ought not to be eaten. Properly used in small amounts, salt is a valuable nutrient and can enhance the flavor of a food without being perceived as "the taste of salt." The taste of salt varies with the food with which it is combined. Does salt taste the same on grapefruit or watermelon as it does alone or on an egg or a potato? While acting as a healthful nutrient in small amounts as a seasoning for food, taken alone in high doses it can be lethal, as is the case with almost any substance. Dosage can cure. Dosage can kill. Dosage can make a poison, a food, or a remedy. (See Paracelsus, p. 485)

MSG or monosodium glutamate $(C_5H_8NaNO_4)$, is another example of a substance that is harmless when ingested in small amounts as a natural compound in certain edible plants, but potentially harmful in isolation or in concentrated doses. MSG occurs in mushrooms and a number of other edible plants that cause no negative reactions due to their natural MSG content. But when MSG is synthetically produced and added to foods as an artificial flavor enhancer, it can become a mild poison manifesting as burning sensations throughout the body, mental anxiety, and chest pain. Toxic reactions to MSG are referred to as the "Chinese restaurant syndrome" since it has traditionally been a common condiment in Chinese cooking.

There are many compounds in oils that, by themselves, are potentially toxic, but when combined in balance and synergy with other compounds, as they are in natural oils, they are not only harmless, but possess healing powers. Some ingredients normally misbehave when alone, but behave nicely in an oil due to the good influence of their companion compounds. In aromatherapy this is called "quenching." In chemistry this would be called "buffering." For example, 1,8 cineole $(C_{10}H_{18}O)$ is the major ingredient in several species of eucalyptus oils. When 1,8 cineole is isolated and tested under lab conditions, it proves hazardous. Yet eucalyptus oils are among the safest of natural substances and offer great relief for respiratory difficulties and other conditions. (See Table Twenty-Six, p. 367)

Therefore, I do not recommend the book, _Essential Oil Safety_, since it would tend to fill one with fears that have no basis when therapeutic grade oils are used. I have met a number of people who, after reading this book, became confused and afraid to use essential oils, thus depriving themselves and their families of opportunities for genuine healing. If you are using cheap perfume grade oils, such as those sold in most retail stores (which are usually formulated from synthetic oils), then you may need to read and heed this book. But if you are using 100% pure therapeutic grade oils, you don't need it.

Oil of Myrrh: The Rule Breaker

A particularly interesting oil is myrrh. It contains many compounds that are individually toxic, yet myrrh is one of the safest, mildest, gentlest oils in nature. In the _Bible_ (Esther 2:12), Esther is massaged with oil of myrrh every day for six months prior to her marriage to the king. Some aromatherapists of the British school don't believe this actually happened, saying that the _Bible_ must be wrong on this point since studies of the individual components of myrrh suggest it would be quite hazardous to apply undiluted to the skin, especially when repeated day after day.

Myrrh contains more furanoid compounds than any other oil. Furanoid compounds can amplify ultraviolet light and can make an oil phototoxic—i.e., causing sunburn and skin damage when exposed to UV sources following application. Yet myrrh is actually a sunshield, protecting one from the sun. Egyptians used it for that purpose for thousands of years. Myrrh also contains phenols and ketones, compounds which are greatly feared by many aromatherapists of the British school.

Myrrh is also unique in that it contains traces of certain acids, like acetic ($C_2H_4O_2$) and formic (CH_2O_2). Formic acid is the poison that causes the painful burning and stinging from many insect bites. Myrrh also contains up to 3% xylene (C_8H_{10}) which is listed in the top three toxic compounds environmental engineers look for in hazardous waste sites. But as a constituent in myrrh, it is harmless.

Single component studies would contraindicate the use of myrrh except in highly diluted applications. However, those who use pure therapeutic grade myrrh know that despite its intimidating chemistry. It is harmless and possesses many wonderful therapeutic qualities. It was the oil most commonly used by the peoples of ancient times and is mentioned directly or indirectly more than 150 times in the *Bible*. It was a customary ingredient in almost every healing ointment of the *Bible* and a fixing agent in almost every perfume. Myrrh is an ingredient in both the holy anointing oil and holy incense described in Exodus 30 which are both used, by Jews, even to the present day. Myrrh was routinely added, by Romans, Greeks, and Hebrews, to most wines of Biblical times. As the bride-to-be for King Ahasuerus, Esther was massaged with oil of myrrh daily for six months in preparation for her wedding. (Esther 2:12) For more on ancient applications of myrrh, see *Healing Oils of the Bible*, in the bibliography.

Myrrh illustrates how chemical compounds that are dangerous alone can be safe and beneficial in the company of other compounds that mitigate their harsh personalities. Despite all of its unruly and potentially harmful components, myrrh also contains 60-80% terpenes—compounds well known for their coordinating, mitigating, and quenching qualities. (see pp. 381-382 for more on myrrh.)

More British School Books

The next two books are (12) *The Aromatherapy Practitioner Reference Manual* by Sylla Sheppard-Hanger and (13) *Natural Aromatic Materials - Odours & Origins* by Tony Burfield. Dr. Burfield is a thoroughly trained British biochemist and Director of the Atlantic Institute of Aromatherapy-UK (AIA-UK), on the eastern side of the Atlantic Ocean, while Ms. Sheppard-Hanger is Director of the Atlantic Institute of Aromatherapy (AIA-US) in Tampa, Florida, on the opposite side of the Atlantic. (See the Resources at end of the book for AIA contact information.)

Burfield's life-long career of more than 25 years has been with the perfume industry. His book is about aroma, not therapy. It is about the fragrances of oils and their chemistry, not about their therapeutic aspects. He gives no recommendations for clinical applications and makes no comments on the relative safety of oils other than to comment on the toxicity of some isolated components.

Although more qualitative than quantitative, Burfield's book is a gold mine of information on the chemical compounds found in more than 500 essential oils. If you want to learn about the science of fragrance, the sense of smell, how your nose works, and how oils and their scents change upon body contact in reaction to one's personal proteins, Burfield's book is the one. You will learn how to describe the aromas of oils as the perfumers do as "green, fruity, floral, fatty, herbal, animal, woody, spicy, balsamic, earthy, fungoid, chemical, mossy, vegetative, and/or citrus." His personal knowledge and experience with oils and the plants from which they come are encyclopedic, and he is generous in sharing his insights and discoveries. Information on just about any essential oil you would ever want to study can be found in this monumental work. This is a British book I can definitely recommend.

Sheppard-Hanger's training and career as an aromatherapist span more than two decades. She is one of the leaders in the field. Her book contains a goodly amount of quantitative chemistry on more than 350 species of oils along with many suggestions for therapeutic applications. However, like other British-oriented texts, Sheppard-Hanger's book is inappropriately cautious in the application of essential oils applied neat on the skin. While she acknowledges, for example, that natural wintergreen oil is often adulterated with synthetic methyl salicylate, which is a source of toxicity, she characterizes wintergreen in general as "hazardous, toxic, sensitizing, and irritant" as if the natural oil has the same untoward qualities as the adulterated or synthetic versions. As for oral applications, she comments that "this area is usually left to medical professionals." She favors inhalation and massage with base oils containing only 1–5% essential oil. As for "therapeutic grade" oils, she does not define that term the same way we do and comments that "adulterated and semi-synthetic oils appear to work," adding that, in her opinion, "fragrance is more relevant than chemical constituents."

Do Essential Oils Penetrate Skin?

While Sheppard-Hanger says that the "safest and most pleasant method of delivery of essential oils is in the form of massage" with highly diluted oils, she presents a lengthy argument to support the theory that essential oils cannot penetrate skin. According to her, when oil molecules are found inside the body following a cutaneous application, they did not pass through the "skin barrier," but entered through the nostrils by inhalation. This idea dates back more than 200 years when the skin was erroneously thought to be impermeable to virtually everything. We now know skin is more like a sieve, blocking some molecules and accepting others—especially the small lipid molecules of essential oils.

There is good research to prove that percutaneous passage of oils does occur. For example, the books by Buckle, Clarke, Tisserand, and Price, reviewed in this chapter, present considerable research in support of transdermal absorption of essential oils. Carvone, a ketone found in spearmint, dill, or caraway oils, has been detected on the breath and measured in the blood within 10 minutes of application to the skin and is later found in the urine. Linalol and linalyl acetate from lavender oil, eugenol from clove or basil, and 1,8 cineole from eucalyptus have been found in the blood in 20-40 minutes and in the urine within 1–2 hours of skin contact. According to Price, a little essential oil on the skin will eventually "pervade every cell in the body," crossing even the blood-brain barrier.

Sheppard-Hanger has apparently never seen, done, nor received a raindrop massage. In raindrop numerous pure oils are applied neat to the skin where they observably penetrate into the body and can administer healing throughout. (See *A Statistical Validation of Raindrop* in the Bibliography.) Many people have placed oils on the soles of their feet and tasted them on their tongues shortly thereafter. This is often cited as self-verifiable evidence that oils do penetrate skin and travel through the body. In Sheppard-Hanger's rebuttal of this phenomena, she claims that when people taste oils in their mouths that have been applied to their feet, they have simply inhaled the vapors rising in the air from their feet.

There is an inherent contradiction in the opinions of British-oriented aromatherapists such as Sheppard-Hanger who say you should never use essential oils undiluted on the skin because of their dangers, yet believe that essential oils cannot penetrate the skin. If oils cannot penetrate the skin, then why would you need to dilute them?

Despite a great deal of research to the contrary, Sheppard-Hanger does not believe essential oil molecules actually travel through the body upon skin contact. We respectfully disagree. Nevertheless, there is much to be gained from her well-organized text, which took her years to compile, and has clearly been a work of love.

Burfield's and Sheppard-Hanger's texts are both published by the AIA and are used in the training programs and correspondence courses of that Institute. While being encyclopedic in scope, they are expensive, costing around $150 apiece in a loose, spiral-bound form. Unless you are willing and ready to dive deeply into the field, your money will be much better spent on one of the first three texts mentioned (i.e. Higley, Manwaring, or Young) or by purchasing the excellent book by Shirley and Len Price.

Oils During Pregnancy

(14) *Clinical Aromatherapy for Pregnancy and Childbirth* by Denise Tiran was a British book whose title caught my attention. My wife Lee and I have published several books on childbirth-related topics including midwifery, natural childbirth, home birth, breastfeeding, nutrition in pregnancy, hospital obstetrics, parenting, and early infant care. I had hoped Tiran's book would be one I could promote as a good reference on essential oil applications for expectant mothers. However, it turns out to be British to the extreme, inculcating unsubstantiated fears of miscarriages and other prenatal

problems when oils are used during pregnancy. If an expectant parent were to read this book they would probably be afraid to use essential oils at all during pregnancy, and, perhaps, even beyond. (Visit www.CarePublications.net for the Stewart's birth works, as well as other books by David Stewart.)

As an example of the British fear of oils, on page 45 of Tiran's book is a table entitled "Hazardous Essential Oils Contraindicated in Aromatherapy." The table is not labeled just for oils "contraindicated in pregnancy." According to Tiran, these are oils not to be used in aromatherapy at any time for any purpose by anyone—even diluted in a base oil.

The list of some 35 taboo oils bans a few with which I might agree. (e.g. Horseradish, *Armoracia rusticana*, which contains several toxic sulfur compounds and powerful lachrymators or tear duct stimulants. Mustard, *Brassica nigra*, which is also a powerful lachrymator and contains chemicals damaging to the lungs and nasal tissues as well as an ester of cyanide. Bitter almond, *Amygdalus communis*, which contains hydrogen cyanide (prussic acid), a lethal poison. I won't quarrel with Tiran for banning these three oils. However, properly used, they all have potentially therapeutic properties. Unfortunately, she also excludes the use of many good oils like basil, birch, calamus, cassia, cinnamon, clove, fennel, oregano, pine, savory, tansy, thuja, and wintergreen for all purposes when, in fact, all of these oils are beneficial and quite safe when they are of pure 100% therapeutic grade applied with common sense and adherence to a few simple safety precautions. (See Chapter Twelve for more on safety.)

Tiran lists 30 "approved" oils for use in maternity care, detailing their applications as well as their chemistry. Oddly, myrrh (*Commiphora myrrha* or *Commiphora molmol*) is not among her chosen 30, even though pregnant women have used myrrh in a variety of ways for thousands of years (since ancient Egyptian times).

Traditionally, oil of myrrh was inhaled, imbibed in wines, and applied neat to the skin throughout pregnancy by women of the *Bible*, as well as used during labor to massage the perineum to prevent tearing, and diffused under the labor bed to promote confidence and calmness. It was rubbed undiluted on the mother's abdomen following birth to reduce stretch marks and applied to the umbilical cords of newborn babes as a protection from infection. Myrrh was the oil of choice for expectant and new mothers of Biblical times, not only for its physical benefits, but for its emotionally uplifting properties as well. Yet, it is not an oil approved by Tiran in her book.

Tiran's book is counterproductive to the beneficial use of oils. I do not recommend it. As for the safe use and beneficial application of oils in pregnancy, follow the recommendations of the first three books mentioned in this chapter (i.e. Higley, Manwaring or Young).

Be a Recognized Aromatic Science Professional

Many users of essential oils want to obtain a widely recognized credential as a professional in aromatic science and practice. North Americans have several choices in this regard. You can become a Certified Aromatherapist (CA), a Registered Aromatherapist (RA), a Certified CARE Instructor (CCI), or an Integrated Aromatic Science Practitioner (IASP).

There are a number of aromatherapy schools in Canada and the United States that offer you the title of "Certified Aromatherapist" (CA) upon completion of their curriculum. Almost all of these subscribe to the British philosophy of aromatherapy, which we don't recommend. However, there is one offering a C.A. credential that we do recommend.

HTSM: The program we do recommend, which is of the French school and actually uses this book as a text, is Healing Touch Spiritual Ministry (HTSM). HTSM is headquartered in Colorado, but they offer classes throughout North America. Completing their aromatherapy program earns you the right to put "CA" after your name.

HTSM training can also make you eligible to take the Aromatherapy Registration Council Exam (ARC). Successful completion of the ARC exam entitles you to use the intials, "R.A." which stand for "Registered Aromatherapist." (See Resources, pp. 842-845, for contact information on HTSM and ARC.)

The HTMS website is www.HTSpiritualMinistry.com and its email is staff@HTSpritualMinistry.com. The phone is (303) 467-7829.

ARC & NAHA: The Aromatherapy Registration Council (ARC) is a non-profit organization registered in Oregon. Eligibility to take the ARC written exam requires completing a course in aromatherapy approved by the National

Association of Holistic Aromatherapists (NAHA). NAHA and ARC are both of the British school. Except for HTSM, all or most of the NAHA approved schools are British in viewpoint.

The ARC exam is a four-hour test administered twice a year in selected locations throughout the United States. It is 100% multiple choice. There is a non-refundable fee. If you don't pass, you may pay the fee again and try again after a waiting period. The exam is administered by the Professional Testing Corporation (PTC) located in New York City. The phone is (212) 356-0660. For information on examination dates and locations, visit the web site at www.ptcny.com,

Which Books to Study for ARC

The ARC exam is somewhat biased toward the British school of aromatherapy. You need to keep that in mind since the acceptable answers to some of the questions may contradict your knowledge and experience outside of the British frame of mind. This is especially true when it comes to questions of safety and administration of essential oils. In order to pass the exam you need to realize that in some instances you must choose the politically correct answer, even though you know it is factually wrong. Reading this book will enable you to recognize the biased questions and to know how to answer appropriately. You will also need to memorize the Latin botanical names of the most popular essential oils. The exam does not use common names at all.

As for which books to study for the exam (besides this one), the ARC website recommends several, some of which are quite expensive (as much as $150 per copy). Others are difficult to find outside of England. Having reviewed all of the books on the ARC recommended list, I suggest that you not obtain any of them. Instead, I would suggest gaining general knowledge from one of the first three books mentioned in this chapter (Higley, Manwaring or Young) and obtaining a copy of (15) _Clinical Aromatherapy: Essential Oils in Practice_, 2nd ed., by Jane Buckle, R.N., Ph.D. Besides being a thorough and well written resource, Buckle's book will give you the necessary British slant to successfully take the test.

Jane is British born but has an American residence. Her bias is British and so is her publisher—Churchill-Livingston. Jane's book, published in 2003, is easily available through any bookstore in North America. It contains a great deal of good information, including just what you need to know to pass the exam, which is no coincidence. Jane Buckle is a leader in NAHA, a founder of the ARC, an editor of the *Aromatherapy Journal*, and a contributor to the ARC exam. You don't need to spend the hundreds of dollars that I did to obtain all of the books suggested by ARC. Save your money and time and get Buckle's book. It has an excellent short section on chemistry. I agree with most of her book and disagree only with her ultra-conservative precautions, which are British in tone and not quite in line with our suggested healing applications of oils.

CARE. ISHA, and IEWS

The other three places you can earn a widely recognized credential in aromatherapy in North America are the Center for Aromatherapy Research and Education (CARE), the Institute of Spiritual Healing and Aromatheraly (ISHA), and the Institute for Energy Wellness Studies (IEWS).

CARE: Headquartered in Marble Hill, Missouri, CARE offers more than 150 seminars annually throughout the U.S., Canada, and several other countries. The topics covered are Raindrop Technique, Vitaflex, Chemistry, Oils of Scripture, and Emotional Release with emphasis on hands-on skills and practical applications of essential oils. People taking these classes receive five certificates of completion worth 25 hours of continuing education credit. Completion of these 25 hours is the first step toward becoming a Certified Raindrop Technique Specialist (CRTS) or a Certified CARE Instructor (CCI). CARE also offers training and certification in Vibrational Raindrop Technique (VRT) and Animal Raindrop Technique (ART). CARE is certified by NCBTMB and IACET as a continuing education provider. (See glossary)

The CARE website is www.RaindropTraining.com, email is careclasses@raindroptraining.com, with phone (800) 758-8629. Get a copy of the *CCI Handbook*, 128 pp., from the website or by phone for full details of the CARE Certification Program.

ISHA: The Institute of Spiritual Healilng & Aromatherapy offers certificates as a Clinical Aromatherapist and others. ISHA trains students to take the ARC Exam. They are recognized by NCBTMB, and the American Nurses Credentialing Center's Commission on Accreditation. ISHA graduates may apply to become Certified Holilstic Health Practitioners (CHHP).

ISHA Founder and President, Linda Smith, RN, is author of the book, *Healing Oils Healing Hands*, available from CARE. Her book and this chemistry book are both used as texts in ISHA trainings. www.ISHAaromatherapy.com is their website.

IEWS: Credentials earned through the Institute for Energy Wellness Studies (IEWS) are recognized by the Canadian government and 16 other countries of the British Commonwealth. They are located in Brampton, Ontario, Canada (near Toronto). One may become an Integrated Aromatic Science Practitioner (IASP) through IEWS. Among their required texts are this chemistry book from which 32 hours of teaching is offered (4 days), and *Healing Oils of the Bible*. The IEWS website is www.energywellnessstudies.com.

General Chemistry Books

(16) Chemistry: The Central Science
     by Theodore Brown, Eugene LeMay, Jr., Bruce Bursten

(17) Organic Chemistry
     by Francis A. Carey

(18) Theory and Problems of Organic Chemistry
     by Herbert Meislich, Howard Nechamkin, Jacob Sharefkin, and George Hademenos

(19) Organic Chemistry: A Crash Course
     by Herbert Meislich, Howard Nechamkin, Jacob Sharefkin, and George Hademenos

(20) Handbook of Chemistry and Physics
     edited by David R. Lide

As a basis for studying essential oil chemistry, it may be good to have some general chemistry texts on hand, but you won't need them unless you want to dig beyond what is in this book. For beginning chemistry, any introductory college text will do. (16) *Chemistry: The Central Science* by Brown, LeMay and Bursten is a good up-to-date basic text.

(17) *Organic Chemistry* by Francis Carey is excellent but presumes you already have a good background in college chemistry. The book is more than 1,100 pages, 90% of which you don't need to understand essential oils. Carey does love natural compounds, however. There is more about essential oils in his book than in most organic texts.

There are two shorter, more student-friendly texts for organic chemistry. These are from the *Schaum's Outline Series* of books which are available for virtually every college course in science, mathematics, and engineering. They are meant as helpful adjuncts to your regular college textbooks. One is called (18) _Theory and Problems of Organic Chemistry_, which is shorter and more simplified than Carey's classic text. There's an even shorter easier version entitled (19) _Organic Chemistry: A Crash Course_. Both of these are by the same authors, Herbert Meislich, et al. (See bibliography.)

The last reference listed here is the classic (20) _Handbook of Chemistry and Physics_. No chemist or physicist can live without it. First published in 1918 by the Chemical Rubber Company, it is now in its 86th edition. Containing 2,700 pages of fine print, it is the most comprehensive reference on elements, compounds, and their physical-chemical properties in the world. I refered to it many times in writing this book, but you don't need it unless you're really love chemistry. It isn't cheap. It can be over $150 depending on where you buy it.

It is interesting that this wonderful reference is produced by a rubber company since rubber is composed of extremely long chains of isoprene units consisting of five carbons and eight hydrogen atoms each (C_5H_8). As you will learn later in this book, isoprene units are the basic building blocks from which essential oils are fashioned. (See pp. 258-261)

The PDR® Family

(21) PDR® for Herbal Medicines
Chief Editor, Thomas Fleming

(22) PDR® for Nutritional Supplements
Chief Editors, Shelden Hendler and David Rorvik

(23) PDR® for Pharmaceuticals (Physician's Desk Reference)
Chief Editor, David W. Sifton

Many people have heard of the "PDR," otherwise known as _The Physician's Desk Reference_. This is the book that lists all currently available drugs with their indications and contraindications. But did you know that there are more than twenty different PDRs? PDR® is a registered trademark. All PDR's are published by—Thomson Medical Economics, Inc. (also called Thomson PDR Co.), Montvale, NJ. Only three are listed above. Others include _PDR® for Nonprescription Drugs_, _PDR® for Ophthalmic Medicines_, _PDR Nurse's Drug Handbook_, _PDR® Family Guide to Over-the-Counter Drugs_, and even a _PDR® Medical Dictionary_ to enable one to understand the other PDRs. There is also a 1,700 page _PDR® Companion Guide_ to assist physicians in making decisions among various drug choices as well as a *PDR® Electronic Library* on CD-ROM.

The first PDR listed above, (21) *PDR® for Herbal Medicines*, contains 854 large pages of fine print and is a gold mine for the herbalist as well as a good reference on many essential oils. This is true even though the book is presented from an allopathic point of view especially for physicians. In the forward the editors state, "When patients approach you—as they surely will—for advice on the latest herbal 'discovery' to hit the nightly news, we hope that this reference will provide you with all the facts you need to offer sound, rational guidance firmly grounded in fact." Almost 700 herbs are listed, along with color photos of their flowering plants with excellent discussions of therapeutic applications. Over 200 of the herbs are featured as sources of essential oils.

Apparently only one essential oil company participated in compiling this book: viz. AuraCacia of Weaverville, California. Five oils are discussed for which AuraCacia is given as a source of supply: ginger, juniper, myrrh, thyme, and German chamomile.

This book was compiled by physicians and pharmacists (not practicing aromatherapists). It contains some unusual and rare essential oils. Even well experienced aromatherapists may not have heard of some of them. You may be interested in some of the more exotic oils in this tome.

Unusual Essential Oils in the Herbal PDR

Burdock oil (*Arctium lappa*) (common cocklebur)
Cabbage oil (*Brassica oleracea*)
Catnip oil (*Nepeta cataria*) (attracts cats, repels mosquitoes)
Cayenne Pepper oil (*Capsicum annum*)
Echinacea oils (3 species—*purpurea, pallida, angustifolia*)
Garlic oil (*Allium sativum*) (taken orally; too strong to be inhaled)
Green Tea oil (*Camellia sinensis*)
Hops oil (*Humulus lupulus*) (the bitter flavoring of beer)
Horehound oil (*Marrubium vulgare*)
Hydrangea oil (*Hydrangea arborescens*)
Magnolia Tree oil (*Magnolia glauca*)
Marigold oil (*Calendula officinalis*)
Marijuana oil (*Cannabis sativa*)
Parsley oil (*Petroselinum crispum*)
Pimento oil (*Pimenta racemosa*)
Red Clover oil (*Trifolium pratense*)

Rue oil (*Ruta graveolens*) (mentioned in the *Bible*)
Saffron oil (*Crocus sativus*) (mentioned in the *Bible*)
Sassafras oil (*Sassafras albidum*)
St. John's Wort oil (*Hypericum perforatum*)
Sweet Violet oil (*Viola odorata*)
Tulip Tree oil (*Liriodendron tulipifera*)
Wild Carrot oil (*Daucus carota*) (Queen Anne's Lace)
Witch Hazel oil (*Hamamelis virginiana*)

Most of their descriptions of the oils are very thorough in discussing the chemical components they contain. This is a valuable resource in gathering information on essential oil chemistry. The book is also a comprehensive reference for natural fatty oils, like almond, evening primrose, olive, rapeseed, sesame seed, wheat germ, avocado, etc.

From this book you can learn that the volatile components of virgin olive oil that create its distinctive flavor and fragrance are various aromatic monoterpenes which have healing properties. Thus, olive as a cooking oil is unique in that while it is principally a fatty oil composed of large molecules, it also contains tiny volatile molecules as well.

The term "essential oil" is seldom used in the *Herbal PDR.* The editors prefer the term "volatile oil." Some of their chosen common names are also different than those used by most aromatherapists. This includes German chamomile (*Matricaria recutita*) which they call "wild chamomile" and Roman chamomile (*Chamaemelum nobile)* which they call "English chamomile." For this reason, you may have some trouble locating certain oils in the book since it is alphabetized by common names rather than scientific ones. Since herbs and oils have many common names, the importance of using Latin nomenclature becomes evident with this reference. (See pp. 496-501)

The *PDR® for Herbal Medicines* cites thousands of research publications in support of the therapeutic benefits, indications, administrations, precautions, and effects of herbs with their oils. Even though this is an allopathic resource, the commentary is generally positive and objective toward the attributes of essential oils.

Not All Plants Have Oils

One of the things you can learn from the *PDR® for Herbal Medicines* is that not all plants have essential oils. All plants have circulating life-giving fluids, but not all plants have aromatic molecules as a component of those fluids. Even in those that do, the essential oil portion of the plant seldom exceeds 10%. By contrast, the oil bearing portions of herbs that produce fatty oils can contain up to 40%. Some plants, rich in fatty oils, have no appreciable essential oil and vice versa. Some plants have significant amounts of both types of oil. For example, seeds of the Nutmeg plant (*Myristica fragrans*) contain 7-16% aromatic oil while containing 30-40% fatty oil as well,

A common range of essential oil content for plants that yield commercially viable quantities is 1–3%. The resins of Frankincense (*Boswellia carteri*) and Myrrh (*Commiphora myrrha*) typically contain 3-9% essential oils and are relatively high yielding species, but difficult to harvest and rare in habitat.

Some plants with less than 0.1% essential oil content are still gathered wild or cultivated because the therapeutic value of their volatile oils is so great, even though costly to obtain. One of these is Immortelle (*Helichrysum arenarium* or *Helichrysum italicum*) also known as "Helichrysum," "Everlasting," and "Goldilocks." Another is Lemon Balm (*Melissa officinalis*) also known as "Melissa" and "Cure-All." Others include Jasmine (*Jasminum officinale*) which has many names, and Rose (*Rosa gallica, Rosa centifolia,* or *Rosa damascena*). In these last three examples, it takes more than a ton of flowers to produce one pound of oil.

Plants whose vital fluids do not include significant amounts of volatile oils contain water and alcohol soluble components, many of which are also medicinal. In fact, of the nearly 700 plants described in the PDR® *for Herbal Medicines*, only 28% are sources of essential oils, but this percent is not representative of the entire plant kingdom. There are approximately 500,000 plant species on planet earth, only 18,000 (3.6%) of which have the means to produce essential oils. The majority of plants do not contain significant amounts of lipid (oily) compounds.

Among the non-lipid constituents of life-giving plant fluids are the following classes of compounds: saccharides (sugars), starches, glucosides, flavonoids, mucilage, caffeic acids (caffeine), amines, peptides, steroids, alkaloids, alkamides, proteins, amino acids, lectins, tannins, ploynes, lignans, and vitamins,. Some of these compounds exist in small amounts in essential oils. Cassia oil (*Cinnamomum cassia*) contains some saccharides (sugars) and has a strong sweet taste like super red hot candy.

The PDR for Nutritional Supplements

The second PDR listed, (22) <u>*The PDR® for Nutritional Supplements*</u> includes only the products of participating companies, which may not include their most effective brands. Many commonly used brands of nutritional supplements are not included because those companies chose not to participate. The book cites many brands of vitamins, minerals, amino acids, and other products, including colloidal silver, and herbal teas.

The only oils mentioned in this reference are fatty oils, not essential. The fatty oils considered as nutritional supplements all come from seeds or fish. Apparently, these editors do not consider aromatic oils to be food supplements, even though some producers of essential oils label them as such. On the other hand, the absence of essential oils in this book probably has more to do with the unwillingness of essential oil producers to participate. That could change in the future.

Among the fatty oils discussed are borage, evening primrose, flaxseed, black currant seed, garlic, vitamin E, beta carotene, wheat germ, coconut, and various fish oils, including cod liver and shark liver oils. Several of these are used as bases for massage oils containing essential oils. It is interesting to note that among the fatty oils discussed, olive oil, which has been known to be an excellent food and nutritive supplement for thousands of years, is not mentioned. The chemistry of fatty oils is quite different from that of essential oils. Fatty oils do not administer therapy to our bodies on a cellular level because their molecules are too large. (See p. 56)

While the book is for and by allopathic physicians and pharmacists, as are all publications of the Thomson PDR Company, there is a lot of valuable information on specific supplements and minerals contained here you won't find elsewhere. It contains hundreds of scientific citations, including the latest findings on nutrition and cancer, aging, immunity, fitness and other aspects of nutritional supplementation. One potentially useful aspect of this book is an index of possible interactions among vitamins, minerals, food supplements and pharmaceuticals as well as a table of companion drugs that work well with natural products. There is no mention of any harmful interactions between drugs and essential oils. The book lists all Drug and Poison Control Centers in the U.S. Most large libraries have this reference.

The PDR for Pharmaceutical Drugs

(23) _The Physicians Desk Reference_, _PDR®_, or _PDR® for Pharmaceuticals_ is the most famous of the PDRs and is a companion to the _Merck Manual_ (described in the next section). This huge tome (3,550 large pages of fine print) contains more than four times as many words as the _Holy Bible_. The PDR referenced here was published in 2003—the 57th edition. It has been reissued annually since 1946.

The PDR describes every prescription drug available at the time of its publication. All of the information in this publication is provided by the drug manufacturers themselves (with the assistance of their attorneys in all cases).

The PDR does not list over-the-counter medicines. There is another PDR for these drugs. You won't find aspirin in the PDR. Neither will you find anything about essential oils since pharmaceuticals are all synthetic (and patentable) while therapeutic grade oils are all natural (and cannot be patented).

While drugs are to be avoided whenever possible, this is a good reference to have if a doctor prescribes something for you, a friend, or a family member and you want to know the truth, the whole truth, about its benefits and risks. While less than 20% of the book concerns indications, protocols, and possible benefits, more than 80% concerns warnings, contraindications, hazards, precautions, and side effects.

The PDR is all about the medicines that kill over 100,000 people a year in the United States and bring injury and sickness to millions more. The words "heal" or "cure" are nowhere to be found in this book. The bulk of its content (over 80%) is dedicated to the down side of drugs, i.e. all of the ways drugs can do you harm. _Pharmakeia_ is a Greek word used in the _New Testament_ which translates into English as "witchcraft" or "sorcery." It means, literally, "medicine from a pharmacy." (See the book, _Healing Oils of the Bible_, for more on this.)

The PDR contains a fair amount of organic chemistry, but not the kind of chemistry applicable to essential oils. The book lists all of the U.S. Drug and Poison Control Centers. The chemistry of essential oils and that of synthetic drugs are compared and discussed in Chapter Eleven of this book.

U.S. Pharmacopoeia and National Formulary

The anonymous and ominous title (24) given below is not for a book you would ever want to buy. Its 2005 price was over $600. It is known as "The Big Red Book." United States Pharmacopoeia (USP) and National Formulary (NF) were, at one time, separate publications from separate publishers, but are now combined into one book under one institution.

(24) USP28-NF23, 2005
Prepared by USP Council of Experts, Roger Williams, M.D., Chairman, (US Pharmacopoeia Convention, Rockville, MD)

The United States Pharmacopoeia Convention (USPC) was founded in 1830 to establish standards for medicinal preparations of all kinds. At that time, many remedies prescribed by doctors were herbal and included essential oils. In fact, there used to be such things as "USP grade" essential oils. This has not been true for some time, but that is changing.

While the USPC was organized to standardize medical formulas, the National Formulary was an organization to set codes for pharmaceutical additives, colorants, flow agents, binders, syrups, carrier oils, enzymes, flavorings, emulsifiers, and other non-drug substances. Thus, the USPC is concerned with the active ingredients of a medicine while the NF is concerned with the inactive ingredients. The two have now merged their work into one publication and one institution.

The *USP-NF* "Red Book" provides the latest FDA-enforceable standards of identity, strength, quality, and purity for prescription and nonprescription drug ingredients and dosage forms, dietary supplements, medical devices, and other healthcare products. It includes tests, analytical procedures, acceptance criteria, and labeling requirements. The main edition of *USP–NF* is published every November and becomes official January 1 of the next year. Supplements are published in February (official on April 1) and June (official on August 1). *USP–NF* is available in print, online, internet, and CD formats. The current title, *USP28-NF23, 2005*, refers to the 28th edition of the USP, the 23nd edition of the NF, published in the year 2005.

This is a "must have" reference for all drug manufacturers and research labs where the $600 price is no obstacle. *The Physician's Desk Reference* lists all prescription drugs currently in use with indications and precautions, etc. The *USP-*

_NF_ provides the nitty-gritty details that drug manufacturers need in order to comply with U.S. government regulations.

Until the last decade (since 1995), _USP_ standards were almost exclusively about the synthetic, unnatural substances comprising allopathic medicines. For decades, editions of _USP_ standards have contained nothing about essential oils but now deal with a number of herbal products. There is a detailed section (pp. 2059-2183) on standards for dietary supplements, but no essential oils are mentioned. Some of the herbs for which USP standards are defined include red clover, ginseng, ginko, goldenseal, hawthorn, echinacea, feverfew, and St. John's wort.

The 2005 edition mentions "Peppermint Spirit," which is an alcohol tincture containing 10% peppermint oil (_Mentha piperita_). However, the oil is obtained by maceration, not by distillation as would be the case in a true essential oil. Oils obtained by maceration are not pure, but are contaminated with the fatty oil used to extract them. There are also tinctures of ginger root (_Zingiber officinale_) and German chamomile (_Matricaria retucita_). For chamomile, the USP standard specifies that the plant contain no less than "0.4% blue oil" and specifies that the extract (oil) be drawn from the plant by maceration, not distillation. For a tincture of Valarian (_Valariana officinalis_) the USP states that the herb must contain no less than 0.3 volatile oil and must be extracted by solvents such as hexane, acetic acid, or ethyl acetate.

Omissions of natural plant remedies by USP started to change after 1995 when the folks at National Formulary united with the folks at USP and suggested that botanical medicines ought to be something for USP to consider. NF is currently devising standards for growing, distilling, and packaging of essential oils. This could be a good thing.

AFNOR and USP/NF Compared

The problem with AFNOR standards (see pp. 7-8) is that they are only concerned with the final oil and its composition, which can be synthetically manipulated to fit the standard. AFNOR does not concern itself with "how oils come to be."

By contrast, "how products come to be" is the main focus of _USP-NF_. USP-NF standards should detail not only the required chemistry profile of the final oil, but also the manner in which it should be grown, harvested, extracted, and bottled. Therefore, while AFNOR standards do not include the factors that make an oil truly therapeutic, the USP-NF standards of the future, may do just that. When that happens, it will be a first in the world. That will help curb a lot of fraud in the essential oil industry. To learn more, visit www.USP.org.

The British counterpart of *USP/NF*, is "BP" or *British Pharmacopoeia* It currently lists standards for several oils, including clove, eucalyptus, peppermint, and citronella. There is also a "PI" or *Pharmacopoeia Internationalis* published by the World Health Organization (WHO).

The first exhaustive work like the USP/NF Red Book on medicines and their preparations was the *Materia Medica* published in 50 A.D. It was compiled by Dioscorides who practiced herbal medicine in Rome during the reign of Emperor Nero. It was five volumes in size.

Other Useful Books

Every book in the bibliography played a role in the writing of this book, but you don't need to accumulate such a library. The following books can be useful in the study of essential oil chemistry. You might find some of them useful for other purposes. They are as follows:

(25) Merck's Manual of the Materia Medica, 1899 edition
anonymous (Merck & Company)

(26) Merck Manual of Diagnosis and Therapy
edited by Mark H. Beers and Robert Berkow

(27) Molecules of Emotion: The Science Behind Mind-Body Medicine by Candace B. Pert

(28) Natural Home Health Care Using Essential Oils
by Daniel and Rose-Marie Penoel

(29) The Secret Life of Plants
by Peter Tompkins and Christopher Bird

(30) Mosby's Medical, Nursing & Allied Health Dictionary
by Douglas Anderson,

(31) Structure and Function of the Body
by Gary Thibodeau and Kevin Patton

(32) Freedom Through Health
by Terry Shepherd Friedmann

The two *Merck Manuals* listed above (25 & 26) are a century apart in their printing. The first one, (25) *1899 Merck Manual (Materia Medica)* listed here was only 364 small pages in size while the 1999 edition (26) is more than 2,800 large pages. Does this mean we have more diseases today than they did a century ago?

While the modern version focuses on surgery, radiation, and pharmaceuticals, the 19th century edition actually suggests the following essential oils: bitter almond, cajuput, eucalyptus, wintergreen, juniper, mustard, pine, scotch fir, rosemary, sandalwood, and thyme. It also lists castor, cod liver, and olive oils as medicines along with oil of turpentine.

Croton oil (*Croton tiglium*), a strong laxative from a plant related to the castor bean, is also recommended for oral use, but with caution. According to *Merck (1899)*, croton oil can be poisonous for which they recommend antidotes of "opium or cocaine."

Today, oil of bitter almond (*Amygdalus communis*), not to be confused with sweet almond (*Prunus dulcis*), is not used by aromatherapists because of its potentially lethal cyanide content, but it was an oil used by doctors a hundred years ago. The *1899 Merck Manual* lists bitter almond oil as not only being a medicine (if properly prescribed), but also as a "poison." As an antidote, it suggests "ammonia" or "a shot of brandy."

Mustard oil (*Brassica nigra*) is also not used today because its vapors can be damaging to the lungs and nasal tissues, but it was used by doctors of the 19th century. It was recommended by *Merck* to be compounded as a liniment for poultices or compresses "with much water."

In all instances, the essential oils recommended by *Merck 1899* were U.S.P. grade (United States Pharmacopoeia) which may not have been true therapeutic grade oils. USP means the oils could have been manipulated by refining, denaturing, rectification, or adulteration with synthetics to fit a USP profile. USP grade oils were produced by drug companies. Modern editions of USP standards do not include essential oils at this time, but that may change.

(26) *The Merck Manual of Diagnosis and Therapy* is the book used by physicians everywhere to diagnose and prescribe. It contains a description of every disease and condition known to mankind as of its printing in 1999. It has been revised, updated, and expanded seventeen times since its

first printing in 1899. It is not legal to diagnose anyone else outside of your own immediate family unless you are licensed to do so, but this is a useful text to have in the home in order to self-diagnose or to corroborate or understand a doctor's pronouncements, prescriptions, and prognoses. The 1999 edition of the _Merck Manual_ does not recommend essential oils at all.

Merck's Misunderstanding

The only mention of essential oils in the _1999 Merck Manual_ is in the section entitled "Aspirin and Salicylate Poisoning." Doctors call this type of poisoning, "Salicylism." Chemically, the active ingredient in aspirin is acetylsalicylic acid ($C_9H_8O_4$). In over a century of its use, aspirin has been the cause of many deaths and visits to emergency rooms. Natural oil of wintergreen contains 85-90% methyl salicylate ($C_8H_8O_3$). You can see by the two formulas how similar the oil is to aspirin, at least superficially. (See pp. 268-270 for structural diagrams of these two.) The two molecules differ only by one atom of carbon (C) and one of oxygen (O), with the number of hydrogens (H) being the same in both.

For therapeutic purposes, wintergreen oil acts in a way that is similar to aspirin in that it can act as an analgesic for pain relief when applied topically directly to the skin where it hurts. Used in this way, natural wintergreen oil is quite safe. _Merck_ would disagree.

The _1999 Merck Manual_ states the following on page 2273: "The most toxic form of salicylate is oil of wintergreen (methyl salicylate); death has been reported from ingestion of less than a teaspoon in a young child. Any exposure to methyl salicylate (found in liniments and in solutions used in hot vaporizers) is potentially lethal."

Apparently, Merck has changed its mind about wintergreen oil since its 1899 edition. At that time the "recommended dosage was: "5-20 minums of a 5% spirit." Translated into modern language, this means 5-20 drops of a 5% tincture (alcohol solution) of wintergreen oil. The 1899 edition issues no warnings and mentions no untoward effects.

"What's going on here?" you are thinking. "How can wintergreen oil be safe when published medical authorities say it is potentially lethal even when applied in simple ointments or when inhaled from a vaporizer?"

The answer to this is in the chemistry. When the literature doctors read talks about essential oils, it is usually referring to synthetic oils or oils not specifically produced for therapeutic purposes. Such oils can be toxic and harmful. In particular, when allopathic writers refer to "oil of wintergreen" they are not talking about the oil as it is distilled from a plant, they are talking about synthetically produced methyl salicylate, as listed in the _USP-NF_ discussed earlier in this chapter.

Natural oil of wintergreen that has been properly distilled and is unrefined and untampered with is 90-98% methyl salicylate. The other 2-10% of natural ingredients changes everything. Ordinarily toxic compounds (like the 1,8 cineole in eucalyptus) are rendered harmless and beneficial when mixed with other compounds as they are in natural oils. Their toxic tendencies are quenched, buffered, and transformed into good by their companions.

But that's not all there is to it in this instance. While pure methyl salicylate from a laboratory is toxic, methyl salicylate produced by a plant, such as wintergreen (_Gaultheria procumbens_) or birch (_Betula alleghaniensis_), is safe. This is not just because natural methyl salicylate in a whole oil is accompanied by friendly ingredients that quench its toxicity, but the methyl salicylate from a lab is not the same substance as the natural version. Natural and synthetic oil compounds can have the same chemical formulas, but different structural formulas and, thus, different effects upon our bodies.

Only God Can Make an Oil

Isomers are two or more compounds with the same formula but different molecular structures. The formula for methyl salicylate is $C_8H_8O_3$, However, the 8 carbons, 8 hydrogens, and 3 oxygen atoms of this formula (19 atoms total) can join together in many ways thus creating molecules with the same formula, but arranged in different structural shapes with different properties. There are 25 known isomers of the formula $C_8H_8O_3$. Two are very similar to that of natural methyl salicylate, but not quite. When plants produce methyl salicylate, they make a specific single pure isomer—only one of the 25. Laboratories can't do this. When a lab tries to produce a single isomer, they end up with mixtures of two or more isomers, not just one. This is significant because, as we will discuss later, different isomers of the same compound can have entirely opposite properties—some helpful, some harmful. So there is good methyl salicylate and bad methyl salicylate. Humans can make the bad while only God knows how to make the good.

The allopathic version of "oil of wintergreen," referred to by the *1999 Merck Manual* is unnatural and toxic and should be considered dangerous, as they say. But what they say has nothing to do with natural wintergreen which has been used quite safely hundreds of thousands of times in raindrop technique as well as in other simple applications, such as on-site use for arthritis. (See *Statistical Validation of Raindrop*.)

The earlier 1899 edition of *Merck*, that recommends wintergreen oil, was probably referring to a natural distillate with minimal manipulation and may have been a genuine therapeutic grade essential oil, even though it also met USP grade requirements at the time. The 1999 edition is talking about a purely synthetic product, which may be potentially "lethal," as it says. There is a major difference between a synthetic oil and a botanical one.

References such as the recent editions of the *Merck Manual* are what some British aromatherapists and some members of the American National Association of Holistic Aromatherapists can cite as a basis for objecting to wintergreen and its use in raindrop technique. The *Merck Manual* is a wonderful publication for identifying and diagnosing disease—the best publication of its kind. But one must be wary of its prescriptions for treatment.

The Murky Manual

What this means is that just because something is published in what seems to be a reputable scientific resource, does not mean that it is true. In fact, when it comes to reading the literature of scientific medicine, one has to be extremely discriminating not to be misguided into many untruths. Medical research literature is rampant with erroneous, misleading, and self-serving information because most of it is financed by commercial interests (i.e. drug companies) rather than seekers of true healing. With this in mind, consider that Merck is not just a publisher of medical manuals. It is a drug company. One of the world's largest.

Now you can understand why most MDs do not approve of or appreciate essential oils. Their training is against it, from medical school all the way through to the references they use daily. They have been propagandized and manipulated and don't know it. And now you know why I call the "*Merck Manual*" the "*Murky Manual*," because it is not clear in that book what is true and what is not true.

Emotions, Home Health, The Secret Life of Plants

(27) *Molecules of Emotion: The Science Behind Mind-Body Medicine* by Candace Pert does not mention essential oils. However, it is an excellent book to gain an understanding of how oil molecules work through receptor sites at cellular levels. The molecules of hormones, described in this book, function in the same ways as the molecules of essential oils. Dr. Pert is an excellent and entertaining writer who makes the complex simple and the obtuse interesting. As much autobiographical as scientific, you will enjoy reading this book while gaining an understanding of how the 100 trillion cells of our bodies can communicate and work in harmony and how essential oils can assist in restoring and maintaining that harmony.

(28) *Natural Home Health Care Using Essential Oils* by Daniel and Rose-Marie Penoel is as much a poetic essay as it is a scientific treatise on the practical use of essential oils. Daniel Penoel, MD, is one of the world's foremost medical experts on the therapeutic use of essential oils. His practice defines the French model of aromatherapy. While you won't find much chemistry in the book, Dr. Penoel delivers innumerable insights into how humans and oils interact for healing purposes. Rose-Marie is his wife and life-long partner.

(29) *The Secret Life of Plants* by Peter Tompkins and Christopher Bird is one of those books that will change your view of the world forever. While essential oils are not discussed, the insights into how plants function, communicate, and interact with humans will enable you to understand how and why the oils of plants are so effective in conveying their healing powers to people, and how thoughts affect plants and, in turn, their oils. I highly rec-

ommend this book to all users of essential oils. It explains a lot of what truly underlies the chemistry of essential oils and why chemistry, alone, cannot account for all that oils do.

You Need a Good Medical Dictionary

If you have the _Merck Manual_ and/or any of the PDRs, then you will need a good medical dictionary to look up all the big words. There isn't any medical publication you can't read and understand if you have the right dictionary and the patience to use it. You will need a recent edition inasmuch as new discoveries are being made constantly and medical terminology is changing all the time.

We highly recommend (30) _Mosby's Medical, Nursing & Allied Health Dictionary_. It is comprehensive in its coverage, simple to understand, and profusely illustrated with great color photos and drawings—very user-friendly for health care professionals, students, and lay people alike.

One more thing you need—a good physiology book. We recommend (31) _Structure and Function of the Body_, an excellent, easy-to-understand reference on human physiology and bodily functions, including the biochemistry of bodily processes. It is used in many medical schools as a required text—beautifully and profusely illustrated—very user friendly. The content is presented in a manner that even medical students can understand. Comes with a CD.

Aromatherapy in Medical Practice

The book, (32) _Freedom Through Health_ by Terry Friedmann, MD, does not contain much about essential oil chemistry, but contains a great deal about healing applications of essential oils. Dr. Friedmann is a practicing allopathic physician who is also a founder and officer of the American Holistic Medical Association (AHMA). His one-of-a-kind book integrates allopathic medicine with homeopathy, acupuncture, reflexology, herbology, nutrition, vibrational medicine, chiropractic manipulation, and, to a great extent, aromatherapy. It is the best book available in English on applying essential oils with a medical/holistic perspective. Dr. Friedmann has not only successfully used essential oils for years in his practice, but has conducted considerable research into their benefits. This is a practical, how-to-do-it book, not only for health care practitioners, but for the public at large. It is easy to read and contains a glossary for unfamiliar terms. This book is highly recommended for everyone using essential oils.

An Ultimate Book on Essential Oil Chemistry

Before we conclude this chapter, we need to mention one more reference, also written by an allopathic physician. Your education in the literature of aromatherapy would not be complete without it. Thus far, all of the cited references have been in English. This one is available only in French.

(33) L'Aromatherapie Exactement
    by Pierre Franchomme and Daniel Penoel

In English, the title is "Exact Aromatherapy." The subtitle (in English) is "Encyclopedia of Therapeutic Applications of Aromatic Extracts." It is over 500 pages in size. An additional subtitle seen on the cover is "Foundations, Demonstrations, Illustrations, and Applications of the Science of Natural Medicine."

This may be the best book available on the chemistry, biosynthesis, and medical application of essential oils. It was written by two leading world authorities—Pierre Franchomme (a chemist) and Daniel Penoel (a physician). If you don't read French, you may not get much from the text, but a trained scientist can still understand most of the medical and scientific terminology. This is a must reference for serious researchers in the field of therapeutic aromatherapy. It is available from Paris, France, at www.biogessendi.com on the internet.

Congratulations
You Are Now Conversant and Literate

By reading this chapter and browsing the extensive annotated bibliography (which contains information on many additional references not discussed in this chapter), you will have become literate in the literature of essential oil chemistry and related topics without having read a single one of the mentioned works. You will have achieved in a matter of an hour or so what normally would have taken weeks of library research and months of laborious study. That is the purpose of this chapter: to introduce you to a cross-section of published resources from which you may choose a few in which to plunge and deepen your knowledge. In Chapter Three we will plunge into chemistry, itself.

Key Points of Chapter One

1. There are four pathways to take essential oils into your body: lungs, skin, digestive tract, and through the absorbent tissues of body orifices.

2. Hypodermic injection is a fifth pathway by which essential oils may be administered to the body in extreme cases, such as in malignant tumors, but this is reserved for licensed physicians only.

3. There are three schools of thought in aromatherapy: German, English, and French which emphasize inhalation, massage, and oral/neat applications of essential oils respectively.

4. There are two basic types of essential oils: therapeutic and non-therapeutic. Healing is unlikely from non-therapeutic grade oils.

5. A therapeutic grade essential oil has to be grown, gathered, distilled, bottled, and labeled properly to retain its naturally healing properties.

6. Food and fragrance grade essential oils represent 95% of the current market and do not measure up to therapeutic standards.

7. All plants contain vital fluids, but not all plants contain significant amounts of lipid-soluble aromatic molecules (i.e. essential oils).

8. While 28% of the nearly 700 plants tabulated in the Herbal PDR produce essential oils, only 3.6% of all the 500,000 known species of the world contain enough volatile oils in their systems to be extracted and used.

9. The non-lipid (non-oily) portions of plant fluids are also of therapeutic value and provide many herbal remedies.

10. Books we Recommend. (The numbers refer to those given in this Chapter to identify the various books)

General Aromatherapy - 1, 2, 3, 8, 32, 33

EO Chemistry References - 3, 6, 7, 10, 13, 21, 33

ARC Exam Resources - 1, 2, 3, 15

Miscellaneous References - 27, 28, 29, 30, 31

11. Books Not Recommended - 11, 14

12. One of the best books on the chemistry and medical applications of essential oils is available only in French: _L'Aromatherapie Exactement_ by Pierre Franchomme and Daniel Penoel—two of the foremost international authorities on essential oils and their therapeutic uses.

13. Aromatherapy books full of precautions, warnings, contraindications, and lists of forbidden oils, are basing their conclusions on animal and single-component studies and/or non-therapeutic grade oils.

14. Animals studies typically test for lethal levels of a compound or an oil by massive overdosages. This type of research does not validly translate into useful guidelines for normal aromatherapy practice with humans.

15. Single component studies are all invalid when applied to a whole essential oil. Only studies using a complete, natural essential oil can provide information useful for human applications.

16. Studies on the toxicity of adulterated, diluted, or refined oils have no bearing on the safety or potential toxicity of pure therapeutic grade essential oils.

17. AFNOR standards are not a measure of therapeutic quality since AFNOR does not consider the growing, harvesting, extracting, and packaging conditions that produce an oil.

18. USP/NF standards do not address essential oils today, but in the future USP/NF may define standards that are a truer measure of an oil's therapeutic quality than AFNOR.

19. There are many books containing essential oil chemistry. One must be discriminating as to their bias and intent—i.e. for whom, by whom, and from which school were they written?

20. This book is written for the public at large from the viewpoint of the French school of aromatherapy which embraces all of the beneficial modalities in administering essential oils.

♥ CHAPTER TWO
WHAT OILS DO
IN LIVING PLANTS

Essential oils serve the needs of plants before they serve us. What they do for us they have already practiced on plants. Thus, essential oils come to us as experienced helpers and healers. Therefore, it is appropriate to learn a little about how oils function in plants to better understand how they function in us.

In the following chapters we will define things like chemistry, organic chemistry, biochemistry, molecules, frequency, resonance, and a lot of other terms, but let's start with a definition of an essential oil—the central topic in the title of this tome.

What is an Essential Oil?

An essential oil is the volatile lipid (oil) soluble portion of the fluids of a plant containing odiferous compounds produced by steam distillation of vegetable plant matter. Plant matter can be any part of a botanical species including stems, branches, fruits, flowers, seeds, roots, bark, needles, leaves, etc. During the distillation process, the vapors are condensed, collected, and separated from the condensation water. The residual water, containing traces of oil constituents, is called a "floral water" or "hydrosol," and has therapeutic applications of its own.

Essential oils are mixtures of hundreds of compounds. For example, it has been found that orange oil (*Citrus sinensis*) contains 34 alcohols, 30 esters, 20 aldehydes, 14 ketones, 10 carboxylic acids, and 36 varieties of terpenes, including mono-, sesqui- , di- and tetraterpenes. And this is not a complete analysis. In fact, no essential oil has ever been completely analyzed to reveal its every constituent.

Essential oils are so complex, it may never be possible to discover everything that is in even one of them.

With careful distillation at atmospheric pressures and minimum temperatures, the extracted essential oil is very close to that in the living plant except that only the lightest molecules (generally those less than 400 amu*) come through the distillation process. Heavier oil molecules of the living plant remain in the plant mass and can be accessed for therapeutic purposes as dried herbs. Dried herbs do not contain essential oils, except in traces, by virtue of the evaporation (drying) process by which they are preserved. (* See p. 78 for the definition of amu.)

Other names for essential oils include "volatile oils," "etheric oils," "ethereal oils," "aromatic oils," and/or "essences." This last term is more properly applied to extractions from plants other than essential oils—such as absolutes and the Bach flower essences.

By strict definition, essential oils are always a product of steam distillation. Even though the temperatures of steam extraction of a properly obtained essential oil are not excessively high (less than 270° F or 132° C), the heat can cause chemical changes in the oil that produce ingredients not present in the original plant. These are called "artifacts." Chamazulene, the blue color in blue tansy, yarrow, helichrysum, and German chamomile, is an example of an artifact. However, chamazulene is a good artifact with therapeutic benefits that have been thoroughly studied and well documented. (See p. 282.)

When oils are obtained by high temperature, high pressure distillation, (as is done for commercial perfumes and food flavorings), there are many artifacts and many of the subtle healing constituents of an oil are destroyed. Chemical solvents are also customarily used in extracting commercial grade oils that contaminate the oils with unnatural residues. Such oils are not therapeutic grade.

The point is that an essential oil, properly distilled by therapeutic grade standards, is as close to nature as the process will permit, but not totally so.

Absolutes

Absolutes are aromatic oils extracted from plants, but are not considered true essential oils because they are not obtained by distillation but by chemical solvents. This is not the most desirable way to extract the oil of a plant because there are always residues of the solvents left behind which adulterate the oil and may be toxic. Unfortunately, the aromatic essences of some plants cannot survive the heat and hydration of distillation. Extracting them as absolutes is the only practical way to obtain them at this time. A relatively new process called "carbon dioxide extraction" is a promising alternative that leaves no residue, but is not economically feasible at this time. The solvents used are usually ethanol (C_2H_6O), methanol (CH_4O), benzene (C_6H_6), or hexane (C_6H_{14}). All but the first of these are toxic chemicals. Absolutes are sometimes called "essences." Absolutes contain a wider range of molecular sizes than essential oils (up to 700 amu) and can include some fatty oils such as lauric acid.

Among the most popular absolutes are jasmine (*Jasminum officinale*) and neroli (*Citrus aurantium*), extracted from jasmine flowers and orange blossoms, respectively. The vanilla plant (*Vanilla planifolia*) is an orchid with large pods from which the vanilla essence is extracted as an absolute. Tolu or Peruvian balsam (*Myroxylon peiera*) is another absolute obtained from the sap of the tolu tree. Its fragrance is variously described as chocolate, vanilla, cinnamon, and clove. There is also a Peruvian balsam essential oil from the same tree obtained by distillation. Both tolu and vanilla are used mainly in the food flavoring and perfume industries. Tolu essential oil has therapeutic applications as well.

Onycha oil (*Styrax benzoin*) is another absolute oil, popular since the *Old Testament* days of Moses (Exodus 30:34). Onycha has powerful antimicrobial properties and has been used as an antiseptic (called tincture of benzoin) in hospitals for more than 200 years, even to the present day.

Expressed Oils

There are exceptions to the definition of an essential oil as being a product of distillation. These exceptions are the citrus oils. These are produced by the mechanical pressing of citrus peels. Strictly speaking, a citrus oil is not an essential oil, but an "expressed oil." However, it is generally regarded and included as an essential oil. Because citrus oils are expressed at normal living temperatures, they contain some larger molecules than those normally found in distilled oils. Citrus oils are also free of artifacts.

Essential, aromatic oils are vital substances to the life of a plant, which is why they are called "essential." The fatty, non-aromatic oils produced in a plant's seed serve as food for the germinating sprouts of the next generation. Fatty vegetable oils are not essential to the plant that creates them, but are required for the continuation of the species. Such oils are not called "essential."

Fatty Oils

Plants produce two types of oils: (1) Essential oils are found throughout their stems, leaves, roots, seeds, flowers, branches, woody parts, etc. and (2) Fatty oils found only in their seeds. Fatty oils are also called vegetable, carrier, neutral, and/or base oils by aromatherapists. Nutritionists and organic chemists call them "fatty acids." The two types of oils are compared side by side, point for point on the next page.

The structural shapes of fatty oil molecules are shown on page 56. These are the typical forms for molecules of vegetable oils. They are depicted as zig-zag chains with a carbon atom (not shown) at each zig and zag. If you take a look at the many drawings of essential oil molecules in Chapters Nine and Ten, you will see that fatty oil molecules don't look anything like essential oil molecules. Most essential oils molecules contain rings (polygonal shapes) and none of them have long chains. Lauric acid (p. 56) is a fatty oil pressed from the seeds of bay laurel (*Laurus nobilis*), but this same tree is also the source of an essential oil distilled from its leaves.

The next few paragraphs, and the figure on the next page, may not make much sense to you at this time, unless you already have a background in chemistry, but bear with me. After you have read Chapters Three, Four, Five, Six, and Ten, you will understand the remainder of this section on fatty oils

Essential and Fatty Oils Compared

Essential Oils	Fatty Oils
1. Distilled from plant parts.	1. Pressed from seeds
2. Not involved with seed germination and early growth	2. Necessary food for seeds to germinate and sprout
3. Essential to the life processes of the plant	3. Not essential to the life processes of the plant
4. Tiny molecules	4. Large molecules
5. Molecules built from rings and short chains	5. Molecules built from long chains (larger molecular size)
6. Aromatic and volatile	6. Nonaromatic and nonvolatile
7. Circulate throughout plants and in human bodies	7. Do not circulate in plants or in human bodies
8. Can pass thru tissues, cell walls, and cell membranes	8. Do not pass thru tissues, cell walls, and cell membranes
9. Not greasy to the touch	9. Greasy to the touch
10. Do not spoil or turn rancid	10. Can spoil and turn rancid
11. Antibacterial, antiviral, antifungal, antiparasitic, antiseptic	11. Not antibacterial, antiviral, antifungal, antiparasitic, antiseptic

NOTE: In this book, the terms "fatty oil" and "fatty acid" mean the same thing.

quite well and will be able to read the structural shorthand in the following figure quite easily.

The first two oils diagramed on the next page (caprylic and lauric) are saturated. That is, they contain all the hydrogen atoms they can hold. You can tell this at a glance by noting that there are no double bonds between C atoms. The bottom three oils (oleic, linoleic, and linolenic) are all unsaturated to one degree or another with linolenic acid having three double bonds, being the least saturated. You can tell this because it has the most double bonds between C atoms (three of them). Saturated or fully hydrogenated oils are more difficult for our bodies to metabolize. The five oils in the figure illustrate that a lighter oil (such as caprylic or lauric) that is saturated may be less healthy than one that is heavier but unsaturated (like oleic, linoleic, and linolenic).

One hears a lot about about trans fats being bad for you, but no one explains what they are or why they are bad. In every

The Shapes of Fatty Oil Molecules

M.W. = 144

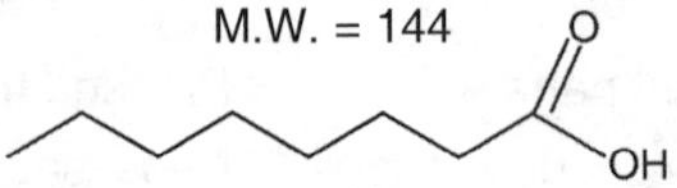

Caprylic Acid $C_8H_{16}O_2$ Coconut, Palm, Olive Oils and Butterfat

M.W. = 200

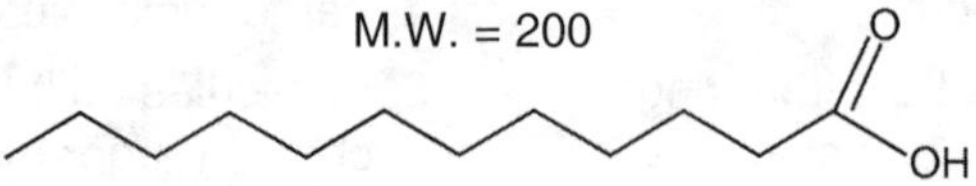

Lauric Acid $C_{12}H_{24}O_2$ Coconut, Castor, Bay Laurel Seed Oils

M.W. = 256

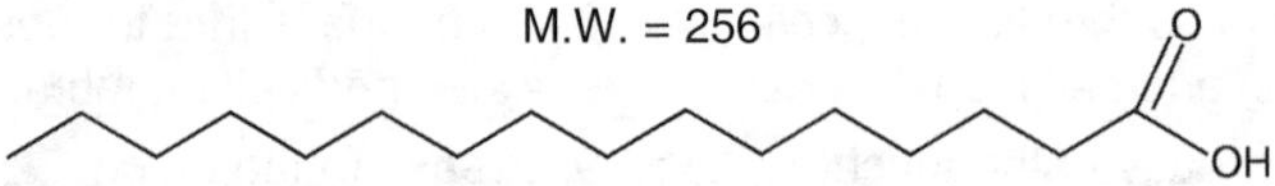

Palmitic Acid $C_{16}H_{32}O_2$ Coconut, Tamanu, Palm Oils

M.W. = 278

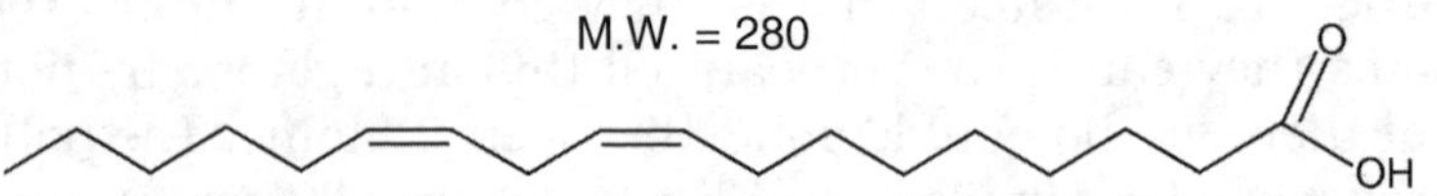

Linolenic Acid $C_{18}H_{30}O_2$ Primrose, Borage, Black Current Oils

M.W. = 280

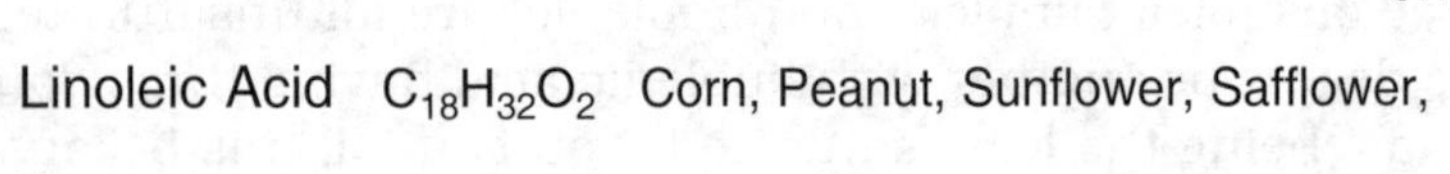

Linoleic Acid $C_{18}H_{32}O_2$ Corn, Peanut, Sunflower, Safflower,

M.W. = 282

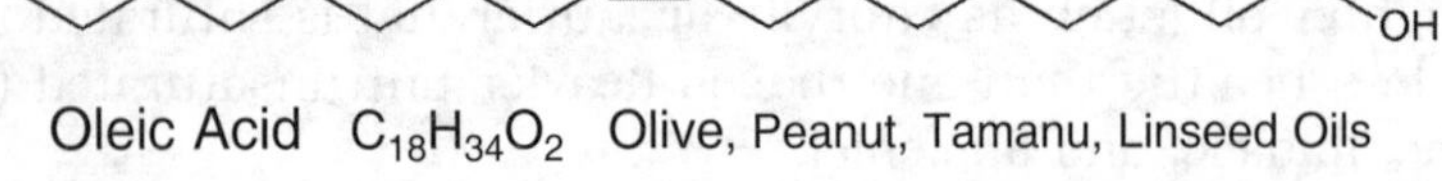

Oleic Acid $C_{18}H_{34}O_2$ Olive, Peanut, Tamanu, Linseed Oils

place you see a double bond in the molecules on the left (the bottom three) there is a hydrogen atom (not shown) attached to the carbon atom at each end of the double bond. When this pair of H atoms are on the same side of the molecule, we have a cis fat. When they are on opposite sides we have a trans fat.

Cis fat molecules are more flexible than trans fat molecules. Since the fats we eat ultimately find their way to our cells, cis fats keep our cells flexible and healthy while trans fats stiffen cell membranes and interfere with cellular function.

Since the hydrogens are not shown in the figures on p. 56 you can't tell if these fats are trans or cis. Produced by nature, they are cis, which is good. Hydrogenated or produced synthetically, they are always trans fats which are more stable and less digestible but have a longer shelf life. "Cis" and "trans" are handy words to keep in mind when you play Scrabble™.

All six of these oil compounds are fatty acids with a methyl radical (CH_3) on the left end and an acid radical (COOH) on the right. They are acids because they have the required carbon with an O atom and OH radical attached (See Table Seventeen, Chapter Ten, p. 314). However, they are very weak acids. That is, they don't easily give up hydrogen ions. (See discussion of acids and pH in Chapter Ten, pp. 338-356.)

When compared to essential oils, vegetable oils are greasy, viscous, non-volatile, and non-aromatic. This is partially because of molecular weight, but mostly because of molecular size (i.e., their length). The molecular weights in atomic mass units (amu) of most essential oil compounds range from 136 amu (for monoterpenes) to 240 amu (for sesquiterpene alcohols) and are non-greasy, low in viscosity, quite volatile, and quite aromatic.

In the six examples shown in the previous figure, caprylic (144), lauric (200), and palmitic (256) acids all have molecular weights within the range of those typical of essential oil compounds. Oleic (282), linoleic (280), and linolenic (278) acids are all slightly heavier than a diterpene (M.W. = 272), which makes them heavier than the heaviest constituents of most essential oils, but they aren't that much heavier. It is mostly their long lengths that give them their slippery, oily characteristics.

By comparison, essential oil molecules are much more compact in size and shape, mostly composed of rings. Even when an essential oil molecule is structured as a chain with no rings (acyclic), the chain is folded accordion-style into a compact size rather than strung out in a long line, as with fatty oils. (See drawings of Triacontane and Squalene, p. 288.) Examples of aromatic acyclic molecules are ocimene, myrcene, α–farnesene, and β–farnesene. (See figures on pp, 274 & 278.) This is an illustration of the importance of molecular shape (rather than atomic composition) in the determination of the characteristics of an oil compound.

While the sizes and shapes of fatty oil molecules do not permit them to penetrate and administer therapy at cellular levels like the molecules of essential oils, there is still some therapeutic value in many fatty oils. Olive oil (*Olea europea*), for example, has been used in various therapeutic applications for thousands of years. There is a whole chapter on this in the book, *Healing Oils of the Bible*. Tamanu oil (*Calophyllum inophyllum*), a fatty oil from the nut of the Polynesian tamanu tree, has been used by natives of the South Pacific as a natural sun screen and skin moisturizer for thousands of years.

The Role of Fatty Oils in Plants

Fatty oils are not essential to the life of a mature plant. They are essential only to sprouts and seedlings. While essential oil molecules easily pass through plant tissue, into and out of cell walls, fatty oil molecules do not. Essential oils circulate throughout all parts of a plant. Fatty oils remain in the seed where they are formed and do not circulate at all. Their purpose is not to sustain the life of the plant that creates them, but to sustain the life of the next generation.

Plants must make their own food by drawing water and minerals from the soil, gases from the atmosphere, and energy from sunlight for photosynthesis. For this they need roots, stems, and leaves, but when a seed is first planted there are no roots, stems, and leaves by which to manufacture fuel and food. So how is a plant supposed to get started? The answer is in the fatty oil of the seed. This is the food upon which the fledgling plant will sustain itself until it can start making its own. Plants consume these oils as food and so do we. We call them vegetable oils. Their properties are quite different than essential oils, and so are their functions.

Let's now discuss what essential oils do in living plants and how these activities actually prepare and train the oils to serve us in beneficial ways.

Plant Metabolism and Nourishment

Essential oils have been called "the life blood of a plant." They circulate through plant tissues and pass through cell walls, carrying nutrition into cells and carrying waste products out.

When essential oils are applied to people, they do the same thing, carrying oxygen into cells and carrying waste products out. In fact, essential oils are one of nature's best body cleansers. They can cleanse our cellular receptor sites of pharmaceutical drugs, petrochemicals, and other disruptors of intercellular communication. They can also chelate heavy metals and other toxins, helping to remove and flush them through the liver, colon, sweat, lungs, and kidneys. They can also increase our ability to absorb vitamins and other nutrients.

Regulators of Plant Functions

Essential oils act as plant hormones, regulating plant functions and orchestrating the production of vitamins and enzymes. They act as messengers and supervisors within the plant that help coordinate and initiate vital plant activities. Essential oils can also do the same when applied to humans. They can act as neurotransmitters, peptides, steroids, hormones, enzymes, vitamins, and other message-carrying molecules (called ligands) which intelligently assist our bodily functions and help to restore or maintain wellness.

Essential oils possess homeostatic intelligence. Homeostasis is that state where every vital biological process within a living organism is functioning as it should. It is a state of perfect wellness. Essential oils always work toward restoring and maintaining balance and homeostasis, first in the plants who create them, and then in the humans who apply them.

To say that an essential oil works toward balance, and homeostasis means that the same oil can work in different directions depending on the needs of the plant or person. Oregano oil (*Origanum vulgare*) will kill hostile microbes while nurturing those that are friendly. Angelica oil (*Angelica archangelica*) can stimulate a uterus to contract or to relax depending on the need. Myrtle oil (*Myrtus communis*) is an adaptigen that can stimulate an increase or a decrease in thyroid activity depending on a person's condition. Drugs are incapable of such intelligent discriminations and act only in preprogrammed directions, like robots, whether beneficial or not.

Protection

Essential oils protect plants in many ways. They kill viruses, bacteria, parasites, and fungi that could harm the plant. They sometimes provide unacceptable tastes or smells that prevent herbivores from eating them to extinction. They repel insects and other pests. (See the example of marigolds, Chapter Ten, p. 333.) Essential oils can even act as herbicides to prevent competing plants from growing too close, placing too much demand on available nutrients.

For example, you may have noticed that desert plants space themselves at a distance from one another. This is because the water supply is very limited. If plants clustered to closely, the available water in that area would be consumed and all of them would die. Desert bushes exude an oil through their shallow root systems for a certain diameter around themselves that prevents the germination of any seeds that could compete with their water supply.

In another example, horn worms are large green caterpillars that love tobacco and tomato leaves. Gardeners who raise tomatoes call them "tomato horn worms." Their green color is such a perfect match with that of the foliage they are almost impossible to see even though they can be quite large, 2-3 inches long and up to half an inch in diameter. One horn worm can devastate a tomato plant, stripping all of its leaves in a day or two unless stopped. Organic gardeners generally try to control the pests by careful inspection of their plants on a daily basis, but if they miss a few days, they can return to a destroyed tomato patch.

It turns out that healthy tomato and tobacco plants have their own defense for the horn worm. When attacked, they emit a volatile oil that blows in the wind and attracts certain species of wasps that will come and kill the horn worms. If there are enough of these wasps in the neighborhood, the problem is solved and both the plants and the gardeners reap the benefits. However, if you are a gardener, I would suggest that you don't wait for the wasps. By the time they arrive (and if they arrive), half of your tomato plants could be destroyed. There may be enough remaining plants to bear fruit to preserve the species, but the objective of a gardener is to maximize the crop, not preserve the species. Why let your gardening efforts go to support the worms?

The oils of the tomato and tobacco plants that attract wasps when they are under attack pose another question. How do the nymphs that lay the eggs that hatch into horn worm caterpillars find tomatoes and tobacco? If you are a gardener, you will never see a tomato horn worm unless you raise tomatoes. The answer is that tomatoes have a certain odor from the oils they continuously emit that can travel for miles on the wind. When a horn worm nymph smells this, they fly upwind until they find your garden.

Another dramatic example of an essential oil used as a protection is the lima bean of South America. The bean plant can fall victim to certain spider mites that chew away on the plant. When attacked by an army of spider mites, the beans release an oil to the wind that attracts a specific species of wasp that feeds on spider mites. With the arrival of the troops of hungry wasps, the problem of the lima beans has been solved.

The examples of the lima beans, tomato, and tobacco plants are not the only ones where plants communicate with animals. There are hundreds of thousands of examples of plant/animal communications and aromatic chemicals usually play a key part in all of them.

When essential oils are applied to humans, they offer us many protections as well. Fortunately, none of the commonly used essential oils attract wasps to people so you don't have to worry about that. In fact, one of the benefits of essential oils is that many of them are effective insect repellents (like lavender or citronella) which not only protect us from mosquitoes, chiggers, and ticks, but are nontoxic to us and have pleasant fragrances as well.

Oils are Smarter than Antibiotics

Essential oils also offer wonderful protection from viruses, bacteria, parasites, and fungi, just as they did in the plants before they were commandeered for our use.

With respect to bacteria, essential oils are particularly valuable. The medical answer to a bacterial attack is to prescribe antibiotics. The problem with antibiotics is that they indiscriminantly kill all the bacteria in our bodies, which isn't good. We harbor many friendly bacteria that help us digest food and engage in other essential bodily activities, without which we can't stay healthy. Hence, when you have gotten over a bacteriologically caused sickness using antibiotics, your immune system has been depressed and your friendly fauna have been diminished. You then need to eat lots of yogurt and other organic, raw foods to build your system back to what it was before the onslaught of the antibiotics. Antibiotics (and most pharmaceuticals) also make your body more acid, which can stimulate the growth of fungi and other organisms in the body—thus trading one form of sickness for another. Essential oils also combat viruses, while antiobiotics cannot.

This is not to say that antibiotics should never be used. There are some situations where their use can help you overcome a severe infection and put you on the road to recovery when no other available means would work. With the crisis past, one must then deal with the negative effects of the antibiotics, but at least the crisis is over and past.

Essential oils have none of these negative side effects. Essential oils have the intelligence to distinguish good bacteria from bad and attack only the bad while nourishing the good. Essential oils can also attack viruses and fungi, which antibiotics cannot. Furthermore, essential oils help alkalize your body, raising it from an acid state prone to sickness, into a slightly alkaline state of balance, which is the natural pH of healthiness.

Just living and breathing around essential oils on a daily basis goes a long way toward maintaining vitality and wellness. The action of essential oils inside the human body is always toward balance, toward the state of homeostasis where every organ and cell is working properly and in harmony. Therapeutic grade essential oils have homeostatic intelligence, something neither synthetic oils nor pharmaceuticals possess.

When God created man and woman, he did not put them in a house. He put them in a garden (Genesis 2:8) where they would be immersed in an atmosphere of essential oils wafting from the vegetation around them, molecules they would breathe 24 hours a day to help keep their bodies balanced and healthy and able to survive for centuries in that state. We don't have to permanently move out of doors and abandon our sheltered, air conditioned homes and environmentally controlled work places to achieve this "Garden of Eden" in a modern world. We can diffuse and wear therapeutic grade essential oils on a daily basis and keep our modern lifestyles while enjoying some of the benefits of Eden at the same time.

Shields from Sunlight and Heat

Essential oils are especially prevalent in desert plants because they help protect the plant from sunburn and dehydration. The larger terpene molecules (especially the tetraterpenes or carotenoids which give colors and pigments to plants) actually lower the frequencies of visible sunlight down to infrared levels and re-emit the energy as heat, thus preventing the plant from damages that can result from certain photochemical transformations in response to light. Platyphyllol, a compound in cajeput oil (*Melaleuca cajuputi*) is such a good blocker of UV light it has been used in commercial sunscreen lotions.

Essential oils also protect plants from dehydration in interesting ways. For example, in the Eastern and Midwestern United States, there are often dry periods of the year, such as late summer or early fall. During these times, when the wind is not blowing, one can often see a haze hovering over the forested hills and valleys in the late afternoons. This haze is not smoke. Neither is it fog. It is a cloud of essential oil molecules emitted by the trees to blanket the forest and reduce evaporation to preserve moisture. That is where the Great Smoky Mountains got their name—not from smoke, but from essential oils.

Solar Amplifiers

While essential oils can protect plants from too much sunlight, in some cases the plants want more sunlight. In this case, the oils act as solar amplifiers. In Chapter Ten we will study furanoids. These compounds have a heterogeneous five-sided ring in their molecular structure called "furan." Its chemical formula is C_4H_4O. This little pentagonal functional group can act as an ultraviolet light amplifier, like a little prism or magnifying glass. The principle place where furanoids are found in essential oils are in the citrus oils, which all come from the rind of the fruit.

Why would nature want to amplify UV light in the skin of a fruit? Answer: To accelerate the ripening of the fruit and maximize its sugar content. Interestingly, when the fruit is fully ripe, the furano-compounds disappear. Hence, if you press the essential oil from the rind of a grapefruit that is not yet ripe, you get furans. If you press the essential oil from the peel of an already ripe grapefruit, you don't get furano-compounds.

How is this significant for people? If you apply citrus oils containing furanoids to your skin, they can amplify UV light when you are in direct sunlight or in a tanning booth. They can cause you to burn and can even produce permanent pigmentation patches in your skin. Such oils are called "phototoxic." So, just to be on the safe side, stay away from sunlight and other UV sources for at least twelve hours after you have applied certain oils containing furans to the exposed parts of your body. As humans, we don't need to accelerate any ripening of our tissues nor increase the sugar content of our bodies. We don't want to be walking grapefruits turning pink. (See pp. 379-383.)

Healing and Repair

When plants are bruised, cut, or damaged, resin flows out of the wound. The essential oils of the resin act as antiseptics to protect the plant from microbial infections and to initiate the healing process.

When humans are bruised, cut, or damaged, our blood flows out, much like the resins in a plant, and also acts to protect us from infections and start the healing process. When we apply essential oils over the wound, they do for us what they did for the plant. They offer additional protection from infection and accelerate the healing process.

Harsh medical antiseptics may cleanse our wounds and kill harmful bacteria, but they do not promote healing. They often retard and interfere with healing. Essential oils, God's natural antiseptics, don't do that.

The Birds and the Bees

One of the most important functions of essential oils in plants is their role in reproduction. Plants are immobile. Some can self-pollinate themselves, having both male and female parts, but most cannot, or if they do, inferior offspring result, reducing the vitality of the species.

Some plants depend on the wind to distribute their pollen to other plants in order to accomplish the fertilization that will ensure the survival of their species. But most plants don't go for this option.

Most plants engage the help of animals—mostly birds and bees. In order to do so, they must communicate to the creature of their choice in such a way that it will do whatever it needs to do to bring pollen from one plant to the ovaries of another so that healthy seed will result.

Communication between plants and animals is by two means: by sight and by smell. The beautiful colors and shapes of flowers may have many purposes, but one purpose is to attract insects or other animals to visit and, in the process, cross-pollinate them. The colors of many flowers are from large terpene oil molecules. The small terpenes—monoterpenes, sesquiterpenes, and even diterpenes—are important constituents of essential oils, especially the first two terpenes mentioned. Tetraterpenes are bigger, are usually not found in aromatic oils, and provide color. You will be introduced to the tetraterpenes, carotene (the orange of carrots) and lycopene (the red of tomatoes), in Chapter Nine.

However, many colors in flowers are not from oily compounds, but from other substances, some of which can be used as pigments, others not. Those that are not pigments are actually light refracting structures that make it appear that a flower is red, purple or blue when, in fact, if you crush the flower petals, there is no red, purple or blue pigment there at all. It is colorless. You may have observed this when mashing a brightly colored flower petal between your fingers and finding no color—your fingers remaining unstained.

Brighter Than Bright

In these cases, the flower has crafted structures that refract or reflect certain colors from the spectrum of sunlight so that what we see is actually an illusion of light. In some cases, these devices of the flowers can actually absorb invisible ultraviolet light from the sun and then re-emit it at a lower visible frequency making the flower appear iridescent, or brighter than the visible sunlight falling upon it. So called "black lights" do this. They emit invisible ultraviolet rays which we cannot see which can be absorbed by various substances and re-emitted in the visible spectrum as fluorescent yellows, greens, and reds.

This property of taking invisible light frequencies and transforming them into visible light frequencies, is applied by manufacturers of laundry products in making "brighteners." Chemicals in a brightening agent actually do this. They absorb UV light and re-emit it at visible levels to make a white shirt appear "brighter than white." Illuminate a freshly laundered white shirt under a black light and you will see what I mean. Just as commercial detergent companies play tricks on our eyes, so do flowers. And we love it.

One of the most interesting ways that plants communicate with animals is how they communicate with us human animals. By their appealing fragrances and alluring shapes and colors, flowers entice humans to grow them, water them, feed them, and nurture them—thus assuring their survival. Just think about it. How many billions of dollars do humans spend each year, not to mention the untold hours of caring people willingly provide, just to grow and maintain flowering and aromatic plants?

How can this be that a passive, immobile plant that produces no consumable fruit can do this—to motivate intelligent human beings to do so much for them? One wonders who is the more intelligent of the two. It is really a matter of mutual benefit and a bit of symbiosis. We humans are not that far from the plant kingdom after all, sharing many of the same compounds and molecules. We are both a part of the universe of God's creation, connected in ways we do not need to understand in order to enjoy.

Pheromones

Color is probably the least of the means by which flowers attract pollinators. Many insect pollinators are color blind or, in many cases, totally blind. The key is smell. Insects carry olfactory sensory organs in many places, not just their noses. Some even on their feet, so they can walk on a surface and smell or taste it at the same time. Common house flies do this.

Pheromones are message carrying molecules (usually ketones, aldehydes or esters) that convey meaning to specific animals or insects. To a male of the species, the meaning is usually that a female is nearby and ready to mate. Some biologists say that every animal species has pheromones, including humans. Cats do, for sure. If you have a female cat and haven't seen a tom cat for months, just wait until she goes into heat and the toms will come visit from miles around. What the male cats pick up is a lactone pheromone released by the female when she is in heat. This is the same compound (nepetalactone) found in the catnip plant (*Nepeta cataria*) and catnip oil, that cats love so much. (We say more about pheromones in Chapter Ten when we discuss aldehydes, ketones, and esters.)

Most people have never seen a cecropia moth (*Samia cecropia*) or a polyphemus moth (*Telea polyphemus*). Both members of the silk worm family (Bombacidae), they are the two largest moths in North America and only come out at night. They are both beautiful to behold. You may see one clinging to the side of your house some night, not too far from your porch light.

These moths are rare and it would not be unusual for there to be only one male and one female of these species to be within a ten square mile area. For them to make a rendezvous would almost seem impossible. Yet, they do find each other, in the dark, and mate. How do they do this? It is by pheromones.

The odor sensing organs of a male moth are in its feathery antennae, which sweep the breezes in search of a certain scent. When the female is ready to mate, she emits a tiny spray of a specific ketone that disperses to the wind. If, on some enchanted evening, a male is downwind and catches even one molecule of the female's pheromone, it immediately gets the message and starts flying against the wind to meet this stranger, never to let her go. And you know the rest of the song. And the species lives on.

Scent as an Expression of Individuality

Most men and women enjoy perfumes, whether they be colognes, after-shave lotions, sachets, or costly potions to titillate emotions. There are perfumes for the morning, for the working day, for occasions of entertainment, for the evening, and for the night. Some people wear different fragrances according to the occasion and the time of day. People usually wear fragrances for a purpose.

Flowers do the same. If you have a rose garden, you may have sampled its floral perfumes individually by putting your nose right into each bloom. If you haven't done this, I recommend it. The first thing you will notice is that every variety of rose has its own distinct signature of scent.

People are like that, too. They pick perfumes that suit their personalities, which is an individual thing for each person. We express our personalities through our choices of the scents we choose to wear. Roses do the same. From an individual rose's point of view, it wants to be a rose that stands out, one that is different from the rest of the bushes and even from every other rose on the same bush. Try smelling several roses on the same bush and you will learn that there is not just one scent associated with that variety, but a suite of scents. While each rose flower shares the common characteristics of its family, it expresses a unique individuality as well.

Another thing you will notice about roses (and many other flowers as well) is that they change their perfumes with the time of day. What they wear in the morning won't be the same as in the afternoon or night. Jasmine, for example, attracts certain night flying insects. Hence, its strongest fragrance is released after midnight and before sunrise. Since the primary purpose of a flower's odor is to attract pollinating insects, adjusting scents throughout the day actually attracts different insects at different times, just as different insects come out at different times from early morning, to late afternoon, to evening, and through the dark of night.

Flower fragrances also change with the aging of the bloom. You will notice in smelling your rose blossoms closely and individually, that what they waft as a new partially opened bud is not the same as that of the mature blossom. Scents are normally not strong in the bud because at that time, the petals are not open and ready for guests and visitors as potential pollinators. It is when they are newly and fully opened that their perfume is the strongest. When a flower ages and its pollination is complete, it loses its scent, its purpose having been fulfilled. All of this is something you can experience in your own rose garden (or someone else's).

A Rose is a Rose is a Rose

The poetess, Gertrude Stein, has aptly said, "A rose is a rose is a rose," (*Sacred Emily*, 1913). It was her attempt to express the unexpressable—the singular beauty, texture, and fragrance of a rose. Rose oil is probably the most expensive of all essential oils and has the highest electro-magnetic frequency (320 MHz). Thousands of pounds of petals are required to distill even one pound of precious oil. Its aroma is physically, mentally, and spiritually ele-vating. Many eyewitnesses to miracles, visions, and spiri-tual manifestations have reported the scent of roses lin-gering about the site of the experience.

Most people cannot afford to purchase rose oil, but you don't have to wait until you buy it to experience it. It is available at no cost to everyone. Just find a blooming rose bush and start inhaling. What you will receive is true, pure, unadulterated rose oil directly from the flower, itself. You will also enjoy the visual beauty of its appearance at the same time. By caressing the flowers gently with your fingers and by letting your nose and face come into contact with the velvet surface of the petals, you will experience the rose with three senses, not just one—sight, smell, and touch. Some people even eat rose petals, thus engaging the sense of taste, taking traces of the oil internally.

This is the way God originally meant for us to enjoy essential oils, by inhaling and contacting them directly from nature the way Adam and Eve did in the Garden of Eden. (Genesis 2:8) In our busy lives, we mustn't forget to stop once in a while "to smell the roses."

The Way to a Bug's Heart is Thru Its Belly

Plants entice insects to visit their flowers in a variety of ways. A common way is by offering a bait and a reward, like food. Pollen, itself, is one of the most common of these food/rewards. Thus, bees are rewarded with a load of pollen they can take back to their hives which they turn into food and honey. Pollen is rich in protein and serves as an excellent food for many insects. In the meantime, much of the pollen they carry is sprinkled from flower to flower, fertilizing them for the future and benefit of the plant species.

The other most common food offered by plants is nec-tar. Nectar is mainly sugar water that collects in the hol-low places in a flower. Plants that produce nectar don't use it themselves. They create it as an enticement for various mobile creatures to come and help them reproduce. Hummingbirds and many butterflies live on nectar. When they come to drink from the pretty flower cups with their long beaks and proboscises, their bodies brush against the anthers (male parts) which bear the pollen. When they alight on the next flower for another sip of their favorite beverage, the pollen dust on their bodies filters down to the pistils (female parts) and into the ovaries to create living seed.

An example of a food offering is given by peonies, which are popular large pink and white flowers of the genus, *Paeonia.* Their name comes from the Greek *Paion,* an epithet for Apollo who used this flower as an herb to cure the wounds of the gods. Peony blooms secrete an oily juice containing saccharides (sugars) that attract sweet-eating ants. As the ants crawl from flower to flower feasting on their favorite dessert, they also act as agents of cross pollination to the benefit of the peonies. But food is not the only thing plants use to entice animals to help them.

Sex in Advertising

Contrary to what you may think, the first to employ sex in advertising were not people. It was plants. In order to attract insects to pollinate them, plants' most common device is to produce oily compounds that imitate sexual pheromones. Thus, they trick either the male and/or the female of a species to visit them and carry pollen from one flower to another.

These imitation pheromones comprise many of the fragrances we love in essential oils which have been the foundation of the perfume business for thousands of years. They are aphrodisiac to many members of the animal kingdom and they are aphrodisiac to us. Plants and flowers have seduced us all, and we love it.

For example, in eastern Kansas, some of the Dakotas, bits of Minnesota, Illinois, Manitoba, Alberta, and Saskatchewan, there lives a rare flower called the western prairie fringed orchid (*Plantanthera praeclara*). It is a stately plant about 1-3 feet high that bears a couple of dozen creamy white flowers. With their beautiful white fringe and delicate fragrance, these flowers stand out against the surrounding grassy prairie. Their survival depends entirely on two species of nocturnal moths the achemon moth (*Eumorpha achemon*) and a variety of sphinx moth (*Sphinx drupiferarum*), both members of the hawk moth family (Sphingidae). These two species are the only pollinators for the western prairie fringed orchid. Its lovely flowers lure no others. The reason is this.

First of all, the fragrance of the flowers (i.e. their essential oils) become more concentrated at night, increasing their scent by several factors over their daytime levels. Their white color is also ideal for seeing in the dim moonlight over the prairie. Hence, they are definitely only interested in night visitors.

The scent that these flowers waft into the night breeze matches that of the sexual pheromones of these particular species of moths. But the factor that restricts their pollinators to only two types of moths is more than scent and night visibility. The nectar of a fringed orchid is found at the bottom of a tubular structure about 2.5 inches long. To sample the nectar, the animal must be capable of reaching to the bottom of the tube. These two types of nocturnal insects are among the few with a proboscis long enough to reach the nectar. Most other visitors would leave the orchid unrewarded and, thus, would not be encouraged to patronize the species.

Even if there are other creatures with the equipment to tap into the orchid's nectar, they would be incapable of pollinating the flowers. The orchids are so constructed that when one of these two moths approach, they provide a runway guide to steer the oncoming insect into just the right position to suck up the nectar. This has to do with the distance between the eyes of these particular moths, which is just right to touch the anthers on either side of the orifice they must locate to find the nectar. When the moth has completed its drink, it flies away with pollen affixed to both eyes. At the next orchid, the pollen grains are brushed onto two receptive structures leading to the ovaries whose location exactly matches that of the moth's eyes.

Only an insect having a head of the right dimensions, and its eyes placed just so, could transport the fringed orchids' pollen from flower to flower. These two species of hawk moth are the only two creatures with a sufficiently long proboscis and properly spaced eyes to match the unique needs of the western prairie fringed orchid.

Such perfect symbiosis between plants and animals makes one realize the infinite planning that continually goes into creation by the Creator. there are literally thousands and thousands of examples of perfect meshing between species, more than we will ever know. There is a fascinating book on this entitled *Tales of Chemistry in Nature* by William Agosta. (See bibliography)

Bees as the First Aromatherapists

Not all orchids invite moths to provide their pollination needs. There are some 600 species of orchids that enlist the aid of bees for pollination. They are called "bee orchids." There is also a corresponding group of bees, called "euglossine bees." These orchids and these bees were made for each other.

Euglossine bees come in about 175 brightly colored species in five genera. They are not like honey bees. They don't live in colonies, nor do they make honey. Their specialty is in collecting fragrance chemicals (i.e. essential oils). They are natural born aromatherapists.

Most flowers will reward their insect pollinators with either a nectar (sugar water stored in the flower's cup) or pollen (a high protein food). However, the group of orchids that euglossine bees pollinate bear flowers with no nectar and no pollen that can serve as food. So there are no sweet or nourishing rewards to entice them to visit. What the flowers do offer are copious quantities of fragrant essential oils that the bees love—the male bees, that is. The female bees could care less and never visit the flowers. This is a case where pollination is exclusively by male bees only.

Among these 600 species of orchids, more than sixty different aromatic compounds have been identified with each plant employing at least a dozen of them in fashioning their particular perfume to entice the male bees. The compounds identified are common to many plants other than orchids. These include 1,8 cineole (found in eucalyptus, rosemary, ravensara, and dozens of other plants), benzyl acetate (found in jasmine, ylang ylang, and Roman chamomile), and α-pinene (found in pine, frankincense, galbanum, the rose of sharon, and hundreds of others).

When a male bee comes to visit an orchid soliciting its attention, it does not look for pollen or nectar. It goes straight for the fragrant oils of the flower. He begins by emitting a blend of his own oils onto the oil droplets of the orchid. The bee's lipid oil gland is in his head and acts as a solvent to facilitate gathering up the orchid's oil secretions. Using brushes on his front pair of feet, he scrubs the plant surface and mops up the mixture until the mopheads on his feet are saturated and unable to hold any more. This takes about 30 seconds. Then, hovering over the petals, he quickly transfers the accumulated perfume to storage containers in his hind legs. Amazingly, the chambers within the hind legs then separate the bees solvent oils from those of the flower and return it to the bee's head for reuse. What remains in the hind leg pouches is pure orchid oil.

After working for a time at accumulating a cache of oil, the bee then begins to act strangely, slipping and falling down, as if he were drunk and out of his head in ecstasy. This may go on for an hour or more, as the bee blissfully enjoys the fragrances it has gathered. It appears that the fragrances that so attract the male bee imitate the sex pheromones of the females.

Meanwhile, the orchid does not let the bee escape without a load of pollen. This it accomplished by a trigger mechanism that shoots a pollen packet at the bee with considerable force, knocking him down, but ensuring that the pollen sticks to his body. Thus the pollen is transferred to the next orchid.

Besides the enjoyment of their mood elevating qualities, what does the male euglossine bee get of his efforts to harvest the essential oils of the orchid flower? Longevity is one of the benefits. Without gathering these fragrances from these flowers, the male bees have shortened life spans and reduced fertility.

Thus, the first aromatherapists were not people. Insects, not humans, were the first to gather and concentrate the oily essences of plants for personal health, pleasure, longevity, hormonal balance, and, perhaps, even for emotional release. Who knows?

Key Points of Chapter Two

1. Essential oils are the volatile oil-soluble portions of the fluids of a plant containing odiferous compounds produced by steam distillation of plant matter.

2. The plant matter may include any part of the plant—roots, stems, branches, leaves, seeds, fruits, or flowers.

3. While, by definition, essential oils are products of distillation, citrus oils, which are produced by cold expression (pressing out of the rinds) are also considered to be essential oils.

4. Essential oils are mixtures of hundreds of compounds and are so complex that, as yet, not one has been completely analyzed for all of its ingredients.

5. The actual oils in living plants contain larger molecules than those that come through the distillation process. Generally, the only oils that compose a significant part of an essential oil are less than 300 amu (atomic mass units) in molecular weight.

6. To access larger plant molecules for therapeutic purposes, one must employ dried herbs which lack the small molecules found in essential oils but which are rich in the large molecules.

7. Essential oils are also called "volatile oils," "etheric oils," "ethereal oils," and "aromatic oils."

8. Essential oils are essential to the vital processes of living plants, which is why they are called "essential."

9. Vegetable oils, pressed from seeds, are not essential to the plants that create them, but are necessary for the continuation of the species and are used to support new seedlings until they have roots, stems and leaves of their own by which to participate in photosynthesis.

10. Vegetable oils are called fatty oils, carrier oils, neutral oils, and base oils by aromatherapists. Chemists call them fatty acids.

11. Steam distillation can alter the chemical composition of the oils so that the constituents in the final oil may not have all been in the living plant. Such constituents are called artifacts.

12. While the task of a distiller is to produce an essential oil as close to the composition of what was in the living plant as possible, not all artifacts are bad. Some are good. Chamazulene is one of the good artifacts highly prized in therapeutic aromatherapy,

13. Oils perform many of the same functions in plants as they do for us. Thus, they come to us as experienced and trained agents for health and healing.

14. Essential oils participate in the metabolism and nourishment of plants and also do so in people.

15, Essential oils regulate plant functions, acting like various types of hormones and ligands, and do the same in humans.

16. Homeostasis is a state of wellness, balance, and proper function within an organism. Essential oils always work toward balance or homeostasis, first in the plants that created them, then in the humans who apply them.

17. Essential oils afford various types of protection to plants such as helping them to fight off viruses, bacteria, parasites, and fungi, and do the same things for people.

18. In fighting off bacteria, essential oils are smarter than antibiotics which are indiscriminate in the bacteria they attack. Essential oils attack only the harmful bacteria in our bodies while they nurture the friendly bacterial flora that assist in our metabolism and provide some of our natural immunities.

19. Essential oils, especially among the plants of the desert, help shield plants from intense sunlight, excessive heat, and dehydration.

20. Essential oils in some citrus rinds amplify ultraviolet light when the fruit is ripening to accelerate the creation of sugars. When the fruit is fully ripe, the furanoid compounds that resonate with UV light disappear from the oil.

21. Oils containing furanoid compounds (like some citrus) may be phototoxic in that if one applies them to the skin and then goes out into sunlight or into a tanning booth, the amplification of radiation by the furanoid compounds can cause sunburn and alterations in the pigmentation of the skin. So don't apply such oils to exposed areas of the skin unless you can avoid sunlight or other UV sources for at least 12 hours. For more on phototoxicity, including a list of phototoxic oils, see the section in Chapter Ten on furanoids. (See pp. 379-383.)

22. When plants are injured, essential oils from within the plant flow to the wound, protecting it from infection like an antiseptic and initiating the healing process. They do the same for people when applied to human wounds.

23. Many fragrances of essential oils are fashioned by plants to imitate sexual pheromones to entice insects to visit them and, thus, carry pollen from flower to flower to produce good seed for the preservation of the species.

24. The first to gather and concentrate the essential oils of a plant were not people, but insects, such as male euglossine bees, who, by anointing themselves with the oils of certain orchids, increase their health, happiness, and longevity.

❤ CHAPTER THREE
BASIC CHEMISTRY MADE EASY

C hemistry is the study of matter and how one kind of matter reacts with another. Matter is anything that has mass (weight) and occupies space. You have mass. I have mass. All God's children have mass, sometimes more than we would prefer to admit. And we all occupy space. Thus, by definition, our physical bodies are composed of matter.

By contrast, light is not matter. It is energy. It has no mass and does not occupy space. You can pass any number of light beams simultaneously through the same region of space without interference. You could not do that with matter. You could not seat a whole room of people in one chair because they each occupy space. The study of energy is physics.

All matter is composed of three kinds of particles.

electrons = e- (negatively charged)
protons = p+ (positively charged)
neutrons = n (neutral, no charge)

Although neutrons are slightly heavier than protons, for practical purposes they have the same mass, which is 1.00 atomic mass unit* (amu). By comparison, electrons are extremely light and small. It takes approximately 1,840 electrons to equal the mass of one proton or one neutron. Therefore, when electrons, protons and neutrons combine to make atoms, the mass of the resulting atom is, essentially, the simple sum of the masses of the protons and neutrons, the electrons being effectively weightless. Despite its

---

* Some medical texts use the term "dalton" instead of "amu" as the unit of measure for atomic and molecular weight. They are synonyms. In this book, we will use the term "amu."

relatively small size and mass, the negative electrical charge on an electron is exactly the same magnitude as the positive charge on a proton—a perfect electrical balance.

When electrons, protons, and neutrons unite to form atoms, the number of protons always equals the number of electrons. This makes atoms electrically neutral and gives them stability. The number of neutrons per atom of a given element can vary, but the number of electrons and protons always remains equal so there is no net charge.

The simplest possible atom is a single electron orbiting around a single proton like this.

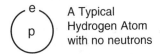

A Typical Hydrogen Atom with no neutrons

This is a hydrogen atom, the lightest of all the elements and represented by a capital "H." Its atomic mass is 1.00 amu (atomic mass unit), the weight of one proton. Hydrogen is thought to compose 90% of all the atoms of the universe and makes up 60%–70% of its total mass. It composes 56% of the sun by weight but less than 1% of the earth's crust. The bodies of plants and animals are about 1% hydrogen by weight.

Theoretically, the next simplest possible atom would be two electrons orbiting around two protons like this.

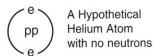

A Hypothetical Helium Atom with no neutrons

This would be Helium, the second lightest of all the elements and represented by the symbol "He." Helium is the second most abundant element in the universe composing about 34% of its total mass. It makes up 44% of the sun, but is rare on earth. Helium is chemically inert and is generally thought to play no role in life processes.

As shown above, its atomic mass would be 2.00, the weight of two protons. However, the drawing shown above is not how helium usually occurs in nature.

Let's now go to Table One (on p. 82 or on the end sheets at the back) and look up helium (element number 2). Notice that the average atomic weight of a sample of helium atoms is not

2.00, but 4.003. Nature does not like helium without neutrons. This is because positively charged protons naturally repel each other and the neutrons are necessary to keep the helium nucleus intact. In fact, all atoms of all elements containing more than one proton must have neutrons to hold them together for that reason. But this is getting into the topic of "strong and weak nuclear forces," which is quantum mechanics and nuclear physics, not chemistry.

Any atom with two protons and two electrons is helium by definition and exhibits all the chemical characteristics of helium, no matter how many neutrons may be present in the nucleus. But a helium atom with neutrons will be heavier than one without. Helium atoms like the one drawn on the previous page do not seem to exist in nature. Most of the helium in the universe contains 2 neutrons per atom with an occasional atom containing 3. If you take a typical sample of helium, weigh it in atomic mass units, and divide by the number of atoms present, your average value will be slightly more than 4 (or 4.003). This number implies if you have 1,000 helium atoms in a bottle, all of them will have 2 neutrons except for three atoms which will have 3 neutrons each. In other words, 99.7% of the time, helium atoms come with two neutrons. So let's redraw our helium atom as it would normally appear with two electrons spinning about a nucleus of two protons and two neutrons.

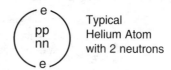

Typical
Helium Atom
with 2 neutrons

This brings us back to hydrogen. If you look at Table One, you will see that the average atomic weight of a sample of hydrogen is not 1.00, but 1.008. This means that some hydrogen atoms weigh more than 1.0 amu. In fact, it means that in a typical sample of 1,000 hydrogen atoms, six of them will contain a single neutron and one will contain 2 neutrons. While adding neutrons makes hydrogen heavier, it in no way affects its chemical behavior. It is still hydrogen in every way, chemically. Let's draw our two new kinds of hydrogen with neutrons.

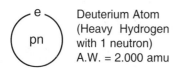

Deuterium Atom
(Heavy Hydrogen
with 1 neutron)
A.W. = 2.000 amu

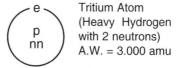

Tritium Atom
(Heavy Hydrogen
with 2 neutrons)
A.W. = 3.000 amu

Heavy hydrogen, consisting of deuterium and tritium, are the ingredients of hydrogen bombs. When the same element comes in more than one variety, where the only difference is in the number of neutrons in the nucleus, the variations are called "isotopes" of that element. Hydrogen comes in three isotopes. However, 99.2% of the time, it occurs as the isotope with no neutrons and an atomic weight (A.W.) of 1.000. This most common form of hydrogen is sometimes called "protium." But that is nuclear physics, not chemistry.

Electricity in Every Chemical Process

We have said at the beginning of this chapter that "chemistry is the study of matter," which is what most chemistry texts say. However, this is not entirely true. Chemistry only studies one aspect of matter. Chemistry is concerned only with the activities of the electrons of the atoms of matter and not the protons or neutrons. Matter, of course, is composed of all three particles. The study of atomic particles as such, including protons and neutrons (and their sub-particles) has been delegated to physicists.

By definition, then, the field of chemistry has only to do with the electrons in the outer shells orbiting the nucleus of the atom. All of the isotopes of hydrogen (protium, deuterium, and tritium) behave chemically in exactly the same way because all of them, though differing in atomic mass, have one electron orbiting the nucleus, which is what determines chemical behavior. All the isotopes of hydrogen make water, H_2O. It is just that deuterium and tritium make "heavy water," but it is still water. Heavy water is a natural part of sea water and natural waters everywhere. The nucleus of an atom plays no role in chemical behavior. Nuclear reactions are the realm of physics, not chemistry.

What has been designated as "a chemical reaction" always has to do with the sharing, stealing, borrowing, loaning, or giving up of electrons between atoms. The number of electrons possessed by an atom is determined by the number of

Table One — Periodic Table of the Elements

Elements Listed in the Order of their Atomic Numbers

Legend:

6	Atomic Number = # of Protons in Nucleus of an Atom
C	Chemical Symbol
12.01	Mean Atomic Weight (A.W.) in amu's (atomic mass units)
	A.W. = # of Protons + # Neutrons in Nucleus of an Atom

1	2	3	4	5	6	7	8	9	10	11	12	13	14	15	16	17	18
1 **H** 1.008																	2 **He** 4.003
3 **Li** 6.941	4 **Be** 9.012											5 **B** 10.81	6 **C** 12.01	7 **N** 14.01	8 **O** 16.00	9 **F** 19.00	10 **Ne** 20.18
11 **Na** 22.99	12 **Mg** 24.31											13 **Al** 26.98	14 **Si** 28.09	15 **P** 30.97	16 **S** 32.07	17 **Cl** 35.45	18 **Ar** 39.95
19 **K** 39.10	20 **Ca** 40.08	21 **Sc** 44.96	22 **Ti** 47.87	23 **V** 50.94	24 **Cr** 52.00	25 **Mn** 54.94	26 **Fe** 55.85	27 **Co** 58.93	28 **Ni** 58.69	29 **Cu** 63.55	30 **Zn** 65.39	31 **Ga** 69.72	32 **Ge** 72.61	33 **As** 74.92	34 **Se** 78.96	35 **Br** 79.90	36 **Kr** 83.80
37 **Rb** 85.47	38 **Sr** 87.62	39 **Y** 88.91	40 **Zr** 91.22	41 **Nb** 92.91	42 **Mo** 95.94	43 **Tc** (98)	44 **Ru** 101.1	45 **Rh** 102.9	46 **Pd** 106.4	47 **Ag** 107.9	48 **Cd** 112.4	49 **In** 114.8	50 **Sn** 118.7	51 **Sb** 121.8	52 **Te** 127.6	53 **I** 126.9	54 **Xe** 131.3
55 **Cs** 132.9	56 **Ba** 137.3	57 **La** 138.9	72 **Hf** 178.5	73 **Ta** 180.9	74 **W** 183.8	75 **Re** 186.2	76 **Os** 190.2	77 **Ir** 192.2	78 **Pt** 195.1	79 **Au** 197.0	80 **Hg** 200.6	81 **Tl** 204.4	82 **Pb** 207.2	83 **Bi** 209.0	84 **Po** (209)	85 **At** (210)	86 **Rn** (222)
87 **Fr** (223)	88 **Ra** (226)	89 **Ac** (227)	104 **Rf** (261)	105 **Db** (262)	106 **Sg** (263)	107 **Bh** (262)	108 **Hs** (265)	109 **Mt** (266)	110 **Uun** (264)	111 **Uuu** (272)	112 **Uub** (277)	113 **Uut**	114 **Uuq** (285)	115 **Uup**	116 **Uuh** (289)	117 **Uus**	118 **Uuo**

Lanthanides (6):

58 **Ce** 140.1	59 **Pr** 140.9	60 **Nd** 144.2	61 **Pm** (145)	62 **Sm** 150.4	63 **Eu** 152.0	64 **Gd** 157.3	65 **Tb** 158.9	66 **Dy** 162.5	67 **Ho** 164.9	68 **Er** 167.3	69 **Tm** 168.9	70 **Yb** 173.0	71 **Lu** 175.0

Actinides (7):

90 **Th** 232.0	91 **Pa** (231)	92 **U** 238.0	93 **Np** (237)	94 **Pu** (244)	95 **Am** (243)	96 **Cm** (247)	97 **Bk** (247)	98 **Cf** (251)	99 **Es** (252)	100 **Fm** (257)	101 **Md** (258)	102 **No** (259)	103 **Lr** (262)

Parentheses around atomic masses mean the values given are approximate.
When no value is given, this element has not yet
been discovered as of 2003.

Table Two
The Ninety-Two Natural Elements

Period	Atomic Number and Name	Symbol	Mean Atomic Wt.	Period	Atomic Number and Name	Symbol	Mean Atomic Wt.
1	1 Hydrogen	H	1.008	5	47 Silver (Argentum)	Ag	107.9
	2 Helium	He	4.003		48 Cadmium	Cd	112.4
2	3 Lithium	Li	6.941		49 Indium	In	114.8
	4 Beryllium	Be	9.012		50 Tin (Stannum)	Sn	118.7
	5 Boron	B	10.81		51 Antimony (Stibium)	Sb	121.8
	6 Carbon	C	12.01		52 Tellurium	Te	127.6
	7 Nitrogen	N	14.01		53 Iodine	I	126.9
	8 Oxygen	O	16.00		54 Xenon	Xe	131.3
	9 Fluorine	F	19.00	6	55 Cesium	Cs	132.9
	10 Neon	Ne	20.18		56 Barium	Ba	137.3
3	11 Sodium (Natrium)	Na	22.99		57 Lanthanum	La	138.9
	12 Magnesium	Mg	24.31		58 Cerium	Ce	140.1
	13 Aluminum	Al	26.98		59 Praseodymium	Pr	140.9
	14 Silicon	Si	28.09		60 Neodymium	Nd	144.2
	15 Phosphorus	P	30.97		61 Promethium	Pm	(145)
	16 Sulfur	S	32.07		62 Samarium	Sm	150.4
	17 Chlorine	Cl	35.45		63 Europium	Eu	152.0
	18 Argon	Ar	39.95		64 Gadolinium	Gd	157.3
4	19 Potassium (Kalium)	K	39.10		65 Terbium	Tb	158.9
	20 Calcium	Ca	40.08		66 Dysprosium	Dy	162.5
	21 Scandium	Sc	44.96		67 Holmium	Ho	164.9
	22 Titanium	Ti	47.87		68 Erbium	Er	167.3
	23 Vanadium	V	50.94		69 Thulium	Tm	168.9
	24 Chromium	Cr	52.00		70 Ytterbium	Yb	173.0
	25 Manganese	Mn	54.94		71 Lutetium	Lu	175.0
	26 Iron (Ferrum)	Fe	55.85		72 Hafnium	Hf	178.5
	27 Cobalt	Co	58.93		73 Tantalum	Ta	180.9
	28 Nickel	Ni	58.69		74 Tungsten (Wolfrum)	W	183.8
	29 Copper (Cuprum)	Cu	63.55		75 Rhenium	Re	186.2
	30 Zinc	Zn	65.39		76 Osmium	Os	190.2
	31 Gallium	Ga	69.72		77 Iridium	Ir	192.2
	32 Germanium	Ge	72.61		78 Platinum	Pt	195.1
	33 Arsenic	As	74.92		79 Gold (Aurum)	Au	197.0
	34 Selenium	Se	78.96		80 Mercury (Hydrargyrum)	Hg	200.6
	35 Bromine	Br	79.90		81 Thallium	Tl	204.4
	36 Krypton	Kr	83.80		82 Lead (Plumbum)	Pb	207.2
5	37 Rubidium	Rb	85.47		83 Bismuth	Bi	209.0
	38 Strontium	Sr	87.62		84 Polonium	Po	(209)
	39 Yttrium	Y	88.91		85 Astatine	At	(210)
	40 Zirconium	Zr	91.22		86 Radon	Rn	(222)
	41 Niobium	Nb	92.91	7	87 Francium	Fr	(223)
	42 Molybdenum	Mo	95.94		88 Radium	Ra	(226)
	43 Technetium	Tc	(98)		89 Actinium	Ac	(227)
	44 Ruthenium	Ru	101.1		90 Thorium	Th	232.0
	45 Rhodium	Rh	102.9		91 Protactinium	Pa	(231)
	46 Palladium	Pd	106.4		92 Uranium	U	238.0

Masses are in atomic mass units (amu). Parentheses imply exact figures not known.

Table Three
Natural Elements Alphabetical by Name and by Symbol

Name	Symbol	Name	Symbol	Name	Symbol	Name	Symbol
Actinium	Ac	Europium	Eu	Molybdenum	Mo	Scandium	Sc
Aluminum	Al	Fluorine	F	Neodymium	Nd	Selenium	Se
Antimony	Sb	Francium	Fr	Neon	Ne	Silicon	Si
Argon	Ar	Gadolinium	Gd	Nickel	Ni	Silver	Ag
Arsenic	As	Gallium	Ga	Niobium	Nb	Sodium	Na
Astatine	At	Germanium	Ge	Nitrogen	N	Strontium	Sr
Barium	Ba	Gold	Au	Osmium	Os	Sulfur	S
Beryllium	Be	Hafnium	Hf	Oxygen	O	Tantalum	Ta
Bismuth	Bi	Helium	He	Palladium	Pd	Tellurium	Te
Boron	B	Hydrogen	H	Phosphorus	P	Terbium	Tb
Bromine	Br	Indium	In	Platinum	Pt	Thorium	Th
Cadmium	Cd	Iodine	I	Polonium	Po	Thallium	Tl
Calcium	Ca	Iridium	Ir	Potassium	K	Tin	Sn
Carbon	C	Iron	Fe	Promethium	Pm	Titanium	Ti
Cerium	Ce	Krypton	Kr	Protactinium	Pa	Tungsten	W
Cesium	Cs	Lanthanum	La	Radium	Ra	Uranium	U
Chlorine	Cl	Lead	Pb	Radon	Rn	Vanadium	V
Chromium	Cr	Lithium	Li	Rhenium	Re	Xenon	Xe
Cobalt	Co	Lutetium	Lu	Rhodium	Rh	Ytterbium	Yb
Copper	Cu	Magnesium	Mg	Rubidium	Rb	Yttrium	Y
Dysprosium	Dy	Manganese	Mn	Ruthenium	Ru	Zinc	Zn
Erbium	Er	Mercury	Hg	Samarium	Sm	Zirconium	Zr

Symbol	Name	Symbol	Name	Symbol	Name	Symbol	Name
Ac	Actinium	Er	Erbium	Mo	Molybdenum	S	Sulfur
Ag	Silver	Eu	Europium	N	Nitrogen	Sb	Antimony
Al	Aluminum	F	Fluorine	Na	Sodium	Sc	Scandium
Ar	Argon	Fe	Iron	Nb	Niobium	Se	Selenium
As	Arsenic	Fr	Francium	Nd	Neodymium	Si	Silicon
At	Astatine	Ga	Gallium	Ne	Neon	Sm	Samarium
Au	Gold	Gd	Gadolinium	Ni	Nickel	Sn	Tin
B	Boron	Ge	Germanium	O	Oxygen	Sr	Strontium
Ba	Barium	H	Hydrogen	Os	Osmium	Ta	Tantalum
Be	Beryllium	He	Helium	P	Phosphorus	Tb	Terbium
Bi	Bismuth	Hf	Hafnium	Pa	Protactinium	Te	Tellurium
Br	Bromine	Hg	Mercury	Pb	Lead	Th	Thorium
C	Carbon	I	Iodine	Pd	Palladium	Ti	Titanium
Ca	Calcium	In	Indium	Pm	Promethium	Tl	Thallium
Cd	Cadmium	Ir	Iridium	Po	Polonium	U	Uranium
Ce	Cerium	K	Potassium	Pt	Platinum	V	Vanadium
Cl	Chlorine	Kr	Krypton	Ra	Radium	W	Tungsten
Co	Cobalt	La	Lanthanum	Rb	Rubidium	Xe	Xenon
Cr	Chromium	Li	Lithium	Re	Rhenium	Y	Yttrium
Cs	Cesium	Lu	Lutetium	Rh	Rhodium	Yb	Ytterbium
Cu	Copper	Mg	Magnesium	Rn	Radon	Zn	Zinc
Dy	Dysprosium	Mn	Manganese	Ru	Ruthenium	Zr	Zirconium

protons in the nucleus, which must always be the same as the number of electrons. While chemistry is still defined as "the study of matter" on a gross macroscopic scale, it is a study that is confined and restricted to only certain aspects of matter. With this in mind, let's refine the definition of chemistry as viewed from a submicroscopic atomic scale:

Chemistry is the study of electrical exchanges between atoms involving only their shells of electrons and is not directly concerned with activities involving their nuclei.

Throughout any chemical process, from beginning to end, there are adjustments of electrons between atoms, while their nuclei remain constant and unchanged. Thus, atoms of hydrogen (H) and oxygen (O) may combine to form water, H_2O, but the atoms retain their identity even in the resultant compound. Hydrogen atoms are still hydrogen atoms and oxygen atoms are still oxygen atoms because in their nuclei, nothing has changed. Each oxygen atom, even when joined to a hydrogen atom, still has 8 protons in its nucleus, no more and no less. Likewise, hydrogen retains its identity, too, retaining its single proton in each nucleus regardless of what elements to which it may be attached.

When compounds of two or more atoms break up, the component atoms return to their previous elemental forms. All of the electrons that were shared, stolen, borrowed, loaned, or contributed when the atoms were united as a molecule of a compound, are returned and restored back from whence they came. Thus, when water is decomposed, its molecules disintegrate back into atoms of the hydrogen and oxygen gases they were before.

Lavoisier's Law

Antoine Laurent Lavoisier (1743-1794) is considered to be "The Father of Chemistry." Lavoisier recognized the manner in which elements combine to make compounds and the manner in which compounds can then break up to allow their elements to be free or to recombine to make different molecules of different compounds.

Lavoisier summarized it as follows: "Nothing is lost. Nothing is created. Everything is transformed." He considered the atom to be a constant in nature and that no new elements could be created or existing ones destroyed. No matter what, the atom would not disappear. If it should separate from one molecule, it could be found unchanged in another.

This concept is called "Lavoisier's Law" and defines the boundaries of the science of chemistry. These boundaries are arbitrary and artificial and do not define the limits of matter and its behavior, as was once thought. This bounding concept became the limit of official science for 200 years—to the end of the 19th century.

Conservation of Matter and Energy

Lavoisier's Law is a corollary to the Law of The Conservation of Matter, which says Matter can be neither created nor destroyed. It can only be transformed. The Law of The Conservation of Energy parallels that of matter, viz. Energy can be neither created nor destroyed. It can only be transformed. (This is also called "The First Law of Thermodynamics.")

With the turn of the 20th century came the discovery of natural radioactivity. There are natural elements, such as radium, radon, and uranium, that spontaneously transform into other elements by giving off alpha particles, beta particles, neutrons, and gamma rays. Thus, some atoms were not found to be constant in nature, as Lavoisier had postulated and as two centuries of scientists had believed.

This discovery did not change the definition of chemistry as it was practiced, however. It simply brought into existence a couple of new fields: i.e. nuclear physics and quantum mechanics and, eventually, a new hybrid field called "nuclear chemistry."

These new developments in physics revealed a seeming violation of Lavoisier's Law. Matter could be destroyed and turned into energy and vice versa. The Laws of Conserving Matter and Conserving Energy had to be modified to say that "matter and energy are equivalent." In fact, they are different forms of the same thing. We can thank Einstein for this. ($E = mc^2$ Energy = mass x speed of light squared)

Chemistry, however, remains defined as it was in Lavoisier's day. Thus, in their "study of matter" chemists choose not to include processes in which one element transmutes into another or where energy and matter are transformed one into the other. (See p. 655.)

It is important to keep the above comments in mind when dealing with chemists or chemistry since the official "chemical" view of matter and its behavior is only part of the picture. Some schooled in the philosophy of Lavoisier's Law erroneously think that when it comes to biological processes, the chemical view can account for everything.

Are Doctors 300 Years Behind?

Keep the foregoing comments in mind when you deal with allopathic doctors and career biologists because these professionals, by their limited academic exposure, are usually wedded to chemistry in the 17th century fashion of Lavoisier. Their entire concept of life processes is a chemical one. They call it "biochemistry." Even mental and psychological phenomena are regarded by many doctors as mostly, if not totally, attributable to chemistry. Even the well known electromagnetic properties of human physiology are largely ignored, unrecognized, and/or unused by most physicians. In their minds, due to their restrictive training, chemistry (by Lavoisier's definition) can account for virtually everything. Hence, they prescribe chemical treatments (drugs) to all manner of disease almost exclusively.

While chemistry is a vital part of life processes, such processes do not completely follow the laws of chemistry, as we shall learn, and neither do the processes by which essential oils bring healing to our bodies, minds, and souls. God's view of matter—what it does, and how it relates to us as whole beings—extends far beyond the confines of chemistry as defined by scientists today. (This idea will be expanded later in Part Three of this book.)

Elements: Natural, Synthetic, and Theoretical

Elements are simple substances that cannot be broken down by chemical means into any other substance. Each atom of any element contains a specific number of protons designated by its atomic number. There are 92 natural elements, another 22 created in laboratories, and 4 theoretical ones yet to be made or discovered. Table One (p. 82) lists all of the elements—natural, synthetic, and theoretical.

Table Two lists the 92 natural ones beginning with hydrogen, the lightest, and ending with uranium, the heaviest. They are numbered from 1 to 92 according to the number of protons in the nucleus (or the number of electrons in orbit). These sequential numerals are called "atomic numbers." They are shown at the top of each little box for each element in Table One.

Thus, all of the atoms of the first element, hydrogen (H), have one proton (and one electron) each. All of the atoms of the second element, helium (He), have two protons (and two electrons) each. All of the atoms of the third element, lithium (Li) have three protons (and three electrons) each. And so forth. You can tell how many neutrons are in a typical atom of any element by subtracting the atomic number (number of protons) from the atomic weight (the sum of the numbers of protons and neutrons).

For example, helium (He) has an atomic number of 2, but an atomic weight of slightly more than 4. (See Table One, p. 82 or the end sheet at the back of this book.) Since $4 - 2 = 2$ a typical helium atom must have 2 neutrons.

Lithium (Li) has an atomic number of 3 and a mean atomic weight of almost 7. Since $7 - 3 = 4$ a typical lithium atom must have 4 neutrons.

Carbon (C) has an atomic number of 6 but its atomic weight is about 12. Since $12 - 6 = 6$, most carbon atoms must have 6 neutrons.

By applying the same arithmetic, we can deduce that most nitrogen (N) atoms have 7 neutrons, most oxygen (O) atoms have 8 neutrons, and most fluorine (Fl) atoms have 10 neutrons.

The importance of understanding the atomic weights of the elements will become evident later when we talk about what makes an oil aromatic or odorless, thick or thin, what makes its fragrance or therapeutic action long-lasting or short-lived, and what makes it able to pass through the skin and blood-brain barrier or not.

Table Four
Elemental Composition of the Earth's Crust
(In Percents by Weight)

Element	Symbol	Percent
1. Oxygen	O	49
2. Silicon	Si	26
3. Aluminum	Al	8.1
4. Iron	Fe	5.0
5. Calcium	Ca	3.6
6. Sodium	Na	2.8
7. Potassium	K	2.6
8. Magnesium	Mg	2.1
9. Titanium	Ti	0.44
10. Hydrogen	H	0.14
11. Phosphorus	P	0.12
All other elements		0.10

Adapted from Principles of Physical Geology by Arthur Holmes, 1965

Elements Essential to Life

Considering the relative abundance of the elements available to living organisms at our planet's surface, oxygen (O) is at the top of the list constituting 49% of the earth's crust, 21% of the earth's atmosphere, 90% of the weight of the oceans, 88% of the mass of plants, and 76% of our body weight. Silicon (Si) ranks second which, with oxygen, comprises 75% of the earth's rocks and soils, mainly as SiO_2 (Silicon dioxide) which occurs naturally as crystalline quartz, sandstone, and common sand. The vast and innumerable beaches of the world, with few exceptions, are composed of grains of silica or silicon dioxide.

Table Five
Elemental Composition of Living Matter
(In Percents by Weight)

Element	Symbol	% in Plants	% In Animals
1. Oxygen	O	88	76
2. Carbon	C	3	16
3. Nitrogen	N	0.3	3
4. Hydrogen	H	1	1
All other elements		7.7	4

Adapted from *Encounter With the Earth* by Leo Laporte, Canfield Press, San Francisco. 1975.

As the earth's composition goes, aluminum (Al) ranks surprisingly in third place. It is the most abundant metal on earth (Table Four). However, Al plays no known role in life processes and although it is found in almost all igneous rocks and in all of the clays of the world, it is tightly bound in stable mineral compounds that prevent it from becoming available to participate in biological processes.

Compare Table Four with the relative amounts of the four elements (Table Five) that compose over 90% of the weight of plants and animal bodies. Of these, only oxygen and hydrogen are abundant enough to be listed in the top ten elements available on earth, while the essential elements, carbon and nitrogen, are not. However, the earth's atmosphere is about 2% carbon dioxide and 75% nitrogen.

After O, C, N, and H, (Table Five) the next seven most abundant elements in the human body are Ca, P, Cl, K, S, Na, and Mg (in that order), all in amounts of less than 0.5%, but they are all vital. Phosphorus (P) is a good example. Besides teeth and bones, there is one P atom on every nucleotide unit in the DNA. Without it we would have no cellular intelligence. The remaining 17 elements that play a role in life processes are all present in traces (less than 0.05%), including iron (Fe)—essential to carry oxygen in our blood. Fe and P point out how critical a trace element can be, making the difference between life and death.

It is similar with therapeutic grade oils. Their healing

power can be from trace components, some of which are yet to be identified. This is why it is so crucial to grow, distill, and package an oil with the intent of preserving its composition as closely to nature as possible. The slightest tampering with an oil can upset its delicate balance and destroy or reduce its curative capacity.

For example, galbanum oil (*Ferula gummosa*) has been used since pre-Biblical times and was part of the holy incense mentioned in Exodus 30:34. A trace constituent, pyrazine ($C_4H_4N_2$), representing less than 0.1% of the oil, accounts for its powerful earthy fragrance and contributes to its therapeutic qualities.

Table Six
27 Elements Needed by the Human Body
(Listed in Order of Atomic Weight)

Hydrogen	H	Lithium	Li	Boron	B
Carbon	C	Nitrogen	N	Oxygen	O
Fluorine	F	Sodium	Na	Magnesium	Mg
Silicon	Si	Phosphorus	P	Sulfur	S
Chlorine	Cl	Potassium	K	Calcium	Ca
Vanadium	V	Chromium	Cr	Manganese	Mn
Iron	Fe	Cobalt	Co	Nickel	Ni
Copper	Cu	Zinc	Zn	Germanium	Ge
Selenium	Se	Molybdenum	Mo	Iodine	I

Adapted from the *Handbook of Chemistry and Physics*, David Lide, Editor, CRC Press, 2003
PDR for Nutritional Supplements, Hendler & Rorvik, Editors, Thomson PDR Co., 2001
Dr. *Whitaker's Guide to Natural Healing*, Julian Whitaker, Prima Publishing, Rocklin, CA 1995
The Merck Manual, 17th edition, Mark Beers & Robert Berkow, editors, Merck Labs. 1999
Prescription for Nutritional Healing by Balch and Balch, Avery Publishing, NY, 1990

So far as we know, not all of the 92 natural elements are essential to life or serve any beneficial purpose in living processes. Going down the Periodic Table (or the list of Table Two), there are only 27 elements thought to be necessary in the human body. They are tabulated in Table Six in the order they appear in the Periodic Table. Of these 27 elements, 95% of our body weight is due to only three of them, namely, carbon, nitrogen and oxygen. These are elements 6, 7, and 8 in the Periodic Table, respectively.

Actually, most of the atoms in the human body are hydrogen, but since H is so light it does not contribute significantly to body weight. Of the first 20 elements in the Periodic Table, all but five of them (helium He, beryllium Be, aluminum Al, neon Ne, and argon Ar) are necessary for human life. It may eventually be discovered that one or more of these are also essential in some small way as yet undetected.

While He, Ne, and Ar are chemically inactive, this is not to say they could not play a role in life processes via their subtle energetic properties. Chemistry is not all there is to life. (See Part Three, pp. 612-737, for more on that.)

In any case, life depends mostly on the lighter elements, not the heavy ones. In fact, most of the really heavy elements (atomic weights greater than 130) are considered toxic.

For example, element #80 (mercury, Hg) has an atomic weight of 200 and is a major source of heavy metal poisoning, which we get from dental fillings, vaccinations, and some fish. This is where essential oils can be extremely valuable in that many of them can chelate heavy metals out of our bodies. By our normal processes of elimination, it can take decades or even a lifetime to cleanse them from our systems. Helichrysum (*Helichrysum italicum*) and cardamom (*Elletaria cardamomum*) are examples of oils thought to have heavy metal chelating power. (See books by Higley, Manwaring, or Young for more on this.)

You might want to put a small check by each of the 27 elements of life where they are listed in Table One to designate them as minerals involved in life processes. This short list may be because we don't know everything about the human body just yet. Some say that actually all 92 natural elements are utilized in bodily functions and we just haven't detected their presence nor discerned their purposes as yet. Sea water contains all 92 natural elements and some say they are also all contained in wheat grass. (See Harting & Bergstrom on these points.)

You may want to take note of some of the elements not listed in Table Six as "needed" or "beneficial-for-life": Al (aluminum—as in cookware), As (arsenic—as in poison), Cd (cadmium—as found in coffee), and, of course, Kr (krypton—

which is pertinent only to Superman©). Arsenic is actually a necessary trace mineral for some animals, such as goats, but not for humans.

Be (beryllium) occurs in minerals and gemstones and is what makes an emerald green. Isolated, it has a sweet taste and has many applications for alloys and solid state electronics, particularly in the space industry. When it was first isolated in a lab, almost a century ago, its sweet taste was used by scientists and technicians to identify its presence. Unfortunately, these early researchers soon found it to be highly toxic. Fortunately, beryllium is not found free in nature and our bodies don't seem to need it.

So far as we know today, except for molybdenum (Mo), A.W. = 95.94 and iodine (I), A.W. = 126.9, no element with an atomic weight greater than 79 amu is chemically usable by the human body. By comparison, the heaviest natural element is Uranium (U) with A.W. = 238.

The Surprising Roles of Trace Elements

Among the elements that do serve a useful or essential purpose for our lives, several of them may surprise you. Most of these would be toxic, even deadly, in higher doses, but as traces they are necessary for life. Given next is a partial list identified by atomic number, element name, and symbol. (The information in this section was compiled and paraphrased from these six sources: Balch & Balch, Hendler & Rorvik, Beers & Barkow, Lide, Kervran, and Whitaker—See Bibliography.)

#3 Lithium (Li) Lithium is the lightest of all metals. With a density half that of water, it floats. It does not occur free in nature. It is found in nearly all igneous rocks and is found in traces in most soils. It is an element in the waters of many mineral springs. It is silvery in appearance like the other alkali metals sodium and potassium. It has the highest specific heat of any substance known. It is used in alloys, heat transfer applications, dry cells, and storage batteries. In biological processes it acts in an enzymatic fashion to facilitate the formation of many organic compounds. As a physiological trace element it plays a role in the orderly transmission of nerve signals throughout the brain and body and may play a role in fertility. As a behavioral element, it has been observed by sociologists that geographical areas with little or no lithium have higher rates of violent crime. Small doses of lithium carbonate (Li_2CO_3) are prescribed as a medicine to calm manic, hyperactive patients, as mentioned in the PDR. For the small traces of lithium you need, eat fish, milk, eggs, alfalfa, potatoes, beets, and other root crops and drink the waters of mountain springs or deep wells.

#5 Boron (B) is used in laundry products, as an igniter for rocket engines, in the fiberglass industry, and to provide a beautiful green color in fireworks. We need it to assimilate calcium in healthy bones and regulate blood pressure. It also plays a role in hormonal balance and regulating the menstrual cycle. It is found in leafy vegetables, fruits, nuts, grains, and unpeeled apples.

#9 Fluorine (F) is the most reactive of all elements. Most substances, even water, will burst into flame in the presence of pure fluorine gas. It has been used as a rocket propellant. As hydrofluoric acid (HF), eats glass and ceramic and is used as an etching compound. HF is also used to frost the insides of light bulbs. Its most abundant form in nature is fluorspar, an attractive purple crystal. It plays a role in kidney and endocrine function as well as longevity. A deficiency can lead to tooth decay and osteoporosis, but when ingested in quantities beyond trace amounts, it can cause mottled teeth, and has been associated with Down's syndrome and cancer. All the fluorine you need can be obtained by simply drinking a variety of teas and eating seafood. Traces of fluorides are also found in coffee.

#12 Magnesium (Mg) is a light metal that burns with a dazzling white flame. It provides the sparkle to sparklers and other types of fire works. It is the eighth most abundant element on earth and is an element in dolomite, a type of limestone that occurs around the world. Magnesium is vital to enzyme activity and to every major biological process, including the production of cellular energy, the synthesis of proteins, and in bone and tooth formation. It is also necessary to maintain the proper electricities and electrical fields of the body. A deficiency interferes with nerve transmission and muscle impulses. It supports cardiovascular function and participates in bone formation. As an alkaline metal, it aids in maintaining proper body pH balance. Magnesium is found in most foods. Rich sources include apples, apricots, bananas, brown rice, figs, garlic, kelp, millet, blackeyed peas, salmon, tofu, nuts, green leafy vegetables, and whole grains.

#14 Silicon (Si), the most abundant of the solid elements, occurs in sand, quartz, rock crystal, agate, amethyst, flint, jasper, granite, asbestos, feldspar, and clay (just to name a few), but is never found free in nature. Silicon constitutes about 47% of the composition of glass and is the backbone of the solid-state electronics industry. Thus the name, "Silicon Valley," for the area around San Jose, California, where electronic industries abound. It is necessary for bone, blood vessels, and various connective tissues (collagen) as well as healthy nails, skin, and hair. Silicon counteracts the toxic effects of aluminum in our bodies and aids in the prevention of Alzheimer's disease. For silicon, eat alfalfa, beets, brown rice, bell peppers, soybeans, leafy green vegetables, radishes, and whole grains. Human breast milk also contains silicon to help build baby's bones. Horsetail, an herb available in health food stores, is a rich source of silica (SiO_2). Taking horsetail as an herbal tea accelerates healing of broken bones and connective tissue. This is because Si is easily biotransmuted into usable calcium by our bodies. (See Part Three.)

#23 Vanadium (V) is a bright, white, soft and ductile metal used to make spring steel, various ceramics, and superconducting magnets. Vanadium is needed for cellular metabolism in making bones and teeth. A vanadium deficiency is linked to cardiovascular and kidney disease, impaired reproductive ability, and increased infant mortality. Vanadium salts have insulin-like properties and have been studied as replacements for insulin. It is found in fish, vegetable oils, and olives, as well as green beans, black pepper, mushrooms, dill, red meat, and radishes.

#24 Chromium (Cr), that shiny metal seen on car trim and truck bumpers, is needed for sugar metabolism and in the synthesis of cholesterol, fats, and protein. A chromium deficiency can result in glucose intolerance, degeneration of the nerves, and weakness of the muscles. To intake sufficient chromium, eat organic foods, especially whole grains. Also found in spices such as black pepper and thyme, as well as in mushrooms, brown sugar, coffee, tea, beer, wine, liver, and brewers yeast.

#25 Manganese (Mn) is widely distributed throughout the earth in the form of oxides, silicates, and carbonates. Large quantities of manganese nodules have been discovered on the floor of many oceans. Alloyed with aluminum, antimony, and copper, it forms a powerful magnet. Manganese is responsible for the true color of amethyst and is used as a drying agent in black paint. Minute quantities are needed for protein and fat metabolism, healthy nerves, and a healthy immune system. It helps regulate blood sugar. It is needed to utilize vitamins B and E as well as in the production of enzymes. The best food sources are avocados, nuts, seeds, seaweed, spinach, blueberries, peas, beans, pineapple, spinach, egg yolks, and herbal teas.

#26 Iron or Ferrum (Fe) is the fourth most abundant element in the crust of the earth and composes most of the earth's core. It is responsible for most of the colors in rocks, soils, and minerals and is the principle source of the earth's magnetism. As for humans, we only need a trace, but it is a trace we must have to live. It is the source of our bioenergy by its ability to carry and release oxygen to our cells via red blood cells. This unique ability is because iron has two principle valences or states of oxidation—2 and 3. (See the next chapter for an explanation of valence.) Too much iron is quite toxic. Here, again, is an example of a substance that is nurturing and therapeutic in minute amounts but harmful and damaging in larger amounts. Adequate iron intake by pregnant mothers is vital to the healthy growth of the unborn child. The best dietary sources of iron are legumes, green vegetables, and, for babies, human breast milk. Other good sources include almonds, avocados, beets, blackstrap molasses, brewer's yeast, dates, egg yolks, parsley, peaches, pears, prunes, pumpkins, raisins, clams, and soybeans. The iron in grains, breads, and cereals is not well absorbed. Milk, cheese, snack foods, and soft drinks are not good sources of iron.

#28 Nickel (Ni). Americans are familiar with nickel as the metal in their five-cent coin. As an element from outer space, it is found in most meteorites and is a key element in identifying them as such. Slightly magnetic, nickel is used in making alnico magnets (an alloy of Al, Ni, and Co). It is also alloyed with iron to make stainless steel, bullet-proof armor, and burglar-proof vaults. Finely divided nickel is used as a catalyst to hydrogenate vegetable oils. Nickel plays a role in processing vitamin B in our bodies as well as the regulation of normal growth. Nickel may participate as an enzyme in adrenal and thyroid function. Too much nickel can be toxic. Possible sources of nickel overdoses are from acid foods in stainless steel cookware and hydrogenated oils. It is found in most vegetables, but particularly in nuts, beans, peas, grains, and chocolate. Don't worry, you're not going to get too much nickel through chocolate. Nickel does not accumulate in the body and is easily excreted through the kidneys.

#29 Copper or Cuprum (Cu), that uniquely reddish metal that makes up most of the wiring in our homes, is needed for proper infant development in the formation of bone, blood cells, and healthy nerves. It is also involved in healing processes and in the coloring of skin and hair. Deficiencies can result in glucose intolerance, high cholesterol levels, heart disease, and neurological problems. You can get it from eating almonds, avocados, beans, peas, molasses, broccoli, garlic, lentils, mushrooms, radishes, raisins, seafood, liver, oysters, or soy beans.

#30 Zinc (Zn) Zinc is a bluish-white metal. When combined with copper as an alloy, it forms brass. Brass is mentioned 124 times in the *Bible*. It is first mentioned in Genesis 4:22 in association with Tubal-Cain, a seventh generation descendant from Adam who was an instructor in molding and creating artifacts from brass. Besides brass, it is an element in typewriter metal, German silver, and aluminum solder. It is used in the manufacture of paints, rubber products, cosmetics, pharmaceuticals, floor coverings, plastics, printing inks, soap, storage batteries, textiles, and other products. It is necessary for healthy prostate function and in the growth of the reproductive organs. It is required for protein synthesis, promotes a healthy immune system, facilitates healing of wounds. and is needed to maintain proper vitamin E concentrations in the blood. Zinc-deficient animals require 50% more food to gain the same weight as an animal supplied with sufficient zinc. A zinc deficiency can also reduce one's sense of taste and smell. Dietary zinc is found in poultry, oysters, seafood, brewer's yeast, lamb chops, lima beans, pecans, pumpkin seeds, sardines, sunflower seeds, and soybeans.

    #32 Germanium (Ge) is a versatile semiconductor used in triodes, diodes, transistors, computer chips, and fiber optics. In our bodies, germanium is an oxygen carrier that protects us from cancer, arthritis, food allergies, elevated cholesterol, and chronic viral infections. Deficiencies can alter the mineral composition of the bone and affect the DNA of bone tissue. It can be found in aloe vera, comfrey, garlic, wheat bran, leguminous seeds, ginseng, shiitake mushrooms, onions, wolfberries, NingXia Red® juice.

    #34 Selenium (Se) is a metal that can convert light into electricity and alternating current into direct current. It has been used extensively for photoelectric cells, rectifiers, photographic exposure meters, and for solar cells to convert sunlight into electricity. In our bodies it is a powerful antioxidant, electrically zapping free radicals. It stimulates the production of antibodies when we need them, participates in pancreatic function, and protects us from cancer. It helps regulate thyroid function and helps in the utilization of vitamin C. A deficiency results in muscle weakness. Find it in brewer's yeast, broccoli, brown rice, chicken, garlic, liver, seafood, wheat germ, and most vegetables.

    #42 Molybdenum (Mo), A.W. = 95.94, has many uses including the hardening of alloys for nuclear reactors and airplane parts, as well as a catalyst in petroleum processing. It is rare, almost as rare as gold, yet it is an essential trace mineral for most plants, as well as for many bacteria and ourselves where it plays a role in some of our necessary enzymes, enabling the body to use nitrogen in building protein. Low molybdenum levels are associated with mouth and gum disorders, cancer, sexual dysfunction in older men, and shortened life spans. Too much molybdenum (which would be hard to get naturally) interferes with copper levels in the body. A Mo deficiency leads to headaches, nausea, disorientation, and tachycardia (racing heartbeat). To maintain a healthy level, avoid processed foods and eat beans, whole grains, legumes, peas, and dark leafy vegetables.

#53 Iodine (I). There are only two elements we need on the 5th level of the Periodic Table: Molybdenum (Mo) and Iodine (I). Iodine has an atomic mass of 126.9 amu and is the heaviest element our body can use. Toxic in concentrated doses, when dissolved in ethyl alcohol (tincture of iodine) it is used as an antiseptic. It is also used in photography. It is essential for thyroid function and participates in the energy control mechanisms of our body. It is also a vital trace element in proper fetal development. A deficiency causes a swollen thyroid condition called goiter. Available iodine is geographically dependent. Many inland areas remote from oceans have no iodine. Besides goiter, deficiencies of iodine lead to growth retardation and brain dysfunction in children. Iodine deficiency is the leading cause of preventable mental deficit in the world. It is found in sea foods, sea salt, eggs, and milk. A trace is all we need.

So there you have it. For all the elements available in nature, only 27 seem to be needed for us to live, most in minute amounts. We don't need anything heavier than iodine, which is number 53 on the chart. There are no elements on levels 6 and 7 necessary for life processes. Most elements below iodine on the table are heavy metals, unnecessary and toxic. Human and plant life depend on the lighter elements, mainly C, H and O—the very same elements that comprise the main ingredients of essential oils.

God's Plan for Creation in a Table

The purpose of this chapter is to lay a foundation of general chemistry upon which you can build an understanding of the science of essential oils. I want you to appreciate the orderly arrangement of the 92 natural elements and how all of them boil down to simple combinations of three things: electrons, protons, and neutrons.

In fact, after electrons and protons everything is based on hydrogen atoms—the simplest, most numerous atoms of the universe. A neutron is really a collapsed hydrogen atom. When an electron orbiting a proton falls into the nucleus, the two opposing electrical charges perfectly cancel and a neutron is born, slightly heavier than a proton.

With this in mind, the next heaviest element, Helium, consists of two protons, two electrons, and two neutrons. From this we can see that Helium, with an atomic number of 2 and an atomic weight of 4, is actually fashioned from four hydrogen atoms, two of which collapsed to make neutrons. (See Part Three of this book.)

God's plan for creation is based on simple building blocks (hydrogen atoms) from which the richness and elegance of our complex world has been made. The forms of his creation tell us something about himself, as stated in Romans 1:20, "Ever since the creation of the world, God's eternal power and divine nature, invisible though they are, have been understood and seen through the things he has made."

Considering the elegance of the Periodic Table, Psalm 23:5 comes to mind, "Thou preparest a table for me..." The Periodic Table is a work of divine genius. Scientists discovered and described it, but God made it. You will notice that there are seven levels in the table. Some say this corresponds to the "seven heavens." (See Harting and Bergstrom.) I don't know about that. What scientists know is that the general chemical characteristics of the elements repeat themselves seven times in ascending atomic weights.

What Makes the Periodic Table Periodic?

The periodic table is a listing of elements in order of their atomic numbers, 1 to 118. This corresponds to listing them by their atomic weights from the lightest (H), to the heaviest natural element (U) to the heaviest theoretical element (Uuo).

Listed as they are in the Periodic Table, all elements that line up in a vertical column have similar chemical characteristics. Hence, if you know something about how one element behaves, you know something about every other element in that column, above and below.

The first scientist to fully articulate the periodicity of elemental properties was a Russian, Dmitri Ivanovitch Mendeleev (1884-1907), who published his discovery in 1869. In his paper he predicted the properties and existence of three elements as yet unknown: #21 Scandium (Sc), #31 Galium (Ga), and #32 Germanium (Ge). When element #101 was created in a laboratory in the 1960s, it was named "mendelevium" in his honor.

As you read the Periodic Table from left to right, top to bottom or read down the list in Table Two, certain chemical characteristics repeat themselves. Things that repeat themselves are said to be "periodic." In the case of chemistry, there are seven periods, levels, or cycles of repetition among the elements. The first period has only two elements, H and He. The second period (next level down on the Periodic Table) contains eight elements, Li, Be, B, C, N, O, F, and Ne. The third period starting with Na also has eight elements while the fourth and fifth levels each have 18 members.

Meet the Families

The elements can be considered as belonging to various families with common family traits as follows:

- **Metals:** Look at Table One again. All of the elements on the extreme left are metals starting with the first column headed by hydrogen (H) and the second column headed by beryllium (Be). Yes, that's right. Hydrogen is a metal. It is just that at ordinary temperatures it evaporates into a gas, but at very low temperatures (–434° F or –259° C) it becomes a solid that is quite metallic in nature and appearance with a density about 30% heavier than water. However, under normal living conditions, hydrogen behaves as a nonmetal—its metallic properties being manifest only in the artificial lifeless cold of a laboratory or, perhaps, in the extremes of dark, frigid outer space. In this book we will consider it as a gaseous nonmetal.

- **Non-Metals:** All of the elements on the extreme right of the Periodic Table are non-metals. This includes carbon (C) and Nitrogen (N) and the columns headed by O, F, and He. All of the elements under He are gases.

- **Transition Elements:** The elements in the middle of the periodic table are all transitional in some way. Some are metallic in nature while others are called "metalloids" because they have characteristics of both metals and non-metals. There are six metalloids: B, Si, Ge, As, Sb, and Te.

- **The Alkali Metals:** In the first column, the seven metals, H, Li, Na, K, Rb, Cs, and Fr, all have a common characteristic. They all have a strong desire to give away one electron from their outermost shell. In chemistry we say that all of these elements have a "valence" of 1, which is why they all behave similarly in a chemical reaction. As a family, these seven are called the "Alkali Metals."

- **The Alkaline Earth Metals:** These start with the second period and comprise the second column. There are six elements in the Alkaline Earth Metals family: Be, Mg, Ca, Sr, Ba, and Ra. Every one of these has a strong desire to give away two electrons, which is why the elements in this column all react in a similar fashion. The reason these elements and the metals listed above are tagged with alkali and alkaline names is because the effect of their presence in an aqueous solution is to raise pH, reduce acidity, and raise alkalinity. Elements that readily donate electrons can neutralize acids. The presence of sufficient stores of K, Na, Mg, and Ca in our bodies is crucial for maintaining a healthy pH. This is why we need to eat plenty of fruits and vegetables which are the natural sources of these elements. (See pp. 347-349.)

- **The Noble Gases:** Going over to the extreme right side of the Periodic Table, the known elements in that column are all gases: He, Ne, Ar, Kr, and Xe. They're all hermits and introverts. They want to keep the electrons they have and have no desire for electrons from anyone else. In chemistry we say that all of these elements have a valence of 0. They are the wall flowers at the party, the unsocial ones, the ones who won't mix, and are never given to marriage. Unwilling to give or take in any relationship, they are all chemically inert.

- **The Halogens:** The next column to the left of the noble gases, headed by fluorine, are anything but inert. There are five elements in this column: F, Cl, Br, I, and At. This is the "halogen" family. Their compounds are called "halides." All of the halogens have a common personality trait: They are all hungry for an electron. Just one electron. They will greedily grab it from wherever they can get it.

- **The Chalcogens:** The third column from the right is headed by oxygen (O) and includes O, S, Se, Te, and Po. Their common family trait is that they, like the halogens, are also starving for electrons, but whereas one electron will satisfy a halogen, it takes two to satisfy a chalcogen. Oxygen (O), sulfur (S), and the other elements in this family are said to possess a "valence" of 2.

Inter–Family Dynamics (Boy Meets Girl)

When elements of the same family get together with no outsiders present, not much happens. Close blood relatives are not supposed to become romantically involved and don't usually intermarry. For example, you can mix all of the Halogen children together and they will maintain their individual elemental forms without combining to make compounds. There is no chemistry between them.

But when different families get together, exciting things happen. When any member of the Halogen family (who are all looking for that one electron) meets anyone of the Alkali Metal family (who are all eager to give up one electron) it is love at first sight! They form an instant union, creating a stable compound. The Alkali Metal gets to give away its electron and the Halogen eagerly takes it. Both are happy.

Similarly, when members of the Alkaline Earth family meet up with any member of the Chalcogen family, they are immediately attracted and proceed to form a bond. The Chalcogens are looking for two electrons and every member of the Alkaline Earth family has two electrons they want to donate to some deserving atom. Members of these two families will readily join in chemical matrimony any time they have the opportunity.

The chemical combinations between Alkalis and Halogens or between Alkaline Earth elements and Chalcogens are all monogamous. One atom of an Alkali pairs up with one atom of a Halogen and only one atom of an Alkaline Earth joins with one atom of a Chalcogen. These simple one-partner marriages are the exception.

Bigamy and Polygamy

When it comes to marriages between elements, polygamy is the rule. Monogamy is the exception. For example, if a member of the Chalcogen family (who wants two electrons) meets with some of the Alkali Metals who have only one electron to give up, the Chalcogen will unite with two of them to satisfy its appetite. Thus, you can have H_2O or hydrogen oxide (aka water) or Na_2S (Sodium sulfide), where the oxygen (O) and sulfur (S), in these respective examples, have each married two spouses. This is chemical bigamy.

There can also be chemical polygamy, where many different atoms join together, sometimes by the hundreds. Group matrimony between many elements creates large molecules—including proteins, fatty oils, and DNA—that serve many essential life functions.

Copper, Silver, and Gold

As an example of the periodicity of the elements, look at the column under element 29, copper (Cu). Directly below is element 47, silver (Ag), and below that is element 79, gold (Au). These three metals exhibit similar metallic properties. For example, all three are excellent conductors of electricity and all are valued for their attractive appearances for jewelry and other ornamentation. All three are coinage metals throughout the world, prized for thousands of years in the minting of metallic money.

The man-made element 111, Unununium (Uun), falls directly below gold in the table and was first created on December 20, 1994, in Germany. Only three atoms were detected, each with 111 protons and 161 neutrons and lasting only a split second. Of course, this was not enough quantity or time to determine its chemical and physical properties. If a sufficient quantity of sufficient half-life can be made to study, it is expected to have properties similar to gold and its other cousins in the table directly above. And, no, its name has not been misspelled. It is pronounced Un-un-un-ium. There are three "Uns." This strange name is actually its atomic number (111) in Latin.

The Lazy Gases

Another illustration of the periodicity of the table is found in the extreme right-hand column. These are called the "noble gases," but they should be called the "lazy gases" or the "antisocial gases." Helium (He), Neon (Ne), Argon (Ar), Krypton (Kr), Xenon (Xe), and Radon (Rn) are all chemically inert. They don't combine with any other element to make any compound. Because of its nonreactivity, helium is used to fill lighter-than-air balloons instead of hydrogen, which was formerly used. Pure hydrogen is explosively dangerous while helium is 100% safe. Helium couldn't explode if it wanted to.

Element 118, to be called Ununoctium (Uuo), was thought to have been created in June 1999, but the physicists at the Lawrence-Berkeley National Laboratory later retracted their claim because neither they, nor anyone else, could repeat their original results. In any case, when Ununoctium has been created, with its 118 protons and 118 electrons, scientists can predict with confidence that, because of where it falls on the periodic table, it will be chemically inert like all of its inactive relatives above, and will probably be a very dense gas. Its odd name is actually its atomic number (118) in Latin.

Practical Applications of the Periodic Table

Compounds are combinations of elements. Not all elements will combine with all other elements. They have preferences, the same as people. Some people get along with others. Some don't. Some elements, such as hydrogen (H), will combine with virtually everything, but others, like helium (He) and neon (Ne), don't combine with anything. Others are just choosy. Calcium (Ca) will combine with chlorine (Cl) or Sulfur (S), but not with sodium (Na) or potassium (K) unless certain other elements join in to make up the compound.

Chemists and physicists make use of the Periodic Table all the time as part of their work. They couldn't get along without it. Examples of how drug companies use the Periodic Table to create new drugs are given in Chapters Ten and Eleven. But what practical use can you make of it without being a scientist engaged in the field? Here is how.

Sodium (Na), an alkali metal, easily combines with Chlorine (Cl), a halogen, to make NaCl, or table salt, where every molecule of salt contains one sodium and one chlorine atom locked together in an intimate embrace. Now look at the vertical column (on the extreme left) in which sodium (element 11) is found. Every element in that column is also an alkali metal and can potentially replace sodium in its embrace with chlorine to form a new marriage and a different compound. Among the possibilities are HCl (hydrochloric acid), LiCl (Lithium chloride), and KCl (Potassium chloride, a substitute for table salt in low sodium diets). RbCl (Rubidium chloride), CsCl (Cesium chloride), and FrCl (Francium chloride) are also possibilities.

While lithium serves a beneficial purpose in human life processes in small quantities, too much can upset the balance of sodium and potassium in our bodies. Physicians prescribing lithium for certain psychotic conditions (manic depressive) are cautioned by the PDR to carefully monitor the serum sodium and potassium levels of the patient. This potential toxicity of lithium is because it is an alkali metal that can chemically replace Na or K anywhere in the body and disrupt normal physiological processes.

Radioactive cesium (Cs-137) is a waste product of nuclear reactors and finds its way into the environment. If your body comes into contact with Cs-137, it can replace sodium or potassium atoms wherever they occur in your body fluids or tissues and deliver carcinogenic (cancer-causing) radiation wherever it lodges.

Getting back to our table salt, NaCl, if we keep the sodium and look over in the chlorine column on the right of the table we have fluorine (F) above with bromine (Br) and iodine (I) below. These are all halogens. This means that if we have NaCl (Sodium chloride), we can also have NaF (Sodium fluoride), NaBr (Sodium bromide), or NaI (Sodium iodide). When an element like sodium (Na) takes a liking to any member of the halogen family, it will like them all.

Iodine is essential to thyroid function. But what if exposure to fluorine through fluoride toothpaste or exposure to chlorine through chlorinated drinking water caused the iodine in your thyroid to be replaced by fluorine or chlorine? Would this not disrupt your thyroid function and affect your energy levels?

As another example, notice that in the second column on the left, magnesium (Mg) is above calcium (Ca) which is above strontium (Sr). Magnesium and calcium are both essential minerals, but strontium is not. Radioactive strontium (Sr-90) is a waste product of nuclear power generation and is found in the atmosphere throughout the world. Sr-90 can replace calcium in your bones and teeth, thus delivering harmful radiation to your body for as long as it is present.

So now you have a useful tool in the Periodic Table. By understanding its implications, you can determine what elements will replace others in your body—either to your benefit or to your harm.

Fragrance, Therapy, and Molecular Weight

The Periodic Table gives the atomic weights of every element. In round figures, the mass or weight of a proton or neutron is 1 amu (atomic mass unit) while that of an electron is effectively zero. The atomic weight of an element is simply the sum of the number of protons and neutrons in the nucleus of an atom of that element.

For a hydrogen atom, this is easy. There is only one proton and no neutrons. Hence, its atomic weight is 1 amu.

Carbon atoms (C) normally have six protons and six neutrons so its atomic weight is 6 + 6 = 12 amu.

Nitrogen atoms (N) normally have seven protons and seven neutrons giving an atomic weight of 7 + 7 = 14 amu.

Oxygen atoms (O) typically have eight protons and eight neutrons with an atomic weight of 8 + 8 = 16 amu.

Now don't get the idea that the number of protons and neutrons in an atom are typically equal. For most elements, the numbers are different. For example, fluorine (F) atoms have 9 protons and 10 neutrons, potassium (K) atoms have 19 protons and 20 neutrons, while iron (Fe) atoms have 26 protons and 29 or 30 neutrons.

When atoms unite to form a molecule of a compound, the weight of the molecule is simply the sum of the atomic weights of its constituent atoms.

For example, the chemical formula for water is H_2O, meaning that each molecule is made up of 2 hydrogen atoms attached to 1 oxygen atom. The atomic weight of hydrogen is 1.0 amu, while the atomic weight of oxygen is 16 amu. To find the molecular weight of water, simply add the weights of 2 hydrogens and 1 oxygen as shown in the following equation:

$$(2 \times 1) + (1 \times 16) = 2 + 16 = 18 \text{ amu}$$

Thus, we find the molecular weight of water to be 18 amu, which is very small—much smaller than the molecules of essential oils.

Given next are three types of larger molecules, found in essential oils. See if you can figure out their molecular weights just for fun.

• **Phenols and Phenylpropanoids** are classes of compounds very common to essential oils. The formulas for phenylpropanoids vary. The simplest and smallest one is $C_9H_{12}O$—meaning that each molecule is made up of 9 carbon atoms, 12 hydrogen atoms, and 1 oxygen atom. The atomic weight of carbon is 12 amu, that of hydrogen is 1 amu, and that of oxygen is 16. To find the molecular weight of this phenylpropanoid, simply add the weights of 9 carbons, 12 hydrogens, and 1 oxygen like this.

$$(9 \times 12) + (12 \times 1) + (1 \times 16) = 108 + 12 + 16 = 136 \text{ amu}$$

Thus, we find the molecular weight of this phenylpropanoid to be 136 amu—considerably heavier and considerably larger than a molecule of water. However, most other phenols and phenylpropanoids have somewhat heavier molecular weights. Oregano and thyme oils are mostly phenylpropanoids while anise, fennel, basil, and tarragon are rich in phenolic ethers.

• **Monoterpenes** are a class of compounds found in every essential oil. The formula defining a hydrocarbon monoterpene is $C_{10}H_{16}$—meaning that each molecule contains 10 carbon atoms and 16 hydrogen atoms. The atomic weight of carbon is 12 amu while that of hydrogen is 1. To find the molecular weight of a simple monoterpene, add the weights of 10 carbons and 16 hydrogens like this.

$$(10 \times 12) + (16 \times 1) = 120 + 16 = 136 \text{ amu}$$

Thus, we find the molecular weight of a monoterpene hydrocarbon to be 136 amu—which is also considerably heavier and considerably larger than a molecule of water and (by coincidence) exactly the same as the smallest phenylpropanoid molecule just described. Oxygenated monoterpenes are somewhat heavier than 136 amu. Frankincense and cypress oils are mostly monoterpene

hydrocarbons.
- **Sesquiterpenes** are yet another class of compounds very common to essential oils. The formula defining a hydrocarbon sesquiterpene is $C_{15}H_{24}$—meaning that each molecule contains a unit of 15 carbon atoms and 24 hydrogen atoms. To find the molecular weight of a simple sesquiterpene, add the weights of 15 carbons and 24 hydrogens like this.

$$(15 \times 12) + (24 \times 1) = 180 + 24 = 204 \text{ amu}$$

Thus, we find the molecular weight of a simple sesquiterpene to be 204 amu—significantly heavier and larger than a phenylpropanoid or a monoterpene molecule and almost 12 times as heavy and 12 times the size of a molecule of water. Oxygenated sesquiterpenes are somewhat heavier than 204 amus. The oils of sandalwood and myrrh are mostly sesquiterpenes—some oxygenated and some not.
- **Molecular Weight** (M.W.) has a direct bearing on the behavior of essential oils because molecular weight affects the viscosity, volatility, and biological half-life of an oil. However, M.W. is not the only determining factor. Molecular shape and size also play key roles in determining viscosity and volatility. (See fatty oils Chapter Two. pp. 54-57. and comparison of triacontane and squalene in Chapter Nine, p. 288.)
- **Viscosity** is the thickness of a liquid. Molasses and honey are more viscous than rubbing alcohol or water. Sesquiterpene oils are more viscous than monoterpene oils. (Compare frankincense with myrrh.)
- **Volatility** is the ability of a liquid to vaporize or evaporate. Rubbing alcohol is more volatile than water, i.e. a dish of alcohol will evaporate faster than a dish of water. Monoterpene oils are more volatile (and more fragrant) than sesquiterpene oils. (Compare sandalwood with cypress)
- **Biological Half-Life** is the amount of time it takes for 50% of an amount of an essential oil to remain aromatically active, as a fragrance, or therapeutically active in the body. The larger the molecular weight, the longer an applied oil will maintain its fragrance, the longer will be its therapeutic action, and/or the longer it takes to be metabolized and

eliminated from the body. (NOTE: Please don't confuse "biological half-life" with "radioactive half-life," which is a term in nuclear physics applied to the decay of certain elements.)

Volatility and viscosity are related to each other in an inverse way. The more viscous an oil, the less volatile. The more volatile an oil, the less viscous.

Volatility and viscosity are related to half-life in that the less volatile and more viscous the oil, the longer will be its biochemical half-life. Myrrh, sandalwood, and other viscous oils, have long half-lives. Viscous oils are often blended with lighter, more volatile and aromatic oils (like frankincense or hyssop) to extend their half-lives.

Volatility and viscosity are directly related to fragrance because we can't smell a substance unless its molecules can vaporize into the air we breathe. You can't smell a solid. You can't smell a liquid. Your nose can only detect molecules in a gaseous or vaporized form. Small light molecules vaporize into the air more easily than large heavy ones and, thus, usually have stronger fragrances that can permeate an entire room with only a few drops.

It is a matter of energy. It takes more energy to toss a large or heavy molecule into the air where it can be experienced as an odor. Whereas the kinetic energy in an essential oil molecule is sufficient to lift it into the atmosphere at room temperature. If enough heat is applied, any substance can be vaporized, even heavy metals. But we should never use heat to vaporize an essential oil since temperatures above 160° F can cause the oil to separate, break down, and alter its chemistry. Common cooking oils (olive, peanut, corn, lard, bacon grease, butter, chicken fat, etc.) are composed of larger, long-chain fat molecules and do not vaporize at room temperature like essential oils. Hence, they have little or no smell until heated in a skillet.

The Power of Being Small

At normal temperatures, substances with molecules too large to vaporize are odorless. For example, you can't smell a protein. They are odorless (unless heated). Their molecules are too heavy—weighing thousands and even millions of amus. You won't find them in essential oils. Proteins produce odors (usually unpleasant) only when they decompose since the process of decay is where large molecules break down into smaller ones. For example, your body eliminates excess proteins through your sweat glands continuously, but there is no body odor from them until they remain long enough to start decomposing. That's why we bathe regularly.

Essential oils are composed entirely of light-weight molecules compact in size. The larger molecules in a plant are too heavy to pass through the distillation process by which essential oils are extracted. They are left behind in the plant mass. If you want to apply the large molecules from a plant, you use dried herbs which, by their drying, have lost 95% of their small molecules but have retained all of their large ones. To apply large molecules for therapeutic purposes, you make a tea, a poultice, a pill, a solution, a tincture, or a capsule from the dried portions of the plant.

All of the molecules in an essential oil vaporize at room temperatures and, thus, can easily pass into our olfactory system. Not all are detected as a fragrance since, for some molecules, we have no receptor sites in our noses that register their presence as such. Nevertheless, all of the molecules of an essential oil can enter our bodies through the nose and from there can go directly into our blood stream via the lungs or directly into the central brain.

All of the molecules of an essential oil can convey benefits to us, even those that have no detectable odor. You don't have to be able to smell an oil or an oil constituent for it to bring you benefit. In fact, you don't need to have a sense of smell at all. All you need to be able to do is breathe. All essential oils are aromatic—some faint, some mild, some strong, and some more pleasant than others.

All essential oil molecules are volatile because their dimensions are small and their atomic weights are all less than 500 amu. In fact, most are less than 300 amu. Any oil with a molecular size less than 500 can penetrate human skin, follow nerve paths, traverse the meridians, pass through the blood-brain barrier, and administer therapy at cellular levels, including the level of cellular memory or DNA.

It is the tiny molecular size and weight that makes oils so effective in dealing with the roots of disease at inter- and intracellular levels. Larger molecules can't do that.

The Science and Art of Blending

The effectiveness of essential oils can be enhanced by combining them in special ways. We won't be teaching how to make oil blends here, because that could be a book in and of itself. But there are some basic principles you need to know as a part of understanding the chemistry of essential oils and how they work. Here are some fundamentals.

• Heavier, larger molecules normally produce thicker (more viscous) oils that are less aromatic (less volatile).

• Lighter, smaller molecules normally produce thinner (less viscous) oils that are more aromatic (more volatile).

• Larger, heavier oil molecules (more viscous and less volatile) are absorbed into the body more slowly and are metabolized more slowly, remaining in the body longer periods of time.

• Smaller, lighter oil molecules (less viscous and more volatile) are absorbed more quickly into the body but are metabolized more readily, remaining in the body for shorter periods of time.

• When oils with small, light molecules are blended with oils with large, heavy molecules, the fragrance of the oil with the light molecules lasts longer and they remain in the body longer when absorbed. In other words, the company of larger molecules extends the biological half-lives of smaller molecules so that they last longer as a fragrance and work longer in your body as a therapeutic agent. The term, "half-life" refers to the amount of time for our body to metabolize half of the quantity of oil ingested or applied to the skin. Heavier oils that help extend the working life of a more volatile oil are called "fixatives" or "fixing oils."

In creating blends, aromatherapists make use of this information. Light aromatic oils (top notes) are combined with heavier oils (middle notes) and heavy oils (base notes). The art of blending oils is like composing a piece of choral music with a harmonic balance between sopranos, altos, tenors, and basses.

For example, eucalyptus, lemon, and basil are top notes, carrying the soprano parts, because they are dominated by small molecules. Geranium, lavender, and marjoram provide middle notes, singing alto and tenor, because of their medium sized molecules. Patchouly, jasmine, sandalwood, and myrrh sing the bass notes with their large molecules.

As we calculated earlier, phenylpropanoids, monoterpenes, and sesquiterpenes have molecular weights of 136, 136, and 204 respectively, with sesquiterpenes being the heaviest and largest of these molecules. These classes of compounds make up the famous PMS trio or "triple whammy" of essential oil compounds. We will talk about that later in Chapter Nine, but for this discussion let's focus on volatility and viscosity and give some real examples.

Thyme, cinnamon, oregano, clove, and peppermint oils are all very strong in their aromas. All of these are rich in phenylpropanoids, which are small molecules. Frankincense and lavender are mainly monoterpenes (another small molecule) in one form or another and also have relatively strong aromas. All of these oils are fairly thin and will pour from a bottle through a dropper cap quite readily. Their half-lives in and on our bodies are measured in minutes and hours.

An exception to this are the citrus oils. They are also mainly monoterpenes (d-limonene) but have relatively mild fragrances—not for lack of volatility on the part of d-limonene, their main constituent, but because d-limonene registers with our olfactory system as being only mildly fragrant to almost odorless. Citrus oils also contain up to 6% in tetraterpenes ($C_{40}H_{64}$, M.W. = 544 amu) which have no fragrance because of their large molecular weights. The tetraterpenes in citrus oils extend the half-lives of the monoterpenes and other lighter compounds that largely comprise their makeup.

Myrrh and sandalwood are mostly sesquiterpenes and are very mild in their fragrances. Jasmine, patchouly, and onycha oils also contain diterpenes (A.W. = 272) which are heavier than sesquiterpenes. These oils also have mild fragrances. All of these oils pour very slowly through a dropper cap. Their half-lives in and on our bodies are measured in hours, perhaps even up to a day or more.

Myrrh Makes It Last Longer

For thousands of years, even to the present day, myrrh has been used by perfumers to blend with more volatile oils to make their fragrances last longer. By the same token, virtually all of the therapeutic ointments mentioned throughout the *Bible* contained myrrh so that the oils blended in the ointment would exert their healing properties for longer periods of time in the body. The use of myrrh as an ingredient in Biblical ointments was so universal that the Greek word for ointment (*muron*) is also the Greek word for myrrh. Myrrh is a "fixing oil," one of the most popular of all time.

As for fatty oils like corn, pure olive, safflower, grape seed, castor bean, soy bean, primrose, borage, linseed, cottonseed, etc., these are always composed of larger, and usually heavier, molecules than those of essential oils. Thus they are almost odorless at room temperatures and are much thicker than essential oils. Fatty oils used as a blending base can lengthen the half-lives of essential oils, retarding their rate of absorption when applied to the skin (as in a massage oil) and retarding their rate of absorption in the body when taken orally. (For more on vegetable oils, including structural diagrams, see Chapter Two.)

If you have any of the essential oils just mentioned on hand, go check them out. The textures and fragrances of essential oils that register with our senses usually reflect the invisible, sub-microscopic structures by which their molecules are fashioned, and which only God can see.

The Oil Blot Test

Essential oils are often blended with fatty oils such as olive, grape seed, sweet almond, jojoba, wheat germ, etc.

This is a good practice when you want to create a massage oil or an oil with unusually long-lasting qualities. Examples of such oils would be Valor™ and Exodus II™ which contain mostly essential oils in bases of almond and olive oil, respectively. The holy anointing oil used by Moses (Exodus 30:23-25) was 82% essential, but also contained a carrier of virgin olive oil. When applied to the skin, the tiny molecules of essential oil of such a blend penetrate in a slowly timed fashion while the large fatty molecules of the mixing oil remain outside on the surface.

Not to be confused with terminology, you need to know that the term "base oil" is applied by aromatherapists both to fatty oils used as a mixing base for essential oils as well as to pure essential oils with the larger, heavier molecules.

The fact that fatty oils slow the absorption rates of aromatic ones can come in handy in an emergency. If an essential oil accidentally gets into an eye or on other sensitive areas of the body, don't try to dilute the burning with water. That will only drive the oil in faster and increase the pain because oil and water don't mix. Unpleasant burning can also sometimes result if oils, such as oregano, thyme, wintergreen, or peppermint are applied neat to the skin, as they are in raindrop technique. In these instances, a quick application of a fatty oil, any fatty oil, will slow down the absorption rate and stop the burning.

Some inexpensive brands of "essential oils" are actually fatty oils with essential oil added, which may not be clearly defined by the label. To find out if an oil blend contains fatty components, you can do two things. First put a little on your fingers and feel it. If it feels greasy and leaves a residue on your skin, it contains fatty molecules. A pure essential oil never feels greasy and leaves no residue.

You can also apply the blot test. Put a drop of oil on some absorbent paper. After a time, an essential oil will evaporate without a trace while a fatty oil will leave a grease spot. The exceptions to this are essential oils with color. Most are colorless, like water, but some have a tint (like German chamomile (*Matricaria recutita*) or blue tansy (*Tanacetum annum*) which may leave a stain behind.

However, stains left on blotting paper from essential oils will not be greasy.

Like an Essential Oil

A thorough study of general chemistry would involve most of the elements in Tables One and Two, which would require many thick text books, many college courses, and many hours in a laboratory. This book has distilled from the vast mass of chemical information only the relevant materials you need to understand essential oils.

Essential oils are concentrated extracts representing only a small percent of the total plant mass. This book is like an essential oil. It has been lovingly and carefully distilled to produce a powerful concentrate, a small percent of the total volume of material from which it was derived. With this book you won't need the many texts, the many courses, and the many hours in a lab to gain what you want. But, like an essential oil, this is a concentrate and you may have to take it "a drop at a time," being sure you have absorbed, assimilated, and metabolized what you have read before you go on. For those trained in chemistry years ago, this chapter will be a refresher.

Now here is the good news. We are through with general chemistry. This chapter is it. I wanted you to gain an appreciation of how all the elements relate to each other through the arrangement of the Periodic Table. But now we are ready to move on.

By persevering to the end of this chapter you have sped through several years of high school science and undergraduate chemistry and are now ready to jump right into graduate school to tackle organic chemistry, biochemistry, and, from there, to jump right into the science of how essential oils work. We will conclude this chapter with a summary of the important terms and concepts:

Key Points of Chapter Three

1. Chemistry is the study of matter and its interactions. Matter is anything that has mass and occupies space.

2. Matter is made of atoms which are composed of electrons (–), protons (+), and neutrons. Almost all of the weight (mass) of an atom is in the nucleus of protons and neutrons.

3. An atom can be visualized as a miniature solar system with a nucleus of protons and neutrons at the center (like the sun) and electrons orbiting at various distances around the nucleus (like planets).

4. Chemistry, as it is defined, is concerned only with the interactions between atoms and their shells of electrons that orbit the nuclei. Nuclear processes fall within the realm of physics, not chemistry.

5. An atom is the smallest unit of an element that retains the properties of that element. Atoms contain equal numbers of protons and electrons, thus making them electrically neutral.

6. The atomic number of an element is the number of protons (or its equivalent number of electrons) in an atom of that element.

7. The atomic weight (A.W.) of an element, stated in atomic mass units (amu), is the sum of the protons and neutrons in an atom of that element.

8. Some texts use the term "dalton" instead of "amu" as the measure for atomic and molecular weight. They mean the same thing. In this book we will use "amu." John Dalton (1766-1844) was an English school teacher who never finished grade school, himself, but began teaching at the age of 12. He is honored by chemists and physicists as the first to propose and develop the atomic theory of matter in the years 1803-1807. Hence, the adoption of his name for the unit of measure in the masses of atoms.

9. The Periodic Table of Elements is a list of elements in order of their atomic numbers starting with hydrogen (#1) which has 1 proton. There are 92 natural elements ending with uranium (#92) which has 92 protons.

10. Lavoisier's Law, formulated in the 1700s, states that "In a chemical reaction nothing is lost. Nothing is created. Everything is transformed." This statement defines the boundaries of scientific endeavor that fall under the definition of chemistry.

11. Lavoisier's Law does not define all possible reactions and interchanges between atoms and molecules. It simply defines the limits of what chemists choose to include in their field of study.

12. The current paradigm of conventional medical practice is almost totally chemical, limited by Lavoisier's law. Hence, the vast majority of treatments prescribed by physicians are chemicals (drugs).

13. Life processes are not entirely governed by the laws of chemistry. Neither is the behavior of essential oils. Herein lies the fallacy of modern medicine.

14. While there are 92 natural elements on the earth, 99.9% of those that comprise this planet (by weight) consist of only ten of them: O, Si, Al, Fe, Ca, Na, K, Mg, Ti, H, and P—in that order. In terms of the number of atoms, however, hydrogen outnumbers them all, comprising over 90% of earth and the universe by atomic count.

15. In terms of numbers of atoms, the human body is made mostly of hydrogen. In terms of body weight, we are composed 99% of only four elements: 76% oxygen (O), 16% carbon (C), 3% nitrogen (N), and 1% hydrogen (H). In terms of molecules, a fertilized human egg is 95% water while the human adult body is 70% water. Hence, from conception to death, humans are mostly H_2O.

16. Elements are simple substances that cannot be broken down by chemical means into any other substance. Each atom of any element contains a specific number of protons designated by its atomic number.

17. Of the 92 natural elements, only 27 are known to play essential roles in human life. They are, in order of their atomic numbers (i.e. increasing atomic weights): H, Li, B, C, N, O, F, Na, Mg, Si, P, S, Cl, K, Ca, V, Cr, Mn, Fe, Co, Ni, Cu, Zn, Ge, Si, Mo, and I.

18. Trace constituents are responsible for some of the most important functions in the human body just as some trace compounds provide the most important actions of essential oils.

19. Most of the elements necessary for human life would be toxic in large doses. Iron, for one, can be quite toxic, but, as the provider of bioenergy through our blood cells, it is absolutely essential. This illustrates a basic maxim of toxicology: Dosage is everything. Everything is toxic. Everything is therapeutic. It all depends on dose. This maxim applies not only to the necessary elements that comprise our physical existence, but applies also to the compounds of essential oils and their usage.

20. All 27 elements necessary for human life are found in the upper portion of the Periodic Table and are, therefore, among the lightest of the elements, all but two (Mo and I) are less than 79 amu in atomic weight (A.W.).

21. Iodine (I) is the heaviest element necessary for human life. Most heavy elements are toxic to people.

22. Elements can be classified as: metals, non-metals, transition elements, alkali metals, alkaline earth metals, noble gases, halogens, and chalcogens. The elements that make up essential oils (C, H, O, S, N) are all non-metals—including H, which is metallic in extreme cold, but non-metallic at the temperatures of living processes.

23. Elements in the same vertical column in the Periodic Table have similar chemical characteristics and can replace one another in compounds.

24. Molecules are the smallest units of a compound that retain the properties of that compound. The molecules of compounds are combinations of complete atoms, which are electrically neutral.

25. The molecular weight of a compound is the sum of the atomic weights (in amu) of all of the atoms that form a molecule of that compound.

26. Molecular weight (M.W.) affects the viscosity and volatility of an oil and has a bearing on the behavior of the oil. Molecular size and shape also influence the viscosity and volatility of an oil.

27. The half-life of an essential oil is a biiological term that refers to the amount of time it takes for half of the oil applied, or ingested, to evaporate, be absorbed, or be metabolized by our bodies. The half-life of an element is a a term used in nuclear physics to indicate the amount of time 50% of a radioactive element sample will decay. In physics the term refers to a nuclear reaction. In aromatherapy it refers to a biochemical reaction.

28. Big molecules make thicker oils (more viscous) with mild fragrances (less volatile) that metabolize slowly and last longer in and on the body (long half-lives).

29. Small molecules make thin oils (less viscous) with strong fragrances (more volatile) that metabolize quickly and last shorter times in and on the body (short half-lives).

30. In the science and art of creating oil blends, oils composed of large heavy molecules are called "base notes" and oils made of light tiny molecules are called "top notes." Those in between are called "middle notes."

31. Oils composed of larger molecules (like Myrrh and Sandalwood) are sometimes called "fixatives" or "fixing oils," because when blended with lighter more volatile oils, they make them last longer as a fragrance or therapeutic agent.

32. A good blend will contain a mixture of essential oils with a variety of molecular sizes, from small to large.

33. Blends can sometimes be more effective for certain purposes than an oil used as a single because blends usually contain a wider variety of molecular shapes, weights, types, and sizes.

34. Fatty oils are blended with essential oils to create massage oils which are mild in their effects, to retard the rates of absorption, to extend the activity times of essential oils, and to stop burning when essential oils applied neat irritate the skin or accidentally get into eyes or on other sensitive areas of the body.

35. Fatty oils are also used in some inexpensive brands of aromatic oils to add more volume to the product without clearly identifying the presence, species, or percent of the fatty oil used. One can identify the presence of fatty oils mixed with an essential oil by the blot test.

❤ CHAPTER FOUR
THE
CHOSEN ONES

Chapter Two was a survey of the 92 natural elements that compose our planet and universe, as well as the 22 laboratory elements and four theoretical elements yet to be discovered. Lucky for you, it is not necessary to comprehend all 118 elements on the Periodic Table, or the 114 known elements, or the 92 natural elements, or even the 27 elements of living organisms. For essential oil chemistry you only need be concerned with five, at the most. Is that good news or what? I call them the "CHOSN Ones," chosen by God from which to build life in a billion forms (along with a few other elements, of course). All five play roles in essential oils—some major, some minor, They are as follows:

Carbon	C
Hydrogen	H
Oxygen	O
Sulfur	S
Nitrogen	N

The elements, C, H, O, and N, comprise 96% of our body weight with S as an essential minor element along with Ca, P, Cl, K, Na, and Mg. But these last six elements are not found in essential oils.

Atomic models of the CHOSN elements are shown on the next page. As you can see, there is a considerable difference in size and weight between hydrogen (with one proton and no neutrons, A.W. = 1) and sulfur (with sixteen protons and 16 neutrons, A.W. = 32). Oxygen, as you can see, is exactly half the size and weight of sulfur.

The CHOSN Ones have some things in common. They

Carbon Atom
6 Protons
6 Neutrons
6 electrons
A.W. 12.00

Nitrogen Atom
7 Protons
7 Neutrons
7 electrons
A.W. 14.00

Oxygen Atom
8 Protons
8 Neutrons
8 electrons
A.W. 16.00

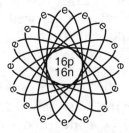

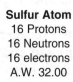

Sulfur Atom
16 Protons
16 Neutrons
16 electrons
A.W. 32.00

Hydrogen Atom
1 Proton
1 electron
A.W. = 1.00

Atomic Models of the CHOSN Ones

---

all belong to a minority class (viz. non-metals). While most of the elements in the Periodic Table are metals, the CHOSN Ones are all non-metals. We are including hydrogen as a nonmetal here, even though it is technically a metal and manifests all the metallic properties at extremely low temperatures. However, it behaves as a non-metallic gas at the temperatures in which it participates in life processes. Except for liquid mercury (Hg) and gaseous hydrogen (H), all metals are solids at room temperatures. Metals all have a recognizable appearance that reflects light in a certain way referred to as "a metallic luster." Metals can be hammered into sheets (malleability) stretched into wires (ductility), and readily conduct both heat and electricity.

As non-metals, the CHOSN Ones do not conduct electricity. Neither do they conduct heat very well. S and C are solids at normal temperatures, but neither has the appearance or texture of a metal, nor are they malleable or ductile, The other three, H, N and O, are all gases. All five are relatively light in atomic weight, ranging from 1 to 32 amus, and they all occur in the top three levels of the Periodic Table—H on the first level, C, N, & O on the second, and S on the third.

Right away you will recognize a major difference between the chemistry of mechanical robots and living human beings. Robots are built mainly from metals. People aren't.

The CHOSN Ones also have characteristics not in common. Looking at the Periodic Table you can see that H (#1), C (#6), N (#7), and O (#8) are each at the top of four different vertical columns. Thus, they are each a head of a different family of elements.

This means that these four elements each have different chemical personalities, different appetites for electrons, different preferences for companions, and different habits of expression. It is these differences that facilitate the unceasing variety of life forms on earth.

Sulfur and Oxygen: The Radical Cousins

Sulfur is located in the Periodic Table directly below oxygen in the same column. This means that sulfur and oxygen are cousins, members of the same family—the Chalcogen family. As relatives they have similar likes and dislikes and can readily exchange places with each other in chemical compounds.

For example, both O and S team up with H in the same way. They both like to hold hands with two hydrogens as in H_2O or H_2S. The first compound is water, of course, while the second is a stinky gas (hydrogen sulfide), better known as "rotten egg gas."

If we remove an H atom from H_2O and H_2S, we end up with two partial molecules which are written as OH and SH. These are called "radicals." Radicals are partial molecules. Radicals are always hungry and eager to complete themselves. They will readily steal electrons from other molecules or aggressively attach themselves to whatever they can find to satisfy their unsated appetites and desire for companionship.

When an OH radical is attached to a molecule, we call that compound an "alcohol." When an SH radical attaches itself to a molecule, we call that compound a "thiol." Thiols can be changed into alcohols and vice versa by simply trading S atoms for O or O atoms for S. Essential oils contain hundreds of different alcohols as major constituents, and many thiols as traces. When thiols are present, they usually dominate the fragrance of the oil.

The Scent of Grapefruit

The major portion of any essential oil (99.99%) is composed of only three elements—C, H, and O—but the other two members of the chosen ones, S and N, sometimes contribute key roles. For example, the distinctive fragrance of grapefruit oil (*Citrus paradisi*) is due to a sulfur compound, 1-p-menthen-8-thiol ($C_{10}H_{18}S$). Also known as thioterpineol, it occurs in a tiny trace amount—less than one part per billion (ppb). One ppb is equivalent to five drops in an olympic swimming pool. In numeric form, that is an infinitesimal 0.0000001%. Yet its presence dominates the scent of grapefruit.

While grapefruit oil is 86-92% d-limonene, that is not what you smell. d-Limonene, in any concentration, is experienced as a faint orange-like aroma. Amazing as it seems, one molecule in a billion of the sulfur compound in grapefruit is so strong that it overcomes the d-limonene and is easily picked up and distinguished by our sensitive noses. (Strong odors are a characteristic of most sulfur compounds, which are also found in onions and garlic.)

Check it out. If you have a bottle of grapefruit oil handy, take a whiff and experience a molecule or two of that sulfur compound. You can impress your friends by saying, "Hmmm . . . I believe there is a trace of 1-p-menthen-8-thiol in this oil."

The other citrus rind oils (bergamot, orange, lemon, tangerine, mandarin, and lime) are all more than 50% d-limonene, like grapefruit, yet they each have different fragrances and different therapeutic properties determined by their minor and trace constituents. Grapefruit, for example, has been shown to be effective against skin cancer. It can also dissolve fat tissue and has been used to assist in weight loss and reduce cellulite. Unlike the other citrus oils, grapefruit is also a topical anesthetic. Put a drop on your tongue and it will go numb. This is due to nootkatone (0.1-2%), a compound unique to grapefruit. These therapeutic properties are not due to its main ingredients, but come from its minor and trace compounds like 1-p menthen-8-thiol and others.

Another fascinating property, unique to the aroma of grapefruit is it ability to make women appear younger than they are. In one study, when men were asked to estimate the ages of women wearing grapefruit scented perfume, they underestimated by an average of six years. So ladies, add six years of youth to your life by simply applying grapefruit oil. Now be careful. Grapefruit oil is phototoxic. So don't apply it to your skin and expose yourself to sun or ultraviolet light. (See pp. 379-383 on phototoxicity.)

Grapefruit is an illustration of why an essential oil needs to be harvested and produced as close to nature as possible without tampering with even the least of the ingredients.

Sulfur Makes Its Presence Known

Sulfur compounds probably occur in most essential oils, but usually in concentrations of only one part per million (ppm) to less than one part per billion (ppb). Such low concentrations are beyond what can be detected by gas chromatography—which is the customary means of analyzing essential oils in a laboratory. Hence, in trying to determine if an oil is natural or synthetic, the usual laboratory procedures may not be able to tell. If all of the major compounds are present in the synthetic version, the absence of all of the trace compounds can go undetected. Nevertheless, when present even in small quantities, sulfur compounds almost always noticeably affect the fragrance of an oil. In many cases, a little sulfur plays the distinguishing role, as in the case of grapefruit just discussed. This is why the human nose can be a better detector of fraudulent oils than a laboratory machine.

Except for a few oils, sulfur compounds are rarely a major constituent. Where sulfur compounds do compose a major portion of the volume of an oil, their pungent properties are so overwhelming as to make them unsuitable for common usage. Among these are garlic oil (*Allium sativum*), onion oil (*Allium cepa*), horseradish oil (*Armoracia rusticana*), and mustard seed oil (*Brassica nigra*). It's the sulfur compounds in an onion that make you cry. Garlic and onion oils are safe and beneficial taken internally, but irritate the eyes and nose when inhaled or brought near the face. Horseradish and mustard oils are generally avoided in aromatherapy because they are powerful lachrymators (stimulating tear ducts like tear gas), can be damaging to nasal membranes, can burn the skin, and can have other harsh consequences.

As a ubiquitous trace element among essential oils, the reason sulfur does not comprise a large percent of the volume of most oils is because it is a much larger atom than C, H, or O—being twice the size of oxygen, two and a half times that of carbon, and 32 times the size of hydrogen. (See atomic diagrams at beginning of this chapter.) Its larger atomic weight makes it less able to create molecules light enough to pass through the distillation process and participate in volatile oils. However, as mentioned above, when sulfur compounds do exist in oils they can dominate the character of the oil even when present in small amounts.

Sulfur compounds are most often found in plants of the families of Liliaceae, Rosaceae, and Asteraceae (also known as Compositae). Liliaceae (lily family) includes hyacinth, tulip, onions, and garlic whose sulfurous odiferous oils are not candidates for sweet perfumes, mouth washes, or breath fresheners. The flowers of hyacinth and tulip are better known for their color and beauty while onions and garlic are in greater demand for their mouth-watering flavor and aroma in foods.

Rosaceae (rose family) includes many species of roses with a variety of pleasing fragrances from floral, spicy, and minty to fresh and fruity. More than a dozen trace compounds of sulfur have been identified in rose oil. This demonstrates that sulfur compounds, which usually have strong odors, are not necessarily unpleasant. The fragrances of rose are among the most highly prized in the perfume industry.

Asteraceae (aster/daisy family) includes Anise (*Pimpinella anisum*), echinacea (*Echinacea purpurea*), (German chamomile (*Matricaria recutita*), Roman chamomile (*Chamaemelum nobile*), goldenrod (*Solidago canadensis*), helichrysum (*Helichrysum italicum*), blue tansy (*Tanacetum annuum*), and Idaho tansy (*Tanacetum vulgare*). All of these oils have distinct odors—some sweet, some bitter, some earthy, some medicinal. Asters and daisies are flowers more valued for their beauty and herbal benefits than for their fragrances.

One member of the mint family (Labiatae) contains a sulfur compound. The plant is peppermint (*Mentha piperita*). The compound is mint sulfide ($C_{13}H_{21}S$). It is one of the ingredients that distinguishes peppermint from spearmint.

Sulfur may also play a role in color inasmuch as red flowers seem to have higher concentrations of sulfur than white or other colors.

Nitrogen Plays Minor Roles

Most essential oils contain traces of nitrogen compounds, but you never find nitrogen as a major element in any oil. One reason for this is because organic nitrogen compounds tend to be water soluble, and do not always mix well with oils. Nevertheless, some of the stronger and unique odors in oils are due to the presence of small amounts of nitrogen compounds.

For example, the characteristic fragrances of ylang ylang (*Cananga odorata*), jasmine (*Jasminum officinale*), petitgrain (*Citrus aurantium*), distilled from orange tree leaves, and bergamot (*Citrus bergamia*) are due to small concentrations (1-2%) of a nitrogenous ester—methyl anthranilate ($C_8H_9NO_2$). In coriander oil (*Coriandrum sativum*), the characteristic fragrance is due largely to minor quantities of pyrrole (C_4H_5N) and pyrazine ($C_4H_4N_2$), both nitrogen compounds. Pyrrole is head of a family of compounds containing a pentagonal ring of 4 Cs and 1 N (C_4N). Pyrazine is a member of the diazine family characterized by a hexagonal ring of 4 Cs and 2 Ns (C_4N_2).

An even more interesting case is indole (C_8H_7N) and scatole (C_9H_8N), which are also members of the pyrrole family. These two compounds are both decay products of proteins that contribute to the stench of dead animals. These are real "bad boys." They are also found in feces and contribute to the stink of it, although pure isolated indole can smell like strong moth balls. Scatole gets its name from "scat," a term for animal droppings, in which it is found. Amazingly, indole and scatole are found in many favorite flowers such as jasmine and orange blossoms as well as several species of *Narcissus* (including jonquil, daffodil, crocus, and tazetta). Quantities of up to 3% are found in the highly prized absolute oil of jasmine. In concentrated samples or when mixed with proteins or amino acids, their odors are horrible. In dilute quantities, and in the company of essential oil compounds, their scents become pleasantly floral. In fact, indole is sometimes included in formulas for patented perfumes where it adds pleasant support for the desired fragrances.

This is an illustration of how concentration is important in one's olfactory response to an aromatic substance. Too much or too little can make all the difference. This also illustrates how specific compounds behave differently depending on their company. When the influence of other compounds in an oil cause a "bad boy" to behave, this is called "quenching." These factors are why testing an isolated component of an oil is not a valid way to determine how that compound will behave in the oil nor is it a valid way to determine the characteristics of the whole oil as blended and balanced by nature.

Other examples of oils where nitrogen compounds contribute character to the fragrance include carrot seed (*Daucus carota*), angelica (*Angelica archangelica*), clary sage (*Salvia sclarea*), celery (*Apium graveolens*), galbanum (*Ferula gummosa*), hyacinth (*Hyacinthus orientalis*), lavandin (*Lavandula x hybrida*), parsley (*Petroselinum crispum*), rosemary (*Rosmarinus officinalis*), spike lavender (*Lavandula latifolia*), and vetiver (*Vetiveria zizanioides*).

In general, nitrogen compounds are found in oils from the plant families of Oliaceae, Lamiaceae (also known as Labiatae), and Apiaceae (also known as Umbelliferae). Oliaceae (olive family) includes jasmine and olive. Apiaceae (parsley family) includes angelica, carrot, celery, coriander, galbanum, and parsley. Lamiaceae (mint family) includes clary sage, lavandin, rosemary, and spike lavender.

Nitrogen may also play a role in color. White flowers, such as jasmine, neroli, and hyacinth, contain more nitrogen than flowers of other colors.

Nitrogen Prefers a Backstage Part

While nitrogen never plays the lead role in the many performances of essential oils, it plays a major role in the creation of some of the most important ingredients in essential oils. Here is how.

Nitrogen is a necessary ingredient in amino acids which are the building blocks of the thousands of proteins that comprise our bodies and make them function. Without nitrogen, not only would our bodies cease to work, there would be no body at all. The same is true in plants.

In plants, nitrogen-containing compounds are involved in the manufacture of essential oils. The raw materials from which oils are made include amino acids. However, when the final product is finished and the oil is complete, nitrogen almost completely disappears.

When it comes to essential oils, most of the time nitrogen atoms behave like the prop managers, set builders, and makeup artists who do all their work before the show begins, setting the stage and preparing the actors and actresses to produce the play, working right up to curtain time, but who then retreat backstage not to be seen by the audience nor involved in the actual performance.

To Make a Phenylpropanoid

The fact that amino acids are among the raw materials from which the compounds of essential oils are made has led some to mistakenly conclude that amino acids are often found in the finished oil. You may have heard it said that "essential oils contain amino acids." But that is generally not true, except for possible trace amounts. An exception to this is cumin oil (*Cuminum cyminum*) in which a trace of an amino acid has been detected, but which usually oxidizes out in time. Amino acids are always a part of a plant's manufacturing processes because they create the enzymes that catalyze organic reactions. But amino acids are rarely a part of the end product.

For example, phenolics and phenylpropanoids are among the most important classes of essential oil compounds. They cleanse receptor sites, eat up free radicals, and protect us from viruses and harmful bacteria. The oils of anise (*Pimpinella anisum*) thyme (*Thymus vulgaris*), oregano (*Origanum compactum*), cinnamon (*Cinnamomum verum*), clove (*Syzygium aromatica*), peppermint (*Mentha piperita*), fennel (*Foeniculum vulgare*), basil (*Ocimum basilicum*), bay laurel, (*Laurus nobilis*) ravensara (*Ravensara aromatica*), tarragon (*Artemisia dracunculus*) and tea tree (*Melaleuca alternifolia*) are all rich in phenolics and/or phenylpropanoids.

There are a variety of formulas for phenylpropanoids. One of the simplest of them is $C_9H_{12}O$—which is the union of 9 C atoms, 12 H atoms, and 1 O into a single molecule. In making a phenylpropanoid, the plant starts by making an amino acid—either phenylalanine ($C_9H_{11}NO_2$) or tyrosine ($C_9H_{11}NO_3$). A phenylalanine molecule contains 9 C atoms, 11 hydrogens, 2 oxygens, and 1 atom of nitrogen while a tyrosine molecule is the same except for an extra oxygen. Even in amino acids that require nitrogen atoms, the molecules are still predominantly composed of C, H, and O atoms. Of the 23 or 24 atoms in a phenylalanine or tyrosine molecule, only one is nitrogen.

Starting from a phenylalanine molecule, the plant removes the nitrogen (N) and 3 hydrogens (H) in the form of NH_3 which may be released to the atmosphere as ammonia gas, deposited in the soil for other plants to use, or recycled by the plant for other purposes. NH_3 is water soluble. This leaves behind a molecule of cinnamic acid—$C_9H_8O_2$ —composed of 9 carbon atoms, 8 hydrogens, and 2 oxygens. The plant then removes an oxygen (O) atom from each molecule of cinnamic acid and releases them into the atmosphere. Simultaneously, with the help and supervision of certain enzymes, it hydrogenates the acid molecules with four hydrogens each to create $C_9H_{12}O$—a phenylpropanoid with two common names. One is "p-cuminol," so named because it is found in cumin oil (*Cuminum cyminum*). The scientific name is 4-isopropyl-phenol. This compound is also found in most species of eucalyptus oils (*Eucalyptus sp.*) where it has the common name of "australol," named after Australia from where eucalyptus trees originate. (See Chapter Six for a diagram of what this molecule looks like.)

As you can see, the nitrogen was lost along the way, but it was there in the form of an amino acid at the beginning of the process. As to why plants choose an amino acid (containing N) as the raw material to make a phenyl-propanoid (which contains no N), only God knows. It seems that there should be a way to do it without starting with a nitrogenous molecule. But who are we to question the Great Chemical Engineer who devised the process. "For my thoughts are not your thoughts, nor are your ways my ways, says the Lord." (Isaiah 55:8)

Plants understand a lot that we do not. There is wisdom in the vegetable kingdom that exceeds our own. That's why the great botanists speak to plants and listen in order that they may learn from them and receive revelations of God's nature from what he has made. (Job 12:8; Romans 1:20)

Phenylalanine and tyrosine, themselves, are manufactured by the plant from simple sugars which it transforms into carboxylic acids to which it adds the necessary nitrogen to make an amino acid. The sugars are manufactured in the leaves of the plants through photosynthesis —a process utilizing the frequencies of sunlight to combine molecules of water H_2O and carbon dioxide CO_2 to create carbohydrates. Nitrogen comprises 78% of our atmosphere, but plants cannot utilize atmospheric nitrogen directly. The nitrogen necessary to make phenylalanine and tyrosine is made available to the roots of the plants by certain "nitrogen fixing" bacteria that live in the soil.

When plants transform phenylalanine into cinnamic acid, they may choose not to make phenylpropanoids at that point. They may choose to create esters, coumarins, lignans, flavonoids, and other compounds—all with the nitrogen missing when the final product is made.

Plants have the intelligence to make whatever substances they need whenever they need them as a dynamic 24-hour-a-day activity. In the process they create thousands of compounds as ingredients for their essential oils.

Plants as Miniature Oil Factories

You can begin to see from this simple discussion of how plants manufacture the constituents of oils, that they are remarkable chemical factories continuously producing numerous substances in ways that no laboratory has ever been able to duplicate or, in many cases, to even analyze. What plants do to create an essential oil is even more amazing when you realize that, not just one or two, but, hundreds of compounds are manufactured and blended by the plant to produce a single oil.

Even when a laboratory does duplicate a natural organic formula, the synthetic versions of organic compounds are not quite the same as those produced directly by God's intelligence manifesting through his plant kingdom. The natural and the synthetic versions may have the same chemical formulas, but not all of the same characteristics as manifested in a therapeutic grade oil. Contrary to popular belief, chemical formulas are not a complete description of a compound.

As you will learn later in this book, there are factors in natural oils and their components that cannot be explained by chemistry alone. You will also learn that plants are able to perform feats of physics, never before seen or duplicated in a lab, that seem to contradict the natural laws currently believed by scientists.

Essential oils are more than simple products of the materialistic laws thus far perceived and adopted by scientists. They are also the products of spiritual laws which are far more encompassing than most scientists can currently envision. In describing our limited faculties St Paul commented in I Corinthians 13:9,12: "For we know only in part, and we prophecy only in part...For now we see through a glass darkly..."

But light is coming and science will some day break out of its box of smoked glass that so dims its view of the universe that surrounds us. We shall speak more on this in Part Three.

The Elements and Their Appetites

Most elements have a desire for companionship. Some atoms are more social than others. Some, like the noble gases, are solitary people who prefer to remain separate from all other elements, seeking the company of no one. Some atoms prefer a one-on-one relationship with a single partner while others like a party, preferring the company of two, three or four companions. This desire on the part of an atom is called "valence."

While we don't intend to get into a detailed explanation of how and why elements have valence, suffice it to say that it has to do with the configuration of the outer shells of electrons in their atoms. Each layer of electrons around a nucleus has a limited capacity—it can only hold so many. When a shell is nearly full, that atom will seek to complete it by finding additional electrons somewhere. When a shell is nearly empty, that atom is willing to release one, two, or three electrons and donate them to other atoms who express a need. Thus, elements who lack a few electrons and seek them are eager to associate with elements who want to give them. Hence, when we place a numerical value on valence, that number represents the number of electrons per atom that element seeks or is willing to give. For more details on this, look it up in any chemistry book. The valences of the Chosen Five (C,H,O,S, and N) are as follows:

Carbon	(C)	4
Hydrogen	(H)	1
Oxygen	(O)	2
Sulfur	(S)	2
Nitrogen	(N)	3

Notice how sulfur and oxygen have the same valence (2). Remember that they are in the same vertical column in the Periodic Table. In fact, every element in that column has a valence of 2. Similarly, every element in the first column, under hydrogen, has a valence of 1, all those under nitrogen have a valence of 3, and all those under carbon have a valence of 4.

Now you can begin to understand why elements that stack up in the same column in the Periodic Table all manifest similar chemical behaviors. Their social appetites are the same. In other words, generally speaking, elements of the Periodic Table in the same vertical column have the same valences.

Judging from the valences given, you can see that carbon has the largest craving for company. Carbon is the most social of all elements that compose living organisms and comprise essential oils. Carbon and its personality is the real key to the remarkable versatility of essential oils.

Memorize the valence numbers given above. Do this and you will soon be working advanced problems in organic chemistry and it will be fun. Just remember those numbers. Here is how it works.

Cartoon Chemistry

Imagine a hydrogen atom whose valence is 1 to be a tiny person with one arm and one little hand to grab with. It would look like the cartoon below.

Now imagine oxygen and sulfur atoms to be little people with two arms and two hands that look like this.

Note the family resemblance between O and S, each with their two arms outstretched. You can tell they're cousins.

Now imagine nitrogen with three arms and hands, and carbon with four arms and hands. They would look like this.

Using the knowledge you have now gained about valence, how many hydrogens will it take to satisfy an oxygen atom? Answer: two. When they join up, here is what you get. (Note: Their hands are invisibly joined in the middle of the bonds and are not shown.)

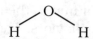

And what do we get? We get H_2O. Water. Everyone's happy. The oxygen is happy because its two hands are full and the two hydrogens are happy having each filled their one hand. Happy atoms joining hands in friendship with all their bonds satisfied is what makes a molecule. Since they are in the same family, substituting S for O in the molecule above will also work. You get H_2S (better known as "rotten egg gas") which looks like this.

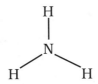

You can remember these two, H_2O and H_2S, as "H_2Okay" and H_2Stinky."

Note that the bonding angle between the two hydrogens in the water molecule, H_2O, is close to 120°. That's one-third of a circle. This is why crystals of frozen water are often shaped like a pair of superimposed equilateral triangles—i.e. like a hexagon or a six-pointed star? Now you know why snow flakes are either six sided or composed of triangles. However, bonding angles in water can change in response to prayers and thoughts, producing different crystalline structures when frozen. (See Part Three.)

Having figured out a couple of combinations, let's try another. How many hydrogens would it take to make a nitrogen atom happy? Answer: three. When they join up, here is what you get.

$$\begin{array}{c} H \\ | \\ N \\ \diagup \quad \diagdown \\ H \qquad H \end{array}$$

And what do we get? We get NH_3. Ammonia gas. If you have ever changed a baby's wet diaper, you've probably smelled it. You can also smell it around a barn where cattle feed. It is one of the waste products in urine, a breakdown compound from protein. Ammonia is a happy molecule. The Nitrogen has satisfied its demand for a partner to hold with each of its three arms. The three hydrogens are happy having each linked their one arm with one of nitrogen's three arms. (Actually, if urine has a strong smell of ammonia, it is usually a sign of eating an unbalanced diet with too much protein.)

Now that we know how valences work, let's try another. How many hydrogens will it take to satisfy a carbon atom? Answer: four. When they join up, here is what you get.

$$
\begin{array}{c}
\text{H} \\
| \\
\text{H} - \text{C} - \text{H} \\
| \\
\text{H}
\end{array}
$$

And what is it? It's CH_4 - A molecule of methane gas. If you have ever noticed the odor of rotting leaves or decaying vegetation in a swamp, you've smelled it. It is also the main ingredient in the gas released by animals (including humans) who eat leafy plants and vegetables as a waste product of digestion. Methane is a happy molecule. The carbon is satisfied with four partners holding onto its four hands and the four hydrogens are satisfied since in each instance, their one arm is engaged.

Let's try one more. How many oxygens will it take to satisfy a carbon atom? Answer: two. When they join up, here is what you get.

$$O = C = O$$

This is carbon dioxide—CO_2. When we breathe in oxygen, we exhale carbon dioxide which is what plants want to breathe. When plants breathe in carbon dioxide, they exhale oxygen. We depend on each other to sustain life. Carbon dioxide is a happy molecule, but something different has happened in this case. The four arms of the carbon atom are satisfied in pairs with two arms grasping one oxygen atom and the other two carbon arms grasping the other oxygen. The two oxygens are satisfied, too, even though in each case, their pair of arms is grasping the same atom. These are called "double bonds." Notice, that unlike the bonds in water, where the angle between the two hydrogens was about 120°, here the angle between the two oxygens is 180°—a straight line.

In the four molecular examples before carbon dioxide, there were no double bonds. Interesting things can happen with molecules containing double bonds. In the chemistry of oils, molecules with double bonded carbon atoms, are said to be "unsaturated." Oil molecules with no double bonds are said to be "saturated." When you "hydrogenate" (add hydrogen atoms) to an unsaturated oil, you change double bonds into single bonds. Saturated oils tend to be thicker, more viscous, and often solid at room temperature (like margarine). Thus, saturated oils are more likely to clog our arteries when ingested. Now you know the difference between a saturated oil and an unsaturated oil. (See Chapter Two, discussion on fatty oils, pp. 54-57.)

And Then There Were Three

Of the five chosen ones, this book will focus mainly on C, H, and O. The chemistry of essential oils is almost entirely the mutual chemistry and family relationships of these three players.

Sulfur is essential to life, but in oils, as a percent of total volume, it's rarely a major element. Its atomic weight of 32 (double that of O) makes it difficult to form molecules small enough to pass through distillation. When an S compound is present in an oil, it usually dominates the fragrance, even in tiny amounts. Grapefruit oil (*Citrus paradisi*) will testify to this, as mentioned earlier in this chapter. The distinctive scent of grapefruit is due to a trace of one sulfur compound. By contrast, the powerful odor of garlic (*Allium sativum*) is from several sulfur compounds that make up a significant portion of the oil—the main ones being diallyldisulphide $C_6H_{10}S_2$ and allicin $C_6H_{10}OS_2$. These two are so strong their vapors can make you cry, which is why essential oil of garlic is taken orally and not inhaled.

As for N, it is never a major element in any oil. This is mainly because organic nitrogen compounds tend to be water soluble which don't mix well with lipid (oily) molecules. Nitrogen compounds (amino acids), which are the building materials for every living cell, can be used as raw materials to make oil molecules. When this happens, the N is usually discarded along the way.

The Chemistry of Essential Oils Made Simple

We started Chapter Two with a monster of 92 to 118 elements that define the scope of chemistry. (Table One) We then narrowed it down to 27 as being necessary for human life. (Table Six) By the beginning of this chapter we had eliminated all but five. Now we step down one more level and reduce the chemistry of essential oils to just three elements—C, H, and O. The further we go into the chemistry of essential oils, the simpler it gets. How about that for getting a break?

In fact, let's define the chemistry of essential oils right now in the fewest possible number of words:

> The chemistry of essential oils consists of simple hydrocarbons, oxygenated hydrocarbons, and their isomers.

That's it. That statement summarizes this whole book in a sentence. We have not yet defined the terms of that statement so you can understand it, but make note of it. As you read on, it will gradually become clear to you how accurate, complete, and appropriate that statement is. Before you finish this book, you will understand and appreciate how that brief statement is "The Chemisty of Essential Oils Made Simple."

Key Points of Chapter Four

1. 96% of the human body is composed of C, H, O and N with S as an essential minor element. These are the "CHOSN Ones." They all play roles in essential oils, some major, some minor,

2. The CHOSN Ones are all non-metals, occur at the top of the Periodic Table, and are among the lightest of elements, H, O, and N are gases. C and S are solids.

3. An element consists of atoms all with the same number of protons in their nuclei.

4. A compound consists of molecules all with the same assortment of atoms in the same structural arrangement.

5. Complete molecules are made of complete atoms with equal numbers of protons and electrons which makes them electrically neutral.

6. Radicals are incomplete molecules which are unbalanced and aggressive toward other molecules.

7. OH and SH are radicals. Molecules containing OH radicals are called alcohols. Molecules containing SH radicals are called thiols.

8. Traces of S are found in many essential oils, but usually not in concentrations greater than 1 ppm to 1%.

9. Oil compounds containing S, even in trace amounts, usually dominate the fragrance of that oil. Grapefruit oil is an example of a trace sulfur compound dominating the character and fragrance of an oil.

10. Oils with large proportions of S compounds include garlic, onion, horseradish, and mustard. All of these oils are too strong for safe use in inhalation aromatherapy.

11. While S compounds tend to have strong odors, they are not all unpleasant. Rose oil with one of the most pleasant and uplifing fragrances of all, contains more than a dozen S compounds in trace amounts.

12. The fragrance and/or the healing properties of an oil may not be due to its main ingredients, but due to its trace compounds.

13. To produce a therapeutic grade essential oil it must be harvested and produced as close to nature as possible without tampering with even the least of the ingredients.

14. N is found in traces in many oils, but never as a major compound.

15. When plants transform nitrogenous compounds into oil compounds, N is usually discarded along the way leaving only a hydrocarbon or oxygenated hydrocarbon to be found in the oil.

16. N compounds tend to have strong odors and noticibly contribute to the character of the fragrance in an oil. Jasmine, neroli, cumin, coriander, and galbanum are oils whose fragrances are partially due to nitrogen compounds.

17. Indole, a by–product of protein decomposition, is a nitrogen compound that smells like feces, when isolated from the oils that contain it. In trace amounts in the company of oil compounds that quench its unacceptable behavior, it has a pleasant floral fragrance. It occurs in jasmine, orange blossom (neroli), and narcissus oils.

18. Normal laboratory procedures do not measure or detect trace compounds in an oil, but the human nose can tell. This makes the human nose better able to distinguish between a synthetic oil and a natural one than even the most sophisticated laboratory equipment.

19. Amino acids are generally not found in oils because they easily oxidize or react with other components in the oil and disappear in time. One exception to this is cumin oil in which traces of amino acids have been found.

20. Amino acids such as phenylalanine and tyrosine are raw materials from which plants make certain compounds (phenylpropanoids) in essential oils, but the N atom in the amino acids disappears along the way and is not found in the finished oil.

21. One reason nitrogen compounds are seldom found in essential oils is because they tend to be water soluble and usually don't mix well with oils.

22. The chemical formula of a compound is written as a list of symbols for the elemental atoms it contains with little numbers written as subscripts indicating how many of each atom is contained in a molecule of that compound.

23. The international symbol for each natural element consists of one or two letters of the alphabet, the first of which is capitalized, as in H, He, Li, Be, B, C, N, O, Fl, Ne, S, P, Cl, Kr, etc.

24. The behavior and characteristics of an essential oil compound is not fully described by its chemical formula.

25. The desire on the part of an atom to link up with other atoms making compounds is called "valence" represented by a numeral. The higher the valence, the greater the number of partners that can be held by that atom.

26. The valences of the CHOSN ones are as follows: Hydrogen = 1, Oxygen = 2, Sulfur = 2, Nitrogen = 3, Carbon = 4.

27. Elements in the same vertical columns of the Periodic Table generally have the same valences. Elements with the same valances behave similarly toward other elements in forming compounds.

28. Of the CHOSN five, H, C, O, and N represent four different families of elements while S is a member of the same family as O. Oxygen and sulfur have similar chemical characteristics and can substitute one for the other in compounds.

29. Oil molecules with double-bonded carbon atoms are called "unsaturated." Oil molecules with only single-bonded carbon atoms are called "saturated."

30. Hydrogenation is a process where the double bonds in an oil molecule are changed into single bonds by the addition of hydrogen atoms.

31. Saturated oils are thicker, more viscous, and often solid at room temperature. Saturated oils are more difficult for our bodies to metabolize and assimilate when ingested.

32. Of the five CHOSN elements that play major roles in life processes, trace amounts of S and N are present in most essential oils, but C, H, and O are the main elements forming the bulk of an oil with C being the most prevalent element by weight and H by quantity of atoms.

33. The chemistry of essential oils consists of simple hydrocarbons, oxygenated hydrocarbons, and their isomers.

♥ CHAPTER FIVE
ORGANIC CHEMISTRY MADE EASY

Organic chemistry was originally defined to be the study of compounds created by life processes. The word, "organic," comes from a Latin root, *organum*, meaning "to organize." Living things take the disorganized and give it form and function. For example, we breathe many kinds of molecules, drink a variety of liquids, eat all manner of foods, taking everything imaginable into our physical vehicles. Yet out of this chaos, our body's innate intelligence can organize this random mixture of molecules into well defined structures and functions—viz. our cells, organs, tissues, and our remarkably synchronized bodily processes.

Natural processes that produce higher levels of organization seem to violate the Second Law of Thermodynamics which states that "natural processes in a closed system will always tend toward greater degrees of disorder." Life, in all of its forms, appears to be an exception to this law. If our bodies were purely mechanical/chemical entities, then they should follow the same scientific laws as the inanimate world. But life processes do not quite follow the same the set of laws as inanimate matter. There are other laws and principles, beyond physics, chemistry, and materiality, that govern living forms and their myriad manifestations. The human body is a self-healing creation.

To appreciate the significance of this fact, consider an inanimate vehicle like an automobile. If a car worked like a human body, you could feed all manner of solids, liquids, and gases into its fuel tank and air filter and the vehicle would sort everything into its proper place—creating lubricating oils where there are bearings, coolant for the radiator, cleaning fluid for the windshield washers, acid for the battery, brake fluid for the brake lines, fuel to the engine, electricity to the headlights, and be able to renew its coat of paint, repair dents and scratches, and maintain all of its other parts on a continuous basis.

By contrast, so long as we are alive, human bodies are self-repairing, self-healing, self-regulating, Divinely endowed vehicles gifted to us for our earthly sojourns. Meanwhile, motor vehicles possess no innate intelligence and no life force, which is the intelligent organizing consciousness within all living things. Automobiles follow the Second Law of Thermodynamics. From the first day they are driven they start disintegrating by the natural processes of normal wear and tear, rust and weather, aging and fatigue. Eventually, they cease to function, unable to be driven any more. When discarded, they slowly decompose back into their elements, losing their form and structure, disbursed into the air, the soil, and the waters of the earth—one molecule after another.

When our spirits depart for the next world, our bodies act the same as the bodies of automobiles. A human body without life obeys the same laws of thermodynamics as any other inanimate object, disintegrating inexorably into nature's elements, returning to formlessness and chaos. "For dust thou art, and unto dust shalt thou return." (Genesis 3:19) But as long as a body is occupied by a living spirit, it rises above the natural laws of chaos, the laws of increasing disorder, the laws of entropy and thermodynamics.

When Does Organic Mean Organic?

While organic chemistry was originally supposed to be the study of the compounds of life, it was not long before scientists came to realize that carbon was the basis of all compounds created by living processes. Hence, today organic chemistry is defined as "the study of carbon compounds." This puts a whole new twist on the field, since today we have thousands of carbon compounds created in laboratories, synthesized outside of the natural processes of living organisms—yet they are called "organic."

Now that scientists call all carbon compounds "organic" regardless of their origin, this poses a terminology problem for the public. For example, all petrochemicals (substances derived from petroleum) are carbon compounds. This means that pesticides, herbicides, fungicides, motor fuels, industrial solvents, pharmaceuticals, paints, disinfectants, cleaning fluids, plastics, styrofoam, and thousands of other products that define modern living can be called "organic" since virtually all of them are composed of carbon-based molecules.

Carbon is the most versatile of all the elements and the only one capable of forming long chains and complex ring structures with itself. Its versatility makes it not only ideal as a building material for innumerable living forms, it is also ideal for innumerable industrial products, as well.

However, this is not what you are thinking when you see the word "organic" on a package label. As a member of the consuming public, you would normally assume that the designation "organic" means the product (or its ingredients) were produced free of herbicides, pesticides, chemical fertilizers, hormones, antibiotics, etc. But to an organic chemist, the term means only that the product contains carbon compounds, most or all of which could be synthetic. To a chemist, the term does not necessarily mean that petrochemicals and/or pharmaceuticals were absent from their production. Fortunately, as of October 2002, the U.S. Federal Government has adopted a law that legally defines the phrase "Certified Organic" to mean what consumers think it should mean.

When Does Natural Mean Natural?

To the public, the term "organic" also implies that the product was grown in healthy soil under sunlight with access to a clean atmosphere—not synthesized indoors in a lab. In other words, a product labeled as "organic" is also assumed to be "natural," which is to say that it was "grown" in some fashion, not engineered in a factory on a chemical assembly line. However, in today's competitive market, even the word "natural" is abused.

The U.S. Federal government permits the word "natural" to be used on a label if the product consists of compounds that can be produced by nature even though the content of that particular product may have been produced entirely in a chemical factory. They equate the product of a natural living plant with that of a human manufacturing plant. (They both come from plants. Right?)

If chemistry completely described the therapeutic and/or nutritional properties of a substance, this might be valid. But it doesn't. There is a vitality and a life force in the compounds produced by living processes that are absent from those produced in a dead environment like a drug lab or a pharmaceutical plant. This is crucially important when it comes to essential oils that are intended to be used for healing.

There are thousands of examples of products labeled as containing "natural" ingredients when, in fact, their tastes are totally manufactured in a lab. One of the most common examples has to do with fruit flavors in drinks, candies, chewable vitamins, and fragrances in shampoos, soaps, and body lotions. Most fruit flavors and fragrances are formed from combinations of esters, a class of chemical compounds found in most essential oils and discussed in Chapter Ten of this book. Thus, the taste of bananas, watermelon, cantaloupe, peach, blueberry, raspberry, apple, orange, lime, papaya, kiwi, and just about any fruit can be imitated by assembling the right esters. Methyl anthranilate is an ester found in minor amounts in many essential oils which is also a natural compound in grapes and cherries. Synthetic methyl anthranilate is frequently used to produce beverages and confections, combined with a little color, and labeled as a "grape" or "cherry" product containing "natural flavorings."

Two compounds with the same chemical formula and molecular structure, one from a laboratory and one created by nature, may be chemically identical, but are therapeutically different. What scientists create and what God creates have different spiritual templates and different subtle energies. Chemical formulas alone do not completely describe a compound. (See Part Three.)

Why Natural Oils Heal and Synthetic Ones Don't

When we use therapeutic grade essential oils they manifest an ability to organize. They can bring healthy order to a confused and sick organ, tissue, or person, dispelling disease and restoring balance to our systems. This organizing power is what the term "organic" originally meant. Order is harmony. Health is harmony. Disorder is disharmony. Sickness is when our bodies or minds are in disharmony or out of resonance with truth. The power to bring order to disorganized systems in our bodies on the part of an essential oil is evidence of the intelligence, vitality, and life force with which the oil was imbued when it was fashioned in the living plant. Just as life processes do not behave according to the law of entropy, which brings disorder, neither do essential oils.

By contrast, such harmonizing powers are absent from oils created synthetically and are greatly reduced in natural oils adulterated with synthetic ingredients or diluted with petrochemicals. Artificial oils follow the natural law of entropy, the law of increasing disorder. That is why they lack the healing powers manifested in pure therapeutic grade essential oils. Let the buyer beware. Study your labels carefully and read between the lines. Know your producer and your supplier. This is especially important in the purchase of therapeutic grade essential oils.

The Simplest Hydrocarbons

We have summarized the chemistry of essential oils at the end of the previous chapter as "simple hydrocarbons, oxygenated hydrocarbons, and their isomers." What is a hydrocarbon? The word reveals its meaning. A hydrocarbon is a compound of just two elements: hydrogen and carbon. Thus, the term "hydro + carbon."

Now don't confuse "hydrocarbon" with "carbohydrate." Hydrate means "water" or H_2O. Carbohydrates are compounds composed of carbon atoms and water molecules. Carbohydrates include sugars, starches, cellulose, and glycogen. For example, the chemical formula for the simple sugars, glucose and fructose, is the same for both—$C_6H_{12}O_6$—which can also be written as $C_6(H_2O)_6$. In the latter form, you can plainly see that glucose and fructose molecules consist of the union of 6 C atoms with 6 molecules of H_2O or water. Thus, the term "carbo + hydrate." There are carbohydrates in some essential oils, but only traces. Carbohydrates are usually water soluble and don't mix well with oil compounds.

The simplest possible hydrocarbon would be to start with one carbon atom and let it team up with as many hydrogen atoms as it chooses to accept. Remember from Chapter Four that C has a valence of 4 while H has a valence of 1. With this information you can predict that given the opportunity each atom of C will grab four H atoms forming CH_4—which is a hydrocarbon called methane, an odiferous gas resulting from the decomposition of vegetable matter, as mentioned in the previous chapter. (See Table Seven, next page.)

The next simplest hydrocarbon would be to start with two atoms of C holding hands together as a team. How many H atoms do you think a pair of carbons could grab and hold on to? If one C holds 4, you might guess two Cs would hold twice as many, or 8. But the answer is 6, not 8. The resulting hydrocarbon formed is C_2H_6—called ethane. The reason for this becomes clear when you draw pictures of the molecules. as seen in Table Seven. You can see by the picture that the two carbons each occupy one of their four hands to hang onto each other. This leaves only three free hands apiece to grab hydrogens, which adds up to six. Ethane is a colorless, odorless gas, one of the compounds found in natural gas. It is narcotic, toxic, and asphyxiating in high concentrations. It is used commercially as a fuel and a refrigerant.

As a young cowboy, Will Rogers (1879–1935), who became a famous humorist and actor, nearly died of ethane poisoning in a San Francisco hotel room when the gas light blew out. Rushed to a hospital not breathing and with no heartbeat the doctors finally gave up their efforts to resuccitate. Turning over what they thought was a dead body to a group of medical students to practice on, the students tried unconventional means and brought him back to life.

The next simplest hydrocarbon would be a chain of three C atoms which can join up with eight atoms of H with a formula like this—C_3H_8. This is propane—a gas commonly used as a fuel to heat homes and small businesses and to run specially adapted cars and trucks.

Next is a chain of four carbons united with ten hydrogens to make butane—C_4H_{10}—a volatile liquid fuel used in lanterns, camping stoves, disposable lighters, and butane torches.

Following the same pattern, we have a hydrocarbon with a five-carbon chain called pentane, one with a six-carbon chain called hexane, one with seven called heptane, and one with eight, we all know, called octane. There is also nonane with nine carbons, decane with ten, etc.

Table Seven
The Alkane Series of Hydrocarbons

CH_4　　Methane

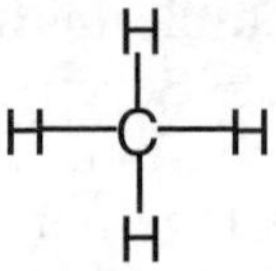

```
      H
      |
  H—C—H
      |
      H
```

C_2H_6　　Ethane

```
   H   H
   |   |
 H—C—C—H
   |   |
   H   H
```

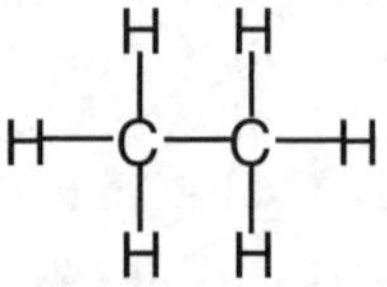

C_3H_8　　Propane

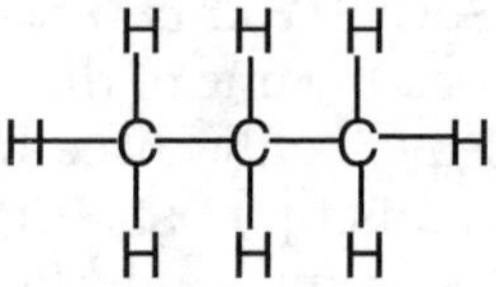

```
   H   H   H
   |   |   |
 H—C—C—C—H
   |   |   |
   H   H   H
```

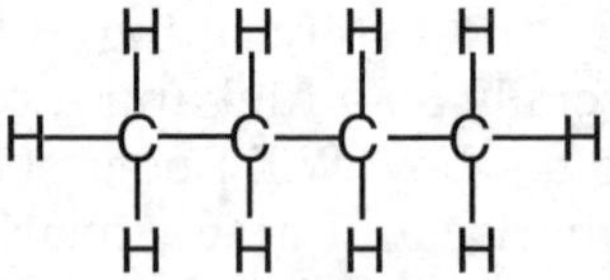

C_4H_{10}　　Butane

```
   H   H   H   H
   |   |   |   |
 H—C—C—C—C—H
   |   |   |   |
   H   H   H   H
```

C_5H_{12}　　Pentane

```
   H   H   H   H   H
   |   |   |   |   |
 H—C—C—C—C—C—H
   |   |   |   |   |
   H   H   H   H   H
```

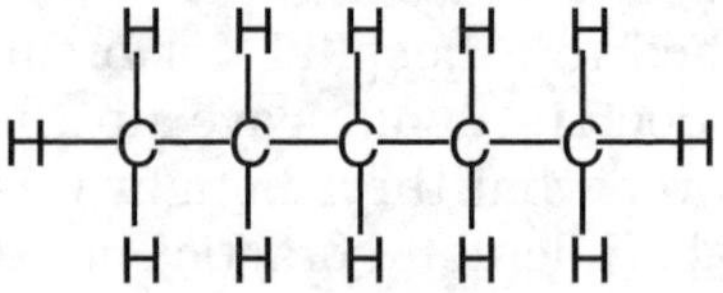

C_6H_{14}　　Hexane　　　(a six carbon chain . . .)

C_7H_{16}　　Heptane　　(a seven carbon chain . . .)

C_8H_{18}　　Octane　　　(an eight carbon chain . . .)

Nonane, Decane, Undecane, Dodecane, Tridecane, Tetradecane, Pentadecane, etc....

C_nH_{2n+2}　　General Alkane Formula *

* Take the number of carbon atoms (n), multiply by 2 and add 2, (2n+2) to get the number of hydrogen atoms in a molecule of an alkane. The names of all alkane hydrocarbons end in -ane.

Octane (C_8H_{18}) is the main ingredient in gasoline. When you go to the gas pump, you see grades like 87, 89, or 93. This means that that particular grade of fuel is approximately 87%, 89% or 93% octane with other compounds making up the difference. These other compounds include other alkanes like pentane, hexane, heptane, or nonane, which do not burn in your engine as well as octane. Gasoline also contains small amounts of benzene, xylene, and toluene—all very toxic substances. Gasoline is not a single compound. It is a mixture.

Kerosene is also not a compound, but a mixture of alkane hydrocarbons with formulas from $C_{12}H_{26}$ to $C_{15}H_{32,}$ (from dodecane to pentadecane). The molecules that make kerosene are heavier and larger than those in gasoline. Hence, kerosene is not as volatile as gasoline, and not as explosive, hence, safe enough to burn in household lamps.

All of these compounds are members of the alkane family of hydrocarbons. They all start with a chain of carbons holding hands who then take on as many hydrogens as they can with their remaining free hands. The limit of the number of carbons that can make such a chain is not known. Beside pentadecane (15 C chain) mentioned in Table Seven, there is every possibility up to icosane (20 C chain), pentacontane (50 C chain), hectane (100 C chain) and beyond.

Notice that all members of the Alkane family have names ending in "-ane." When you see the name of a compound, even one you never heard of before, if its official name ends in -ane, you know it is probably an alkane. If you know the meaning of the Latin or Greek prefix (pent-, hex-, hep- oct-, etc.) then you will know its formula just from the name. Whenever possible, the names given to organic compounds are designed to reveal their formulas.

International Union of Pure and Applied Chemistry

The business of naming compounds has been delegated to the IUPAC (International Union of Pure and Applied Chemistry). Their conventions are called "The IUPAC Rules." By following IUPAC guidelines, if you develop or discover an entirely new organic compound with no name, you can follow the IUPAC rules and give it a name that reveals its composition and its relationship to other compounds. Understanding and applying IUPAC rules makes the study and understanding of organic chemistry much easier. In fact, since there are literally millions of known organic compounds, without a logical system of nomenclature, it would be an unmanageable body of information. We will make use of these rules throughout this book.

The Family Formula for an Alkane

The composition of all alkanes fit a pattern given by a mathematical formula C_nH_{2n+2}. What the formula says is that for an alkane, if you take the number of carbons (represented by n), multiply by 2, and then add 2, you will get the number of hydrogens.

Let's give this scheme a test. The first alkane, methane, has one carbon. In other words, n=1. If we apply the formula, 2n+2, we get 2 x 1 + 2 = 2 + 2 = 4. This results indicates that the single C atom in a molecule of methane should be bonded with 4 atoms of H, which it is.

Let's give it another test. There are 3 carbons in propane. In this case, n=3. When we apply the formula, 2n+2, we get 2 x 3 + 2 = 6 + 2 = 8. Hence, the 3-carbon chain in propane should have 8 hydrogens, which it does.

Try the formula with pentane, hexane, heptane, and octane. You will find the formula is always true for any alkane. Try this one just for the heck of it: How many hydrogens does a hectane molecule have (hectane has a 100 C chain)? What is 2 x 100 + 2 ?

Oil and Water Don't Mix

Alkanes do not dissolve or mix with water. In fact, no hydrocarbon dissolves or mixes with water. This is a universal property of hydrocarbons.

The physical state of an alkane at room temperatures depends on its molecular weight. The first one, methane, has 1 C and 4 H atoms. The molecular weight of carbon is 12 and that of hydrogen 1. Hence, 12 + 4 = 16, which is a very small molecule. Methane is a gas at normal temperatures, and a very smelly one, too.

The first three alkanes are all gases: methane, ethane, and propane. Butane is a liquid at room temperature. Its molecules have 4 C and 10 H atoms and its molecular weight is 4 x 12 + 10 = 58, which is still a pretty small molecule. Butane is cigarrett lighter fluid, volatile and highly flammable liquid. Pentane is also a liquid, as is hexane, heptane, nonane, and octane. In fact, the alkanes are all liquids from butane through henicosane, $C_{21}H_{44}$, Henicosane, a viscous oil, has a molecular weight of $21 \times 12 + 44 = 296$. In this range of alkanes, from C_4 to C_{21}, we find gasoline, kerosene, diesel fuel, furnace fuel, and various lubricants.

Docosane ($C_{22}H_{46}$) is the next alkane after henicosane, and has an atomic weight of 310. Docosane through pentatriacontane ($C_{35}H_{72}$) are waxy solids, including paraffins from which candles are made. Beyond pentacontane you get the heavy compounds that make up tars, asphalts and thick gooey roofing compounds.

Tje first eight alkanes (methane through octane) are all high energy fuels. Octane, C_8H_{18}, the principal compound of gasoline, has an atomic weight of only 114, smaller than a phenylpropanoid or a monoterpene. Hydrocarbon molecules less than 500 amu can pass through human skin and the blood-brain barrier. What do you think happens when you wash your hands in gasoline or breathe its fumes?

Do Essential Oils Contain Alkanes?

The answer to the question in the subheading above is "yes, but not much." There are small amounts of methane ethane or propane in some oils, but not much. Undecane ($C_{11}H_{24}$), dodecane ($C_{12}H_{26}$), and hexadecane ($C_{16}H_{34}$) can be found in ginger oil (*Zingiber officinale*), but not much. The aromatic oil containing the most alkanes is rose, which we will discuss in the next section.

There are several alkane alcohols in essential oils like decanol ($C_{10}H_{22}O$), nonanol ($C_9H_{20}O$), octanol ($C_8H_{18}O$), heptanol ($C_7H_{16}O$), and hexanol ($C_6H_{14}O$) in lemon oil and butanol ($C_4H_{10}O$) in ginger. There are also several alkane aldehydes in essential oils like octanal ($C_8H_{16}O$) in rose, lavender, and citrus oils, decanal ($C_{10}H_{20}O$) in coriander, lemongrass, and mandarin oils, and hexanal ($C_7H_{14}O$) in clary sage. However, except for traces, alkanes hydrocarbons are not found in the vast majority of essential oils.

Alkanes occur frequently throughout nature. Beeswax,

for example, is a mixture of heavy alkanes, but beeswax is not an aromatic oil. Many fruits, like apples, pears, plums, and oranges have a waxy coating to prevent the loss of water, as do many leaves. This natural wax is composed of larger alkane molecules with chains of 28 C atoms and more. Tobacco leaves contain an alkane wax, called triacontane ($C_{30}H_{62}$), with a molecular weight of 422. (See p. 288.) But these molecules are too big to easily pass through the distillation process. They are generally not found in essential oils. So why are we studying the alkane family?

General chemistry books usually end with an introductory chapter on organic chemistry and a discussion of alkanes— the simplest of hydrocarbons. Organic chemistry books usually begin with a discussion of alkanes, since they are the easiest to comprehend. Through the alkanes you can begin to appreciate the possibilities provided by carbon atoms by their unique ability to link up with each other to create molecules of all sizes and shapes and how essential oils can contain hundreds of different compounds from only two or three elements. Understanding alkanes and their myriad structural variations will also help you to understand how and why synthetic organic compounds are not the same as natural ones. The names of alkanes also introduce us to certain prefixes used throughout organic chemistry such as "methyl," "ethyl," "propyl," and "butyl." (See pp. 153-155.)

Rose's Affair with the Alkane Family

Rose oil (*Rosa damascena*) is unusual in many ways and contains the highest known concentration of alkanes in an essential oil. Rose oil can be up to 19% alkanes while all other aromatic oils contain less than 1% (See Table 37.) The oil of rose petals contains at least ten different alkanes ranging from C_{18} to C_{25}. They are as follows: 0.2% octadecane ($C_{18}H_{38}$), 10% nonadecane ($C_{19}H_{40}$), 1.0% icosane ($C_{20}H_{42}$), 0.4% henicosane ($C_{21}H_{44}$), 0.3% docosane ($C_{22}H_{46}$), 0.8% tricosane ($C_{23}H_{48}$), 0.2% tetracosane ($C_{24}H_{50}$), and 0.4% pentacosane ($C_{25}H_{52}$). These compounds range in molecular weight from 254 to 352, which are heavier than many essential oil molecules, making them less volatile. In fact, several of these are paraffins and waxes, not because they are so heavy, but because of their long molecular shapes. The sizes and weights of these molecules provide long-lasting qualities to the fragrance and therapeutic action of the oil. Rose oil also contains traces of decanol ($C_{10}H_{22}O$) and nonanol ($C_9H_{20}O$)—both alkane alcohols, M.W. = 158 and 144, respectively, weights that would be volatile and aromatic. Altogether, alkanes average about 11% of a typical rose oil. This may not sound like much, but as discussed in Chapter Four concerning grapefruit oil, even trace amounts of some compounds can have a significant influence on an oil's fragrance and action. However, 11% is no trace amount. Any concentration over 1% is considered a major ingredient. If you have ever felt a rose petal, it feels waxy, velvety and smooth. Those are alkanes. You will also note a waxy background in the scent of a rose bloom as well as in rose oil. Those are the fragrances of volatile alkanes.

Rose is unique among etheric oils in many ways. It is the only essential oil with this many kinds and quantities of alkanes. Rose notes are the foundation of many fine fragrances, such as Chanel No. 5®, Paris®, and Eternity®. Rose oil has the highest known electromagnetic frequency (320 MHz) of any natural substance. Its spiritual and healing qualities have been recognized and applied for thousands of years. One wonders to what extent rose's affair with the alkane family determines its unusual and highly prized properties.

Meet Methyl, Ethyl, Propyl, and Butyl

Methyl: CH_4 represents a molecule of methane, balanced and complete, with one carbon holding 4 H atoms. Take one hydrogen away and you get CH_3 —a partial molecule, unbalanced and incomplete with a hungry hand ready to grab something. (See cartoon on the next page) This is the ubiquitous "methyl radical." Radicals are incomplete molecules looking for something to which to attach themselves in order to satisfy their unfulfilled appetites. When a molecule has a CH_3 radical incorporated into itself, the scientific name of that compound will include "methyl." Even though she is a radical, Methyl must be very attractive because she has been invited to participate in hundreds of thousands of compounds. Anytime you read of a compound with "methyl" in its name (like methyl salicylate or methyl chavicol) you know that there is a methyl radical integrated into that molecule. If there are two, then "dimethyl" will be in the name. If three, then "trimethyl," etc.

Whenever you see "methyl" in a name, know there is a single C atom bonded with three H atoms that is part of that molecule. (Sometimes there may only be two H atoms, but it is still called "methyl.") When you see "methyl," think "one carbon."

Methane	Methyl
Molecule	Radical
CH_4	CH_3
◀◀	▶▶

Ethyl: C_2H_6 represents a molecule of ethane, balanced and complete, based on a two-carbon chain saturated with 6 H atoms. Take away one hydrogen and you get C_2H_5 — a partial molecule, unbalanced and incomplete. This is the famous "ethyl radical." When a molecule has a C_2H_5 radical incorporated into itself, the scientific name of that compound will include "ethyl."

Even though she, too, is a radical, Ethyl is very popular. She (like her sister Methyl) has also been invited to participate in hundreds of thousands of compounds. Anytime you read of a compound with "ethyl" in its name (like ethyl alcohol) you know that there is an ethyl radical integrated into that molecule. If there are two ethyl radicals attached, then "diethyl" will be in the name, like diethyl ether (p. 161). If three, then you will find "triethyl," etc. Tetraethyl lead molecules ($C_8H_{20}Pb$) are lead atoms (Pb), with four attached ethyl radicals (C_2H_5). Years ago it was put in gasoline (called "ethyl" or leaded gas) to improve performance and increase engine life until it was found to be a Class B Poison. It is now illegal as a gas additive. If there are many ethyls in a formula, then you see the name "polyethyl." There is a very useful and extremely large molecule called "polyethylene" from which we make film, clear plastic, various containers, and insulation.

So remember, whenever you see "ethyl" in a name, you know there are two C atoms, usually coupled with five H atoms, as part of that molecule. (Sometimes there may be less than four H atoms, but the radical is still called "ethyl.") When you see "ethyl," think "two-carbon chain."

Propyl: C_3H_8 represents a molecule of propane, based on a three-carbon chain saturated with 8 H atoms. Take away one hydrogen and you get C_3H_7 —a partial molecule. This is the "propyl radical," also a popular unit found in thousands of molecules. When a molecule has a C_3H_7 radical incorporated into itself, the scientific name of that compound will include "propyl."

So anytime you read of a compound with "propyl" in its name (like propylene glycol), you know there are three C atoms bonded with several H atoms that are part of that molecule. If there are two propyl radicals attached, then "dipropyl" will be in the name. If three, then "tripropyl," etc. Compounds containing propyl radicals in their formulas are sometimes referred to as "propanoids."

So remember, whenever you see "propyl" in a name, you know there are three C atoms, usually joined with seven H atoms, as part of that molecule. (Sometimes there may less than seven H atoms, but the radical is still called "propyl.") When you see "propyl," think "three-carbon chain."

Butyl: C_4H_{10} represents a molecule of butane, based on a four-carbon chain saturated with 10 H atoms. Take away one hydrogen and you get C_4H_9 —a partial molecule. This is the "butyl radical." She must be radically beautiful since she is a sought-after partner in thousands of compounds. When a molecule has a C_4H_9 radical incorporated into itself, the scientific name of that compound will include "butyl."

So anytime you read of a compound with "butyl" in its name (like butyl rubber) or methylbutyldiene (p. 255), you know there are four C atoms bonded with several H atoms as part of that molecule. If there are two butyl radicals, then "dibutyl" will be in the name. If three, then "tributyl, " etc.

So remember, whenever you see "butyl" in a name, you know there are four C atoms, usually joined with nine H atoms, as part of that molecule. (Sometimes there may be less than nine H atoms, but the radical is still called "Butyl.") When you see "butyl," think "four-carbon chain."

Now you have met Methyl, Ethyl, Propyl, and Butyl—the radical sisters. These names will be used throughout the rest of this book. Now you know what these names mean.

Oxygenated Hydrocarbons

We have summarized the chemistry of essential oils as simple hydrocarbons, oxygenated hydrocarbons, and their isomers. What is an oxygenated hydrocarbon? The word reveals its meaning. An oxygenated hydrocarbon is a compound of three elements: hydrogen and carbon (which make a hydrocarbon) with one or more oxygen atoms attached.

The alkane series is a perfect set of hydrocarbons by which to illustrate the process of oxygenation. Oxygenation creates new compounds with entirely different chemical and physical properties.

Table Eight on the next page takes the first four hydrocarbons in Table Seven and shows them as oxygenated hydrocarbons. What we have done is to insert an oxygen atom between the carbon and hydrogen on the right end of the methane, ethane, propane, and butane molecules as shown in Table Seven. This will work because the valence of oxygen is 2. In this arrangement, one arm of the O clings to the C on one side while the other arm holds onto the H on the other. The C attached to the O still has its 4 arms occupied, H has its 1 arm engaged, and O has its 2 hands full. All valence requirements are met. Everyone is satisfied. This is a happy molecule. But what a difference adding one oxygen atom makes!

Note that in the molecular diagrams of methanol and ethanol shown on the opposite page, the bond between O and H is represented as a fine line connecting the two to show the bond between them, but this is not normal notation. The O and the H are usually depicted simply as OH, as shown for propanol and butanol.

You can think of OH, by itself, as a water molecule (H_2O) that has lost a hydrogen. OH is thus seen as a partial molecule. Therefore it is a radical. It is called the "hydroxyl radical." The hydroxyl radical is a very popular fellow, indeed, and a rascal as well. He is found in literally billions

	Table Eight			
	Alkane Alcohols			
CH_4O	Methanol	H—C—O—H (with H above and H below the C)		Methyl Alcohol
C_2H_6O	Ethanol	H—C—C—O—H (with H above and below each C)		Ethyl Alcohol
C_3H_8O	Propanol	H—C—C—C—OH (with H above and below each C)		Propyl Alcohol
$C_4H_{10}O$	Butanol	H—C—C—C—C—OH (with H above and below each C)		Butyl Alcohol

and billions of compounds and whenever he is there, he can them into alcoholics.

The Alkanes Become a Family of Alcoholics

Notice what happened when the alkanes (methane, ethane, and propane) were oxygenated by an OH on one end, as seen in Table Eight. They all used to be flammable gases. Now they are alcoholic liquids. Any hydrocarbon with a hydroxyl radical (OH) is classified as an alcohol. Notice also that their names no longer end in -ane, as they did before oxygenation. They now all end in -ol. These are the IUPAC rules for alcohols. There are countless varieties of alcohols. The four diagrammed in Table Eight are the simplest and lightest.

Alcohols are quite different from alkanes. While alkanes do not mix with water, these four alcohols easily mix with water in all proportions. They also dissolve oils. Most perfumes containing essential oils are over 90% ethyl alcohol. Some of the heavier alkane alcohols (such as hexanol, heptanol, octanol, nonanol, and decanol) are oily in nature, do not mix with water, and naturally occur in essential oils in small amounts. As for methanol, ethanol, and propanol, none of them are found in essential oils except when oils are diluted or adulterated for commercial purposes.

Methyl alcohol (or methanol) is also known as "wood alcohol" because it can be produced from wood chips. It is highly toxic. During the days of Prohibition in the U.S., during the 1920s, the corn whiskey made by bootleggers (owners of illegal distilleries) sometimes produced spirits contaminated with wood alcohol. Those who unwittingly drank the tainted liquor either died or went blind. Methyl alcohol is also produced in our bodies when we ingest aspartame (Nutrasweet®), which has resulted in vision problems for some. Think of methyl alcohol as a marriage between two radicals—methyl and hydroxyl.

Ethyl alcohol (or ethanol) is also known as "grain alcohol" because it can be distilled from grain. Ethyl alcohol is what makes beer, wine, whiskey, and other alcoholic beverages alcoholic. While not toxic in the usual sense, it is inebriating and is certainly considered a toxin by our livers. Ethanol comprises the greater portion of perfumes in which fragrant oil compounds have been dissolved. Ethanol may also be familiar to you as a fuel extender blended with gasoline. Think of ethyl alcohol as a marriage between two radicals—ethyl and hydroxyl.

Propyl alcohol (or propanol) is a marriage between the two radicals—propyl and hydroxyl. This alcohol may sound familiar to you, but is it? We will discuss this in the next section under isomers.

Butyl alcohol (or butanol) is a clear, toxic liquid. It is an industrial solvent and paint remover—employed for many purposes. Think of butyl alcohol as a marriage between the two radicals—butyl and hydroxyl. Butyl alcohol occurs in concentrations up to 1% in ginger oil (*Zingiber officinale*). Butanol, by itself, is harmful to humans. It can cause headaches, blurred vision, dermatitis, auditory nerve damage, and hearing loss. But as a constituent in ginger oil, under the quenching influ-

Isopropyl
Alcohol

$$H-\underset{\underset{H}{|}}{\overset{\overset{H}{|}}{C}}-\underset{\underset{OH}{|}}{\overset{\overset{H}{|}}{C}}-\underset{\underset{H}{|}}{\overset{\overset{H}{|}}{C}}-H \qquad C_3H_8O$$

ence of sesquiterpenes and monoterpenes, it becomes harmless and therapeutic.

Isomers

As stated before, <u>the chemistry of essential oils consists of hydrocarbons, oxygenated hydrocarbons, and their isomers</u>. What is an isomer? If you know some Greek, the word, itself, reveals its meaning. The word "isomer" comes from *isos*, meaning "equal" or "the same" and *meros*, meaning "parts." In other words, isomers are molecules with the "same parts" (same atoms) but different configurations (arrangements of the atoms). That is to say, isomers are compounds with the same chemical formula, but with differently structured molecules.

Now let's go back to propyl alcohol. The name sounds familiar because you have probably used rubbing alcohol, which is isopropyl alcohol. Go back and look at the molecular diagram of propyl alcohol in Table Eight. We have attached the OH to a carbon at one end of the molecule. What if we attached it to the middle carbon instead, as shown at the top of this page?

Propyl alcohol and isopropyl alcohol are isomers. They have the same formula (C_3H_8O). Both have "propyl" in their names, indicating that both contain a C_3H_7 radical. But they aren't the same shape. And they aren't the same in physical or chemical characteristics either.

Dangers of Diluted Oils

Compared to propyl alcohol, rubbing alcohol has superior cleansing properties and is safer and less toxic. While they are both liquids and both have the same molecular weight (60 amu), isopropyl or rubbing alcohol is less dense, has a lower boiling point, and has a stronger smell than propyl alcohol (which is almost odorless).

By comparison, propyl alcohol has a lower flash point and is more flammable. Propyl alcohol is also a suspected carcinogen while isopropyl alcohol is not. The flashiness and flammability of propyl alcohol has created a serious hazard in some countries (like Taiwan) where essential oils are often diluted up to 90% in propyl alcohol and sold as if they were pure essential oils.

Many people don't know the difference between a pure essential oil and a diluted one. A number of people have been severely burned when propanol tinctures of essential oils are put on hot light bulbs, in shallow dishes over a candle, or in an oil lamp. Because so many people have been seriously burned, some Taiwanese officials are pushing for a national ban on essential oils in their country, not realizing that the problem is not with the oils but with the adulterating alcohol.

The terms, propyl and isopropyl alcohol, are considered quasi-scientific names, more for the public than for scientists, although scientists use them. According to IUPAC rules, the official scientific names for these two alcohols are 1-propanol and 2-propanol. 1-propanol is also called n-propyl alcohol where the "n" means the "normal" or first isomer. The name "1-propanol" (propyl alcohol) indicates that the OH is attached to a #1 carbon (one of the carbons on either end). The name "2-propanol" (isopropyl alcohol) indicates that the OH is attached to the #2 carbon (the middle carbon). In technical terminology, the prefix, "iso," in a compound name implies that a radical or functional group is attached to the middle of the molecule. You can see from the previous structural diagram that this is so with isopropyl alcohol.

There are only three isomers of propanol and none for methanol or ethanol, both of which can be structured in only one configuration.

The First Anesthetic

While the two isomers of propanol are different, they are also somewhat similar. With butanol, $C_4H_{10}O$, we can gain a fuller appreciation of how extreme the differences can be

Diethyl
Ether

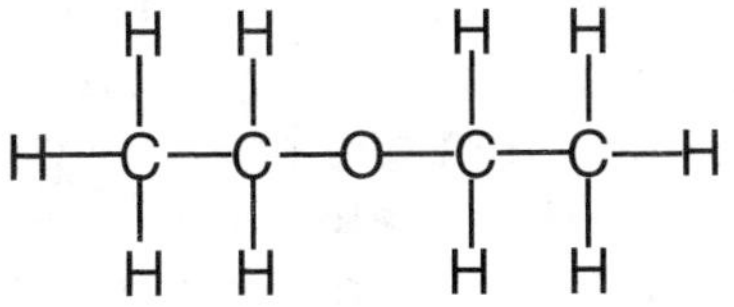

$$H-\overset{\overset{\displaystyle H}{|}}{\underset{\underset{\displaystyle H}{|}}{C}}-\overset{\overset{\displaystyle H}{|}}{\underset{\underset{\displaystyle H}{|}}{C}}-O-\overset{\overset{\displaystyle H}{|}}{\underset{\underset{\displaystyle H}{|}}{C}}-\overset{\overset{\displaystyle H}{|}}{\underset{\underset{\displaystyle H}{|}}{C}}-H$$

$C_4H_{10}O$

between isomers of the same compound.

Given in Table Eight we have what is called 1-butanol or n-butyl alcohol. This is considered to be the "normal" isomer with the OH attached at one end. Instead of the end of the last C, as it is shown in the table, you can also arrange the OH on the bottom or top of the same carbon. This is called 2-butanol. Or you can move the OH to one of the middle carbons and get 3-butanol. This makes three isomers of butanol, all alcohols. But there is another isomer of $C_4H_{10}O$ and it is not an alcohol.

Oxygenating an alkane does not always make it into an alcohol. Only when the O atom is inserted between an H atom and a C atom do you get an alcohol—as was done in 1-, 2-, and 3-butanol and in all the examples of Table Eight,

What if we inserted an oxygen between the two middle C atoms of butane? That would work. All the valences would be satisfied. We'd still have the same formula as all the other butyl alcohols, viz. $C_4H_{10}O$, but we wouldn't have the O connected to an H atom. There would be no OH radical anywhere. Instead, the O would be connected to two carbons. It would look like the model shown above. What we have now is an O atom between two hydrocarbons each with the formula C_2H_5. If you refer back to the section on ethyl a few pages back, you see that C_2H_5 is an incomplete molecule of ethane. It is the "ethyl radical." We have two of them here with an O atom in the middle.

This compound might be called "isobutanol" or "isobutyl alcohol," indicating that butane has been oxygenated in the middle of the molecule. But this name is misleading because this compound is not an alcohol, even though it has the same formula as the three butyl alcohols previously mentioned.

When you have two hydrocarbon groups with an oxygen in between connecting the two, you have a class of compounds called "ethers," not alcohols. By placing an O atom between the two middle C atoms, as we have above, we have divided butane (C_4H_{10}) into two ethyl radicals (C_2H_5). We don't have a "butyl" compound any more. We have a double "ethyl." Its proper name is "diethyl ether." "Diethyl" means literally, "two ethyl radicals," while "ether" means "two hydrocarbons joined by an O atom." We will study more about ethers in Chapter Ten. The properties of ethers are very different than those of alcohols.

Butyl alcohol was described briefly a few pages back as a clear, toxic solvent. The isomers, 1-, 2-, and 3-butanol, are all clear, toxic solvents with isomeric differences, but similarities as well. But diethyl ether is not similar. This is the famous anesthetic called "ether" that has been used by medical doctors since the late 1700s. It became famous when Queen Victoria of England (1837-1901) was the first to use it as an inhalation anesthetic for childbirth in the 1850s. It is no longer used as an obstetric anesthetic because it is dangerously depressing to the baby and because storing ether in emergency rooms is an explosion hazard. Instead of an anesthetic, it is currently available in aerosol cans as a starter fluid for gasoline engines available in most hardware, farm supply, and automotive stores.

So you can see how drastically the properties of a compound can change from one isomer to another even though they all have the same formula, but different structural arrangements. The isomers of a given formula can differ so much that they don't even belong to the same chemical families, as in the example of butanol and ether.

This is a crucial point in understanding essential oils and especially in understanding the differences between natural compounds and synthetic ones. Nature produces only certain isomers which, in laboratories, often cannot be reproduced. Laboratories can produce compounds with the same chemical formulas as natural ones, but usually not as the same isomers. Essential oils with synthetic components are never the same as those produced by nature for several reasons. A major part of why labs cannot replicate nature has to do with isomers. Plants, under God's supervision, are capable of feats of chemical synthesis no human can match in even the most sophisticated of scientific facilities.

Shortening the Shorthand

In Tables Seven and Eight, and in the structural diagrams of isopropyl alcohol and diethyl ether in the previous pages, the H and C atoms are explicitly shown. While it is useful to represent hydrocarbons this way for some purposes, drawing in all the little C and H symbols is cumbersome and unnecessary most of the time. Organic chemists have developed a shorthand for representing linear carbon chains that makes them much easier to draw yet still conveys the same information. (See Table Nine on the next page.)

The shorthand is this. Scientists simply draw a zig-zag line of sawteeth stipulating that at each angle and at the end of each line is a carbon (not shown). Thus, it is easy to count the C atoms and identify their locations by simply counting the sawteeth points and the two ends of the jagged line.

As for the H atoms, we apply the fact that every carbon requires the filling of four bonds since its valence is 4. To deduce the number and locations of H atoms, simply count the bonds visibly converging at each carbon location and subtract from 4 to get the number of hydrogens that must be there to satisfy the valence requirements. At each sawtooth point where a C atom is located, there are two bonds converging from each side of that location so there must be 4 - 2 = 2 H atoms invisibly present. Likewise, at the end of each line where a C atom resides, there is only one bond from one side at that location so there must be 4 - 1 = 3 H atoms invisibly present.

This scheme works only when you have at least three carbons in a chain. Hence, you cannot represent methane or ethane this way, but you can represent propane and all of the rest of the alkanes. For methane and ethane, scientists draw molecular models like those in Table Seven.

Table Nine
The Alkane Series in Structural Shorthand

C_3H_8	Propane	
C_4H_{10}	Butane	
C_5H_{12}	Pentane	
C_6H_{14}	Hexane	
C_7H_{16}	Heptane	
C_8H_{18}	Octane	
C_9H_{20}	Nonane	
$C_{10}H_{22}$	Decane	

Study Table Nine and see if you can tell how it contains the same structural information as Table Seven from propane to pentane, but this time the molecules are depicted without explicitly writing in the Cs and Hs. Because this method of representing carbon chains take so much less space, Table Nine is also able to show some additional molecular models for hexane to decane, not found in Table Seven. We will be using this manner of representing structural formulas throughout the rest of this book.

Playing with Legos®

Because they are very small molecules, there are only two isomers of propanol and none of methanol or ethanol. The larger the molecule the more atoms it contains and the more possibilities exist for isomers. Think of it this way. Legos® are popular, colorful, interlocking children's building blocks. If I provided each person in a group with an identical set of say, 3 blue, 5 yellow, and 8 red Legos®, and asked them each to build something (without looking at anyone else's work), would any two persons build the same exact thing? No, they would not. They would all be working with the same formula (i.e. 5 yellow (Y), 8 red (R), 3 blue (B)—16 total) which in chemical notation could be written $Y_5R_8B_3$. Yet, even in a group of, say, 100 people, the odds are overwhelming that no two would be exactly alike.

In fact, in this simple example of only 16 Legos® in three colors, there are an unbelievable number of possibilities: 20,922,789,888,000 to be exact. That is more than 20 trillion! Now you can understand why children can play with Legos for hours and days without ever getting tired of them. The playtime possibilities are endless.

Now let's explore the possibilities of organic molecules constructed from atoms, which are God's Legos®. You may think of the yellow, red, and blue Legos as representative of carbon, hydrogen and oxygen atoms, respectively.

Isomers Without End

We have depicted the alkanes in Table Seven as linear chains. For the first three—methane, ethane, and propane —the configurations shown in Table Seven are the only ones possible. There are no isomers of these alkanes.

With butane (C_4H_{10}), however, there are two possibilities or two isomers—butane and isobutane—where the first is a long molecule and the second forms of a cross.

There are 3 isomers for pentane (C_5H_{12}), 5 for hexane (C_6H_{14}), 9 for heptane (C_7H_{16}), 18 for octane (C_8H_{18}), 35 for nonane (C_9H_{20}), 75 for decane ($C_{10}H_{22}$), 4,347 for pentadecane ($C_{15}H_{32}$), 366,319 for icosane ($C_{20}H_{42}$), and a whopping 62,491,178,805,831 isomers for tetracontane ($C_{40}H_{82}$).

That's over 62 trillion possibilities for one compound and there are alkanes of higher orders and large molecules of other families with even greater numbers of isomers.

Now you can see how God can create life with all of its infinite variations and inscrutable complexities from only a few elements, mainly carbon, with the help of hydrogen, oxygen, nitrogen, sulfur, and a few others. But the key is carbon.

An Element of Love

God said, "Let us make humankind in our image, according to our likeness." (Genesis 1:26) God must have had lots of fun playing with the chosen Legos® of his creation—the atoms of carbon, hydrogen, oxygen, sulfur, and nitrogen that comprise his countless life forms, giving unique personalities to each of his creatures, no two exactly alike, each imbued with a special image of himself, a spark of his own divinity. God must love his work and he must love his creation just as much. "And God saw everything that he had made, and, indeed, it was very good." (Genesis 1:31)

In Romans 1:20 we read, "Ever since the creation of the world, God's eternal power and divine nature, invisible though they are, have been understood through the things he has made." God chose carbon as his basic building block for the living forms he has made while essential Oils are 70-80% carbon. Invisible though they are, you can gain a glimpse of God's nature through atoms of carbon.

Carbon is the most versatile of all the elements, capable of forming more compounds of more variety than any other. Even in its elemental state, carbon exists in at least three very different forms: (1) There is diamond (the hardest substance known and one of the most precious), (2) There is lampblack (an amorphous, formless black dust with many practical uses, including a base for black ink). And (3) There is graphite (that wonderful writing material in pencils we call "lead"). Carbon has long been a facilitator of expressions of love as the gem stone of choice in lover's rings, as the inks of printed poetry, and as the penciled lines of hand-written letters of affection.

Carbon is the most useful, humble, and loving of all the elements, willing to accept and embrace virtually every other element as friend and partner—participating in compounds without limit. Always willing to take a back seat, carbon is willing to provide the support structure by which other more active atoms can do their work.

Carbon is willing to take on whatever roles are necessary to maintain life in whatever organisms it happens to serve at any given time. It is willing to contribute to any vital task—from metabolism, assimilation, circulation, and motor activity, to reproduction and respiration. Neither is carbon too good to participate in lowly janitorial duties of clean up, detoxification, and disposal of waste.

All of our hormones, enzymes, proteins, tissues, our blood, our lymph, our sweat, our tears, and even the DNA, itself, are composed of carbon compounds. Carbon compounds are part of every human process expressed through the body—including our mental, spiritual, and emotional activities.

Of the elements that compose God's healing oils, carbon is by far the main ingredient. In fact, by weight, 70-80% of every essential oil is carbon. The miraculous properties of volatile oils are, to a major extent, due to the properties of carbon.

Carbon dust has no form and is not considered a thing of beauty or value, but rather something to be rejected and swept away, like the unwanted soot in a chimney. And yet, lowly carbon is the best absorber of toxic chemicals, heavy metals, allergens, and pathogenic microbes known. Activated carbon is used as a filter in many air and water systems and is a prime antidote for many poisons. Overdoses of many pharmaceutical drugs can be neutralized by oral administration of activated carbon. Poultices of carbon ashes have been applied in many cultures for many centuries to withdraw the venom of insect, snake, and spider bites.

The peoples of the *Bible* used ashes, often accompanied by fasting, in many purification rituals to cleanse themselves from physical, emotional, and spiritual toxins. When Job was afflicted with boils, he "sat down among the

ashes," which was an ancient way to treat boils and to alleviate, absorb, and eliminate wastes from the body. (Job
2:7-8) Chewing on a blackened burnt stick is an old fashioned way to mitigate the pain of a toothache while swallowing powdered wood ashes with water has long been a
folk treatment for nausea or diarrhea from food poisoning
or the flu. Activated charcoal is available in tablet form for
oral administration in most drug and health food stores.

Thus, humble carbon has always been willing to take
the sins of the world upon itself as a willing sacrifice in
order to save us from our iniquities, alleviate our pains,
and shield us from the harm that could befall us from the
pollutants we encounter. In Isaiah 53:2-5 we read: "He has
no form or comeliness; and when we shall see him there is
no beauty that we should desire him. He is despised and
rejected...and we esteemed him not. Surely he has borne
our griefs, and carried our sorrows...He was wounded for
our transgressions, he was bruised for our iniquities: the
chastisement of our peace was upon him; and with his
stripes we are healed."

The essential role that carbon plays in creating and
maintaining life is all the more remarkable when you realize that carbon is not among the most abundant substances on earth. In fact, it is not even listed in the top ten
elements. (See Table Four.)

In I Corinthians 13:4-7 we read, "Love is patient; love is
kind; love is not envious or boastful or arrogant or rude. It
does not insist on its own way; it is not irritable or resent-
ful; it does not rejoice in wrongdoing, but rejoices in the
truth. Love bears all things, believes all things, hopes all
things, endures all things." You could almost replace the
word "love" with "carbon" in this scripture and it would
still be true.

God selected carbon as his fundamental atom for creating all forms of life, including our human hearts, brains,
and bodies. Carbon is the principal primordial dust from
which our physical forms were created as stated in
Genesis 2:7: "God formed man from the dust of the
ground."

According to Romans 1:20, God's nature can be seen and understood through the things he has made. The harmony and love of God seems to be expressed in the qualities manifested in the humble atoms of carbon. God's omnipresence is conscious in those atoms. According to I John 4:16, "God is love, and those who abide in love abide in God, and God abides in them." The more fully we grasp the nature of carbon the more fully we grasp the nature of God.

Key Points of Chapter Five

1. Organic chemistry was originally defined as "the study of compounds created by life processes."

2. The root meaning of "organic" is "that which can organize," i.e. that which brings order from chaos.

3. Inanimate matter obeys the Second Law of Thermodynamics, also known as the Law of Entropy, which says that "natural processes in a closed system will always tend toward greater degrees of disorder."

4. Living processes do not follow this law. They tend toward greater degrees of order, not disorder.

5. When scientists realized that all compounds created by life processes were based on carbon, the definition of organic chemistry changed to "the study of carbon compounds."

6. Thus, all carbon compounds are now called "organic," even those created synthetically in laboratories that have never before existed on earth and are not produced by living processes.

7. This poses a problem for consumers when they see the word "organic" on labels. To a consumer this means natural, no chemicals, etc. while to an organic chemist it only means "carbon compound."

8. Pesticides, herbicides, and most of the chemicals that define modern industrial living are carbon compounds and are, therefore, organic by the chemist's definition.

9. Petrochemicals are hydrocarbons derived from crude oil or petroleum.

10. The word, "natural," by U.S. Federal standards, can be applied to anything produced by nature or to any chemical that exists in nature, but which can also be produced in a lab. Thus, many synthetic substances are legally labeled as natural.

11. Therapeutic grade essential oils are imbued with organizing powers (i.e. life force). Synthetic oils are not.

12. Hydrocarbons are compounds of only two elements: hydrogen and carbon. The simplest hydrocarbons are the alkanes whose general formula is C_nH_{2n+2}.

13. The scientific and semi-scientific names of organic compounds are designed to reveal their chemical formulas and structures, as well as how they relate to other organic compounds of a similar formula or form.

14. The International Union of Pure and Applied Chemistry (IUPAC) is the agency that sets the guidelines for naming organic compounds. These guidelines are called "The IUPAC Rules."

15. By IUPAC rules, the names of alkanes end in -ane while the names of alcohols end in -ol.

16. Hydrocarbons are not water soluble, but they are lipid soluble (will dissolve in oil).

17. Alkanes are not major components of essential oils, but understanding them helps one to better understand the compounds that do make up essential oils.

18. Rose oil is different from most essential oils in many ways, including the fact that, unlike any other oil, it averages about 11% alkanes. All other oils either have no alkanes or less than 1%. This may be one reason rose manifests many characteristics unique among aromatic oils.

19. Incomplete molecules of the alkanes—methane, ethane, propane, butane—give rise to the important radicals, methyl, ethyl, propyl, and butyl which are common components of the molecules of essential oils.

20. Hydrocarbon molecules containing propyl radicals are called propanoids, an important class of compounds found in many essential oils.

21. Oxygenated hydrocarbons are hydrocarbon molecules with one or more attached oxygen atoms.

22. Alkanes can be oxygenated into alcohols, the four most common are methyl alcohol (wood alcohol), ethyl alcohol (grain alcohol), isopropyl alcohol (rubbing alcohol), an isomer of propyl alcohol, and butyl alcohol.

23. The lightest alkane alcohols—methyl, ethyl, and propyl—are not natural compounds in essential oils, but some of the heavier alkane alcohols are. Light alcohols are used to dilute essential oils for perfumes and for profit.

24. Isomers are different compounds with the same elements in the same proportions (i.e., same chemical formula) but arranged in different configurations.

25. The bigger the molecule (i.e., the larger the number of constituent atoms) the greater the number of possible isomers.

26. There are trillions and trillions of isomers possible with alkanes and the hydrocarbons or oxygenated hydrocarbons that comprise essential oils.

27. The isomers of a given formula often fall into different families of compounds and may exhibit extreme variations in their properties from one isomer to another.

28. Laboratories can synthesize compounds with the same chemical formulas, but not necessarily with the same structural formulas or isomers.

29. Essential oils containing synthetic compounds do not have the same therapeutic properties as oils created by nature even if their components have the same chemical formulas.

30. Carbon is the most versatile of all the elements. Its personality and characteristics are what dominates and determines all life forms as we know them. Carbon is what accounts for the infinite and unending varieties of life that exist on earth.

31. Carbon is an element of love. The more fully we grasp the nature of carbon the more fully we grasp the nature of God. (See Romans 1:20 and I John 4:16)

♥ CHAPTER SIX
LORD
OF THE RINGS

C arbon is the key to the chemistry of living things and to the chemistry of essential oils as well. We have seen, in the previous chapter, how carbon can form chains—long, short, simple, and complex—creating trillions of different molecules. But one of the most amazing abilities of carbon we have not yet mentioned.

In 1825 a heretofore unknown compound was found that was a puzzle to the scientists of that time. They figured out its formula, but could not figure its structural form. Its stable and unique properties suggested many industrial applications. It dissolved fat and made an excellent base for varnishes and lacquers.

The compound was first isolated from the fuel burned in gas lamps as well as from the pleasant smelling balsams of several kinds of trees including onycha (*Styrax benzoin*), a Biblical oil. In 1834 it was synthesized in a lab by mixing benzoic acid with lime. Because of this, they called it "benzene." Its formula is C_6H_6.

The problem was this. According to the level of scientific understanding at that time, six hydrogen atoms would not be enough to fulfill the appetites of six carbons and form a stable compound with properties like benzene. The valence of carbon is 4 and the valence of hydrogen is 1. So how can 6 hydrogens bond with 6 carbons and occupy all of the available bonds? For example, in the alkane family discussed in the previous chapter, it takes 14 hydrogens to satisfy the 6 carbons in a hexane molecule (C_6H_{14}). It just didn't add up.

Then comes a German scientist named August Kekule— 1829-96 (pronounced KAY-ku-la). He was one of the first to realize that carbon atoms formed chains to which other elements, such as H, O, S, and N, could attach themselves. He was among the first to visualize the limitless possibilities of molecules built on skeletons of carbon chains. Kekule had started college as a student of architecture. Visualizing structures in three dimensions was his special talent and interest. He never became an architect, but his life work in chemistry helped define the structural architecture of carbon molecules as we know them today.

Dancing Snakes

When Kekule first encountered C_6H_6, he was stumped like all of his colleagues. For more than 40 years scientists had puzzled over benzene without success. One evening, as he sat with a pen and note pad contemplating the mysteries of carbon and the benzene molecule, he had a vision. The year was 1866.

"I turned the chair towards the fireplace and began to doze," he wrote. "Atoms danced before my eyes. I saw repeated apparitions of similar kind, now distinguished as larger units of various shapes. Long rows, frequently joined more densely; everything in motion, twisting and turning like snakes. And behold! What was that? One of the snakes caught hold of its own tail and mockingly whirled round before my eyes. I awoke, as if by lightning. I spent the rest of the night working out the consequence of this hypothesis."

From that dream Kekule realized that carbon atoms could make not only chains (like snakes - see pp. 56 & 164), but could also make rings (like snakes biting their tails). He then drew a picture of a ring of six carbons, forming a hexagon with alternating double bonds. And behold! This arrangement satisfies the valence requirements of every atom in the formula C_6H_6. The enigma of benzene had been solved.

Kekule's diagram of the benzene molecule is shown on the next page and is one of the most fundamental and useful concepts of organic chemistry even to the present day. Kekule's epiphany is all the more remarkable when you realize that in his day the concept of an atom with a nucleus of protons and neutrons with electrons in orbiting shells had not yet been expressed. These concepts were not to be articulated until after the turn of the century, decades after his death.

Kekule won a Nobel Prize for his work and in 2005 the U.S. Postal Service issued a stamp in his honor featuring both a picture of himself and of a benzene ring.

The
Benzene
Ring

C_6H_6

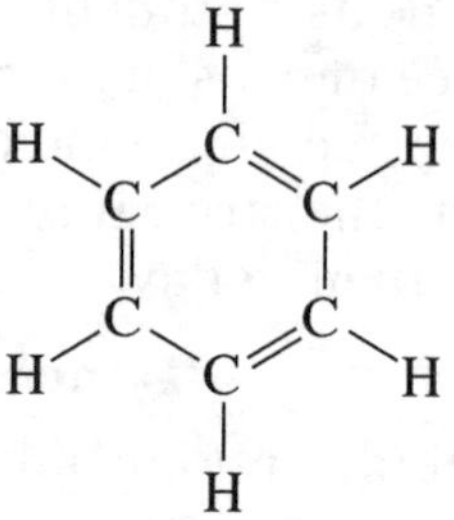

Aromatic Rings

Since Kekule's time, with the help of modern technology such as magnetic resonance imaging, electronic refractometry, mass and infrared spectrometry, we now know that carbon forms not only six-sided rings, but polygons of many sizes and shapes including 3-, 4-, 5-, 7-, 8-, and 9-sided rings, and more. Some rings are flat and some are twisted into all manner of three-dimensional shapes. There are already trillions of possibilities when carbon atoms simply link up in chains. When carbon forms rings to build molecules, the possibilities become even more astronomical, mounting into the trillions of trillions.

Carbon ring compounds play major roles in the compositions of every essential oil. Because of their prevalence in natural fragrances, they are called "aromatic rings" by chemists, even though some of them have no aroma detectable by the human nose.

The benzene ring diagram above has the locations of the six carbons (C), the six hydrogens (H), and the double bonds written in. A double bond, as depicted above, is where two arms of a carbon atom are holding onto the same atom, which, in this case, is another carbon. Since this ring occurs so frequently as a part of other larger molecules, a shorthand has been developed to represent it without writing in the Hs and Cs. It is drawn as a simple hexagon with alternating double bonds.

Three C-atom locations, with 3 bonds meeting at each location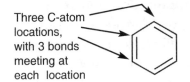

Benzene Rings Shown in Shorthand

Here is how you read formulas from structural diagrams like those shown above. Visualize a C atom at the apex of each angle (six of them). Notice that 3 lines (representing bonds) meet at each apex where a C atom is invisibly located. Since each carbon atom has a valence of 4, it requires that 4 bonds be satisfied. Therefore, there must be another bond (not shown) for the C at each corner of the hexagon to be satisfied. Since hydrogen has a valence of 1, one H atom bonded with each of the six carbon will satisfy the fourth necessary bond.

Stated another way, take the three bonds in the diagrams above converging at each C atom in the hexagon and subtract from the valence of C (which is 4) to deduce the number of H atoms invisibly attached to that carbon. Look at each of the six apexes and imagine one carbon (C) there. Note that there is a double bond and a single bond converging from two sides at each corner of the hexagon. That adds up to three bonds shown for each carbon. Since C has a valence of 4, we subtract what we see (3 bonds) from 4 to deduce the number of H atoms that must be attached there. (4 - 3 = 1) Thus, there are six carbons in the hexagon with one hydrogen atom at each apex, which makes C_6H_6. By the shorthand above, we have reduced the number of written strokes, but have still preserved all of the information that was contained in Kekule's original diagram on the previous page.

In this way, the chemical formula of a hydrocarbon can always be deduced from its structural diagram even though the Cs and Hs are not visibly shown. You will increase your skill in reading this shorthand later when we start getting into more complicated molecules, but at this time we have something more important to discuss.

Where Oil Frequencies Come From

Notice that we have drawn two hexagons to represent a benzene molecule. The only difference in the two is where the double bonds are located. But which one is right? The answer is both are right and neither is right.

Electrons are normally wedded to a particular atom and do not easily escape. They just keep spinning around and around the same nucleus. Each carbon atom has six electrons in its outer shells while each hydrogen atom has but one. (See atomic diagrams at the beginning of Chapter Four.)

When six carbons and six hydrogens join together to make a molecule of benzene C_6H_6, the electrons are no longer associated with a particular atom any more. They become "delocalized." That is, they are no longer confined to the orbits of a single atom, They can now roam all over the ring. They aren't "free electrons," just "non-localized." They are still confined to the molecule, but they now have a much larger neighborhood in which to move and explore.

Therefore, in the two drawings of a benzene ring shown in the previous page, the truth is that we don't know where the double bonds are located since they are actually oscillating continuously with certain frequencies. Therefore, in recognition of the fact that a benzene ring has no stationary bonds in the traditional sense, the shorthand representation is a hexagon with a circle in the middle, like this:

Symbol for
a Benzene Ring with
Non–Localized Electrons

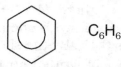

C_6H_6

Non-localized electrons are "shared" with other atoms of the molecule. In their new found freedom, they zip around the ring, visiting the various homes of the neighborhood at megahertz frequencies (millions of times per second). This is one of the sources of electromagnetic frequencies that have been measured in association with therapeutic grade essential oils. The additional energy carried by the electrons dashing around the molecule (as compared to what they had when tied to a single atom) is called the "resonance energy" of the molecule. The back cover of this book depicts an aromatic ring (benzene) as a nebulous hexagonal cloud with a spectrum of colors to represent the range of electromagnetic frequencies and intensities present in such a molecule. In this state, the concept of particles (electrons, protons, and neutrons) composing matter no longer makes sense. Instead we have an energy form—a waveform. The wavelike nature of benzene and other functional groups with aromatic rings or resonant bonds leads directly into relativity and quantum physics which takes us to a hybrid field of science called nuclear chemistry—a blend of both chemistry and physics. The wavelike properties of aromatic rings also lead beyond chemistry and physics into the the nature of consciousness itself, including both our consciousness and that of God. But we won't go there until Part Three. For more on this, read *Transcendental Physics* by Edward R. Close, Ph.D. (See bibliography.)

Vibrating, non-localized electrons are not only found in benzene, but in carbon rings of many types and sizes. In fact, non-localized electrons are present in all "covalent" bonds where electrons are "shared" between atoms. Hence, electromagnetic resonance energy is present in many organic molecules, not just the ones containing benzene rings. (See pp. 716, 741-42)

A Spectrum of Frequencies

Electromagnetic frequencies are measured in units of cycles-per-second (cps) which are called "Hertz" (abbreviated as "hz") in honor of the German physicist who first described and discovered radio waves—Heinrich Rudolph Hertz (1857-1894). There are a variety of sources of vibrational frequencies within the molecules of essential oils. In fact, there is a whole spectrum of frequencies within every organic molecule and the larger, more complex it is, the greater the spectrum.

Every time a pair of atoms forms a bond to create a compound, there is a measurable frequency associated with that bond. For example, double bonds between carbon atoms have been measured to vibrate at frequencies between 49 and 68 mega-megahertz. One megahertz (Mhz) is a vibration of one million times per second (10^6 hz). A mega-mega hertz (MMhz) is a million-million times per second or, in other words, a trillion times per second (10^{12} hz). A double bond between a carbon atom and an oxygen atom measures to be 51-53 MMhz while a single bond between a carbon and an oxygen is only 30-39 MMhz.

Visualize chemical bonds like rubber-bands stretched between pairs of atoms which can be strummed like a guitar string to produce a musical tone. Each bond between each pair of atoms in a molecule can produce different pitches producing a spectrum of frequencies like the spectrum of the 88 diatonic tones that comprise a piano keyboard spanning seven octaves. Strumming the bonds of a molecule is exactly how our bodily cells and organs access the vibrational qualities of an essential oil. In fact, modern physicists are now thinking that the whole universe is composed of tones like those of a vibrating violin string. They call it the "String Theory."

Table Ten gives the frequency ranges of the electromagnetic spectrum. By comparison, the sonic spectrum of sound frequencies audible to human ears ranges from 10 cps (10 hz) to 20,000 cps ($2x10^4$ hz).

Table Ten
The Electromagnetic Spectrum
(Frequencies are given in cps or hertz)

ELF waves (Extremely Low Frequency)	10^0 hz
TV waves (Video)	10^3 hz
Radio waves (Audio)	10^6 hz
Microwaves (including cell phone transmissions)	10^9 hz
Infra red (IR - Experienced as Heat)	10^{12} hz
Visible Light (Red, Yellow, Green, Blue, Violet)	10^{14} hz
Ultraviolet Rays (UV - Cause of Sunburn)	10^{15} hz
X-Rays	10^{18} hz
Gamma Rays	10^{21} hz
Cosmic Rays	10^{24} hz

• Exponentially expressed numbers can be written out as a 1 followed by the number of zeros indicated by the exponent. Hence, in the case of cosmic rays, whose exponent is 24, the long version would be a 1 with 24 zeros: 1,000,000,000,000,000,000,000,000. Thus, one can appreciate the value of the mathematical shorthand of writing these astronomical numbers in exponential form.

Expressed as numbers with names, 10^0 = units, 10^1 = tens, 10^2 = hundreds, 10^3 = thousands, 10^6 = millions, 10^9 = billions, 10^{12} = trillions, 10^{14} = hundreds of trillions, 10^{15} = quadrillions, 10^{18} = quintillions, 10^{21} = sextillions, and 10^{24} = heptillions.

Harmonics and Beat Frequencies

When the pitch of a middle C (257 hz) is played or sung, you can tell what instrument sounded the tone and/or whose voice was the singer. When a clarinet, a guitar, or a piano all play the same note, you can tell which instrument played it. Yet they all played the same pitch. How can this be when the frequency of the pitch heard is the same in all cases—257 cycles-per-second.

This is because the frequency we hear as pitch is not the only frequency present in the sound. A single vibrating piano or harp string actually sends forth a spectrum of pitches ranging from the fundamental (257 hz) to a range reaching up into the kilohertz range of thousands of cps. The additional pitches other than the fundamental are called "harmonics." We hear the fundamental frequency as pitch (middle C) and the rest as color or timbre, which combines in our ears as sounds we can identify as different voices or instruments. (The technical term, timbre, is pronounced "TOM-burr.")

When you have many frequencies emitted from the same source, our ears usually identify a fundamental as pitch and hear the rest as harmonics that color the tone. Harmonic frequencies usually occur in even multiples of the fundamental like double, triple, quadruple, quintuple, and so forth. When two frequencies are slightly different and are not even multiples of one another, they can alternately reinforce and cancel one another to produce a new frequency different than either of them and much lower. These are called "beat frequencies." In this way, one could play a middle C (257 hz) simultaneously with another pitch slightly higher (say 260 hz) and the two would vibrate together to produce a much lower beat frequency that could be as little as 10 hz or even less.

Thus, even though the individual bonds between atoms of a molecule vibrate at mega-megahertz frequencies (10^{12} hz), when combined they can form beat frequencies that are much slower, like in the Mhz range (10^6 hz). From these beat frequencies, acting as fundamental harmonics, we get measurable values like those in Table Eleven on page 182.

Coherence and Incoherence

When you have a mixture of hundreds of varieties of molecules each capable of a variety of frequencies, it could be chaos. It could be like a badly out-of-tune piano where the frequencies of the strings are not in harmony with one another according to the pitches of the diatonic scale of half steps, whole-steps, fourth, fifths, and octaves. The standard musical scale (also called the chromatic or tempered scale) upon which we compose all of our music is mathematically based on the 12th root of the number 2. This is referred to by scientists as a "logarithmic scale." The tempered scale for tuning instruments was developed by Johanne Sebastian Bach (1685-1750)—a genius in both music and math, and a devout man of God.

A badly out-of-tune piano possesses a spectrum of frequencies incapable of producing pleasant harmony and true music. Such a body of disharmonic frequencies is called "incoherence," like a dysfunctional family that manifests no peace.

Amazing as it may seem, the hundreds of varieties of molecules in a typical therapeutic grade essential oil do not form an incoherent mass. They do not produce chaos. Their many frequencies are tuned in mathematical precision like the logarithms of a musical scale to make music for our bodies, minds, and souls. When natural compounds are blended by God to create a healing oil, the molecules, imbued with God's word, respond to one another and adjust their frequencies into the coherence of a finely tuned instrument. The molecules of a therapeutic grade essential oil form a harmonious, coherent, functional family designed and intended to serve us and heal us according to the highest will of their creator and our creator who is one and the same—God.

Now do you understand why modifying a therapeutic grade oil by removing some of its constituents, by adding synthetic ingredients, or by adulterating it with solvents can upset or destroy the subtle and delicate harmony that God has so lovingly prepared for us?

Now do you understand why a non-therapeutic grade oil might carry dissonance, incoherence, and disharmony in its molecular makeup and, thus, carry no healing power and, perhaps, carry harm?

Now do you understand how and why a compound that is potentially harmful when acting alone can behave beneficially within the balanced environment of an essential oil as it adjusts its vibrations to play in harmony with the rest of the family of compounds that define that oil?

Think of therapeutic grade essential oils as symphonies of molecular music composed by God to sing health and harmony to us, his children. All we have to do to receive the benefits of his aromatic compositions is to acquire and develop the art of music appreciation in using the oils with and by his direction as the master conductor of the music that heals our bodies and feeds our souls.

The Significance of Frequency

When molecules of essential oils are inhaled, swallowed, applied to the skin, or internalized into your body in any way, they resonate with your bodily tissues at the frequencies intrinsic to their molecular spectrum as well as their resultant harmonic and beat frequencies. This increases your own natural electromagnetic vibrations and restores coherence to your electric fields to produce healing and maintain wellness. Frequency resonance is only one of more than six processes by which oils can heal and benefit your health. (See *Healing Oils of the Bible* for more.)

In the book, *Reference Guide to Essential Oils*, by Higley and Higley, (see bibliography), there is an excellent discussion of the frequencies measured in oils. *Healing Oils of the Bible* is another book that discusses this and includes a list of specific oils and their fundamental frequencies. Due to the sensitivity of the instrumentation used to obtain the data of Table Eleven, their absolute values are not important. What is important are the relative values and that they fall within the megahertz or radio-frequency range.

What is clear is that one should maintain a certain level and spectrum of harmonic vibrations within his or her body to maintain health. When your fundamental electromagnetic frequencies fall below certain levels of intensity or lose certain portions of the normal spectrum, you become susceptible to colds and flus. If they fall even lower, you become susceptible to more serious diseases. If they fall too low, you die.

Table Eleven
Fundamental Frequencies of People and Things
(Frequencies are given in Megahertz)

Healthy Human Brain	71–90 Mhz
Healthy Human Body (overall)	62–68
When you have cold symptoms	58
When you have flu symptoms	57
When you have candida infection	55
When you have Epstein Barr syndrome	52
When you have cancer	42
When you begin to die	25
Processed or Canned Foods	0
Fresh Produce (depending on how fresh)	10–15
Dry Herbs	12–22
Fresh Herbs	20–27
Therapeutic Grade Essential Oils	52-320

Adapted from *Reference Guide to Essential Oils* by Connie & Alan Higley 2002 The data published here was obtained by Bruce Tainio of Tainio Technology, Cheny, Washington. For more information visit www.tainio.com. Also see *Freedom Through Health* by Terry Friedmann, MD, where he discusses the healing frequencies of essential oils.

What can we do to help elevate and tune our electromagnetic frequencies and keep them high and coherent? The types of food we eat make a difference. Our thoughts also make a difference, depending on whether they are habitually positive or negative, peaceful or dissonant. Our emotions matter, too, where love, faith, calmness, humility, joy, and peace elevate our vibrations while hate, fear, anxiety, bitterness, unforgiveness, pride, resentment, jealousy, envy, depression, or restlessness can pull us down and make us susceptible to sickness. Even the types of people we regularly associate with can raise or lower our personal vibrations and increase or decrease our subtle inner harmony. Dramatic differences can be made with essential oils which have the highest most coherent measured frequencies of all natural substances.

Oils Respond to Words, Thoughts, and Prayer

We respond to the thoughts and prayers of others, whether we are aware of it or not, and so do essential oils. In some of Bruce Tainio's work, discussed in Higley's book, essential oils were measured before and after being bombarded with negative thoughts. Their frequencies went down by 12 MHz. When positive thoughts were aimed at the oils, their frequencies went up by 10 MHz. When the oils were prayed over, their resonant frequencies went up by 15 MHz. Oils amplify intent. And intent will move molecules of oil to where they can best serve to heal. That is why prayer and anointing with essential oils work so well when combined together. (See Part Three.)

One reason it is impossible to exactly duplicate the numbers in experimental measurements of oil frequencies (such as those of Tainio) is that the thoughts and attitudes of the experimenter are part of the experiment. Thus, if a skeptical or negative scientist tried to duplicate such measurements, he or she would fail. Their thoughts and attitudes would sabotage their attempt.

"Paranormal" is a term referring to phenomena thought to be outside the realm of material science and/or the perceptions of our five physical senses. Within the science of parapsychology, it has been known for many decades that scientists who disbelieve and want to disprove paranormal phenomena can seemingly succeed in doing so while those who believe in the authenticity of the paranormal can perform experiments that verify its existence and provide data to describe its parameters. This is called the "experimenter effect." In this case it is also called the "sheep-goat effect" where sheep (believers) tend to get positive confirming results while goats (non-believers) tend to get negative disconfirming results. Of course, documentation of the "sheep-goat effect" is, in fact, a verification that the paranormal exists and that psychology and physics, mind and matter, spirit and body, are connected and do interact.

Evidence of Things Not Seen

We believe in many things we cannot see. Take the wind, for example. Jesus once said, "The wind blows where it chooses, and you hear the sound of it, but you do not know where it comes from or where it goes." (John 3:8)

If you sit quietly on a hill when the air is calm, sometimes a sudden breeze will arrive, but you don't know of its existence until it strokes your face, brushes your clothing, or rustles the neighboring trees. You can not see it coming and you cannot see where it goes when it ceases to touch you. Even so, invisible as it is, it still affects us.

Have you ever studied the flutter of a flag flapping in the wind? It ripples in a vibratory fashion with traveling waves that roll from the pole to its outer edge. The flag is manifesting a visible spectrum of vibrations with specific frequencies in time and space, yet the causes of the vibrations are unseen. The agent that energizes the flag to wave is an invisible force manifesting as the motion of the flag. The invisible wind creates a visible display before your eyes through the instrument of the flag tethered to a pole.

The frequencies exhibited by the movement of the flag are partly intrinsic to the flag, itself—its weight, its size, its shape, its material, and its flexibility. But the frequencies are also partially determined by the velocity, direction, and nature of the wind. Essential oils are like flags with intrinsic frequencies of their own, but when energized by our bodily and spiritual forces they vibrate with a spectrum of frequencies that are a unique combination of ourselves and the oils.

To Believe or Not to Believe

The rules of the scientific method dictate that as a scientist "One must prove before one can believe." But in some forms of research, where experimenters cannot separate themselves from the measurements, the operative rule is the opposite: "One must believe before one can prove." This leads us directly into the nature of faith and its impact on us and the world about us.

In Hebrews 11:1, we read, "Faith is the substance of

things hoped for, the evidence of things not seen." In science, "substance" is matter and "evidence" is hard data. This scripture implies that if you possess a true faith that comes from direct experience with God, that faith, in and of itself, constitutes a form of substantive proof, a valid verification of your vision of things unseen and undetected by the five physical senses. Such faith is tangible evidence of a deeper reality existing in spirit that may not yet be manifest in material form. Hebrews 11:3 continues, "The worlds were prepared by the word of God, so that what is seen was made from things that are not visible." God has created us and the manifested universe, visible and audible through our eyes and ears, from his unmanifested word (subtle vibration) that we can neither see nor hear physically. (John 1:1) Yet by faith we can gain direct and certain knowledge of his unspoken mysteries as certain as the proofs of science. But we will reserve further discussion of that topic for Part Three of this book.

From an experiential and empirical viewpoint, it is clear to those in an anointing, healing ministry, that prayer makes oils work better and oils make prayer work better. One can work without the other, but prayer and oils are both more powerful when combined. Thus, in Mark 6:7-13 and James 5:13-16, we are directed to pray and anoint with oils for healing. Prayer and oils are both prescribed by scripture along with the associated laying on of hands that is part of the anointing process. And as for scriptural authority for you to anoint, pray, and heal, I Peter 2:4-9, states that true believers are "a holy priesthood." (See *Healing Oils of the Bible* for more on this.)

The Power of Prayer on Plants by Franklin Loehr is also a good source for this kind of information. Loehr found results with living plants that parallel those of essential oils measured by Tainio. Plants respond appropriately to thoughts, both negative and positive, as well as to prayer. Loehr was both a research chemist and a pastor. Loehr's work showed that even the bonding angles of the water molecule are altered by prayer and thought. His book contains a great deal of scientific data, carefully controlled and meticulously documented. Another book with this kind of data is *The Secret Life of Plants* by Tompkins and Bird. Yet another book, *Messages From Water* by Emoto, presents considerable evidence of the same kinds of responses in water molecules, almost as if they possess some form of cognitive consciousness. (See biblio-graphy.) As we shall discuss in Part Three, there is more to essential oils than mere chemistry. (See *Quantum Physics, Essential Oils, and the Mind-Body Connection* by Stewart available at www.RaindropTraining.com.)

How Frequencies Heal

Here is how the frequencies of oils work to heal us: Specific oils have many frequencies. When we say that an oil has "a frequency," what we are referring to is the "fundamental harmonic" of that oil.

Fundamentals and harmonics were discussed earlier in this chapter. When you play a specific note on a piano, like middle C, the frequency you hear as its pitch and register is 257 hz. But that piano note actually contains many frequencies. You just don't hear them as pitch. (Pitch is a particular position on the twelve-tone chromatic scale—a, b, d#, etc. Register is the octave—middle-c, high-c, low-c, etc. The vibration of 257 hz that enables us to identify the pitch and register of a middle-c is only the "fundamental harmonic" of that tone. The remaining frequencies in the vibration for middle-c give it color or "timbre." (which is pronounced "TOM-burr")

Hence, we could hear a middle C played by a piano, a clarinet, a trumpet, an oboe, or a violin. Yet, even though it was the same pitch and register in all cases, we could easily tell which instrument was playing the note. That's timbre. In fact, if ten different people sang the same note, we could identify the person in each instance since every human voice has a different spectrum of harmonics (timbre). Human voice is so unique for each person that a vibrational analysis of a voice will identify the person to whom it belongs as precisely as a set of fingerprints. It's called "voice printing" and is used for identification in sensitive secure top secret facilities.

The pitch of a note is what we hear as the "fundamental." The color or flavor of the note (whether it is instrumental or vocal, etc.) is from the other frequencies in the note. These are called "harmonics" or "overtones."

Oils, vegetables, herbs, animals, and people all have fundamental mechanical, sonic, and electromagnetic frequencies. They also emit and resonate with hundreds of harmonics that give them personality and set them apart as distinguishable and unique. There are also beat frequencies that vibrate at much slower rates than the harmonics, overtones, and fundamentals.

Each species of essential oil has a fundamental frequency and a series of harmonics, just like the tones of a musical instrument. When you blend two species of oils, you have created a musical interval. When you blend three or more oils, you have created a chord. When you layer one oil after another in time, you are creating scales, arpeggios, and melodies with the notes of essential oils. When you do a raindrop session on a person with its seven species of oils and its one or two blends over an hour, you have performed a symphony with the recipients body and spirit as part of the score.

When you hear different performers play music, some sound good and some don't. Some produce resonant coherent frequencies that blend in accord in a pleasing and harmonious way while others produce dissonant incoherent frequencies in discord that are unpleasant and disturbing. Some sounds make us feel good, full of peace, joy, love, and a sense of well-being. Others make us feel uncomfortable, anxious, depressed, and out of sorts. Did you know that when birds sing daily over your garden, things grow better. The frequencies of bird songs promote plant growth, which is one reason why bushes and trees invite them to come nest in their branches.

Resonance

Resonance occurs when two things vibrate in unison at the same principal frequency or frequencies. For example, you can place a violin on one side of a room with its four strings of different pitches exposed and free to vibrate. Then play the G-string on another violin across the room. The G-string on the other side of the room will begin to vibrate in unison with the string played, while the other three strings remain silent. The G-string of the remote violin will hum in resonance with the G-note that was sounded across the room, even though it was never plucked or bowed. That is resonance. This is sometimes called "sympathetic vibration." It is also called "vibrational energy transfer" since the energy of the string that was played is transferred to the receiving string of the same pitch. The energy is not transferred to the strings tuned to pitches other than G. They would not be stimulated to respond because they are "out of tune" and "unsympathetic" with the energizing source.

The great Italian opera singer, Enrico Caruso (1873-1921), was able to break glass goblets with his voice. He could match the tone of a piece of crystal so perfectly that singing with enough force he could shatter it to pieces. It was resonance that shattered the glass, not just volume. If he sang another note than that of the fundamental frequency of the glass, it would not break no matter how loudly he sang.

Essential oils work in a similar fashion. The various organs, tissues, and cells of your body inherently possess certain pitches or fundamental frequencies. Oil molecules that resonate at the frequencies of, say, your pancreas, will administer therapy there. Oil molecules that resonate with the brain will administer therapy there. Oils that do not have the frequencies of your pancreas or brain will not resonate for these organs, but will transfer their energies to other body parts and tissues in harmony with them. Because each essential oil is imbued by God with a unique spectrum of frequencies or timbres, they selectively administer to specific body parts according to their spectra. This is why some oils work best for muscles, others for nerves, others for bones, some for the mind, some for the emotions, etc. Aromatic oils transfer their healing to the various aspects of our being according to the music in their molecules—composed by God, himself.

What happens when we are in contact with or in the presence of living, therapeutic, vibrating essential oils is this: Ourselves, our spirits, our minds, our bodies, our organs, our tissues, and/or our cells can each resonate with the spectrum of healing harmonics of the oils while the sickness in our bodies does not. In other words, when healing takes place, our bodies resonate at frequencies where health and balance is restored and disease cannot exist.

There is a book entitled *Cymatics*, by Hans Jenny, a Swiss physician and research scientist, that has to do with the effect of sound vibrations on both living and inanimate matter. One of the insights gleaned from Jenny's research is that each organ of the body makes sound at specific frequencies. It is not sound that most people would hear with the unassisted ear, since the amplitudes are too small, but there are measurable sonic vibrations associated with each part of our bodies. Dr. Jenny and a fellow researcher and physician, Dr. Peter Manners of England, have determined what these frequencies are in many bodily organs. When an organ malfunctions, they found that the organ no longer emitted its healthy frequencies. They found that by aiming specific, audible, high intensity frequencies of sound at those organs they would be restored back to health. In other words, the sick organs, which were "out of tune" and in a state of dissonance would, by coming into resonance with the healthy frequencies of the sound generator, come back into a state of wellness and vibrate, once again, at their proper frequencies.

On a much higher yet more subtle level of energy, that is what essential oils do. That's how they work—by resonance at various levels, with organs and cells and even with our thoughts and feelings. They don't resonate with the toxins in our bodies, which is why they stir them up and drive them out. Oils are also out of phase with negative emotions, which is why they dislodge forgotten traumas and help us to resurrect them into our conscious mind where we can deal with them and resolve them.

When something vibrates at many dissonant frequencies, it is said to produce "chaotic or incoherent frequencies." When something vibrates in harmony with itself with no dissonances, we say that it produces "coherent frequencies." Therapeutic grade essential oils produce coherent frequencies that are naturally tuned to pitches that mean health to our bodies. Pharmaceuticals and synthetic oils do not.

Why Essential Oils Work so Well

How is it that therapeutic grade essential oils resonate with all the right frequencies to address our mental, spiritual, emotional, and physical needs? Is it an accident? A coincidence? It goes back to Genesis Chapter One.

"In the beginning when God created the heavens and the earth, the earth was a formless void and darkness covered the face of the deep..." In other words, there was chaos, incoherence, and dissonance.

"Then God said Let there be light; and there was light" In other words, God spoke his creation into being, He vibrated it into being, He imbued it with his Word. And what is light, but a spectrum of frequencies?

Continuing in the Book of Genesis, we find the phrase, "And God said..." at least seven more times as the prelude to his every act of creation.

On the third day of creation (Genesis 1:9-13) we find the same process: "And God said Let the earth put forth vegetation: plants yielding seed, and fruit trees of every kind on earth that bear fruit with the seed in it. And it was so...And God saw that it was good." In other words, God imbued the plants and their oils with his very vibrations, his intelligent Word.

Current scientific thinking says that the universe was apprently created in a split second from a great explosion. This is the so called "Big Bang Theory" of creation, It is based on the astronomical observation that all of the stars and galaxies of the universe seem to be traveling away from a common point, as if everything started with a big bang or explosion from that point.

Of course, an explosion in the traditional sense could not create the order as is seen in the universe from the systematic arrangements and motions of countless heavenly bodies down to the fine structures of atoms and molecules, not to mentioin the order of living processes. Explosions create chaos and disorder in conformance with the second law of thermodynamics. You could not go to a used auto parts lot containing junk cars of every description, sufficient to build an entire car from their parts, and detonate a ton of dynamite there in hopes that a perfect automobile would be assembled in midair from the explosion.

So the Big Bang Theory, presented as some sort of supernova or cosmic explosion cannot be true. However, the Big Bang theory does lead us to a truth. Instead of referring to a chaotic explosion, it could refer to the boom of God's voice speaking creation into existence, imbued with all of the intelligence and order of his nature. (See Part Three.)

The first lines of the Gospel of John speak the same truths. "In the beginning was the Word, and the Word was with God, and the Word was God. . ." The universe is dynamic with the Word, the vibrations of God, the conscious presence of God. Those who are in resonance with that truth see God, feel God, and know God's presence in everything they see and touch around them. Those who are not in resonance with that truth are blind to see God's handiwork in anything. John spoke of this blindness when he wrote, "And the light shown in darkness and the darkness comprehended it not." (John 1:5) Experiencing the Divine is not a function of the intellect or a simple matter of belief. It is a matter of resonance. God's grace is received through attunement, humility, and spiritual receptivity—which is resonance with his will.

If, as it says in Romans 1:20 and Psalm 19, that God has revealed his nature in what he has made, then surely his making of healing oils reveals his love and concern for us. He has created medicines whose molecules sing sonorous songs of healing to our very cells resounding with his grace—if only we will attune ourselves to receive it.

Phenols

Among the many active constituents of oils are a class of compounds called "phenols" or "phenolics." The phenol molecule is a benzene ring (C_6H_6) configured with a hydroxyl radical (OH) as shown below.

The Phenol Molecule
(An Oxygenated Hydrocarbon)

(Formula = C_6H_6O)

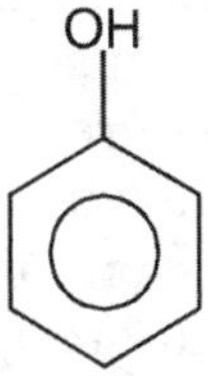

Phenol is an oxygenated hydrocarbon. You may recall from the previous chapter that when an OH radical is attached to a hydrocarbon molecule, it makes it into an alcohol. When alcohols are given names, they are supposed to end in -ol. Phenol is an alcohol. It has a hydroxyl group attached. Its name ends in -ol. But phenol is a very special compound with properties different from any other alcohol.

Among its differences, phenol forms a weak acid when mixed with water and, for that reason, it is also called carbolic acid. It was introduced as a hospital antiseptic and antibacterial solution by Joseph Lister in 1865. Phenol is used industrially in making dyes and plastics. It is also a topical anesthetic in many commercial sore throat sprays. Camphophenique® is a popular nonprescription ointment available at drug stores and groceries that you simply apply where it hurts or itches. The main active ingredients in Camphophenique® are camphor (11%) and phenol (5%).

While benzene is highly toxic, phenol is relatively harmless. Benzene is not found in any essential oil, but phenol is found in minor concentrations (<1%) in several oils such as cassia, cinnamon, and ylang ylang. However, as a functional group, phenol plays a major role in many oils, including oregano, thyme, and mountain savory.

Functional Groups

Up to now we have been using the word "radical" to designate an incomplete molecule eager to join another in order to complete itself. In Chapter Five we mentioned hydroxyl, methyl, ethyl, propyl, and butyl radicals as examples. You can understand why an incomplete molecule would be hungry to find a partner since it has unsatisfied bonds.

However, there are also many complete molecules, such as benzene and phenol, that are quite satisfied as they are but which can also act like radicals in that they will join with others to create new molecules. Complete molecules willing to unite with others are called "functional groups."

While no essential oil contains benzene as a compound, as a functional group, the benzene ring is one of the most popular among the constituents of volatile oils. Because of its popularity with fragrant compounds it is sometimes called an "aromatic ring." There are other aromatic rings besides benzene with more or less than the six sides of a hexagon. Compounds containing such rings are called "aromatic" even when they have no aroma. One of the characteristic features of essential oils is the abundance of aromatic rings in their composition.

Beyond the social circles inhabited by essential oils, the benzene ring is probably the most popular functional group in all of organic chemistry, forming an untold number of compounds, many of which we could not live without. This is pretty amazing for a compound that, by itself, can be a deadly poison. As examples of compounds vital to your life built of benzene rings, consider cholesterol, pregnenolone, and all of the necessary steroid hormones, including the estrogens and androgens that determine sex. These are all built of aromatic rings attached together—four in each molecule, to be exact. (See Chapter Eleven, p. 401)

Phenol is built on benzene and is quite content to just be itself as an aromatic alcohol. Phenol, like benzene, can also act as a functional group. Compounds containing a phenol molecule are referred to as "phenolics." However, often they are simply called "phenols."

The most common phenols in essential oils include ter-pinen-1-ol-4 (in tea tree and marjoram oils), thymol (in thyme and mountain savory oils), carvacrol (in oregano and catnip oils), and eugenol (in clove, cinnamon, basil and bay laurel oils). Other oils rich in phenols include calamus, anise, fennel, wintergreen, birch, and tarragon, (See Table Forty-Eight for a complete list with percents.)

Phenols in oils carry many benefits crucial to healing, but need to be applied with care and common sense. Some of them are very strong and can irritate the skin or create inflammation to the sensitive tissues of the mouth or face.

Phenols in essential oils are thought to be antiseptic and antibacterial, and may boost the immune system in various ways. Oils containing phenols have also been used in sup-port of the nervous system and in treatments for depres-sion. Phenolic oils cleanse cellular receptor sites.

Diphenols

Some compounds in essential oils are diphenols. This means that they contain a benzene ring with two OH rad-icals attached, not just one as in a regular phenol. The diphenol molecule can act as a functional group. This cre-ates another type of phenolic compound which, in some cases, can manifest the properties of phenols in greater strength because it contains two oxygen atoms instead of one. The toxins in poison ivy are diphenols and can be allergens. (pp. 466-470) The diphenol molecule can look like the one shown below where the OH radicals are attached to adjacent carbon atoms. The OH radicals can be attached to other C atoms of the ring as well.

The Diphenol Molecule
(An Oxygenated
Hydrocarbon)

(Formula = $C_6H_6O_2$)

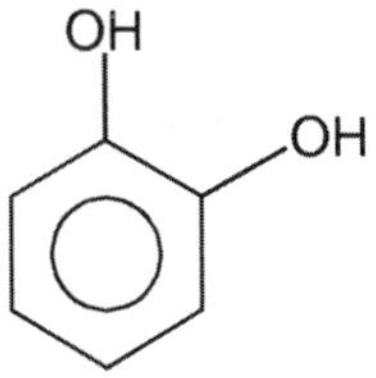

The toxic compound in poison ivy oil is a diphenol (toxicodendrol) which is discussed in Chapter Twelve. Diphenols are not uncommon, but are usually not a main ingredient in essential oils. Except for toxicodendrol, they are not harmful. Lemon mint oil (*Monarda citriodora*) and Fern oil (*Monarda menthaefolia*) both contain thymoquinol, a harmless diphenolic compound. Both of these are found, quite safely, in perfume fragrances. Allylpyrocatechol, found in onions and garlic oils, is another diphenol containing sulfur with an odor strong enough to bring tears to the eyes.

Phenylpropanoids

One of the most important phenols found in essential oils contains a propyl radical (a 3-carbon chain). The propane molecule C_3H_8 has eight hydrogen atoms while the propyl radical has only six or seven (C_3H_6 or C_3H_7). It is an incomplete propane molecule. (See section on alkanes in Chapter Five.) When a molecule contains both a phenol molecule and a propyl radical it is called a "phenylpropanoid."

In the three diagrams of a phenylpropanoid molecule on the next page, phenol is represented by the hydroxyl radical (OH) attached to the top of a benzene ring (hexagon with a circle). The propyl radical is shown as a 3-carbon chain attached to the bottom of each ring. The scientific name for this compound ($C_9H_{12}O$) is 4-isopropylphenol. There are two common names for this compound. One is "p-cuminol" and the other is "australol." It is found in cumin oil (*Cuminum cyminum*) and most species of eucalyptus (*Eucalyptus sp*). The fact that this compound has more than one common name illustrates why scientists prefer scientific names, since they are unique and contain structural information not found in common names. The scientific name for this simple phenylpropanoid is "4-isopropylphenol." The manner by which p-cuminol (or australol) is manufactured by the plant from an amino acid is discussed in Chapter Four.

Phenylpropanoids are compounds that cleanse receptor

The Simplest Phenylpropanoid
p-cuminol or australol (also 4-isopropylphenol)
Found in Cumin and Eucalyptus Oils

Example of a Phenylpropanoid Molecule
Diagrammed Three Ways • Formula = $C_9H_{12}O$

sites—an essential and crucial step in the process of healing and the maintenance of wellness. While all phenylpropanoids have a benzene ring, an OH, and a propyl radical, their formulas vary. Eugenol ($C_{10}H_{12}O_2$), carvacrol ($C_{10}H_{14}O$), and thymol ($C_{10}H_{14}O$) are phenylpropanoids found in oils of clove, oregano, and thyme respectively. Eugenol is also found in basil and cinnamon oils.

Reading Structural Formulas

The phenylpropanoid model above is shown three ways for a purpose. The first one (on the left) shows the 3-carbon propyl chain explicitly as CH_3CHCH_3 or C_3H_7. The last one (on the right) contains all the same information, but in shorthand notation.

The second version (middle) omits explicit representation of the H atoms, but you can figure out the number of Hs without showing them by noting the number of bonds connecting with each C. In the central C of the propyl radical, three bonds are shown converging at that site—one from the top and two from the sides from underneath. Since the valence of C is 4 and only 3 bonds are shown, there must be 1 hydrogen unshown (4 - 3 = 1). In the two lower Cs, at the bottom end of each line, only one bond is seen for each. Since each C must each fulfill 4 bonds and only 1 is shown, there must be 3 unshown Hs with each of these (4 - 1 = 3). Hence, writing in the Hs, as in the first diagram, is unnecessary since their number can always be deduced from the number of bonds converging on any particular C location.

The last diagram (on the right) is the shorthand form we use the most. In this one, all of the symbols (C) for the carbon atoms are omitted, but they are represented in another way. In structural diagrams of organic molecules, the positions of a carbon atom are represented by every corner, the apex of every angle, every junction of lines, every intersection of lines, and by the ends of every line (or double line) not occupied by anything else. (See Chapter Five, Table Nine.)

In the third diagram, we have the six Cs of the phenol represented by the six corners of the hexagon while the three Cs of the propyl radical are represented by (1) the conjunction of three lines below the ring and (2) by the bottom ends of the two lines extending downward at angles.

Hence, without writing in the symbol C anywhere, we can count the angles, conjunctions, and end points to get the number of Cs. There are 9 Cs in this molecule. By reading the diagram we know how many Cs there are and where each is located. From the number of lines drawn as bonds, we can deduce the number and locations of Hs, also. The only thing that needs to be explicitly shown is the hydroxyl radical at the top.

Oxygen, sulfur, nitrogen, and atoms of any other element, except H and C, are always explicitly shown in molecular diagrams. Only H and C are represented invisibly. Hence, with a minimum of writing and drawing, we can represent the shape of an organic molecule and reveal its formula without writing in all the symbols for C and H. We will use these skills later in reading other molecular diagrams in this book. Such diagrams are also referred to as "structural formulas."

How Structural Formulas Are Determined

No one has directly seen a molecule of an essential oil, at least not in a way acceptable within today's understanding of science. Some scientists, like August Kukele, seemed to have an extrasensory gift that enabled them to see living, vibrating molecules, but such subjective perceptions are not yet accepted as scientific observations. Since small molecules, such as those in essential oils, are too small for even the most powerful microscopes, you might wonder how scientists know their shapes.

The analytic techniques of modern chemistry can determine chemical formulas without much difficulty. But once you have the formula in numerical form, the next task is to determine the structure or structures that correspond to that formula.

The basic analytic tool to determine the main compounds of an essential oil is the gas chromatograph (GC). There is also the so called high performance liquid chromatograph (HPLC), the gel liquid chromatograph (GLC), and the thin layer chromatograph (TLC). What these instruments do is to separate the components of an oil into individual compounds so the percents of each can be determined. Only the main ingredients can be measured in this way. Not the trace compounds. There is a lot of skill, art, and subjective judgment that goes into the interpretation of a chromatogram. It isn't all science. There is plenty of room for error. Some labs and some scientists do better than others in achieving a reliable analysis.

To determine structural formulas, chemists have other tools. The mass spectrograph (MS) is a main one. Nuclear magnetic resonance (NMR), infrared spectral analysis (IR), ultraviolet spectral analysis (UV), and enantio-selective gas chromatography (ESGC) are other sophisticated tools to determine structural shapes of molecules. In the case of MS, molecules are bombarded with high energy electrons and burst into pieces. The pieces are then analyzed to determine the shape of the molecule from which they broke free. In the case of IR and UV spectral analysis, molecules are bombarded with infrared and/or ultraviolet light. By studying the wavelengths absorbed, information about the shape and structure of the molecule can be gleaned. NMR uses high energy magnetic fields to determine things like bonding angles in a molecule. ESGC provides a means of recognizing the relative abundances of various chiral isomers and is one of the principal ways labs can tell a synthetic oil from a natural one. (Chiral isomers are discussed in the next chapter.) Nature produces only certain isomers in certain ratios that labs generally cannot duplicate. ESGC can tell if an oil has a natural mix of isomers or one that could only have come from a lab.

The bottom line is that there has been an incredible amount of technological effort, mathematical deduction, intuition, serendipity, patience, money, and sweat that has gone into the determinations of the structural formulas we know today. The thousands of structural formulas catalogued in tomes like *The Handbook of Chemistry and Physics* and *The Merck Index* represent millions of hours over many decades by thousands of dedicated researchers and technicians the world over. This book owes a debt to all of these men and women who, for the most part, will never receive the credit they deserve.

God's Legos®

As we have said before, "essential oil chemistry can be summarized as simple hydrocarbons, oxygenated hydrocarbons, and their isomers." Now you know what hydrocarbons, oxygenated hydrocarbons, and isomers are and have seen examples of some of their possibilities.

We have learned that carbon compounds form the microskeletons of all organic molecules. Carbon can form long bones (chains) as well as a variety of hollow structures (rings). Attaching and arranging these skeletal elements in various ways, we have literally trillions of possibilities. There is plenty of flexibility and variability in the carbon atom to express every life form in all the detail, complexity, and individuality God may choose to manifest. Carbon atoms are God's Legos®.

Key Points of Chapter Six

1. When benzene was first isolated and its numerical formula was determined as C_6H_6 in the early 1800s, its structure remained a mystery for more than forty years.

2. The German scientist, August Kekule, was the first to solve the mystery of the benzene ring by insights he gained through a dream of dancing snakes.

3. Benzene rings are six sided polygons with a carbon at each corner and one hydrogen attached to each carbon.

4. Benzene (C_6H_6) is highly toxic and, as a compound, is not found in any essential oil, but as a functional group it is a structural component of numerous essential oil molecules in which form it is therapeutic and beneficial.

5. Carbon can also form 3-sided, 4-sided, 5-sided, 7-sided, 8-sided, 9-sided rings, and more.

6. Carbon rings are also called "aromatic" because they are so prevalent in natural fragrances, including essential oils. Because a compound contains "aromatic rings" does not always mean it has a detectable fragrance.

7. When carbon forms rings (or any other covalent bond) the electrons that were formerly associated with one specific atom become non-localized and can move within the molecule.

8. Non-localized electrons give a molecule resonance energy which is energy in excess of what the molecule would have had with localized electrons.

9. Organic molecules possess a spectrum of natural frequencies that come from their different bonds as well as their shape and structure.

10. One of the ways essential oils can heal is to elevate our bodily frequencies to healthy levels and tune us into harmony by sympathetic vibration or resonance.

11. Resonance is when two entities vibrate in unison. The healing vibrations of essential oils are transferred to us by resonance.

12. We hear the fundamental harmonic of a musical note as pitch, but we hear the other frequencies in that tone as timbre or color. In this way, we can distinguish different instruments playing the same pitch.

13. When something emits a spectrum of inharmonious frequencies, we say it is chaotic or incoherent. When something emits a spectrum of harmonious frequencies, we say it is ordered or coherent.

14. Therapeutic grade essential oils resonate with coherent frequencies which enables them to bring order back to a disordered, diseased body or mind.

15. The universe was spoken into creation by God and his vibrational words. What he has created is imbued with his consciousness and his Word.

16. In order to see God in his creation and to receive the blessings he has hidden in the things he has created, including essential oils, one must be receptive, i.e. they must be able to resonate at God's frequencies.

17. Those that are in tune (i.e. resonate) with God's creation see and experience him in everything everywhere. Experiencing life in this manner provides a solid and real basis for true faith.

18. Phenol is a compound comprised of a benzene ring (C_6H_6) with an attached hydroxyl radical (OH) with the formula C_6H_6O. Phenol is an alcohol with peculiar properties different than other alcohols. Phenol is an oxygenated hydrocarbon.

19. There are some oils containing minor portions of phenol as a compound, but no essential oil contains benzene as a compound. However, thousands of therapeutic molecules are contained in essential oils that incorporate a benzene or phenol molecule into their structure as a functional group.

20. Radicals are partial molecules that seek to unite with another group in order to complete the demands of their unfulfilled valence bonds. We have discussed hydroxyl, methyl, ethyl, propyl, and butyl radicals which form countless varieties of compounds in essential oils.

21. Functional groups are complete molecules that act as radicals in that they can unite with other groups or molecules to make new compounds. Benzene and phenol are both functional groups that form many different compounds in essential oils.

22. Compounds containing a benzene functional group (C_6H_6) or any other ring are called "aromatic." Every essential oil contains aromatic molecules.

23. Compounds containing a phenol functional group (C_6H_6O) are themselves called "phenols" or "phenolic." Essential oils with phenols are known for their antimicrobial properties as well as their support of the immune and nervous systems.

24. When a compound contains a phenol functional group (C_6H_6O) and also a propyl radical (C_3H_7), it is called a phenylpropanoid. Phenylpropanoids and other phenolic compounds cleanse receptor sites at cellular levels—an essential process for healing and maintaining health.

25. Oils rich in phenols and/or phenylpropanoids include thyme, oregano, clove, marjoram, cinnamon, cassia, calamus, fennel, anise, basil, and tarragon.

26. In the shorthand for reading and writing structural formulas for organic compounds, the symbols for C and H are omitted whenever possible.

27. In a structural formula, the number and locations of C atoms can be determined by the angles, conjunctions, intersections, and ends of lines or double lines,

28. The numbers and locations of H atoms in a molecular diagram can be deduced by the number of lines representing bonds that converge at any particular carbon site. The number of bonds plus the number of hydrogens at that point must always add up to 4.

29. It took humankind until the 19th century to figure out that the secret compounds of life are chains and rings. Man can try to imitate God's creations in factories and labs, but in the end, only God is Lord of the Rings. We must learn to respect that in order to receive their benefits.

♥ CHAPTER SEVEN
BIOCHEMISTRY
MADE EASY

There are an estimated 100 trillion cells in your body and each has six gigabytes of memory. That is more memory than all the computers in the world today. The intelligence of even a single cell is astronomical since every cell contains information on every other cell and part of the body. The fact that every cell contains a copy of the master DNA blueprint is the basis of cloning where a complete living animal, with all the diversity of its tissues and organs, can be generated from a single cell.

The aggregates of cells that form our bodies are like holograms. A hologram is an image of light that looks like a solid three-dimensional form, but it is just light projected into space that only appears to be solid. A hologram is truly three-dimensional in that one could walk completely around it and see every side of what appears to be a solid 3-D figure.

The most remarkable property of a hologram is that if you were to cut out a small piece of the holographic film, you could project another hologram from that piece complete in every detail, the same as the original. In fact, if you were to cut the film into 100 pieces, each piece would be capable of projecting every detail of the original uncut film.

This is because every part of a hologram contains the whole image of the projection just as every cell in your body contains the whole image of your body. In fact, there is a verse in the *Bible* where Jesus says, "If your eye be single, your whole body will be full of light." (Matthew 6:22) Is it possible that this enigmatic statement is a hint that we are, in fact, walking holograms of light, projected into a material universe? Projections of the light of God?

In fact, in Genesis 1:3-4, we are given more than a hint as to the nature of the universe. God's initial statement, speaking the worlds into existence, was "Let there be light."

Protons, neutrons, and electrons (i.e. the physical world of gross matter) came from light, the first manifestatioin of God's creation. It appears that underlying all material creation is a template of subtle light of which the physical is but a mirror and a reflection. Therefore, since every part of a hologram contains every part of the whole, when you touch one part of your body, you touch it all. Essential oils are captured photons of subtle light that address our holographic body on an energetic level, as well as chemical.

We will pursue this further in Part Three. If you want to read more, see Dr. Richard Gerber's wonderful book entitled, *Vibrational Medicine.* (See bibliography.) The point we want to make here is that our bodies are not what they appear to be and the amount of intelligence necessary to keep our bodies alive and smoothly functioning on a daily basis is beyond astronomical and beyond the physical.

100 Trillion Employees

If you consider your 100 trillion cells to be your employees who work for you and do your bidding, how is it that such a massive number of workers can function in harmony most of the time? Even when you are sick, over 90% of your body still functions as it should, keeping you alive and working to heal you. It is an amazing thing that there could be such harmony among so many. If only the six billion inhabitants of earth could live in such accord.

If you have ever been an employer or a supervisor of even a small number of workers you know that unless there is good communication between everyone with lines of responsibility clearly drawn—job descriptions clearly spelled out, and all tasks clearly assigned—there is chaos. When workers fail their assignments, the company also fails.

So how does your body keep 100 trillion employees so well coordinated that they can execute billions of complex life-sustaining functions continuously every day for a lifetime without us ever giving them the slightest thought? Part of the answer lies in biochemistry.

Is Biochemistry an Objective Science?

Mosby's Medical Dictionary defines biochemistry as "the chemistry of organisms and life processes." This is different from organic chemistry. As discussed in Chapter Four, organic chemistry was originally concerned with the compounds created by life processes, but not the processes themselves. Today, organic chemistry has been redefined as the study of carbon compounds whether originating from life processes or not.

In any case, organic chemistry is a laboratory science that studies compounds outside of a live environment. Biochemistry is a life science that studies live processes by which chemical compounds are created and employed by living organisms. Organic chemistry is the study of the chemical products of life in a lifeless environment while biochemistry is the study of chemical reactions in a living environment.

Hence, biochemistry is an incredibly more complex and difficult topic than organic chemistry because it is next to impossible to study a natural, undisturbed living process. The very act of trying to observe the chemical behavior of a live organism will disturb its natural course and alter the process so that what we record, in a scientific fashion, is not a true observation of untouched nature.

In other words, it is impossible for a biochemist studying a living process not to become part of the observation and experiment. Thus, the first rule of the scientific method, which says "the experimenter must be independent of the experiment and the observations made must be replicatable by others independent of who makes them," is broken by the very nature of the subject matter. In order to effectively find the answers they seek, biochemists must become intuitive scientists.

We will discuss the scientific method at greater length in Part Three, but for now our interest is in how essential oils participate as biochemical agents in our bodies. As for the biosynthesis of essential oil compounds in plants, the best resource I know of is in French, *L'Aromatherapie Exactement* by Franchomme and Penoel—both intuitive scientists.

How Cells and Organs Communicate

Our bodies have at least three internal communication systems: the nervous system, the endocrine system, and the cytokine network. When there is an urgent or simple task and one part of your body needs to communicate with another, messages are sent by wire. This is your nervous system. Call this your email system. It works very much like the internet.

For example, if you step barefooted on a sharp rock, your foot sends a message that reaches the muscles of your leg in a split second telling them to tense up and jerk your foot off the object of pain immediately. This is a simple situation requiring a simple motor command that was delivered by a simple electrical signal. But what if the message is more complex like, "digesting a pizza" or "processing a soda pop," "stopping a hemorrhage," "destroying a cluster of cancer cells," "fighting off a virus," "dealing with difficulties at work," "preparing to fight a bear," or "growing from a child to an adult?"

For these your body has other communication systems. When complex responses are required, messengers are actually dispatched between cells or body parts carrying coded information. Your endocrine system works this way. Call this your FedEx® system. The countless hormones and other ligands that circulate throughout your body are couriers that carry vital information from one organ to another in an elaborate system of intracellular communication. There are peptides, steroids, neurotransmitters, vitamins, enzymes, antibodies, and a variety of information carrying molecules employed by our bodies. Many of these are dispatched and coordinated by the endocrine glands of the body. As a group such molecules are called "ligands." Ligands can communicate through cell membranes and talk to the DNA.

The endocrine system consists of a finite set of organs called "ductless glands" that discharge hormones directly into the blood stream. The known endocrine organs are as follows: thyroid and parathyroid (in the throat area), hypothalamus, anterior pituitary, posterior pituitary, and pineal (in the brain), pancreas (just above the spleen on the front and left side of the abdomen), adrenal glands (just above the kidneys), and the gonads (ovaries in women or testes in men). The heart may also be an endocrine gland.

The secretions of endocrine glands are called "hormones." Hormones are only one of several types of ligands that serve to coordinate the myriad functions of the body.

The Cytokine Network

The body's third communication system is the cytokine network. The prefix "cyto" means "having to do with a cell," and the suffix "kine" is from the Greek word *kinein* which means "to move." We get our word "kinetic" from this Greek root. Cytokines are low-molecular weight proteins that act as intercellular messengers moving back and forth between cells on a continuous or as-needed basis—24 hours a day. There are countless millions of types of cytokines—enough to communicate whatever information is needed for cells to work together in cooperation, harmony, and synchronicity. Cytokines from mothers are passed to their babies through breastmilk and help build the infant's immunities.

In one way, the cytokine network operates like the endocrine system in that message-carrying molecules are sent back and forth between cells. The difference is that the cytokine network involves every cell in the body as a source of ligands. There are no specific glands or organs that can be seen, counted, or dissected in gross anatomy, as with the endocrine system. The cytokine network of bodily communication is invisible to the naked eye because it functions on a microscopic scale that only cells can see.

Another difference between the cytokine network and the endocrine system is that the ligands of the ductless glands work globally throughout the body via the circulatory system while the cytokine network works locally in the tissues between neighboring cells. Hormones can move rapidly from head to toe with a few beats of the heart, as anyone knows who has experienced a "rush of excitement" or felt the rapid flush of embarrassment or anger as one becomes "red in the face."

Since cytokines are not usually released directly to the blood stream (like hormones), they do not carry their messages far from their origins as hormones can. You might say that hormones are national government officials that deal with the whole country while cytokines are municipal, county, and state officials that deal with restricted regions of the country.

The cytokine network is not well understood by either scientists or physicians at this time. The study of its functions is a biochemical subspecialty called "cytochemistry" which must be carried out under a microscope. Since cytochemistry involves living processes, it's a nearly impossible task since to study any living process under a microscope is to disrupt its natural function and destroy its living environment. For instance, how does one observe kidney function at microscopic levels in a living human being?

The truths sought by cytochemists are, in fact, beyond the capability of present day scientific methods. Here is where intuitive science can come to the rescue. But as yet, intuitive science is not openly understood, practiced, or accepted by left-brained scientists. That deficiency in the development of scientific methodology is in the process of changing, as we speak. (See Part Three for more on this.)

So there you have it. Our 100 trillion cells, and the organs they comprise, work by at least three means of communication—nerves, endocrine glands, and cytokines. Essential oil molecules support, enhance, and mesh with all of these systems in ways that are beneficial physically, emotionally, and spiritually.

Who Controls the Biochemistry of Our Bodies?

It appears that most, if not all, cells participate in the cytokine communication network. At this time, cytokines are best known and best understood in their coordination of immune functions. Interleukins, interferons, and lymphokines are types of cytokines that manage the immune system. They train and direct B-cells, T-cells, and macrophages to search out and destroy hostile invaders such as viruses, bacteria, fungi, cancer cells, and alien proteins.

More than a dozen different interleukins have been identified. Interleukin 2 is the cytokine your body needs to instruct the immune system on how to recognize cancer cells and other enemies of physical wellbeing. Without interleukin 2, your phagocytes, B-cells and T-cells, which would normally attack and kill cancer cells, will misjudge them as friendly and allow them to live and multiply. Interleukin 2 levels are reduced with overproduction of cortisol, a necessary steroid hormone that regulates many bodily functions. The right amount of cortisol is healthy. Too much can lead to sickness and even death.

Overproduction of cortisol, and the concomitant reduction of interleukin 2, can result from a variety of emotional and spiritual factors. These include chronic anger, fear, anxiety, bitterness and stress around any issue. Attitudes of unforgiveness, revenge, hatred, repressed rage, a poor self image, or inability to deal with a significant loss or trauma can increase cortisol and reduce interleukin 2, thus setting up conditions favorable to cancer.

With a properly functioning immune system, getting cancer is impossible. God has given us control over our immune systems by how we think, feel, and live. The molecular and cellular activities in our bodies may be chemical, but control of that chemistry is ultimately in the spiritual nature of our lifestyles.

Here, again, because of the emotion–releasing qualities of essential oils, they can be of great assistance in getting at the true roots of diseases in general and cancer in particular. (See *New Insights into Cancer* by Wright, *Healing Oils of the Bible* by Stewart, and *Essential Oils Integrative Medical Guide* by Young, in the Bibliography.)

To Digest a Danish

So how does this all work? For example, how is it that when your eyes, your taste buds, and your olfactory nerves sense a hot sweet fresh cinnamon roll that they quickly inform your liver, pancreas, and salivary glands that they should prepare to deal with an onslaught of carbohydrates about to hit the tummy?

The system works like this. The organs of your brain (pituitary, hypothalamus, pineal gland, amygdala, diencephalon, etc.) release hormones among themselves in order to discuss the situation. Then one or more of these cerebral glands sends hormones to prepare the mouth and others to the liver which, in turn, sends other ligands to the pancreas, which then sends messengers back to the liver and to the stomach, the brain, the intestines, the heart, the lungs, etc. etc. Meanwhile, the cells within these various organs are engaged in continuous chatter, through their ceaselessly circulated cytokines, in order to assure the smooth and effective delivery of all necessary services, products, and functions. As a result of all of these memos and messages carried back and forth between organs and glands, your whole body gets ready to digest a sweet roll and will do so successfully in a manner that is highly coordinated and efficient. All the enzymes and digestive juices are called into place to make it happen, along with the necessary rhythmic contractions of the digestive tract to move the food along its way into and out of the body. Such coordination is communicated by hormones, cytokines, and other ligands of which your body creates untold thousands every day to fit every situation, as the needs arise.

The Hormonal Alphabet

One of the most interesting classes of hormones are the peptides. Peptides are chains of amino acids that form words and sentences that cells can understand. Peptides communicate through receptor sites and pass information through cell membranes to speak directly with the DNA. There are 20 amino acids utilized by the human body. Consider them as 20 letters of a molecular alphabet. The variety of messages that can be written by such an alphabet is without limit, numbering in gazillions. Just think how many words we have made in the English language with our simple 26-word alphabet. There is no limit. The only restriction with peptides is that the words, sentences, or phrases must be less than 100 characters each in order to maintain a size small enough to circulate through the body and reach the cells. When 100-200 amino acids are linked we call that a polypeptide, an intermediate substance on the way to becoming a protein. When more than 200 amino acid molecules join together we call that a protein. Even the smallest proteins are more than 1500-2000 amu in molecular weight, which is why they have no odor and cannot pass through the body like the molecules of essential oils. Short peptide chains carrying their messages pass through our bodies all the time, transferring information from one organ to another all day long.

While hormones may not travel with the speed of an electrical impulse, like the signals carried by nerves, they can still travel pretty fast. Just think how long it takes you to feel your temper rise when someone or some thing provokes you. That feeling of the rush of anger is the sweep of hormones through your body which, for some people, can travel from head to foot in seconds. If you want to dig into this fascinating field more deeply, the book, *Molecules of Emotion* by Candace Pert, Ph.D., is an excellent treatise on how hormones work as agents of communication throughout the body. (See bibliography.)

Receptor Sites Explained

The question is this: How does a hormone with a message intended for the thyroid or the heart, or any other body part, deliver its message to the right place? In other words, how does a hormone secreted directly into the blood stream migrate to the right organ and, in turn, be recognized, accepted, and understood by that organ as a legitimate courier of necessary information?

It works like this. On the surface of every cell are little portals or doors that allow message carrying ligands to pass or not pass. These are called receptor sites. There are thousands of these on each cell. Each door has a lock and only the right key will fit. Hormones carry keys that will fit only certain doors that belong only to the cells to which they are to deliver a message.

Once a hormone is released into the blood stream, it has to find the specific organ to which it has been addressed. Does the ligand have to search the whole body by trial and error to locate its intended destination? The answer is no. Ligands hum little songs and so do the cells or organs for whom they are intended—and the two songs are in phase and harmony with each other. When the free ligand circulating in the blood stream begins to resonate with the melody of its target tissue, it is drawn toward it so that it does not have to search the whole body to find its place. Ligands are vibrationally guided to their proper destinations, passing all other tissues on the way. If a ligand should approach the wrong cell, its key will fail to open the lock and the cell will direct it to go elsewhere. The ligand will then pass on, whistling its happy tune, until it finds a cell with music in harmony with its own. When the ligand has found its correct receiver, it opens the lock and passes information to the DNA, the intelligence of the cell.

At that point, the DNA may simply store the information for future use, write a ligand of response to be sent to some other part of the body, or it may take action, instructing its inner parts to manufacture various biochemicals, produce heat, turn on or shut down certain functions, assimilate nutrients, eliminate wastes, release antibodies, accelerate your heart rate, prepare your body to take flight, or engage in some other activity.

More Complex than a Major City

We won't be discussing the intricacies of intercellular activity very much in this book. Suffice it to say that what goes on inside of a cell is even more complicated that what goes on outside. We often see drawings of a "simple cell" as a bit of protoplasm with a nucleus and a few simple primitive organelles. Don't let these simple pictures fool you. Most human cells are so complicated that drawing a picture of all of their parts would be impossible.

The infrastructure of a single cell is more complex than that of a major city with all of its streets, bridges, railroads, pipelines, electric lines, phone lines, water pipes, sewer tunnels, factories, businesses, homes, parks, schools, fire stations, police stations, government offices, service agencies, libraries, and churches, etc. The intelligence and complexity of a human cell is even greater than we suggested at the beginning of this chapter. Scientists have barely scratched the surface of understanding the microbiology of inner cell activities.

As for now, let's focus mainly on what goes on between cells and outside of cells. They communicate by sending molecular messengers to each other. These messengers can be of a variety of molecules, including hormones and cytokines. A general term for information-carrying molecules is "ligand." Ligands carry keys that fit only the locks of the receptor sites on the cells to which they are intended to carry their messages. It only takes seconds for a burst of hormones to sweep through the body and find its intended destinations. Once the messages have been delivered, the body usually sends the spent hormones to the liver to be metabolized and eliminated through the colon, kidneys, sweat glands, and/or the lungs as the case might be. This is an ongoing process that takes place billions of times a day, whether waking or sleeping, every day of our lives. When such processes cease, we die.

Right and Left Handed Carvone

Shown below are two models of a compound called carvone. They are a pair of isomers—same formula, different structure. Notice where they are alike and where they are different. They are almost alike. Their difference is not great. Invisible (in chemical shorthand) at the end of the vertical line at the top of each hexagon is a CH_3 group. This is a methyl radical. Attached to the bottom of the ring is a 3-carbon chain with a CH_3 group on the single bond side and a CH_2 group on the double bond side. When combined with the C atom in the middle, you have a C_3H_5 group represented in scientific shorthand. This is a propyl radical. So we have a benzene ring with methyl at the top and propyl at the bottom. We could call this compound methylbenzylpropane, but it prefers to be called carvone.

Right and Left Handed Carvone • A Chiral Pair

Spearmint Oil
(*Mentha spicata* -
A Member of the
Mint Family)
45-55% l-carvone
$C_{10}H_{14}O$

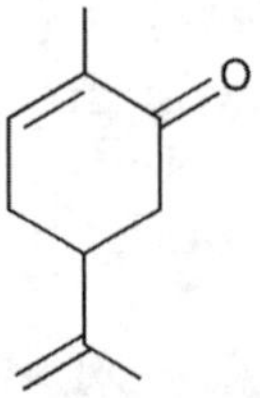

l-Carvone
(levorotary)
Left-Handed

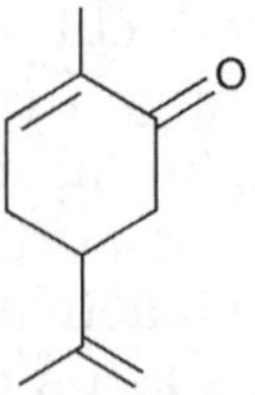

d-Carvone
(dextrorotary)
Right-Handed

Dill Oil
(*Anethum graveolens* -
A Member of the
Celery Family)
35-45% d-carvone
$C_{10}H_{14}O$

If you count up the C, H, and O atoms implied in the short-hand of these line drawings, you will get the formula $C_{10}H_{14}O$.

These compounds are definitely propanoids since they both incorporate a propyl radical. The propyl is also attached to a ring, like a phenylpropanoid. But this is not a phenylpropanoid because the ring has no OH radical attached. Without the OH the ring isn't a phenol. The double-bonded O makes it a ketone. We haven't mentioned ketones yet, but ketones have some properties that are the same as phenols, including the ability to cleanse receptor sites. We will learn about ketones in Chapter Ten. Ketones usually have interesting fragrances.

Dill Candy, Spearmint Pickles

Carvone can teach us something truly amazing about our bodies. The two molecules shown on the previous page have exactly the same chemical formula and are almost exactly the same in structure except for one thing. The propyl units hanging from the bottoms of the two rings are twisted 180° from one another. If you imagine that the double bond sides are fingers and the single bond sides are thumbs, then you can see a right hand and a left hand hanging down from each molecule with the thumbs facing inward.

Isomers such as these that come in right and left hand-ed pairs are called "chiral molecules." The term, chiral, comes from the Greek root, *cheir*, meaning "hand." From the same root we have the words, "chirographer," one skilled at handwriting, and "chiropractor," one who prac-tices therapy with their hands. The Latin prefixes "levo-" and "dextro-" (abbreviated l- & d-) mean "left" and "right," respectively. The "rotary" part refers to the way these mol-ecules are analyzed in polarized light where they are rotat-ed either left or right to distinguish the structures. That is a technical point beyond where we want to go in this book.

Now here is the amazing part. Your nose is so sensitive that it can tell which way the propyl unit is turned, right or left. Take a bottle of spearmint oil and one of dill and, without looking at the labels, see if you can tell the difference by smell alone. Of course you can. They don't smell anything alike. Would you like some spearmint pickles? Probably not. Would you like to chew some dill gum or eat dill candy for a breath freshener? I doubt it. Yet these flavors and aromas are from the same compound—carvone. The only difference is whether the double bond on the bottom points to the right or to the left.

So how is it that your nose and your taste buds are so smart that they can detect something so slight as the turn of a functional group on a molecule so small that even the most powerful microscopes can't see it? Here's how.

Your Amazing Receptor Sites

Your nose has millions of cells with billions of receptor sites, each designed to receive only certain molecules according to their shapes. Can you put a right hand into a left glove? Or vice versa? No. Not really. Likewise, you have receptor sites that accept only right-handed carvone (d-carvone) and those that accept only left-handed carvone (l-carvone). When the left-handed receptor sites are stimulated, they send a message back to the brain that says "spearmint." When the right-handed receptor sites are stimulated, they send the brain a message that says "dill." (It might say "caraway," too, since the composition of caraway oil [*Carum carvi*] is also about 40% d-carvone.) Thus, the detection, identification, and distinguishing of different oils by our brain and sensory systems is a biochemical process.

But how can such a slight difference in a molecule, like the simple turning of one part, make such a major difference? The taste and fragrance of spearmint and dill are not alike at all. No one would ever confuse the two. The therapeutic effects of these two oils are also quite different.

Dill oil is antispasmodic, antibacterial, an expectorant, and a stimulant. It was rubbed on the bodies of gladiators in Roman times because emotionally it reduced anxiety and nervousness so they would fight better. Dill may also help normalize insulin levels, lower glucose levels, promote milk flow in nursing mothers, and support pancreatic function. When diffused in combination with Roman chamomile it can help calm fidgety children. (Now, there's an idea for elementary teachers.)

Spearmint is anti-inflammatory, antiseptic, calming, stimulates the gallbladder, and promotes menstruation. It may also help with acne, soothe the intestines, help with depression, relieve sore gums, help bad breath, promote easier labor in childbirth, and assist in appetite control and weight loss. Spearmint may also help to open and release emotional blocks and bring about a feeling of balance and well-being.

You can see that the physical and emotional responses to d- and l-carvone are not the same. It is not only the receptor sites in our noses and taste buds that can readily tell the difference, there are receptor sites all over our bodies, in all the organs, that can respond to these oils. In all cases—whether it is the pancreas, the liver, the stomach, or the brain—your body can tell one carvone from the other and reacts differently to each.

It is interesting to note that monkeys and rats can also tell one carvone from another. Rats prefer d-carvone (dill) while monkeys prefer l-carvone (spearmint). How does this line up with your preferences?

It's Not Always the Main Ingredient

Of course, we cannot attribute all of the properties of dill and spearmint oils to carvone, even though it constitutes the main ingredient in both oils and is definitely responsible for their tastes and fragrances. Some of the differences and similarities of these two oils also have to do with the fact that they also contain well over 100 other compounds—including 15-25% d-limonene for both oils. Limonene has its own therapeutic properties.

Like carvone, limonene also comes as a chiral pair of isomers with d-limonene being the one found in citrus oils and l-limonene in the oils of evergreens. The fragrance of right-handed d-limonene is a very faint hint of fresh orange while that of left-handed l-limonene is a definite pine-like smell with a hint of mint. While the major contributor to both the fragrance and therapeutic action in dill and spearmint oils appears to be due to its main ingredient, carvone, we need only refer back to our example of grapefruit oil in Chapter Four where the major contributor to fragrance and therapeutic action was a trace compound and not the main ingredient.

Keys to the Heart of a Cell

Carvone is a small molecule. It's molecular weight is only 152 amu. The difference between l-carvone and d-carvone is only slight. So how does such a small difference in such a small entity evoke such a big difference in the responses of our body, mind, and emotions? Here's how.

Look at the drawings of the two keys shown below. They are almost identical, cut from the same master blank. But they aren't quite the same. Notice the tooth on the left key that is missing from the key on the right. Otherwise they are the same. Only one tooth difference. Will this slight difference in the keys make a difference in what they do? Absolutely. The one on the left may start the ignition to a brand new Lexus® automobile, open the door to a plush mansion, or fit a cash box with a million dollars, while the other one may fit in the same locks, it won't turn or open them. Let's say that the key on the right fits an old farm tractor that no longer runs, or turns the lock on an empty tool shed, or opens a box full of rubber bands and rusty paper clips. See what a slight difference can make in two nearly identical keys.

The point is this. The tiniest difference in a key completely alters what it will or will not open. It is the same with the two carvone molecules. One is left-handed, the other right. Can you put your left hand into a right hand glove? Not very well. Yet the two gloves of a pair are almost

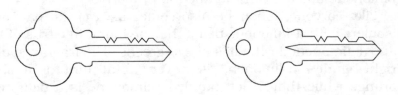

Will These Two Keys Open the Same Locks?

identical except that they are mirror images of one another to match the mirror images of our hands.

Chiral molecules, like l- and d-carvone, are also mirror images. The difference in them is slight, but they turn entirely different locks to entirely different sets of organs and tissues. L-carvone communicates with the cells of the pancreas and other organs that have to do with sugar metabolism as well as the glands of lactation in nursing mothers. D-carvone communicates to the cells of the gall bladder, the intestines, and the uterus.

Essential oil molecules are biochemical agents that act like ligands—messengers of information that gravitate to the places in our bodies where their information or presence can be of beneficial use. In this capacity, they can play the roles of hormones, peptides, steroids, neurotransmitters, vitamins, enzymes, cytokines, or antibiotics. They can be balancing, rejuvenating, stimulating, energizing, calming, restoring, facilitating, cleansing, immunizing, detoxifying, mood elevating, soothing, healing, emotionally releasing, and spiritually uplifting depending on what receptor sites they open and what we may have stored in that body region in the form of diseases, toxins, microbes and blocked feelings. Essential oils carry intelligence. They have a life force that goes beyond chemistry. Essential oils molecules are remarkably compatible with human tissue.

More Examples to Play With

If you had a bottle of spearmint and one of dill or caraway and smelled them during the discussion we just had, you had to be impressed how easily your body could tell which way the propyl radical was turned on the carvone molecule—whether to the left or to the right. That is incredibly sensitive. Now you understand how that can be. Either the key fits or it doesn't. One way it slips into the lock and turns easily. The tiniest change and it might not even slide into the keyhole, much less be able to turn the tumblers. The carvone keys that fit the locks on the spearmint receptor sites stimulate those sites and only those sites while the carvone keys that fit the locks on the

Similar Shapes, Different Fragrances

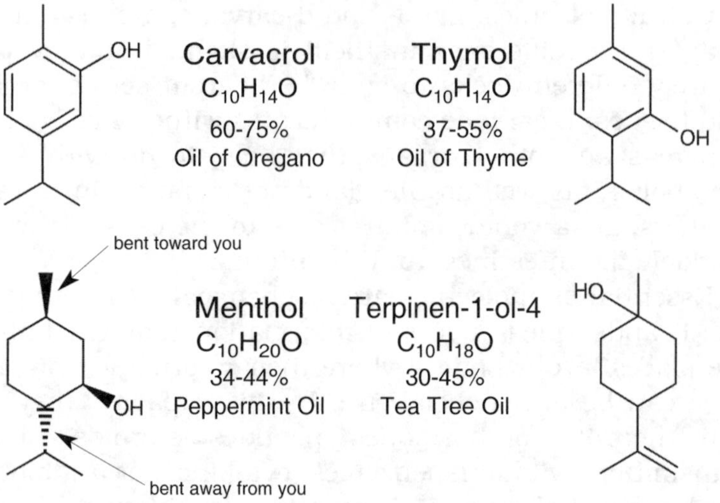

OH **Carvacrol**   **Thymol**
    $C_{10}H_{14}O$ $C_{10}H_{14}O$
    60-75%   37-55%
    Oil of Oregano   Oil of Thyme   OH

bent toward you

        Menthol   **Terpinen-1-ol-4**   HO
        $C_{10}H_{20}O$ $C_{10}H_{18}O$
        34-44%   30-45%
OH   Peppermint Oil   Tea Tree Oil

bent away from you

dill or caraway sites stimulate only those. So your brain receives either one or the other unequivocally. No confusion. It's either spearmint or it isn't.

Shown above are structural diagrams of four molecules. Each is the principle ingredient in a common essential oil: Carvacrol found in oregano (*Origanum compactum*), thymol in thyme (*Thymus vulgaris*), menthol in peppermint (*Mentha piperita*), and terpinen-1-ol-4 in tea tree (*Melaleuca alternifolia*). Right now is a good time to get out bottles of these, if you have them on hand. Sniff each oil and note how well your nose can discern their distinctive odors. (Note: The numbers in the name, terpinen-1-ol-4, identify C atoms where radicals are attached. See numbered template shown later in this chapter. This compound is also called terpinen-4-ol and/or β-terpineol.)

Note the similarity of the shapes of these four molecules, yet your nose knows the difference. What you are smelling in every case are hexagonal rings with a hydroxyl radical (OH) on the side and a propyl radical (C_3H_7) or (C_3H_5) attached to the bottom.

The only difference between carvacrol and thymol is where the OH is connected. Both are phenylpropanoids.

These two are isomers of one another—same formula, different shape ($C_{10}H_{14}O$). Notice that carvone, discussed a few pages back, is an isomer of carvacrol and thymol. Carvone has the same formula ($C_{10}H_{14}O$), but carvone is not a phenol and neither carvacrol nor thymol smell anything like dill or spearmint. Neither do oregano and thyme smell exactly alike. Oregano has a strong, spicy odor (like pizza) while thyme smells mildly herbaceous.

Raindrop facilitators pouring these two oils from a bottle through a dropper cap, have probably noticed that the viscosity of oregano seems to be greater than that of thyme, even though carvacrol and thymol have the same chemical formula. It is common for isomers to have different boiling points, densities, and other physical characteristics even though they have the same molecular weights. As phenols, both carvacrol and thymol are strong antiseptics. In fact, thyme oil is one of the strongest natural antiseptics known and is able to kill over 60 different strains of bacteria, including anthrax. Such an oil in a mouth-could be a great deterrent for tooth and gum disease, as well as flus and the common cold. Unfortunately, most people just won't take the thyme.

Now look at menthol and thymol. They both have their OH radicals attached to the same position, yet they don't smell alike at all. The main difference is that thymol is a flat molecule while the functional groups attached to the aromatic ring in menthol are bent in and out at 90° angles. Peppermint has a strong pleasant minty fragrance while thymol smells more like strong medicine. Tea tree, on the other hand, has its OH attached at the top and has yet another fragrance. See if you can distinguish these four oils with your eyes closed. The differences are determined by which olfactory receptor sites are engaged.

Menthol: The Bent Key

The menthol molecule is interesting. Notice in the diagram in the previous figure that it has no double bonds. The aromatic rings of both carvacrol and thymol have three double bonds. Terpinen-1-ol-4 has one double bond shown in the lower right leg of the propyl group hanging below the ring. Molecules with double bonds are said to be "unsaturated." They have the potential to hold more hydrogens, but don't. When there are no double bonds at all, we say the molecule is "saturated." Saturated hydrocarbons have all the hydrogen atoms they can hold. They are said to be completely "hydrogenated."

Menthol is a saturated essential oil compound. It holds 20 H atoms. Carvacrol or thymol each hold only 14. Terpinen-4-ol is partially saturated (partially hydrogenated) with 18 H atoms. But the distinct fragrance of menthol, which is the identifying feature of peppermint and the smell we associate with innumerable medications containing it, is due to more than its hydrogen saturation.

Note the different symbols in the menthol diagram. The one at the top and the one on the side connecting the OH are both solid black and tapered with the widest end away from the ring. This is chemical shorthand for "bent towards you." The striped symbol connecting the propyl radical at the bottom and tapered with the smallest end away from the ring is shorthand for "bent away from you." These symbols make it possible to represent a three-dimensional molecule on two-dimensional paper.

Hence, the main difference between menthol and the other molecules shown is the fact that the top and side legs of menthol are bent at right angles toward you while the bottom leg is bent 90° into the page. There is a big difference in the fragrance and qualities of menthol when compared to thymol or terpinenol. You would never confuse peppermint oil for tea tree or thyme.

If you think about the keys shown a couple of pages back and realize that each of these molecules is a key that fits only certain receptor sites, then you can understand why bending a part of a key would make such a dramatic difference. The bent key (menthol) would fit totally different locks than the unbent keys (carvacrol, thymol, and terpinen-1-ol-4), even though they are all basically the same shape, cut from the same blank. It is amazing that our sense of smell can so easily tell the bent from the unbent when we are talking about dimensions so small that even the most powerful microscopes cannot see them.

If you want to practice reading structural diagrams, try to deduce the formulas for the four molecules shown in the last figure. The chemical formulas are given, so you already have the answers. Just see if you can come up with the same answers.

Synthetic vs. Natural Menthol

Menthol provides us with a good example of the difference in a synthetic molecule and one produced by nature. The chemical formula for menthol is $C_{10}H_{20}O$. There are actually 19 known isomers of this formula: 14 alcohols, 3 ketones, and 2 aldehydes. Two of these isomers are a chiral pair: l-menthol and d-menthol. The full IUPAC scientific name of l-menthol is 5-methyl-2-isopropylcyclohexanol while that of d-menthol is 3-methyl-6-isopropylcyclohexanol. Personally, I prefer simple l- and d-menthol.

The menthol manufactured by the living peppermint plant (and a number of other plants) is entirely levorotary (left-handed). Its proper short name is l-menthol and is known by a sharp penetrating cold odor that will clear your nose and chest of congestion. The dextrorotary or right handed version, d-menthol, is not produced by any plant. It is not a natural substance. It has a mild woody odor, not at all like l-menthol, and has no decongesting properties. The two menthols (l & d) are shown below.

Drug companies don't like natural products because they cannot be patented (giving them a monopoly). Neither

Right and Left Handed Menthol

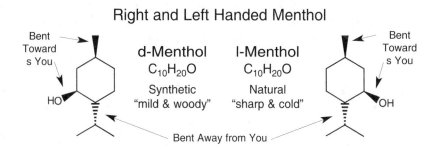

Bent Toward s You

HO

d-Menthol
$C_{10}H_{20}O$
Synthetic
"mild & woody"

l-Menthol
$C_{10}H_{20}O$
Natural
"sharp & cold"

Bent Toward s You

OH

Bent Away from You

can they be mass produced at will. When you grow something, it takes time and you have to conform to nature's
schedule to produce it. Drug companies like synthetics
where they can control everything, including their production schedule and the price.

The problem with trying to synthesize a pure isomer
(like l-menthol) is that it is not easily done in a laboratory
and, in many cases, technologically impossible. Most of
the time, producing an isomerically pure substance
requires the intelligence and participation of a living
organism, like a live plant. When a laboratory tries to
make l-menthol, the result is a mixture of equal parts of
both l- and d-menthol. Chemists call these "racemic mixtures."

Synthetic menthol is commercially produced by taking
a thymol molecule $C_{10}H_{14}O$ (see previous figure), bending
the functional groups at right angles, and saturating the
aromatic ring with six additional hydrogen atoms. This will
result in a compound with the formula, $C_{10}H_{20}O$, which is
the same as l-menthol, but you won't have just l-menthol.
You will have a racemic mixture, which, at best, is only
half l-menthol. And if the lab is not careful, you may even
get some of the other 17 isomers of $C_{10}H_{20}O$ in the mix,
which can include some potentially toxic ketones and
aldehydes. The bottom line is this: If you want the safe,
therapeutic form of menthol in pure form, you must allow
nature to make it in its own time and own way, through
plants. Man and his devices cannot do it.

So when you purchase a product with synthetic menthol, it will contain molecules of l-menthol structured like
the natural levorotary (left) isomer, but it will also contain
molecules of the unnatural dextrorotary (right) isomer
and, perhaps, some of the other isomers of this formula.

Here is the problem. We have receptor sites that can
accept and respond positively to l-menthol, while we do
not have receptor sites that fit d-menthol. Molecules for
which we have no suitable receptor sites cannot be utilized
without side effects, are impossible to metabolize, are dif-

ficult to eliminate, and can gradually accumulate as toxins that lead to disease. Our bodies have problems with all synthetic molecules that do not exist in nature. God did not create our bodies to deal with them.

This is yet another illustration of what happens when commercial enterprises try to substitute an artificial substance for a natural one, and then claim that they are "the same." Manufacturers can state, accurately, that the two menthols have the same formula. They are isomers, but they cannot truthfully claim that the two menthols (one pure levo-, the other a mixture of the two) have the same reactions and benefits in our bodies. They don't. In fact, in the presence of synthetic d-menthol, even l-menthol does not react with our bodies in the same beneficial ways as when it acts alone without the influence and interference of molecular misfits and mischief makers.

Either Ether Will Do

Let's practice our olfactory skills on another pair of compounds before we move on. Phenols are hydrocarbons containing a phenol molecule (C_6H_6O). Phenolic compounds are found in essential oils in a variety of forms, not just as phenylpropanoids. All phenols have the ability to cleanse receptor sites and fight bacteria and viruses. They are also powerful antioxidants that eat up free radicals in our bodies. protecting us from aging and degenerative disease.

Shown below are a pair of isomers of a phenolic ether. One is called anethole, the other estragole. (The names of

Anethole and Estragole: Same but Different

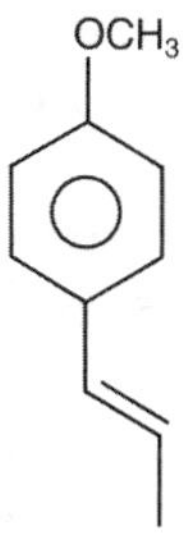

OCH₃	Anethole $C_{10}H_{12}O$	Estragole $C_{10}H_{12}O$	OCH₃
	60-80% Oil of Fennel	75-80% Oil of Basil	
	85-95% Oil of Anise	68-80% Oil of Tarragon	

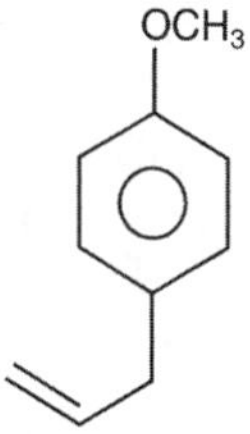

ethers often end in -ole, which we will discuss in Chapter Ten.) These two are isomers—both with the formula $C_{10}H_{12}O$—but they are not a chiral pair. Their only difference is in the angle at which the propyl radical (C_3H_5) is attached at the bottom. Anethole is the main ingredient in the oils of fennel (*Foeniculum vulgare*) and anise (*Pimpinella anisum*). Estragole (also called "methyl chavicol") is the main ingredient in the oils of basil (*Ocimum basilicum*) and tarragon (*Artemisia dracunculus*). The "methyl" of methyl chavicol (estragole) is written explicitly at the side of the O atom as CH_3. As you can see, anethole also has a methyl radical bonded to the O.

If you have any of these oils on hand, get them out and test their fragrances. See if you can tell fennel and anise from basil and tarragon with your eyes closed. Besides the change in position of the double bond, the only other difference in these two molecules is the way the propyl chain is bent, one pointing down, the other twisted to the left. Your nose knows. There is also a little anethole in tarragon. Your nose can tell basil from tarragon this way. These are not the only isomers of $C_{10}H_{12}O$, but are the ones most common to essential oils.

The fact that fennel and anise are both mostly composed of the same ether (anethole), makes them interchangeable in the practice of aromatherapy. The same goes for basil and tarragon, both being largely composed of the same ether (estragole). If you don't have one, but have the other, simply substitute. Either ether will do.

Basil and tarragon are both excellent antispasmodic oils, relaxing to muscles both voluntary and involuntary. They are both antiseptic and antibacterial. Their other ingredients make them somewhat different, however. Tarragon is good for hiccups, allergies, sciatica, and premenstrual pain while basil is a decongestant (because of its 1,8 cineole content) and supports the prostate. Basil can help restore a lost sense of smell, cleansing the receptor sites of the nose. Basil has also been used in Europe for migraines, in India to repel evil spirits, and by women in Italy to attract men.

While predominantly composed of anethole, fennel and anise both also contain 2-5% estragole—the dominant ingredient in basil and tarragon. But the actions of fennel and anise are not like basil nor tarragon. Fennel and anise are both antiseptic and antispasmodic. Fennel stimulates estrogen production, facilitates birthing, increases lactation, promotes digestion, and supports pancreatic function. It also expels worms and parasites. Anise is a diuretic and a stimulant.

So we can see from this example that different isomers of the same compound do different things biochemically in our bodies. We also see that oils that are largely made of the same identical compound may behave similarly, but have their differences due to the other ingredients they don't share. Even so, knowing a little chemistry will enable you to use one oil in place of another when you don't have the one you want on hand.

If you want to practice reading the structural diagrams for anethole or estragole, count 4 hydrogens hidden in the ring and see if you get the answers shown in the drawings.

Useful Eugenol

Before we move on, there is one more important phenol we should consider. Eugenol—$C_{10}H_{12}O_2$. Comparing the picture below with that of anethole and estragole on the shown earlier, notice the similarity between eugenol, anethole and estragole. All three have an OCH_3 group attached to an aromatic ring, except that eugenol has it in a different place. All three have a propyl radical hanging from the

Eugenol
$C_{10}H_{12}O_2$

Clove Oil	Syzygium aromaticum	75-80%
Cinnamon Oil	Cinnamomum verum	20-30%
Basil Oil	Ocimum basilicum	2-10%
Bay Laurel Oil	Laurus nobilis	3-9%
Rose Oil	Rosa damascena	1-2%
Ylang Ylang Oil	Cananga odorata	0-2%

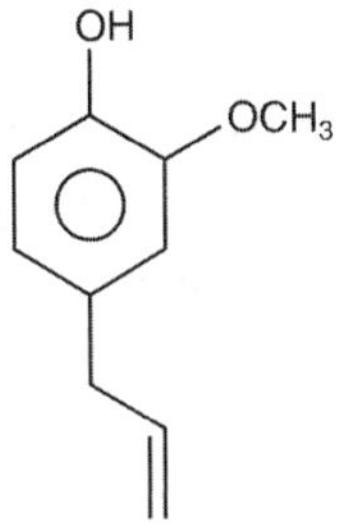

bottom except that eugenol has it hanging straight down like anethole but with the double bond at the end like estragole. The main difference is an extra atom of O at the top making it a phenolic alcohol. Eugenol is a phenyl-propanoid with many wonderful attributes.

Clove contains more eugenol (75-80%) than any other oil. However, clove's characteristic fragrance is not principally due to eugenol but to a saccharide comprising less than 0.1%—methyl-n-amyl ketone. Beside adding a spicy note to the sweet floral fragrances of rose and ylang ylang, eugenol has many unique therapeutic properties. It is highly antimicrobial, antiseptic, and is the most powerful antioxidant known. Jean Valnet, M.D., a French physician who has been called the father of modern aromatherapy, reported that he had found clove beneficial for a variety of purposes including the prevention of contagious disease, arthritis, bronchitis, cholera, amoebic dysentery, diarrhea, tuberculosis, acne, halitosis, headaches, insect bites, nausea, skin cancer, mouth sores, warts, and lymphoma.

The natives of Ternate, an island of Indonesia in the South Pacific, were free from epidemics until the 16th century when Dutch explorers destroyed the clove trees that had grown there in abundance. Many of the islanders died from the diseases that followed because their protector, the clove tree, had been annihilated.

Eugenol's most notable property is as a topical anesthetic. Oil of clove has been used by dentists for centuries to numb gums. Today, 65% of the world's supply of cloves is ground and mixed with tobacco in cigarettes to numb the tongue and "take the bite" out of smoking tobacco.

Blank Master Keys

When you lose the key to your car, you go to the hardware store to have another one made. They will ask you the brand, year, and model of your car and then locate a blank key that fits your ignition. As a blank key, it will slip into the lock of every car of that year and model, but it won't turn until notches are cut to match the tumblers of a particular ignition switch. Countless keys to fit countless vehicles can be cut from the same blank. A blank key is

Templates for Keys: Molecular and Mechanical

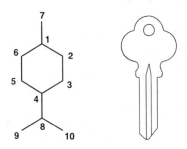

shown above, on the right, ready to be customized to fit any car of your choice.

You probably noticed that the structural diagrams of p-cuminol, carvone, carvacrol, thymol, terpinen-4-ol, and menthol were all similar in shape—like the molecular model next to the key shown above. The molecular shape shown there is a blank master key for countless essential oil molecules that act as ligands (chemical keys) to open or activate specific receptor sites in the cells of plants and people. As you will see throughout this book, this molecular key pattern occurs repeatedly in the structuring of essential oil molecules.

There are ten carbon atoms in this skeletal frame. Because of its frequent occurrence, numbers have been assigned to identify the individual carbons in this structure. The numbers shown by each carbon site are the identifiers for those atoms. These are the numbers you see incorporated into the scientific names of organic compounds to tell you where the methyl, propyl, hydroxyl, oxygen atoms, and other functional groups are attached.

For example, back in Chapter Five we introduced you to p-cumenol (australol), the simplest of phenylpropanoids. Its scientific name is 4-isopropylphenol. The structural formula for cumenol is revealed through its scientific name which, being translated, means that a propyl radical has been attached to C #4 of a phenol molecule. "Iso" means that the propyl (carbons 8, 9 & 10) was attached at the middle C (#8) dangling like a little coat hanger below the ring. Carbon #7, at the top, usually holds three H atoms, making it a "methyl radical" most of the time. Oxygens can be attached to any of the ten carbons in various ways to form different compounds.

Numbering carbons is particularly useful in distinguishing various isomers one from another. There are other blank keys for other families of molecules besides the one just given. Each has their own assigned numbering system. All you need to know is that when you see numbers in the name of an organic compound, they reveal the configuration of the molecule to those who know how to read them. We will refer to this numbered figure again when we get to Chapter Ten, but that is as far as we will go with organic chemistry numbering systems in this book.

Serenades to Cells

"Ligand" is a general term for information carrying molecules that can communicate through receptor sites on the surfaces of cells. We have described ligands as biochemical messengers with keys that open locks of receptor sites. A biochemical messenger, like a hormone or cytokine, will carry only the key that fits the body part for which it is intended. This is how they act at the right place with the right information. Other information containing molecules include vitamins, enzymes, and antibodies.

We have seen that the molecules of essential oils can also behave like ligands, opening certain receptor sites and administering to various organs and body parts. The keys we have used to illustrate our point were mechanical—a piece of precisely shaped metal designed to turn tumblers in a mechanical lock—like a car key in an ignition switch. But the keys carried by ligands and essential oils are not mechanical and neither are the locks on the receptor sites. They are sonic and electromagnetic. They don't work by mechanics. They work by vibrations.

Ligand keys are more like the magnetized plastic cards issued by hotels that let you into your room. Your key opens only your room, and perhaps the back door and a few other places in the hotel, but will not open anyone elses room. Ligands are like that, too. They may have the ability to access more than one type of cell or organ, but none of them are master keys that open everything, like the key of the hotel manager. When you insert the key to open a hotel room door, the lock listens to the magnetic message and either accepts or rejects it. In a similar way, a ligand attaches itself to a receptor site which listens to the message and accepts or rejects it. Thus, a magnetic plastic hotel key is a better analogy for ligands and receptor sites than a hard metal key.

In reality, the cells throughout your body respond to electricity, magnetism, light, and sound as various forms of vibration delivered by a hormone, enzyme, cytokine, vitamin or other ligand. When a peptide or steroid or any other ligand visits a cell with the intent of delivering information to or evoking a response from the DNA inside, it must persuade the receptor site guarding the door to open and allow it to pass. The ligand does so by "singing" a sequence of tones, vibrations, or electromagnetic frequencies. If they resonate in a way that is pleasing to the sentinel at the receptor site, it will smile, open, and invite the ligand to come in and do business. If the little song sung by the ligand does not resonate and the receptionist at that cellular site is not pleased, the site remains closed, signaling the ligand to move on to another place.

Look at it this way. Instead of our organs, tissues, cells, proteins, enzymes, and ligands speaking their lines to one another as in a play, they sing their conversations to one another as in a grand opera. Our bodies are, thus, seen to be works of choral and symphonic beauty, composed and conducted by God, himself.

How Enzymes Work

It is not just the chemistry of a molecule that enables it to open receptor sites and communicate with cellular intelligence. It is the more subtle electromagnetic properties of the molecule that actually transmit the message. This subtle energy is the basis of homeopathy. This is also the means by which enzymes work.

Chemists have always been puzzled over catalysts and enzymes, because these are molecules that have to be present for certain chemical reactions to take place, but don't actually participate in the reaction and are not altered or consumed by it. The thousands of enzymes that work in our bodies are long-term residents, presiding over many processes—digestion, assimilation, regulating body temperature, combating disease, detoxification, management of sperm and egg, etc. Enzymes are engaged in the production of countless hormones and other ligands.

Enzymes are the supervisors of biochemistry. They are biochemical managers. Just as the executives of a company don't actually do the work, their direction and oversight are necessary for the corporate mission to be accomplished smoothly, efficiently, and properly. You can't have just workers. You must also have leaders. Enzymes communicate instructions that other molecules follow to create the biological products and tissues our body needs to function. While standing by to oversee a biochemical process in our bodies, the enzymes croon melodies to the working molecules. When they sing the right songs, on key and in tune, the molecules and cells of our bodies do the right things and keep us healthy. Like directors of a choir, enzymes lead the cells, the molecules, and the functions of our bodies to sing songs together, in the proper tempos, rhythms, and harmonies to make good music. Without intelligent direction and leadership at molecular and atomic levels, our bodies would be full of noise, not music. Dissonance leads to disease.

Therapeutic grade essential oils serenade your cells with songs they want to hear, bringing relief and healing in thousands of ways. They vibrate in tune with your body and its needs, balancing and restoring natural function. Their molecules were made to resonate with your receptor sites. That is how they work and why they work so well, not only on the physical plane, but the mental, emotional, and spiritual as well. That is why aromatic oils have been used throughout the world in the practice of medicine, religion, and daily living for thousands of years. Aromatherapy is a lost art and science whose time has returned.

Conclusion

In Biblical account of creation, God created plants on the third day and human beings on the sixth day. (Genesis 1:11-31) The geologic account of creation postulates the same order events in that plants appeared on earth first, long before people. The molecules of essential oils fit our bodies so well that I can only conclude that he created them with foresight of what we, his children, would eventually need. He knew, before we were ever born, that we would not always follow his health laws of proper exercise, right eating, positive thinking, and spiritual attunement with him and his plans for us.

God knew we would need medicines from time to time. So he created them for us and then gave us a brain and the freedom to find them and figure them out. The molecules of essential oils, crafted by God in the plants he provided for us, tell me that he loved us before he ever created us. That is why the subtitle of this book is "God's Love Manifest in Molecules."

Key Points of Chapter Seven

1. Biochemistry is the study of compounds and chemical processes in living organisms.

2. Organic chemistry studies compounds created by living organisms, but not while the organisms are still living.

3. Today, organic chemistry is the study of carbon compounds whether originating from a life process or not.

4. There are 100 trillion cells in the body and each has six gigabytes of memory.

5. Cellular activities are coordinated by two systems of intercellular communication: Our nervous system and our endocrine system.

6. The nervous system operates by electrical impulses that travel from one body part to another carrying simple information, like email on the internet.

7. The endocrine glandular system operates by sending messengers (called ligands) from one body part to another carrying complex information, like packets delivered by a FedEx® courier.

8. The cytokine network operates by sending information carrying proteins (called ligands) between cells to facilitate intercellular communication.

9. Cytochemistry is a subspecialty of biochemistry that studies the intercellular communication chemistry of cells at microscopic levels.

10. Besides their other properties, essential oil molecules behave like ligands, carrying information to cells, communicating with cellular DNA, in order to bring balance, wellness, and healing.

11 Receptor sites are the doorways on the surfaces of cells through which ligands communicate to the DNA inside.

12. Receptor sites have locks that can be opened only by the right keys. The right ligands and essential oil molecules carry keys that fit only certain cells. This is how hormones and other ligands get to the right places and deliver the right messages.

13. Receptor sites are so sensitive they can detect the most minute differences in a molecule.

14. The chiral pair of isomers, l-carvone and d-carvone, which characterize the oils of spearmint and dill, respectively, illustrate the incredible sensitivity of the receptor sites in our noses.

15. Chiral pairs of isomers are like right and left handed gloves, where the molecules are mirror images of one another and fit entirely different receptor sites with different consequences to our bodies.

16. Menthol is another molecule that comes as a chiral pair. l-menthol is natural. d-menthol is synthetic. Our bodies respond to l-menthol in a positive way, but are not made to handle d-menthol.

17. Just as hardware stores will have a supply of blank keys from which to customize keys to all makes and models of cars, plants also create a supply of blank structural forms from which to customize all manner of molecules.

18. One of the most popular blank keys in molecular biology consists of ten carbon atoms in a structural arrangement with a single C at the top of a hexagonal ring and a chain of 3 Cs attached at the bottom.

19. This particular 10-C blank key has numbers assigned (from 1 to 10) to identify each C atom in the structure. This is useful in writing scientific names for the various compounds and isomers that can be made from this common molecular form.

20. There are many other blank keys in organic chemistry and each has its own numbering system.

21. When you see numbers incorporated into the names of organic compounds, these reveal where the various radicals or functional groups are attached.

22. The manner by which ligands open receptor sites has been compared to a mechanical key. A better analogy would be the magnetic keys used in hotels.

23. Neither ligands nor receptor sites operate mechanically. They operate by vibrations of electricity, magnetism, light, and sound.

24. Hormones, vitamins, enzymes, cytokines, and other message carrying molecules may be said to sing to our cells to communicate their information.

25. Plants, and their oils, were created before people, and the molecules of essential oils fit our bodies so well that it seems that God created them with us in mind, foreseeing that we would need medicines from time to time.

26. Therefore, I can only conclude that God loved us before he ever created us. This is why the subtitle of this book is "God's Love Manifest in Molecules."

❤ CHAPTER EIGHT
CHEMOTYPES &
ENVIRONMENTAL FACTORS

An essential oil of a single plant species typically contains 100 to 400 different chemical compounds. As for essential oils in general, there are thousands of different chemical compounds to be found among them. Because many of these constituents are in trace amounts, there has never been even one essential oil completely analyzed. Thus, the notion of synthetically manufacturing a complete essential oil is out of the question. Chemists have yet to account for all of the ingredients in even one bottle of even one species.

For example, attempts to completely determine the composition of orange oil (*Citrus sinensis*) have, thus far, found 36 different terpenoids, 34 alcohols, 30 esters, 20 aldehydes, 14 ketones, 10 carboxylic acids, plus flavonoids, carotenoids, steroids, coumarins, and a variety of saccharides (sugars). There are more than 150 known constituents. Researchers suspect there may be as many as 200 additional compounds in orange oil in traces as yet to be identified.

Lavender (*Lavandula angustifolia*) is another good example of a thoroughly studied, thoroughly analyzed oil whose constituents have yet to be all discovered. So far chemists have identified more than 50 monoterpenes, at least 10 sesquiterpenes, 10-15 alcohols, 10-15 esters, and at least 5 oxides, 5 aldehydes, 5 ketones, and 5 lactones. There are over 200 known compounds identified so far and scientists suspect that this is only half of the constituents present in lavender.

There are no simple essential oils. They are all complex. While certain compounds are found in many plant oils, like pinene, limonene, and 1,8 cineole, there are many compounds unique to a specific plant and found nowhere else. These include santalol (found only in sandalwood oil), vetivone (found only in vetiver oil), and aristoladiene (found only in spikenard oil). Every plant makes a few compounds unique to itself, unmanufactured by any other.

While there are always seasonal variations in the production of an oil such that no two year's crops will produce identically the same oil, the chemical composition of an essential oil is relatively constant within a single botanical species. However, with some plants significant variations in chemical composition can occur in response to different growing conditions for the same species.

Oils from the same species that have significantly different compositions in response to environmental factors are called "chemotypes." Before we go any further, however, let's define what we mean by "species."

Botanical Families of Oil-Bearing Plants

Plants are classified by botanists into broad categories called "families" according to common visual characteristics. There are hundreds of such families into which the flora of the world are grouped. The Latin names of botanical families are capitalized in regular face type and all end in -ae. In some cases, two different names for the same family are in usage. The most common families of plants that produce essential oils are as follows:

Annonaceae	Ylang ylang family
Apiaceae (or Umbelliferae)	Celery/Carrot/Parsley
Araceae	Cane family
Asteraceae (or Compositae)	Aster/Daisy family
Ericaceae	Heather family
Burseraceae	Frankincense/Myrrh
Cistaceae	Cistus family
Cupressaceae	Cypress family
Geraniaceae	Geranium family
Gramineae (or Poaceae)	Grass family
Lamiaceae (or Labiatae)	Mint family
Lauraceae	Laurel family
Malvaceae	Hibiscus family

Myristicaceae	Nutmeg family
Myrtaceae	Myrtle family
Oleaceae	Olive family
Pinaceae	Pine family
Piperaceae	Pepper family
Rosaceae	Rose family
Rutaceae	Citrus family
Valerianaceae	Valerian family
Zingiberaceae	Ginger family

The family of plants that produces the most chemotypes (variations in oil compositions within the same species) is Lamiaceae (or Labiatae)—the Mint Family. Plants produce chemotypes as an adaptation to survive in a variety of different environments. Some plants are adaptable and some are not. Some species can live in only one special environment, like frankincense and myrrh, while others can grow almost anywhere. The large variety of chemotypes produced by the mints is evidence of their ability to live under a wide range of soil types and environmental conditions. Here are some oil producing members of the mint family:

Basil	(*Ocimum basilicum*)
Clary Sage	(*Salvia sclarea*)
Hyssop	(*Hyssopus officinalis*)
Lavandin	(*Lavandula x hybrida*)
Lavender	(*Lavandula angustifolia*)
Marjoram	(*Origanum marjorana*)
Melissa	(*Melissa officinalis*)
Mountain Savory	(*Satureja montana*)
Oregano	(*Origanum compactum*)
Patchouly	(*Pogostemon cablin*)
Pennyroyal	(*Mentha pulegium*)
Peppermint	(*Mentha piperita*)
Rosemary	(*Rosmarinus officinalis*)
Sage	(*Salvia officinalis*)
Spearmint	(*Mentha spicata*)
Spike Lavender	(*Lavandula latifolia*)
Thyme	(*Thymus vulgaris*)
Vitex	(*Vitex negundo*)

As you can see from the list, mints are not all "minty" in the customary sense of the word as in "breath mint," "spearmint gum," or "peppermint tea," And wintergreen (*Gaultheria procumbens*), which is often referred to as a "mint" and is used to flavor hard candies and mouth washes, is not a member of the mint family at all. The common characteristics that define a botanical family are visual, not a matter of taste or fragrance.

Members of the mint family are easy to identify in the field. A unique and easily visible characteristic they all share is that they have square stems with pairs of leaves that alternate at right angles up and down the stalk. Go out and pluck some peppermint, basil, oregano, or sage from your front yard or herb garden and you will see.

The Mark of a Genus

The scientific names of plants are Latin binomials which are always italicized. The first name is the "genus" and is capitalized while the last name is the "species" and is always written in lower case. The plural of genus is genera.

A genus of the plant kingdom is another broad category of plants, but not as broad as a family. A genus is a subgroup of a family. In the list on the previous page you can see that lavandin, lavender, and spike lavender all belong to the same genus—*Lavandula*. Marjoram and oregano also share a common genus—*Origanum*. Peppermint, pennyroyal, and spearmint share yet another genus—*Mentha*.

While there can be considerable variation between members of a family, plants of the same genus are "generically" similar, clearly marked, and usually recognizable as close relatives.

For example, all members of the *Lavandula* genus have recognizable lavender-like fragrances which are due to high levels of linalol and linalyl acetate in all species of this genus. There are also noticeable variations, mostly to the extent that camphor is present in the oil or not.

Crushed leaves of the two members of the *Origanum* genus listed here, marjoram and oregano, can be used almost interchangeably as a spicy flavoring for pizza. They both contain major amounts of γ-terpinene (5-20%) However, their therapeutic actions are significantly different. Oregano acts as a strong antimicrobial agent due to its phenolic carvacrol content (60-75%). Marjoram contains no carvacrol, but does contain 14-22% terpinen-4-ol, a phenolic compound somewhat like carvacrol, but with less bite. Marjoram consists mainly of monoterpenes (28-60%) which makes it a mild, gentle, balancing oil with hormonal attributes.

Spearmint, pennyroyal, and peppermint are all species of the *Mentha* genus. While easy to distinguish, they all have definite "minty" fragrances. Pennyroyal also has a disagreeable earthy, terpentine-like note. Pulegone is a ketone found in all three of these oils, but occurs only as a low-concentrate compound in peppermint and spearmint (1-5%) while it is the main ingredient in pennyroyal (55-80%). Pennyroyal (*Mentha pulegium*) is one of the forbidden oils in British aromatherapy practice, but is often used in France for a range of conditions—from bronchitis, to liver disfunction, to menstrual problems.

What Makes a Species Is Its Seed

The determining factor that isolates a species of plants into a class of its own is that all offspring of a species come from one kind of seed. Oregano and marjoram are both of the same genus, but you cannot grow marjoram from oregano seed nor oregano from marjoram seed.

The principal determinant of essential oil chemistry is the genetic recipe coded in the DNA of the plant. While oils of most species tend to be relatively constant from crop to crop and year to year with only minor variations, some species can produce significantly different oils from the same seed depending on the place of planting. Chemotypes (differences in oils of the same species because of location) are the result of a plant adjusting its vital fluids in order to survive and meet the demands of different growing environments. Some species can adapt to different situations while others can't. Those that can't adapt produce no chemotypes.

Most oils can be adequately identified by the genus, species, and plant part from which it was extracted—such as seed, stalk, leaf, flower, bud, root, fruit, etc. Pure properly distilled frankincense, for example, that has not been diluted, adulterated, or tampered with (as most is) can simply be identified as *Boswellia carteri*, distilled from the resin of the tree. Its basic chemical composition would not be significantly different whether it was gathered from the Southern Peninsula of Arabia or the Somalian deserts of Northeast Africa. Both of these locations have the same climates, latitudes, and soil conditions. *Boswellia carteri* won't grow anywhere else and produces no chemotypes.

What Is a Chemotype?

With some plants, different geographic locations results in significantly different chemistry in their oils. For such oils, simply naming the genus and species is not enough. One must also identify and name the dominant chemical constituent on the label or at least give the region of its growth. Thus, you sometimes see an extra notation after the scientific name like "linalol CT" or "thymol CT." In this way the dominant chemical compound is identified as a "chemotype" (CT) of that particular species of oil.

Thus, you could take a single packet of seeds, all of the same species, divide them into several groups, and plant them in various places—like on the seashore at sea level, on an inland hillside, on a mountain at high elevation, in a wet climate, in a dry climate, in acid soil, in alkaline soil, in a sunny place or a cloudy place, in the tropics, near the arctic circle, etc. If that particular species can survive in a range of environments and is sensitive to environmental differences, it will usually produce different chemotypes of oil for each location. If the species is not particularly sensitive to environment, then you can get an oil of the same basic chemistry regardless of where it is grown.

Many plants are also sensitive to time of harvest, whether morning, afternoon, or evening, whether before, after, or during blooming, and whether spring, summer, or fall, etc. Thus different chemotypes can arise from the same species, not only for differences in geography, but differences in timing as well.

All of these factors are what make the growing and harvesting of plants for essential oil production a complex art and science. This is why it is important to know your grower and his or her attitude, and level of experience and skill, if possible. For good information on chemotypes, I recommend the books by Burfield, Price & Price, and Schnaubelt.

Variations on Vulgaris

Thyme (*Thymus vulgaris*) is one of the most variable of plants when it comes to chemotypes. We shall use it first to illustrate chemotypes. And by the way, its specific name, "*vulgaris*," does not mean thyme is vulgar, uncouth or nasty in any way. *Vulgaris* comes from the Latin word for "common." It is a popular specific name used for many plants. For example, there's *Berberis vulgaris*, *Beta vulgaris*, *Hordeum vulgare*, and *Tanacetum vulgare*, names for barberry, beet, barley, and tansy respectively. So anytime you see the name, "*vulgaris*" or "*vulgare*," no jokes please. Plants and oils have feelings, too.

The following nine chemotypes are discussed in Price & Price. While the Latin name of the plant is italicized, the name of the chemotype compound is not and the acronym, "CT," can go either before or after the compound:

Thymus vulgaris CT thymol
Thymus vulgaris CT carvacrol
Thymus vulgaris CT linalol
Thymus vulgaris CT thujanol
Thymus vulgaris CT α–terpineol
Thymus vulgaris CT geraniol
Thymus vulgaris CT 1,8 cineole
Thymus vulgaris CT p-cymene
Thymus vulgaris CT phenol

Chemotypes of Thyme

Thymol CT is strongly antiseptic and aggressive to the skin. Cultivated in valleys, this is the chemotype used in raindrop technique. Harvested in the fall it is 60-70% thymol. Harvested in the spring it is a different chemotype, p-cymene CT.

Carvacrol CT is also strongly antiseptic and similar to oregano in its action. Harvested in the spring it is only 30% carvacrol. Harvested in the fall during or right after flowering, it is 60-80% carvacrol. Carvacrol is the main compound in Oregano oil.

Linalol CT is gentle and soothing and is sometimes used in raindrop technique when clients are sensitive to *Thymus vulgaris* CT thymol. Grown at high altitudes, it is fungicidal, parasiticidal, and uterotonic. Linalol is the main compound found in Lavender oil.

Thujanol CT shows no seasonal variation, being about 50% thujanol regardless of when harvested. It is only found in the wild. When cultivated, thyme does not manifest this chemotype. It is hormonally balancing and a stimulant to the immune system.

α–Terpineol CT is obtained by an early spring harvest. It has a slightly peppery smell.

Geraniol CT is grown at high altitudes and harvested in the fall. It has a lemony smell. It is antiviral and cardiotonic. Geraniol is a main ingredient in Geranium oil.

1,8 Cineole CT is 80-90% cineole and has virtually the same properties as *Eucalyptus globulus* which is 70-75% 1,8 cineole. It is analgesic, anticatarrhal, diuretic, expectorant, and an insect repellent.

p-Cymene CT is topically analgesic when applied to the skin and has been found useful for rheumatism and arthritis. This CT must be harvested in the spring just as the plants start budding. In the fall, the chemotype becomes thymol CT.

Phenol CT is the result of high latitude geography. The further north thyme is grown, the higher it is in phenolic compounds. For instance, when grown in Finland, thyme can acquire phenol in concentrations of up to 90%.

Rosemary Chemotypes

Rosmarinus officinalis **CT camphor** is high in camphor, serves as a general stimulant, and works well with other oils. Combined with oil of black pepper (*Piper nigrum*) it can be a powerful energy stimulant. It is grown in Spain and Croatia.

Rosmarinus officinalis **CT 1,8 cineole** is used in some countries for congestion of the lungs and to help eliminate toxins in the liver and kidneys. It is grown in Tunisia and Morocco.

Rosmarinus officinalis **CT verbenon** is the most gentle of the rosemary chemotypes. It has powerful regenerative properties and is popular for skin care. It is grown on Corsica, a French island in the Mediterranean.

Basil Chemotypes

Ocimum basilicum **CT fenchol** is from Germany. It is antiseptic and neurotonic. It has been applied for liver and gall bladder insufficiency.

Ocimum basilicum **CT eugenol** is from Madagascar. It is anti-inflammatory and used for topical relief of pain. There is some eugenol (1-5%) also in the methyl chavicol CT of basil, but not as much.

Ocimum basilicum **CT linalol** is grown in Europe. It is tonifying, antiflatulent, and stimulating to the liver. It has been used for coronary weakness and nervous depression.

Ocimum basilicum **CT methyl chavicol** is grown in several places including Reunion, Comoro, and Egypt. Methyl chavicol CT (also known as estragole CT) is the chemotype of basil used in raindrop technique. It is strongly antispasmodic.

Other Plants with Chemotypes

Melissa or lemon balm (*Melissa officinalis*) comes as CT citral or CT citronellal.

Sage (*Salvia officinalis*) comes in two chemotypes, as CT thujone or CT cineole.

Tarragon (*Artemisia dracunculus*) comes two ways, as CT estragole or CT sabinene.

Valerian (*Valeriana officinalis*) comes three ways, as CT valeranone, CT valeranal, or CT cryptofuranol.

Tarragon and Valerian are the only two plants we have mentioned with chemotypes that are not members of the mint family (Labiatae or Lamiaceae). Tarragon is from the celery/carrot family (Apiaceae or Umbelliferae). Valerian is from the family of Valerianaceae.

Meet the Myrtle Family

One of the most popular and powerful families of oils is Myrtaceae, the myrtle family, with over 3,000 species and 75 genera. Except for clove, oils of the myrtle family all come from leaves. Revelation 22:2 comes to mind: "and the leaves of the tree are for the healing of the nations." While many members of the myrtle family manifest chemotypes according to the geography of their growth, their large variety of oil-bearing species are sometimes confused for chemotypes. The following plants and their oils are all members of the myrtle family:

Eucalyptus citriodora (Lemon Eucalyptus oil)
Eucalyptus dives (Peppermint Eucalyptus oil)
Eucalyptus globulus (Eucalyptus oil)
Eucalyptus polybractea (Blue Mallee oil)
Eucalyptus radiata (Black Peppermint oil)
Melaleuca alternifolia (Tea Tree/Snake oil)
Melaleuca ericifolia (Rosalina/Lavender Tea Tree oil)
Melaleuca cajuputi (Cajuput oil)
Melaleuca quinquenervia (Naiouli/MQV oil)
Myrtus communis (Myrtle oil)
Syzygium aromaticum (Clove oil)

All but the last two species are natives of Australia. Myrtle is native to the Mediterranean and the Middle East while clove is native to the Mollucas Islands of Indonesia. Both myrtle and clove were used by people of the *Bible*, but not eucalyptus or melaleuca.

It is easy to confuse *citriodora, dives, globulus, polybractea,* and *radiata* as being chemotypes of *Eucalyptus*. They are not. They are five individual species. Each of these species of eucalyptus produces its own unique seed and one cannot be grown from the other.

These oils, especially *E. globulus* and *M. alternifolia* (Tea Tree) are among the most popular in the world. When you see an oil that simply says "eucalyptus" without identifying the species, it is probably *globulus* or possibly *radiata*. When you see an oil simply identified as "melaleuca," it is probably *alternifolia*.

There are four genera of the myrtle family represented here: *Eucalyptus, Melaleuca, Myrtus,* and *Syzygium.* Let's consider the chemical properties of these oils one at a time. If you have samples of any or all of these, it is fun to experience their different aromas. The family and generic resemblances are there yet each oil has its own personality and character as well.

Species and Chemotypes of Eucalyptus

There are over 600 species of the genus, *Eucalyptus,* all native to Australia. The medicinal varieties produce oils rich in 1,8 cineole, a compound also known as eucalyptol. The perfume varieties are rich in citronellal. The varieties used for industrial purposes are rich in piperitone and phellandrene. However, even the perfume and industrial varieties have medicinal properties. Eucalyptus leaves constitute the sole food of the koala bear, whose digestive tract is specially adapted to digest the oils of the tree. We shall discuss only five of the 600 species here.

E. citriodora **(Lemon Eucalyptus oil).** 40-80% citronellal. Native to Australia but also grown and harvested in India, China, South Africa, Cuba, Guatemala, Colombia, Egypt, and Madagascar giving rise to several chemotypes. The Brazilian trees produce an aldehyde CT while the trees of Madagascar are high in phenols. Used to perfume linen closets to repel cockroaches and silverfish. It has been used for asthma, athlete's foot, dandruff, herpes, shingles, laryngitis, sore throats, and respiratory infections.

E. dives **(Peppermint Eucalyptus oil).** 35-50% piperitone and 23-30% phellandrene. A native of Australia, it has been imported to Brazil, South Africa, and the Belgian Congo where it is also grown today. There are at least three chemotypes: CT phellandrene (used as an insecticide); CT piperitone (with a minty fragrance); and CT cineole (grown in South Africa and Australia). Dives is strongly antibacterial, can be applied topically, and can be diffused with the cautionary note to avoid direct inhalation too close to the nebulizing nozzle.

***E. globulus* (Eucalyptus or Blue Gum oil).** 60-75% 1,8 cineole. When an oil is simply designated as "Eucalyptus" without identifying which species, *globulus* or blue gum is usually the one intended. Originally from Australia it is also grown in China, Brazil, Portugal, Corsica, and Ecuador. This is the eucalyptus oil most commonly used throughout the world and has many uses. Used for centuries by Australian aborigines to protect and heal wounds, its antimicrobial properties make a popular ingredient for mouthwashes. Combined with pine oil, it is commonly used in household cleaning products, shower gels, and air fresheners. Jean Valnet, MD, found that a 2% solution sprayed in the air will kill 70% of airborne staph bacteria. Eucalyptus oil is still used to disinfect surgical dressings. Vicks® VapoRub® is an over-the-counter medication for relief of respiratory congestion whose principle active ingredients are camphor (5%), menthol (2.6%), and *E. globulus* oil (1.2%). Vicks VapoRub also contains essential oils of cedarleaf and nutmeg and has been popular throughout the world for more than a century.

***E. polybractea* (Blue Mallee oil).** 85-95% 1,8 cineole. A native of Australia, it is also grown in France where a CT cryptone chemotype with a powerful cumin-like odor is produced. Anti-infectious, antiviral, anti-inflammatory, an expectorant, and insect repellent. It has been effective for treating acne. Used as a source for pure cineole which can be separated from the oil by freezing.

***E. radiata* (Black Peppermint oil).** 60-75% 1,8 cineole. Native of Australia. Used extensively for respiratory infections. Next to *E. globulus,* this is the most popular of the eucalyptus oils. While *E. globulus* and *E. radiata* both contain 60-75% 1,8 cineole, *globulus* has a stronger, more astringent smell while *radiata* is mild and more mellow. Some people prefer one over the other. Both are effective for respiratory conditions. There are six known chemotypes of *E. radiata*, but only two are commonly harvested: CT 1,8 cineole and CT piperitone. *E. radiata,* as with all of species of *Eucalyptus* oils, can be used in a humidifier.

Snake Oil and Other Species of Melaleuca

There are over 200 species of the genus *Melaleuca*—all native to Australia. *Melaleuca* is a genus of evergreen trees, many of which like to grow in swampy places. Some species of melaleuca also have chemotypes. The popularity of melaleuca oils has to do with their effectiveness in dealing with many conditions as well as their relative safety. *Melaleuca* oils have been used for extended periods of time without any problems. Applied with common sense there are generally no contraindications. We shall discuss only four of the many species of melaleuca here.

M. alternifolia (Tea Tree or Snake oil). 25-40% terpinen-4-ol and 10-28% γ-terpinene. This is probably the most popular essential oil in the world with innumerable uses. During the settling of the Western United States, pioneer families faced many perils, including rattlesnake bites. Known as "snake oil," the Australian aborigines taught early English settlers that tea tree leaves and their oils could detoxify the site of a snake bite and save a life. Australians ought to know. There are more than 100 species of venomous snakes in Australia—more than any other continent on earth and including two of the world's ten most deadly. When this information became known in America, there was a great demand for the oil among early settlers headed West. Traveling merchants carrying the product were called "snake oil salesmen."

So originally, "snake oil" was an honest and legitimate product. Unfortunately, some traveling salesmen were of questionable character and sold fraudulent merchandise—oils that were diluted or not true tea tree that did not work. Thus the profession and the product acquired a bad name and the term, "snake oil salesman" came to connote a purveyor of fraud. Eventually, it was forgotten that snake oil in the form of *M. alternifolia* was not a fraud, so that today the term, itself, is applied to any medicinal concoction with questionable benefits.

M. alternifolia comes in two chemotypes, both grown in Australia. In the south there is CT 1,8 cineole while in the north there is CT terpinen-4-ol. Even the cineole chemotype is still dominated by terpinen-4-ol, which provides the main fragrance and therapeutic properties we associate with tea tree oil. *M. alternifolia* is also grown in Zimbabwe, Kenya, Vietnam, India, Guatemala, and China.

***M. cajuputi* (Cajuput oil)** 50-70% 1,8 cineole (eucalyptol). Native of Australia, it also grows in India, Java, Vietnam, and the islands of Malaysia and Indonesia. There are two chemotypes: CT cineole and CT methyl eugenol with cineole remaining dominant in both cases. It's high cineole content gives it many of the same qualities as *E. globulus, E. polybractea,* and *E. radiata* with which it works well as a blend. Used for many purposes, including respiratory congestion, asthma, urinary problems, coughs, hay fever, toothaches, bursitis, psoriasis, insect bites, and sore muscles. "Kaju-Puti" is a Malaysian word meaning "white tree." NOTE: According to Burfield, Franchomme, and Penoel, *M. cajuputi* has been confused for another species (*M. leucadendra*) in many publications. *Leucadendra* produces quite a different essential oil that is mostly phenols, including eugenol, which are compounds not found in *M. cajuputi.*

***M. ericifolia* (Rosalina oil)** 34-45% linalol and 10-20% 1,8 cineole. Native to Australia, the high linalol content gives this species of Melaleuca the name of "lavender tea tree oil." Linalol is a major ingredient in lavender oil. There are two chemotypes: CT 1,8 cineole and CT phellandrene. Gentler than *M. alternifolia,* rosalina is used in vegetable carrier oils for body massage.

***M. quinquenervia* (Niaouli, Nerolina, or MQV oil)** 35-65% 1,8 cineole and 6-15% viridiflorol. Native of Australia, it also grows in Madagascar, New Caledonia, and the Florida Everglades. Chemotypes include CT 1,8 cineole, CT methyl eugenol, CT terpinolene, CT nerolidol, and CT viridiflorol. The name, "MQV," refers to the last chemotype which is also called, *Melaleuca quinquenervia viridiflorol* (MQV). Gentle and safe, naiouli oil can be applied liberally and undiluted to the whole body after a morning shower. Possessing hormonal properties (both male and female) it is noted for its hormonal balancing properties (mainly due to viridiflorol). *M. quinquenervia* was transplanted in the Florida Everglades in the early 20th century where it has spread so much it has become a pest. Efforts to check its growth have been unsuccessful. Once it takes root, it refuses to go away. The pollen of niaouli trees is a powerful allergen and is considered responsible for the great increase in allergic conditions in Florida. This fact points to one of the most important qualities of niaouli oil. It is one of the most powerful anti-allergenics in aromatherapy, acting in a homeopathic fashion (i.e., "like cures like").

Oil of Myrtle

Myrtle, *Myrtus communis*, is a native of the Holy Land and the Middle East. It grows in every country that borders on the Mediterranean including Turkey, Morocco, Algeria, Tunisia, France, Spain, Greece, and Italy. It also grows in several other European countries as well as in Russia.

The oil is extracted from both the berries as well as the leaves and branches. Its principal compounds are α-pinene (45-60%) with 1,8 cineole (17-27%). This composition compares somewhat with frankincense oil (*Boswellia carteri*) which contains 28-49% α-pinene. α-pinene is a monoterpene hydrocarbon found in many oils with a pine-like aroma. Oddly, the ancient Greeks compared the fragrance of myrtle oil, not with that of frankincense, but with that of myrrh (*Commiphora myrrha*). Myrrh is rich in sesquiterpenes and contains very little α-pinene. If you have bottles of these three oils, you can make your own comparison. Personally, I think myrtle smells more like frankincense than myrrh, which it should, considering its chemical constituency.

Myrtle oil has been researched by Daniel Penoel, M.D. of France for normalizing hormonal imbalances of the thyroid and ovaries. It also has benefits for decongesting the respiratory system and the sinuses.

The myrtle berry oil has been used as a flavoring for drinks and alcoholic beverages throughout the Mediterranean Area. The myrtle leaf oil has also been used for flavor when the berry oil is not available. There is more α-pinene in the leaf than in the berry.

There are at least two chemotypes: CT 1,8 cineole available from Morocco and Turkey, and CT myrtenyl acetate available from Corsica. The Turkish chemotype has a greater cineole content than the Moroccan version and also has a tinge of anise in its fragrance.

Oil of Clove

Clove was imported from the Mollucas Islands by the Chinese as early as 1000 years before Christ and was imported by traders from the Holy Land during Biblical times. Extracted from the buds and their stems, it is rich in eugenol (75-87%) (a phenol) which is a strong local anesthetic. For centuries, clove oil was the anesthetic of choice used by dentists to numb the gums. It is still widely used for this purpose in many countries. Besides eugenol (77%), the rest of clove oil consists mainly of sesquiterpenes (10%) and esters (12%). Medically, clove has been found to be broadly antiviral, antimicrobial, and antiparasitic. It has been applied for bursitis, herpes, bronchitis, diarrhea, and toothaches. It also repels mosquitoes and clothes moths.

Indigenous to Indonesia, clove is currently cultivated in many places including China, Madagascar, Zanzibar, and Brazil. While eugenol comprises the main chemistry of the oil in all cases, different geographical locations produce different chemotypes including β-caryophyllene CT and eugenyl acetate CT,

Same Plant, Different Parts, Different Oils

While the same species can produce various oil chemistries depending on timing and geographical environment, the very same plant in the same location can produce considerably different oils depending on the plant part used. Hence, one oil may result from the roots, another from the stems and branches, while yet another from the flowers.

An example of this are three popular oils produced from the bitter orange tree (*Citrus aurantium*): Neroli, Orange Bigarade, and Petitgrain. Neroli oil is extracted by solvents from the flowers and is technically an "absolute," not an essential oil. Orange bigarade oil is cold-pressed from the rind of the fruit while petitgrain oil is distilled from the leaves and twigs.

There is considerable contrast in the chemistries of these three oils. Neroli is 35-60% alcohols while orange bigarade is 89-95% monoterpenes and petitgrain is 48-65% esters. Each oil has its own distinctive aroma and unique therapeutic applications, yet all three can come from the very same tree.

Oils vs. Antiobiotics & Antiseptics

The principal determinant of essential oil chemistry is the genetic coding of the plant that produces it. In general, a plant will produce oils with the same suite of chemical constituents regardless of where grown, dutifully following the genetic predisposition stored in its cellular DNA. Such oils can be adequately labeled with the genus and species alone.

However, this is not to imply that two batches of essential oil are ever identical, even when grown from the same species on the same plot of cropland. The compositions of essential oils vary naturally, just as the taste and aroma of wines vary from year to year from the same vineyard. These variations are normal and are not usually so great as to constitute chemotypes. Essential oils are natural products over which humans have only limited control regarding their exact composition. The fact is that no two batches of essential oil are ever identicle in the proportions of compounds present.

This is one of the reasons essential oils have enduring antimicrobial properties that antibiotics and chemical antiseptics do not have. Because commercially produced products are always the same exact formulas, bacteria eventually develop resistance and then they don't work any more. Drug companies have tried to deal with this problem by creating stronger and stronger antibiotics and antiseptics. The problem is that such pharmaceuticals eventually become too toxic to be applied to people.

Vancomycin and methicillin are the two most powerful antibiotics in current usage which are normally prescribed only when the patient is on the verge of death. "Hence," doctors reason, "if the patient dies from the drugs, they would have died anyhow."

Research has shown that oils such as cinnamon, oregano, and tea tree are as effective against resistant strains of bacteria as vancomycin and methicillin, but without any dangers being posed to the patient. Furthermore, oil of onycha dissolved in alcohol is a better antiseptic than any commercially produced antiseptic. Because these are natural products, formulated by God, whose compositions vary with every batch, bacteria will never become resistent to them. Unlike the temporary drugs of today, essential oils will always maintain their antimicrobial properties. Furthermore, essential oils also pose unfriendly environments for viruses, which antibiotics do not.

Make Friends With Your Oil Producer

As you read the information in this chapter, it should have become apparent that the exact chemistry of an oil is determined by more than genetics. It also has a great deal to do with where the oil-producing herb is grown, as well as the manner and timing of cultivation and harvesting, not to mention the manner of extraction.

Even the attitude of the grower can make a difference—whether they are disinterested commercial producers or lovers of plants that shower their fields with kind and positive thoughts and, perhaps, with a little prayer. As we will learn in Part Three of this book, plants and their fluids respond physically and chemically to human thought and human intent.

No individual can afford to routinely submit oil samples for laboratory testing to check their quality. Besides, some of the most important healing attributes of an oil are not measurable by laboratory technology. Therefore, it behooves one to know their grower, their distiller, their packager, and their provider. In the end, obtaining a therapeutic grade essential oil of known species and chemotype is largely a matter of trust. The definitive test is whether or not the oil performs in a satisfactorily therapeutic manner, something you can verify for yourself by direct experience.

Key Points of Chapter Eight

1. The general chemical composition of an essential oil is mainly predetermined by the genetic codes of the plant and only slightly altered by the environment of growth.

2. When genetics is the determining factor in the chemical makeup of an oil, only the genus and species of the producing plant are needed to identify it.

3. In the botanical classifications of plants, families are broad categories, genera are subcategories under families, and species designate a specific plant of a genus.

4. The distinguishing quality of a species is its seed. For example, *Eucalyptus globulus* and *Eucalyptus radiata* are both trees of the same genus (*Eucalyptus*) and share many obvious family characteristics in common. However, you cannot grow *E. globulus* from *E. radiata* seed, nor can you sprout an *E. radiata* tree from an *E. globulus* seed. Although members of the same family and genus, their seed is what sets them apart as species.

5. The scientific names of plants consist of Latin binomials giving the genus and species, both in italics, where the first part is the genus (capitalized) and the second the species (in lower case).

6. Some plants, like *Thymus vulgaris*, while they have their genetic codes for producing oil, can be widely responsive to environment to the point that considerably different chemistry can result from where it was grown, how it is grown, and when it was harvested.

7. When a single species produces oils of significantly different chemistry, depending on environment, genus and species are not sufficient to identify the nature of the oil. Thus, a third identifier is required to indicate its dominant chemistry and to distinguish it from oils of the same species that are different. This identifier is called "chemotype" and abbreviated as "CT."

8. When a single plant species tends to produce markedly different oils in response to different environments and harvesting conditions, you can take a packet of seeds of that species, divide it into several parts and plant them in a variety of altitudes, latitudes, climates, and soils and harvest them at a variety of times from early spring to late fall, morning to night, and you will produce chemically different oils even though they are all from the same species. These are chemotypes,

9. Chemotypes are the result of a plant modifying its vital fluids in order to adapt to its environment. With different environments, different chemistries are necessary for the plant to remain strong and healthy, thus resulting in chemically different oils.

10. Chemotype is to essential oils what vintage is to wines.

11. The mint family, Lamiaceae, includes more species susceptible to chemotypes than any other botanical family of plants. This is an indication of the adaptability of members of the mint family which are found in a wide range of environments throughout the world.

12. Thyme (*Thymus vulgaris*) a member of the mint family, produces more chemotypes than any other known species.

13. Other species that produce chemotypes include Basil, Rosemary, Melissa, Sage, Tarragon, and Valerian.

14. Among the most popular of essential oils are those from the myrtle family (Myrtaceae). These include the *Eucalyptus* and *Melaleuca* oils, both genera of Myrtaceae.

15. There are over 600 species of *Eucalyptus* and more than 200 of *Melaleuca* all native to Australia and all capable of producing essential oils. Many species of *Eucalyptus* and *Melaleuca* produce chemotypes according to geographical location.

16. Of the many species of *Eucalyptus*, only a few are widely employed as essential oils, namely *citriodora, dives, globulus, polybractea,* and *radiata*. Most of these have chemotypes.

17. *E. globulus* is the most popular species of *Eucalyptus* and is usually the one implied when a label simply says "Eucalyptus Oil" without identifying the species. It is also called "blue gum."

18. Of the many species of *Melaleuca*, only a few are widely employed as essential oils, namely *alternifolia, ericifolia, cajuputi,* and *quinquenervia*.

19. *M. alternifolia* is the most popular species of *Melaleuca* and one of the most popular essential oils in the world. It is usually the one implied when a label simply says "Melaleuca Oil" without identifying the species. *M. alternifolia* is also known as "Tea Tree."

20. Snake Oil (*M. alternifolia* or Tea Tree) was popular during the settling of the American West 100-200 years ago for its ability to detoxify a snake bite, a property known to Australian settlers which they learned from the Aborigines.

21. Myrtle (*Myrtus communis*) is indigenous to the countries bordering the Mediterranean, and was used in Biblical times.

22. Clove (*Syzygium aromaticum*) originated in Indonesia, but is grown in several countries today with some resulting variations in chemotypes. All chemotypes of clove are dominant in eugenol, a phenol and local anesthetic.

23. A single plant can produce strikingly different oils depending on the plant part used. The bitter orange (*Citrus aurantium*) is a good example of this. From the fruit peel (orange bigarade), you get a monoterpenic oil; from the flowers (neroli), an alcoholic oil; and from the leaves (petit-grain), an oil of esters.

24. The chemistry of an essential oil begins with its genetic recipe stored in the DNA of the plant, but the final product is a result of the place and manner of growth and harvest, as well as details of distillation.

25. Because growing conditions are never exactly the same from year to year or place to place, each batch of an essential oil is unique, even from the same species. These variations block any possibility for bacteria to become resistant to their antimicrobial properties. This makes oils superior to antiobiotics and synthetic antiseptics, to which bacteria always become resistant, sooner or later.

26. Routinely sending samples of the oils you use to a laboratory for testing is neither economically nor practically feasible.

27. The best thing is to know your grower, your distiller, and your packager. Obtaining a therapeutic grade oil is largely a matter of trust in your producers and providers.

28. The ultimate test of the therapeutic properties of an oil (or the lack thereof) is in your usage. Do they work or don't they work? You are the final judge.

❤ CHAPTER NINE
ISOPRENES,
TERPENES, AND PMS

---

ore than 150 years ago chemists discovered that many organic compounds were built of multiples of a functional group with the formula, C_5H_8. This includes thousands of compounds that make up essential oils. For lack of a better name, they called it an "isoprene unit." It looks like this:

Isoprene Unit
(with C atoms shown)

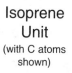 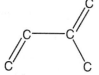

Formula
C_5H_8
(M.W. = 68)

2-methylbutyl-1,3-diene

Reading the Isoprene Formula

In this picture the 5 C atoms are shown explicitly but the 8 H atoms are not. Here's how you figure the hydrogen atoms. Let's start at the top C on the right and number the Cs down to the left 1 through 4. That would make the bottom left C #4. Then let's count the bottom right C as #5. You might want to lightly sketch in these numbers by each C with a pencil. To get the number of H atoms invisibly attached to any particular C, simply subtract the number of bonds shown converging at that carbon from its valence, which is 4.

C #1 has two bonds coming to it. Since 4 - 2 = 2, there must be 2 H atoms attached there.

C #2 already has 4 bonds converging on it so 4 - 4 = 0. There are zero H atoms there.

C #3 has 3 bonds converging on it so 4 - 3 = 1. There is 1 H atom there.

C #4 has 2 bonds attached so 4 - 2 = 2. There are 2 H atoms there.

C #5 has only 1 bond showing so 4 - 1 = 3. There are 3 H atoms there.

Tallying up the H atoms, we have 2 at C #1, 0 at C #2, 1 at C #3, 2 at C #4, and 3 at C #5. Adding them up, 2 + 0 + 1 + 2 + 3 = 8 H atoms total. Thus, our chemical formula for an isoprene unit is C_5H_8.

If you take the first four carbons with their hydrogens by themselves, you see that they make a hydrocarbon chain whose formula would be C_4H_5. Remembering back to Chapter Four where you met Methyl, Ethyl, Propyl, and Butyl, you will see that a 4-C hydrocarbon chain is a "butyl radical." Then if you consider C #5 as a 1-C hydrocarbon unit with the formula CH_3, you have a "methyl radical." Thus, the isoprene unit is a methyl radical attached to a butyl radical.

The scientific name for an isoprene unit is 2-methylbuta-1,3-diene. Here's how it translates: "2-methylbuta" means a methyl radical has been attached to C #2 of a butyl radical. "1,3 diene" means the butyl radical has two double bonds starting at C #1 and C #3.

The placement of the double bonds as shown in the figure on the previous page is not rigid. When molecules are built of isoprene units, the double bonds can shift between any pair of C atoms in the unit. The ability for these double bonds to shift is indicative of another situation like that of the benzene ring where electrons are non-localized. As you may recall from Chapter Five, when electrons become non-local, they generate electromagnetic frequencies and give off resonance energy. In this state, molecules start behaving more like electromagnetic waves than like particles of matter. The isoprene unit is another source of frequencies in essential oils.

As for the name of this unit, you can forget the long scientific name. We will use the simple name of "isoprene" for the rest of this book. But for those of you who are so inclined, I thought you might enjoy some practice reading a structural formula and learning how the scientific names are derived.

In actuality, we never write the isoprene unit in the form just shown. We show it as given below, without writing in the C atoms, where a C is implied at each angle, each convergence of lines, and at the end of each line or pair of lines:

Isoprene
Unit
(without C
atoms shown)

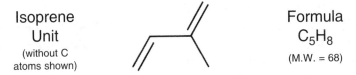

Formula
C_5H_8
(M.W. = 68)

People make jokes about the appearance of the isoprene unit structure. They say it looks like a little horsey galloping along, a doggie running away, a reclining lawn chair, etc. What do you see? How it appears to you is a sort of Rorschach or inkblot test. The isoprene unit in the form given above (without the Cs) may look familiar. If you have ever attended a seminar sponsored by the Center for Aromatherapy Research and Education (CARE) you may recognize it immediately. Here is the CARE logo:

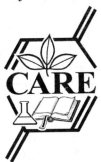

Can you see an isoprene unit in the logo? Can you see two of them? In the CARE seminars where we teach an Essential Oil Chemistry Course based on this book, we sometimes wear a tee shirt with a large copy of this logo on the back. We say, "We are teaching subliminal chemistry."

What Good is an Isoprene?

Now that we have shown you an isoprene unit, what is it good for? That's like asking "What is a brick good for?" The answer would be, "One brick isn't worth very much, but as a building unit, it is priceless." The isoprene unit (C_5H_8) is the basic building unit from which essential oils are made. In fact, the isoprene unit goes way beyond essential oils. This is the most fundamental and frequently found functional group comprising the living tissues of all plants and animals on planet earth.

Molecules built of isoprenes are called "terpenoids." More than 20,000 have been isolated and identified in laboratories, but there are millions of others as yet not studied and unknown. The number of terpenoids far exceeds that of any other class of natural compounds.

Molecules built of isoprene units are implicated in almost every interaction between plant and animal, plant and plant, or plant and microorganism in the world. Isoprenes dominate the chemical ecology of natural products participating in such diverse substances and activities as Vitamin A, Vitamin E, Vitamin K, marijuana, pollination, plant defenses, hormones, and pheromones—those amazing chemical messengers by which moths, mammals, and even humans communicate.

To make molecules, isoprenes link up in two ways: (1) in Chains and (2) in Rings. The first arrangement (chains) is called "acyclic" and the second (rings) is called "cyclic." Some large molecules have both cyclic and acyclic parts. Isoprene units can connect in chains and rings in any number. Natural molecules built of isoprene units start with two or three in a small molecule while the largest molecules contain hundreds and even thousands of isoprenes. As for carbon rings in molecules made of isoprenes, there are 3-, 4- 5- and 6-sided rings, 7-, 8-, and 9-sided rings and beyond. Molecules with one ring, are called "monocyclic." Those with two rings are called "bicyclic," those with three "tricyclic," etc. The possibilities are boundless.

You may notice in the figure below, whereas the basic isoprene unit has two double bonds (called a diene), when they link up, some isoprenes will have only one double bond (on their middle member) and, in some cases, no double bonds at all.

Given below are drawings of two linked pairs of isoprene units, one cyclic the other acyclic. There are also two drawings of three isoprenes linked together—an acyclic chain and a bicyclic molecule. This will give you an idea of how isoprenes can combine to make molecules.

Notice in the drawings that when isoprene units start joining up, the double bonds start shifting around from what we have originally shown. In any case, multiples of the group formula (C_5H_8) remain intact— $C_{10}H_{16}$, $C_{15}H_{24}$, $C_{20}H_{32}$. etc. The isoprene units are in solid lines while the bonds between units are dashed. Can you see all the little horsies and doggies? These models can give you good

$C_{10}H_{16}$

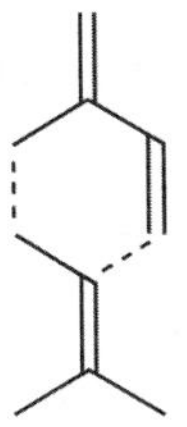

A Monocyclic Molecule formed from 2 Isoprene units

$C_{15}H_{24}$

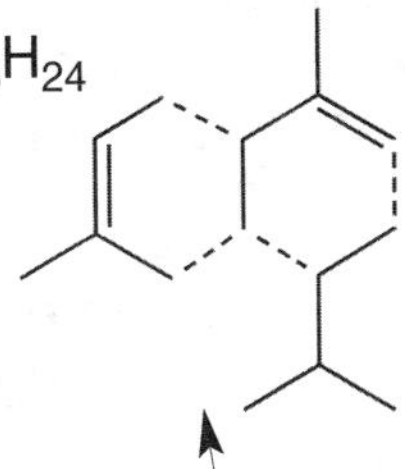

An Acyclic Molecule formed from 2 Isoprene units

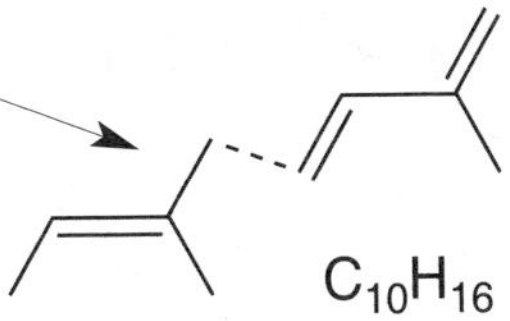

$C_{10}H_{16}$

A Bicyclic Molecule formed from 3 Isoprene units

$C_{15}H_{24}$

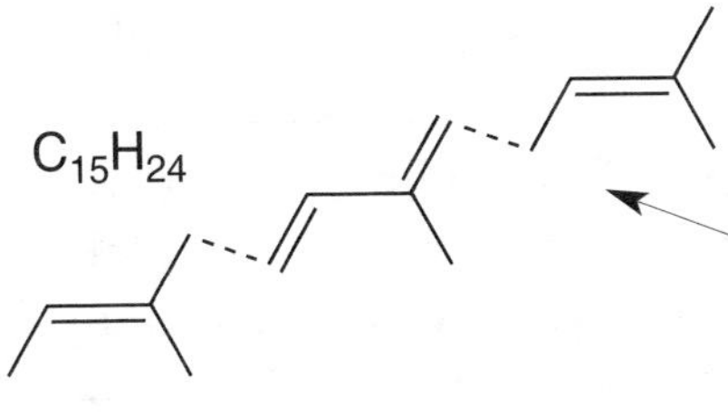

An Acyclic Molecule formed from 3 Isoprene units

practice in reading structural formulas. The answers are
given for each molecule.

Terpenes

The most common class of chemical compounds found
in essential oils are the terpenes and their oxygenated
derivatives. Terpenes are built from isoprene units. Two
isoprene units combined is called a "terpene unit."

2 Isoprene Units = 1 Terpene Unit

Hence, the CARE logo actually has a terpene unit (two
isoprenes) incorporated into its design. Terpenes are
hydrocarbons (composed of only C and H atoms), but they
can be oxygenated into terpene-alcohols, terpene-ethers,
terpene-aldehydes, terpene-ketones, terpene-esters, ter-
pene-oxides, and other varieties of oxygenated compounds. Oxygenated hydrocarbons will be discussed in
detail in the next chapter. For now, let's just focus on terpenes as hydrocarbons.

The table below lists the classes of terpenes found in
essential oils with their hydrocarbon formulas:

Table Twelve
Classes of Hydrocarbon Terpenes
Found in Essential Oils

Name	Terpene Units	Formula	Molecular Wt
Monoterpene	1	$C_{10}H_{16}$	136
Sesquiterpene	1.5	$C_{15}H_{24}$	204
Diterpene	2	$C_{20}H_{32}$	272
Triterpene	3	$C_{30}H_{48}$	408
Tetraterpene	4	$C_{40}H_{64}$	544

The names of the terpenes tell how many terpene units
($C_{10}H_{16}$) are in the molecule. Mono = 1, Di = 2, Tri = 3,
Tetra = 4, while Sesqui = one-and-a-half. You may have
heard of a city or county celebrating their "sesquicenten-
nial." That would be their 150th year (one-and-a-half cen-

turies). The names of hydrocarbon terpenes end in -ene. Names of oxygenated terpenes take on a variety of endings to be discussed in the next chapter.

The five classes of terpenes in Table Twelve are not the only ones. These are just the five with the smallest molecular weights. There are countless numbers of larger terpenes built of larger and larger numbers of isoprene or terpene units. In fact, the word "isoprene" is associated with rubber which is composed of large numbers of isoprenes in chains and grids called "polyisoprenes." One rubber molecule consists of 1,500 to 15,000 isoprene units with a molecular weight ranging from 100,000 to a million amu. These are among the dinosaurs, whales, and monsters of the molecule kingdom.

Only the tiniest molecules are found in essential oils. The five classes of terpenes given in Table Twelve are the only terpenes you will find in aromatic oils. Generally speaking, any molecule more than 500 amu will not pass through distillation, nor through human skin, nor through the blood-brain barrier.

There are an estimated 1,000 different monoterpenes and as many as 3,000 sesquiterpenes found in essential oils. The reason for more varieties of sesquiterpenes is that they are larger molecules with more atoms (Legos®) to play with, which offers a greater number of possibilities for isomers. Diterpenes, triterpenes and tetraterpenes, by their larger molecular size, offer even greater numbers of atoms (Legos®) as possibilities for isomers but they are less common in essential oils. This is because their larger molecular size makes them less able to pass through the distillation process and end up in a volatile oil.

Except for traces, triterpenes and tetraterpenes are absent from distilled oils. Small amounts are found in expressed oils, like orange, lemon, grapefruit, and lime, as well as in oils extracted by solvents such as jasmine and neroli. Expressed oils are pressed from the rind. One of the large molecules in citrus oils is β-carotene ($C_{40}H_{64}$)—a tetraterpene. Tri- and tetraterpene molecules do not contribute to the fragrances of the oils that contain them because they are too large and heavy to be aromatic. However, they do contribute color, weight, viscosity, substance, taste, and various therapeutic qualities to the oil.

Cures in Big Molecules

Other than obtaining them in cold pressed oils, if you want to apply the healing powers of large botanical molecules, you need to eat them as fresh, complete parts of the plant or apply them as dried herbs in teas, poultices, and capsules. Only the smallest healing molecules of plants are captured in volatile oils. Essential oils can address many health issues, but not all of them. Dried herbs, which are missing the small molecules, can supply you with benefits of big molecules not afforded by small ones.

For example, there is an herbal remedy for cancer originating centuries ago among the Anishanake Indians (also known as Ojibway, which was their language). The tea is made from four dried herbs: burdock root (*Arctium lappa*), sheep sorrel (*Rumex acetosella*), Indian rhubarb root (*Rheum palmatum*), and slippery elm bark (*Ulmus fulva*).

The recipe was given to a Canadian nurse in the 1920s by a Native American woman who had been cured of breast cancer using the tea. The nurse was Rene Caisse— pronounced "Rain Case." The tea brewed from these dried herbs came to be known as "Essiac Tea," where "Essiac" is "Caisse" spelled backwards. During her lifetime, Nurse Caisse successfully treated thousands of cancer patients, many under the supervision of medical doctors. The remedy is also known as "Mary's Tea," named for a friend of Rene's (Mary McPherson) who published and widely distributed the recipe.

There are many documented cases of cancer healings from this tea, one of which is personal to me and my wife, Lee. My mother-in-law was diagnosed (by palpation and biopsy) with terminal lymphoma cancer and given six months to live. She started drinking Essiac Tea every day and within two months she was cancer free, confirmed by two physicians. She lived four more years, passing away peacefully and disease free at age 89. Essiac tea has no negative side effects, only positive ones. People drinking the tea for a cancer cure have experience unexpected benefits such as the remission of diabetes.

Essiac Tea contains no essential oils. Only the big molecules are there. In focusing on essential oils, God, who made the oils, does not want us to overlook the other medicines he has designed for our needs. His loving presence is in all of the molecules of his creation—big and small.

Check your local health food store, or go on the internet, and you will probably find the tea or the herbs to brew it, as well as a variety of books and literature on Essiac. We got the actual herbs along with everything we needed to make and store the brewed tea from Cheryl's Herbs in St. Louis, Missouri. Her website is www.cherylsherbs.com, her email is info@cherylsherbs.com, and her phone is (314) 645-2165. She will ship anywhere.

Tomatoes are Red, Carrots are Orange

Except for expressed citrus oils, tetraterpenes are virtually absent from most essential oils. Tangerine oil contains the most—about 8%. (For a complete list, see Table 40.) Tetraterpenes play a special role in the plant kingdom. They are one of the prime sources of color. Most of the compounds in essential oils are either colorless or only lightly tinted because their molecules are too small to absorb, emit, or reflect visible light. The dimensions of the larger molecules of tetraterpenes are compatible with the wave lengths of light in such a way as to produce brilliant colors, providing pigments to thousands of flowers, fruits, and vegetables as well as the brilliant yellows, red, and oranges of fall foliage. Tetraterpenes also provide colors for many insects and animals.

For example, you may have heard of carotene and probably know that it is the orange color of a carrot. It is also the orange color in cantaloupes as well as the yellowish hue in broccoli, spinach, and collard greens. In fact, it is a coloring in many plants, insects, and animals, including humans where it provides the yellow tint to our skin—present more in some races than in others.

The name, carotene, ends in -ene. It is a terpene. A tetraterpene. There are many isomeric variations of carotene. There's alpha-carotene, beta-carotene, gamma-carotene, delta-carotene, and more. Beta-carotene is the famous one. It is often included in natural vitamin and mineral supplements. (See Figure on next page.)

All of your life you have probably heard that carrots are good for your eyes. Your mother was probably the first to tell you this. The scientific basis for this statement is that

Lycopene, Carotene, and Vitamin A

Lycopene Molecule – $C_{40}H_{64}$ – Red

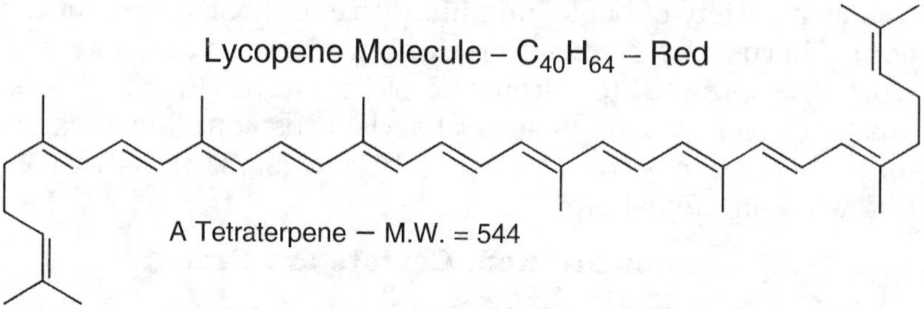

A Tetraterpene – M.W. = 544

β–Carotene Molecule – $C_{40}H_{64}$ – Orange

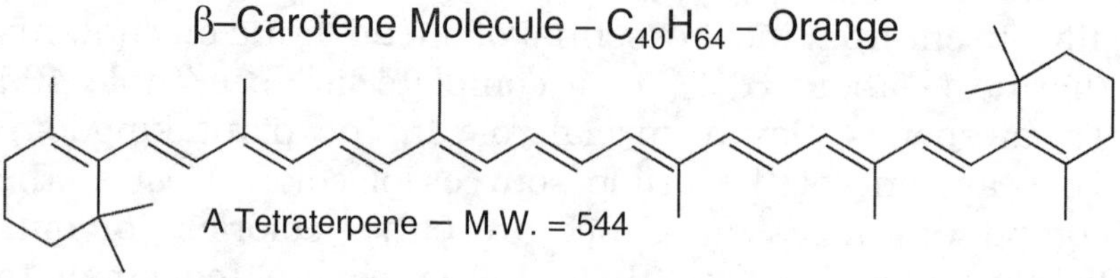

A Tetraterpene – M.W. = 544

Two Halves of a β–Carotene Molecule – $C_{20}H_{32}$ – Colorless

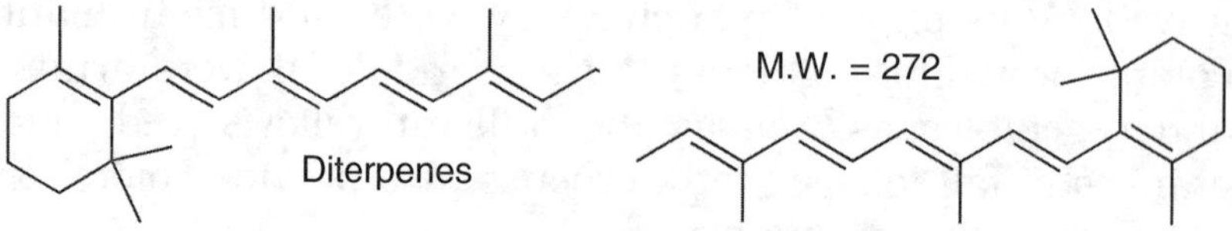

M.W. = 272

Diterpenes

Vitamin A Molecule (Retinol)– $C_{20}H_{32}O$

A Diterpene
Alcohol

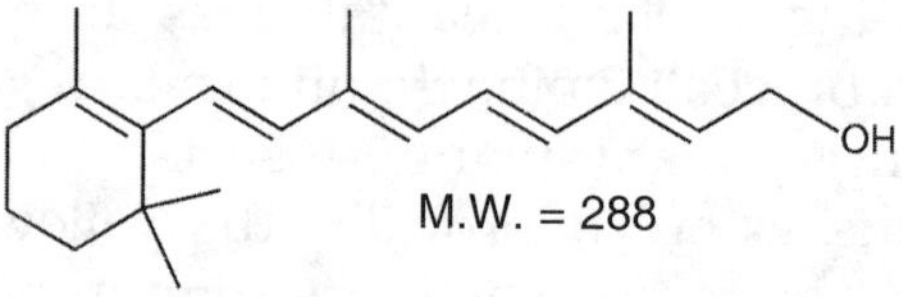

OH
M.W. = 288

beta-carotene ($C_{40}H_{64}$) is a long chain molecule made of isoprene units linked together, head to tail, with a six-sided ring at both ends. It is called a "bicyclic" molecule because of its two rings. When you eat a carrot your body's metabolism divides the long beta-carotene molecule exactly in half to make two identical diterpene molecules ($C_{20}H_{32}$) each with a ring on one end. Your body then adds an oxygen atom to this diterpene transforming it into vitamin A ($C_{20}H_{32}O$). Vitamin A is an oxygenated diterpene known as retinol. Its name suggests its affinity with the retina of our eyes, where vision begins. Vitamin A is necessary for your eyes because it is the raw product and precursor from which your body makes rhodopsin—the protein in our eyes that gives us sight. When a rhodopsin molecule absorbs a photon of light, it sends an electrical message to the base of the brain which we interpret as vision. Now you know why you should eat carrots.

Lycopene is another tetraterpene ($C_{40}H_{64}$) that has been receiving a lot of attention in news and advertising these days. Lycopene is another isomer of carotene. Lycopene is red and occurs in many plants, including ripe tomatoes, watermelon, papaya, pink grapefruit, and red wine. The molecular structure of lycopene is simply a long chain of eight isoprene units connected head to tail in a single line bent at both ends. Lycopene has no rings, like β-carotene, and, therefore, is called an "acyclic" molecule.

Recent studies have found that eating foods containing lycopene help to reduce one's risk of cancer. Hence, it is now common to see ads for multivitamins and natural supplements saying that they contain lycopene.

Both lycopene and carotene are members of a class of compounds called "carotenoids." This class of tetraterpenes absorbs visible light and re-emits it at a lower frequency, dissipating the energy as heat, thereby protecting the plant or animal from any potentially harmful effects associated with sunlight-induced chemistry. Carotene in our skins serves that purpose for us, too, as a protection from too much sunlight.

In the drawings of lycopene, carotene, and vitamin A, see if you can recognize how they are constructed of isoprene units. Lycopene and carotene each have eight isoprenes while vitamin A has only four with an oxygen attached on one end. It's easy to see that six of lycopene's eight little horsies are attached in a line, head to foot with two turned at right angles on the ends—one hanging down on the left and one sticking straight up on the right.

p-Cuminol
$C_9H_{12}O$

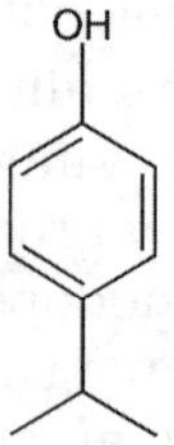

p-Cuminol
showing an
isoprene unit
C_5H_8

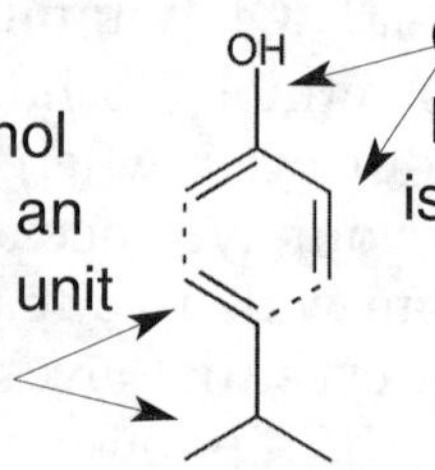

C_4H_4O
Not an
isoprene
unit

While the isomers of monoterpenes and sesquiterpenes number in the thousands, the isomers of diterpenes number in the millions, triterpenes in the billions, and tetraterpenes in the trillions. No lack of possibilities here.

Hemiterpenes

The question may arise as to whether there are such substances as "hemiterpenes." "Hemi" means "half." Half a terpene would be an isoprene unit (C_5H_8). The answer is yes and no. There is no compound consisting of an isoprene unit by itself. However, most phenolic compounds do contain an isoprene unit hidden in their structure. Therefore, some phenols and phenylpropanoids could be called "hemiterpenes."

For example, if you take another look at p-cuminol $(C_9H_{12}O)$, the first phenylpropanoid we introduced back in Chapters Four and Five, you can see the isoprene unit (C_5H_8). See the little horsey running vertically straight down in the figure above? At first, it may appear that the upper part of the p-cuminol molecule is another isoprene unit. It has the same doggie shape. But this is not an isoprene. Instead of a C atom at the head, it has an OH. The formula for the upper portion of this molecule is not the formula for an isoprene (C_5H_8), as in the lower part. Its formula is C_4H_4O.

The reason phenolic molecules with an apparent isoprene unit are not usually called "hemiterpenes," is because, during their biosynthesis, they are not actually built of isoprene units by the plant. They are built from amino acid molecules turned into phenol molecules, propyl radicals, and hydroxyl radicals. It just happens that in the end there is a hidden isoprene, but it was not placed there as a C_5H_8 functional group as is the case when plants build terpenes.

Phenylpropanoids

We will be concluding this chapter with PMS—Phenols, Monoterpenes, and Sesquiterpenes. Remember from Chapter Six that phenols (phenolics) are compounds containing a phenol functional group (C_6H_6O) and that phenylpropanoids are phenols with a propyl radical attached. Propyl radicals are 3-carbon chains with either

Table Thirteen
Phenolic Compounds in Essential Oils

Name	Formula*	Example of an Oil where Found
Anethole	$C_{10}H_{12}O$	Fennel (*Foeniculum vulgare*)
Borneol	$C_{10}H_{18}O$	Citronella (*Cymbopogon nardus*)
Carvacrol	$C_{10}H_{14}O$	Oregano (*Origanum compactum*)
Cinnamal	C_9H_8O	Cinnamon (*Cinnamomum verum*)
p-Cuminol	$C_9H_{12}O$	Cumin (*Cuminum cyminum*)
Estragole	$C_{10}H_{12}O$	Basil (*Ocimum basilicum*)
Eugenol	$C_{10}H_{12}O_2$	Clove (*Syzygium aromaticum*)
Menthol	$C_{10}H_{20}O$	Peppermint (*Mentha piperita*)
Methyl Salicylate	$C_8H_8O_3$	Wintergreen (*Gaultheria procumbens*) and Birch (*Betula alleghaniensis*)
Myristicin	$C_{10}H_{10}O_3$	Nutmeg (*Myristica fragrans*)
Terpinen-4-ol	$C_{10}H_{18}O$	Tea Tree (*Melaleuca alternifolia*)
Thymol	$C_{10}H_{14}O$	Thyme (*Thymus vulgaris*)

* The Molecular Weights of many Phenolic compounds in oils range between 120 and 178 amu, although some can be as large as 232 amu.

5, 6 or 7 H atoms—(C_3H_5), (C_3H_6), or (C_3H_7). They are incomplete propane molecules (C_3H_8).

Table Thirteen (on the previous page) lists a few phenolic compounds found in essential oils, along with examples of some oils in which they are found. (For a more comprehensive compilation of phenols, See Tables 48, 63, 64, and 70 in Part Two of this book.)

Phenols are a very important category of therapeutically active molecules in essential oils that are in a class of their own. They are not terpenes and not generically related to terpenes, even though an isoprene unit may be seen tucked into their structure. Phenolics are assertive and aggressive. Their presence often dominates the flavor or fragrance of an oil. They are warriors who will fight off invading microbes and parasites, while protecting and preserving the friendly flora of our bodies. They are nice fellows to have on your side.

There are a hundred or so varieties of phenolic compounds found in essential oils. Phenols are not as numerous as terpenes but they play key roles in cleansing, stimulating, toning, anesthetizing, and in fighting bacteria or viruses. While terpenes are hydrocarbons, phenolics are oxygenated hydrocarbons. Phenolic compounds in essential oils cleanse receptor sites.

Aspirin and Methyl Salicylate

You have already seen structural diagrams of most of the molecules in Table Thirteen displayed in earlier chapters. However, you have not seen methyl salicylate $(C_8H_8O_3)$, an aspirin-like compound with cortisone-like effects, but without the side effects of actual cortisone $(C_{21}H_{28}O_5)$. Methyl salicylate is a compound found in only two essential oils: birch and wintergreen, which is an anomaly in that birch and wintergreen are not botanically related at all. Birch (*Betula alleghaniensis*) is a member of the birch family (Betulaceae) while wintergreen (*Gaultheria procumbens*) is a member of the heather family (Ericaceae) which includes ledum (*Ledum groenlandicum*) which contains no methyl salicylate in its oil whatsoever. Meanwhile,

Aspirin and Methyl Salicylate Structures

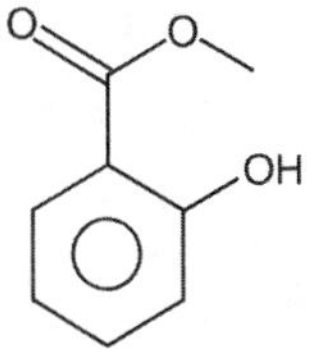

Methyl Salicylate
$C_8H_8O_3$

Comprises 85-99% of
Birch & Wintergreen Oils

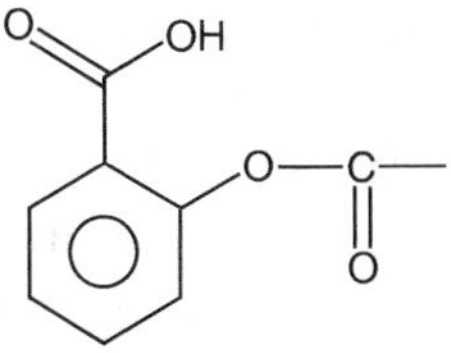

Acetylsalicylic Acid
$C_9H_8O_4$

(Common Aspirin)

both birch and wintergreen oils consist almost entirely of this compound—85-99%.

The structural formulas for methyl salicylate and aspirin ($C_9H_8O_4$), acetylsalicylic acid are shown above. The "methyl" part of methyl salicylate is a CH_3 radical hanging invisibly at the end of the fine line extending to the right at the top at attached to the O atom. There is an invisible CH_3 radical hanging out at the end of the line on the right side of aspirin, also.

Methyl salicylate was discussed in Chapter One in reference to the *Merck Manual*, which considers it to be highly toxic, even potentially lethal. Methyl salicylate is the main ingredient in the oils of birch (*Betula lenta*) and wintergreen (*Gaultheria procumbens*). These oils have an analgesic effect which has been compared to cortisone. (See Higley and Higley) It has also been likened to the effects of aspirin. Its formula is given above for your comparison. Contrary to the common folk lore, aspirin does not occur naturally in any plant. It is not found in willow bark nor willow leaves.

What has been found in willow bark and leaves (*Salix nigra*) is salicin or salicyl alcohol glycoside ($C_8H_{18}O_7$). As you can see, this isn't the formula for aspirin. Methyl salicylate is a lot closer to aspirin than salicin. Salicin was an analgesic enjoyed by Native Americans who chewed willow bark and leaves for relief. The oldest European mention of willow was in 1763 as a treatment for feverish conditions. It was first isolated from the plant in 1829 by a French pharmacist, H. Leroux. However, Hippocrates was familiar with the virtues of willow some 400 years before Christ.

Upon ingestion, salicin converts to salicylic acid which is its real active principle. Salicylic acid is analgesic, fever-reducing, and anti-inflammatory. However, when used over an extended period of time, salicin and salicylic acid are quite damaging to the intestinal tract.

Around 1899, a chemist named Felix Hoffman at the Bayer Company, in Germany, discovered something new. He tried acetylsalicylic acid as an experiment on his rheumatic father who could no longer tolerate salicin. Thus, aspirin was introduced into the medical world.

Besides being a phenol, methyl salicylate is also an ester created in the plant by combining methyl alcohol (CH_3OH) with salicylic acid ($C_7H_6O_3$). Methyl salicylate is one of the most misunderstood compounds in aromatherapy. This was pointed out in Chapter One where it is mentioned that in the British school of aromatherapy, both birch and wintergreen oils are banned and considered unsafe for human use.

More Profitable to Make It than to Grow It

Methyl salicylate is what you taste and smell in wintergreen mints, breath fresheners, and mouthwashes, It is one of the flavorings for root beer. It is the ingredient that gives that delicious and distinctive flavor to birch syrup. Its soothing medicinal properties have put it in demand for many ointments, liniments, and salves.

It is a lot less expensive to produce methyl salicylate as an industrial chemical than to wait for plants to produce it. It is also a lot more profitable to synthesize methyl salicylate in a lab, bottle it, label it, and sell it as oil of wintergreen.

Wintergreen and Birch are both 85-90% methyl salicylate which dominates their fragrances and flavors. However, while the other 10-15% of ingredients may not be important to the food and fragrance industry, they are the ingredients that keep methyl salicylate from being toxic. They are the quenchers that make natural oil safe and effective while the synthetic version is neither safe nor effective.

There is also an isomer problem with synthesizing methyl salicylate. There are 25 isomers of $C_8H_8O_3$. The scientific name for the natural isomer of methyl salicylate found in oils is methyl 2-hydroxybenzoate, where the number "2" refers to the fact that the OH (hydroxyl) part of the compound is attached to the #2 carbon of the benzene ring. Among the 25 isomers of $C_8H_8O_3$, there are two synthetic versions with almost the same structure as the natural one. Their names are methyl 3-hydroxybenzoate and methyl 4-hydroxybenzoate where the OH is attached to the #3 and #4 carbons, respectively.

If you go back to Chapter Seven to the section on Blank Keys, you find a numbering system around the benzene ring where the top carbon is #1, the next one going clockwise is #2, then #3, and #4, etc. Numbers 2, 3, and 4 are the only differences in the names of the three compounds just mentioned and refers to where the OH is connected to the aromatic ring. We can call them methyl-2, methyl-3, and methyl-4 salicylate where methyl-2 is the natural compound with all the benefits found in wintergreen and birch while methyl-3 and methyl-4 are not.

The bottom line is that synthetic methyl salicylate is not isomerically or functionally the same as natural methyl salicylate. Synthetic methyl salicylate does not fit our receptor sites in a therapeutic manner, as does the natural version. Hence, synthetic wintergreen oil is toxic, which is why many aromatherapists are afraid of this oil and refuse to use it. They don't realize that natural wintergreen does no harm and has healing powers.

Monoterpenes

Many oils are composed of mostly monoterpenes including grapefruit (93%), silver fir (92%), and frankincense (77%). (For a more complete list, see Table Forty-Six.) Monoterpenes are one of the most fundamental classes of plant compounds. They contain two isoprene units per molecule and are found in every essential oil— comprising as little as 1% to more than 95% of the oil. While they are rarely responsible for the character, flavor, or distinguishing aroma in an essential oil, they support the flavors and aromas of the other ingredients.

For example, the highly prized oil of rose (*Rosa damascena*) contains only small amounts of monoterpenes (less than 5%) which have little or no fragrance, themselves. However, in the absence of these terpenes, the fragrance of rose becomes noticeably different and not as pleasant.

Monoterpenes are responsible for many benefits. They are supportive and enhance the therapeutic talents of other components. They coordinate the various healing abilities of the many individual constituents and help quench the potentially toxic effects of compounds that could, by themselves, be harmful, turning them, instead, into helpers in the healing process. Monoterpenes are the balancing components of an oil, the organizers and the peacemakers. "Blessed are the peacemakers, for they will be called the children of God." (Matthew 5:9)

There are an estimated 1,000 varieties of monoterpenes in essential oils. Theoretically, they all contain the functional group—$C_{10}H_{16}$—which is one terpene unit or two isoprenes. Some of the most popular monoterpenes, found in hundreds of oils, are given in the Table Fourteen in order of their popularity. The pinenes and limonenes are at the top of the chart. With each monoterpene an example of an oil in which it is found is listed. For a more comprehensive listing, see Tables 46 and 57 in Part Two.

A Master Template for Molecules

Back in Chapter Seven we talked about keys, locks, and receptor sites. It was noted that when you lost your car key and went to the hardware or auto supply store to have a new one made, they would pull out a blank master key that would fit all of the vehicles of your make. From that they would customize a key for your particular car. In that section we drew a picture of a 10-carbon molecular blank key that seems to be a popular pattern in making molecules for essential oils. This 10-carbon pattern was utilized in several phenylpropanoids. It is also a blank key for many monoterpenes, as you can see on page 274. Even the two acyclic compounds, myrcene and ocimene, utilize this template, bending their chains to conform to this shape.

Table Fourteen
Common Monoterpenes in Essential Oils

Name	Formula*	Example of an Oil Where Found
α–Pinene	$C_{10}H_{16}$	Pine (*Pinus sylvestris*)
d–Limonene	$C_{10}H_{16}$	Orange (*Citrus sinensis*)
β–Pinene	$C_{10}H_{16}$	Galbanum (*Ferula gummosa*)
l–Limonene	$C_{10}H_{16}$	Balsam Fir (*Abies balsamea*)
Sabinene	$C_{10}H_{16}$	Juniper (*Juniperus communis*)
Myrcene	$C_{10}H_{16}$	Frankincense (*Boswellia carteri*)
γ–Terpinene	$C_{10}H_{16}$	Marjoram (*Origanum marjorana*)
β–Phellandrene	$C_{10}H_{16}$	Ginger (*Zingiber officinale*)
Camphene	$C_{10}H_{16}$	Spruce (*Picea mariana*)
Ocimene	$C_{10}H_{16}$	Basil (*Ocimum basilicum*)
δ-3-Carene	$C_{10}H_{16}$	Galbanum (*Ferula gummosa*)
p-Cymene	$C_{10}H_{14}$	Thyme (*Thymus vulgaris*)

* The monoterpenes above are listed in order of their popularity. The formula is usually the same for all Monoterpenes and their Molecular Weight is usually 136 amu. Their volatility is high.

Every compound in the chart of structural formulas on the next page is a monoterpene with the formula $C_{10}H_{16}$—except one. P-cymene has the formula, $C_{10}H_{14}$, but is still considered a monoterpene. It is an important constituent in many oils, including several species of eucalyptus and melaleuca, as well as the raindrop oils of oregano, thyme, frankincense*, and blue tansy*. (*in Valor®) Its aromatic

VARIATIONS ON A BLANK KEY
Common Monoterpenes ($C_{10}H_{16}$) in Essential Oils

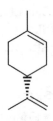 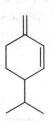 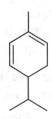 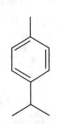

d–Limonene	**l–Limonene**	**α–Phellandrene**	**β–Phellandrene**	**p–Cymene**
Orange	Pine	Dill	Tsuga	Tea Tree, Blue
Celery	Naiouli	Elemi	White Fir	Tansy, Oregano,
Tangerine	Black Pepper	E.dives	Tangerine	Frankincense

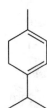 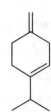 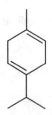 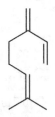 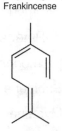

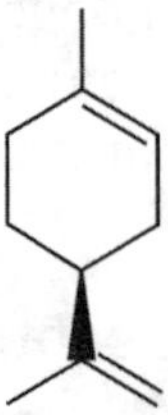

α–Terpinene	**β–Terpinene**	**γ–Terpinene**	**Myrcene**	**Ocimene**
Cumin	Cumin	Lemon	Cypress	Basil
Tea Tree	Tea Tree	Bergamot	Grapefruit	Tarragon
Marjoram	Marjoram	Coriander	Galbanum	Lavender

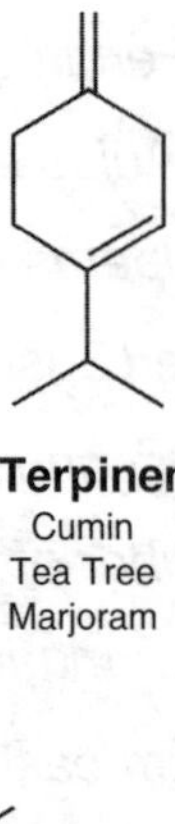

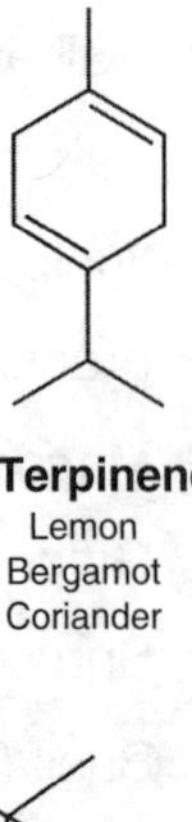

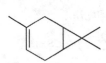

δ-3-Carene	**Camphene**	**α–Pinene**	**β–Pinene**
Pine	Spruce	Myrtle	Hyssop
Spruce, Galbanum,	Juniper, Cistus,	Balsam Fir	Nutmeg
Douglas Fir	Rosemary	Frankincense	Galbanum

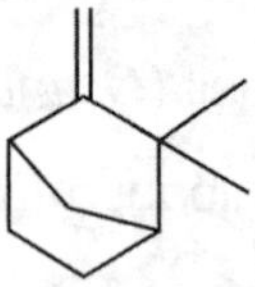

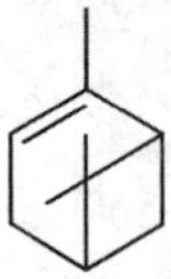

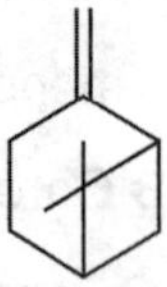

NOTES

The first eight molecules are all monocyclic
    monoterpenes (1 ring)—a hexagon.
Myrcene & Ocimene are acyclic (no rings).
The rest are all bicyclic monoterpenes (2 rings):
    δ-3-Carene—hexagon & triangle
    Camphene—two pentagons
    α & β Pinene—quadrilateral & hexagon
    Sabinene—pentagon & triangle

Sabinene
Vitex
Ravensara
Bay Laurel

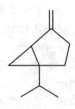

ring with three double bonds is a special source of vibrationally high healing energy. P-cymene is also known for its soothing, analgesic effects.

Deterpenized Oils

The oils of lemon (*Citrus limon*) and celery seed (*Apium graveolens*) are both about 65% d-limonene, a mild mannered monoterpene, but each oil has a markedly different smell and taste due to the other ingredients. If you remove all of the limonene from both oils, the lemon would still smell like lemon and the celery like celery, only about three times as strong. By deterpenizing the oils, you concentrate the ingredients that provide taste and aroma, to which limonene makes no discernable contribution.

Since monoterpenes, in general, are not usually the source of flavors or fragrances sought by the food and fragrance industries they are often removed from food and perfume grade oils. This reduces or destroys the therapeutic value of these oils, not only by the absence of some of its key healing participants, but also because its natural balance has been upset. The balance of oil constituents is a key factor in the therapeutic potential of an oil. The perfume and food industries deterpenize their oils also to make them more soluble in alcohol, sugar syrup, and other dispersants.

Cosmetic manufacturers who like the fragrance of bergamot (*Citrus bergamia*) for their products always want "deterpenized" oil. This is to remove bergaptene, which is phototoxic. Phototoxicity is when a substance applied to the skin amplifies ultraviolet light and can cause sunburn and possible permanent discoloration of the skin. Though its name ends in -ene like a terpene, bergaptene is not really a terpene. It is a furanocoumarin—a class of compounds we will study in the next chapter. Nevertheless, the term "deterpenization" is used when bergaptene is removed from the oil of bergamot. The fragrance of bergamot has been a popular part of both men's and women's colognes and perfumes for hundreds of years. It is also the flavor of Earl Grey Tea.

Fragrance and food people also claim that terpene containing oils will "readily degrade, producing undesirable by-products, which often have a tainting effect on their products." (See Burfield.) While this is not so for true therapeutic grade essential oils left untampered with, apparently it is a problem with the manipulated, rectified, partially synthesized oils of these non-healing industries.

The known shelf life of pure therapeutic grade essential oils containing terpenes is in the thousands of years, as testified by those found in Egyptian tombs. However, monoterpenes can react with or be modified by the other ingredients of a cosmetic, soap, shampoo, mouth wash, syrup, or confection, in ways that degrade these products. Since it isn't the monoterpenes that usually contribute significantly to the taste or smell of interest anyhow, commercial corporations would rather just not have them.

Thus, you can see, that a food or fragrance grade essential oil is really not designed for healing purposes and generally has little or no therapeutic value. Such oils are apparently safe when used in small quantities in commercial products, as they are. However, when such oils are applied by the customary methods of therapeutic aromatherapy, they are not only unlikely to provide any real help, but can actually result in harm.

Oils that have been "rectified," "denatured," "redistilled," "standardized," or "deterpenized" are oils with ingredients removed—usually monoterpenes. They are not therapeutic. Included among their beneficial actions, monoterpenes restore or awaken correct information in the cell's memory and re-establish proper cellular function. An oil without monoterpenes is not a healing oil.

Sesquiterpenes

Oils composed mostly of sesquiterpenes include cedarwood (95%), patchouly (85%), sandalwood (83%), ginger (77%), blue cypress (73%), and myrrh (65%). (See Table Forty-Nine for a more complete list.) Included among their various therapeutic functions, sesquiterpenes delete faulty information in cellular memory.

Table Fifteen
Sesquiterpenes Found in Essential Oils

Name	Formula*	Example of an Oil Where Found
α–Bergamotene	$C_{15}H_{24}$	Fleabane (*Conyza canadensis*)
Bisabolene	$C_{15}H_{24}$	Myrrh (*Commiphora myrrha*)
δ–Cadinene	$C_{15}H_{24}$	White Fir (*Abies grandis*)
β–Caryophyllene	$C_{15}H_{24}$	Black Pepper (*Piper nigrum*)
Chamazulene	$C_{14}H_{21}$	Blue Tansy (*Tanacetum annuum*)
α–Copaene	$C_{15}H_{24}$	Rosewood (*Aniba roseaodora*)
α–Curcumene	$C_{15}H_{22}$	Ginger (*Zingiber officinale*)
γ–Curcumene	$C_{15}H_{24}$	Helichrysum (*Helichrysum italicum*)
Elemene	$C_{15}H_{24}$	Elemi (*Canarium luzonicum*)
α–Farnesene	$C_{15}H_{24}$	Valerian (*Valeriana officinalis*)
β–Farnesene	$C_{15}H_{24}$	G. Chamomile (*Matricaria recutita*)
Guaiene	$C_{15}H_{24}$	Patchouly (*Pogostemon cablin*)
Humulene	$C_{15}H_{24}$	Sage (*Salvia officinalis*)
Longifolene	$C_{15}H_{24}$	Vitex (*Vitex negundo*)
α–Selenene	$C_{15}H_{24}$	Celery (*Apium graveolens*)
α–Ylangene	$C_{15}H_{24}$	Ylang Ylang (*Cananga odorata*)

* The formulas are approximately the same for all hydrocarbon sesquiterpenes and their molecular weights are usually 204 amu. Their volatility is low.

Sesquiterpenes are a fundamental class of plant compounds containing three isoprene units per molecule. They are found in most essential oils—sometimes comprising more than 50% of the oil. While sesquiterpenes don't usually have strong fragrances, some do. Caryophyllene, for example, has a strong woody, spicy odor found in cloves, lavender, thyme, black pepper, vitex, melissa, cinnamon, and ylang ylang. While many sesquiterpene formulas are unique to a single oil, β-caryophyllene is a popular sesqui-

THE STRANGE SHAPES OF SESQUITERPENES
Selected Sesquiterpenes ($C_{15}H_{24}$) found in Essential Oils

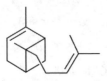

α–Bergamotene
Fleabane
Bergamot

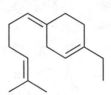

Bisabolene
Myrrh, Ginger
German Chamomile

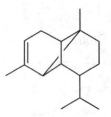

δ–Cadinene
Ginger
Cedarwood
White Fir

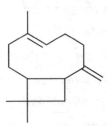

β–Caryophyllene
Black Pepper, Melissa,
Cinnamon, Vitex, Clove,
Mt. Savory, Frankincense
Ginger, Helichrysum,

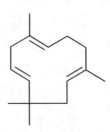

Humulene
(α–Caryophyllene)
Sage, Clove, Hops

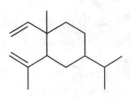

α–Copaene
Rosewood, Frankincense

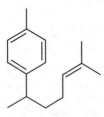

α–Curcumene
Ginger

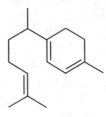

γ–Curcumene
Helichrysum

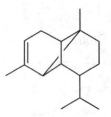

β–Elemene
Elemi, Myrrh, Blue Cypress

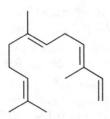

α–Farnesene
Valerian, Ylang Ylang

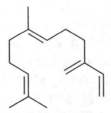

β–Farnesene
German Chamomile

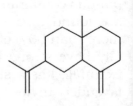

α–Selenene
Celery, Ginger, Blue

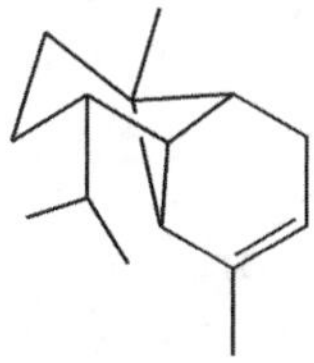

α–Ylangene
Juniper
Birch Bud
Ylang Ylang

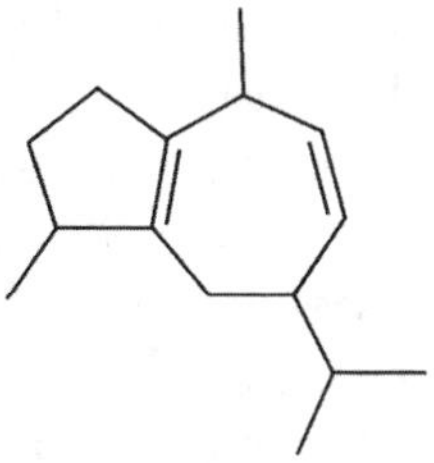

Guaiene
Patchouly
Geranium

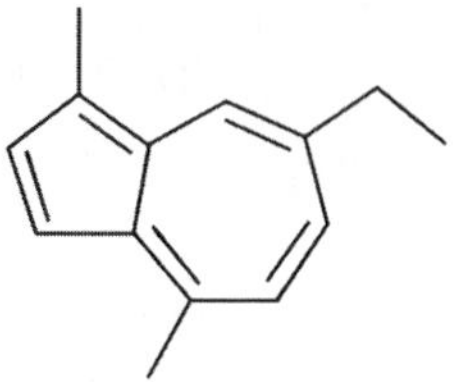

Chamazulene
German Chamomile
Yarrow, Blue Tansy
Helichrysum

terpene and is found in more oils than any other. Sesquiterpenes, in general, are the largest group of naturally occurring terpenes in the world, playing numerous vital biochemical functions in both plants and animals. Farnesene, for example, comprises part of the waxy coating on apple skins, but is also a constituent in several essential oils.

Sesquiterpene molecules are larger than monoterpene and phenylpropanoid molecules and are less volatile. As a participant in an essential oil, sesquiterpenes increase the half-life of smaller light molecules, both aromatically and therapeutically. They are called "fixing" molecules, highly prized by perfumers for making valuable top-note short-lived fragrances linger longer than they could on their own.

So when perfumers deterpenize an oil, they usually don't take out all the terpenes, only the monoterpenes. They often leave in the sesquiterpenes, which sometimes provide the fragrance desired for the perfume blend. When sesquiterpenes are removed, it is because of their poor solubility in alcohol. Modern perfumers and consumers do not want to see cloudy perfumes, which are often in an ethyl alcohol base. They want them to be transparent and clear in the bottle.

Oils like myrrh (*Commiphora myrrha*) and sandalwood (*Santalum album*)—both over 90% sesquiterpenes—have been added to perfumes and healing ointments for their fixing properties for thousands of years before the word "sesquiterpene" was ever coined or its formula known.

While they don't oxidize as readily as monoterpenes, most hydrocarbons will oxidize if exposed to air long enough. A problem with some sesquiterpenes is that when they do oxidize, they tend to resinify—i.e. thicken with air contact. Anyone who has ever had a bottle of pure myrrh has experienced this when the oil left on the threads of the bottle and cap oxidizes. Bottle caps on myrrh become hard to remove when the resinous residue accumulates over time and acts like an adhesive. Wiping off the the glass top and the threads of the cap with each use can minimize this. Cheap versions of myrrh may not have this problem, since they are usually diluted with light petrochemical hydrocarbons. If your bottle of myrrh does not have a resin problem around its lid, it probably isn't pure myrrh.

There are an estimated 3,000 varieties of sesquiterpenes in essential oils. Those with the formula $C_{15}H_{24}$ are hydrocarbons, but any compound containing $C_{15}H_{24}$ as a functional group is considered a sesquiterpene. By oxygenating a sesquiterpene we can create sesquiterpene phenols, alcohols, aldehydes, ketones, acids, oxides, and lactones—all sesquiterpenes. For example, cedarwood oil is composed entirely of sesquiterpenes as hydrocarbons, ketones, and alcohols. Valerian oil contains sesquiterpene aldehydes, acids and lactones in addition to sesquiterpenones (ketones) and sesquiterpenols (alcohols).

Unlike monoterpenes where certain monoterpene compounds occur repeatedly in many different species of oils, sesquiterpenes are often species-specific. Numerous sesquiterpenes are one-of-a-kind only, found in only one species of oil, not copied by any other plant. Examples of include zingiberene, patchoulene, viridiflorene, himachalene, valeranone, and aristoladiene found only in the oils of ginger, patchouly, niaouli (MQV), cedarwood, valerian, and spikenard, respectively. With each sesquiterpene in Table Fifteen, an example of an oil (or the oil) in which it is found is listed. (For a more complete listing, see Tables 49, 65 and 66 in Part Two.)

Learning Greek

We have been using Greek characters and other alphabetic prefixes in this chapter (and some previous chapters), so perhaps we should at least give names to the symbols so you can pronounce them and know what they imply. Here are the Greek and Latin characters we are using in this book, as well as three English letters also used as hyphenated prefixes:

α = alpha
β = beta
γ = gamma
δ = delta
ζ = zeta
χ = chi
d = dextrorotary (right-handed)
l = levorotary (left-handed)
p = para

The first six are Greek letters corresponding to a, b, g, d, z, and c in English. When you see several variations of a compound, like α–Farnesene and β–Farnesene (Table Fifteen) or like α–Terpinene, β–Terpinene, and γ–Terpinene (Table Fourteen), the Greek letters simply mean that these compounds are isomers of one another where the difference in their structures is usually where the double bonds occur. When a double bond is moved, the locations of hydrogens (usually not shown in structural diagrams) also move. So the shape of the actual molecule changes when double bonds are in different locations.

The letters, d and l, stand for Latin prefixes (dextro- and levo-). You have already met these characters in Chapter Six when we discussed right and left-handed isomers. We include it in this list for completeness.

The last one, p = para, isn't Greek or Latin. It's just a plain old English letter "pee" standing for "para," as in p-cymene in Table Fourteen or p-cuminol in Table Thirteen. Para is a prefix that tells organic chemists where a functional group is attached. You will also see prefixes like n = normal, o = ortho, and m = meta, which have meanings to

organic chemists, but we won't use or explain these prefixes in this book.

So from now on, when you see p-cuminol you can say
"para-cuminol." You can speak Greek, too. When you see
α–pinene, you say "alpha pinene." When you see β–pinene,
you say "beta pinene." Or when you see δ–cadinene, you
say "delta cadinene," and know that there is also an
alpha–, beta– and gamma–cadinene—all isomers of
cadinene whose differences are where the double bonds
are located.

Chamazulene Sings the Blues

You may have noticed in Table Fifteen that all of the
compounds listed had the expected sesquiterpene formu-
la ($C_{15}H_{24}$) except α–curcumene ($C_{15}H_{22}$) and chamazulene
($C_{14}H_{21}$). In the case of α–curcumene there is an extra double bond in the ring which eliminates two hydrogens and
increases the resonance energy of the molecule. Found in
ginger oil, α–curcumene is thought to help reduce cholesterol. Although the formula isn't exactly that of a
sesquiterpene hydrocarbon, α-curcumene contains three
isoprene units, which makes it a true sesquiterpene. See if
you can find three little horsies hidden in its structure.

As for chamazulene $C_{14}H_{21}$, the formula is short by a
CH_3 unit (a methyl radical). Even so, it is still classed as a
sesquiterpene or "terpenoid." Note the similarity between
the diagram of chamazulene and that of guaiene next to it.
Guaiene is a true sesquiterpene ($C_{15}H_{24}$). Both of these
compounds are bicyclic, both combining a unique 7-sided
ring with a 5-sided ring.

The truth is that chamazulene is not a compound found
in living plants. It is what we call an "artifact." It is the
result of a natural plant compound that has been altered
by the heat of distillation. Chamazulene is produced by
the alteration of a colorless sesquiterpene molecule (matricene) where it loses a methyl unit (CH_3) during distillation
changing it from $C_{15}H_{24}$ to $C_{14}H_{21}$.

While distillers of essential oils usually do everything

they can to capture the essence of the plant as closely as possible, preserving what was in nature, the distillation process, itself, can slightly change things. This is why distillation needs to be handled carefully at minimum temperatures and low pressures to keep the production of artifacts to a minimum—unless the artifacts are desirable and of therapeutic value, which some are. Some distillers are more skillful and more conscientious than others, which is why it is important to know and trust your distiller.

Chamazulene is deep blue in color and is found in German chamomile (*Matricaria recutita*), blue tansy (*Tanacetum annuum*), Helichrysum (*Helichrysum italicum*) and yarrow (*Achillea millefolium*). Chamazulene has some notable therapeutic qualities and has been the subject of extensive research. It has a high resonance energy. (Note the high number of double bonds in the molecular diagram on page 279.) It is considered to possess anti-allergy and anti-inflammatory properties and to be beneficial to cells and nourishing to skin. It has been found to be a muscle relaxant in animal studies.

In the distillation of German chamomile a high concentration of chamazulene is considered desirable, increasing the value of the oil. The darker the blue color, the better. Hence, distillers of the oil adjust their techniques to maximize the chamazulene content.

Some dishonest oil dealers purchase the cheaper Moroccan chamomile (*Ormenis mixta* or *Ormensis multicaulis*) and add synthetic chamazulene. They then label it and sell it as if it were the more costly German chamomile.

While Moroccan chamomile has its own useful properties, they are not the same as German chamomile. The Moroccan oil is high in santolina alcohol (30-33%), as well as many other alcohols, all of which are absent from the German oil. When presented without fraud, Moroccan chamomile is usually sold by the name of "ormenis oil." Ormenis is said to be good for skin problems such as acne, eczema, dermatitis, and cysts. It has also been used for rheumatism and is supportive of the gall bladder.

There is actually a family of azulene artifacts derived

Table Sixteen
Diterpenes Found in Essential Oils

Name	Formula*	Example of an Oil Where Found
Camphorene	$C_{20}H_{32}$	White Camphor (*Laurus camphora*)
Hishorene	$C_{20}H_{32}$	White Camphor (*Laurus camphora*)
Cembrene	$C_{20}H_{32}$	Pine (*Pinus sylvestris*)
Labdanenol	$C_{20}H_{34}O$	Cistus (*Cistus ladanifer*)
Labdanendiol	$C_{20}H_{34}O_2$	Cistus (*Cistus ladanifer*)
Abienol	$C_{20}H_{36}O$	Cypress (*Cupressus sempervirens*)
Manool	$C_{20}H_{36}O$	Cypress (*Cupressus sempervirens*)
Pimarino	$C_{20}H_{34}O$	Cypress (*Cupressus sempervirens*)
Sempervirol	$C_{20}H_{34}O$	Cypress (*Cupressus sempervirens*)
Totarol	$C_{20}H_{36}O$	Cypress (*Cupressus sempervirens*)
Cupressic Acid	$C_{20}H_{34}O_2$	Cypress (*Cupressus sempervirens*)
Phytol	$C_{20}H_{36}O$	Jasmine (*Jasminum officinale*)
Sclareol	$C_{19}H_{37}O_2$	Clary Sage (*Salvia sclarea*)
Cannabinol	$C_{21}H_{30}O_2$	Marijuana (*Cannabis sativa*)

* Only the first two of these are diterpene hydrocarbons. The rest are diterpene alcohols except for cupressic acid, a diterpene acid and cannibanol, a diterpene phenol. They are all diterpenes, however.

from sesquiterpenes during the distillation process. For example, there is guaiazulene in blue cypress oil (*Callitris intratropica*) and elemazulene in elemi oil (*Canarium luzonicum*). These two compounds are isomers. Their chemical formula is $C_{15}H_{18}$, which has the same number of carbons as a standard sesquiterpene, but is short six hydrogens. In other words, a sesquiterpene has been dehydrogenated and desaturated. When this happens, one additional double bond is added for each pair of hydrogens lost—thus increasing the resonance energy of the molecule—which can improve the therapeutic potential of the oil.

Diterpenes

Jasmine oil absolute contains about 14% diterpenes. A single terpene unit has the formula—$C_{10}H_{16}$. Linking two terpenes together makes a diterpene whose non-oxygenated formula is $C_{20}H_{32}$. Triterpenes ($C_{30}H_{48}$) and tetraterpenes ($C_{40}H_{64}$) are larger molecules than diterpenes and do not pass through the distillation process in creating an essential oil. They are found only in cold-pressed oils such as orange and tangerine and are too large to have aromas. See Table Forty for a list of oils containing di-, tri-, and tetraterpenes.

Diterpenes are among the largest, heaviest molecules found in essential oils produced by distillation. Diterpenes are larger and heavier than mono– and sesquiterpenes, but not too large or heavy to be aromatic and participate in the therapeutic activities of some essential oils. They are not common, however. Table Sixteen lists thirteen diterpene compounds which represent most of the known diterpenes in essential oils. Although there are thirteen compounds, there are only six oils in which they are found. The labdanenols of cistus are also found in cypress. In none of these examples does the occurrence of the compound amount to more than 1-2% percent of the oil except for sclareol, which can be as much as 7% in clary sage oil, cannabinol, which can be up to 10% of marijuana oil, and phytol, which can be up to 15% of jasmine oil.

Also note that only the first three listed in Table Sixteen are hydrocarbon diterpenes. The rest are oxygenated diterpenes, which are all diterpene alcohols except for cupressic acid (a diterpene acid) and cannabinol (a diterpene phenol)—the hallucinogenic ingredient in marijuana. Marijuana oil is used by some physicians and is described in the *PDR for Herbal Medicine*.

White camphor oil goes by several common names such as "Japanese camphor oil," "Chinese camphor oil," "ho leaf oil," or simply "camphor oil." It used to be a major source for camphor ($C_{10}H_{16}O$), before chemists learned to synthesize it more economically in laboratories.

Examples of Diterpene Molecules

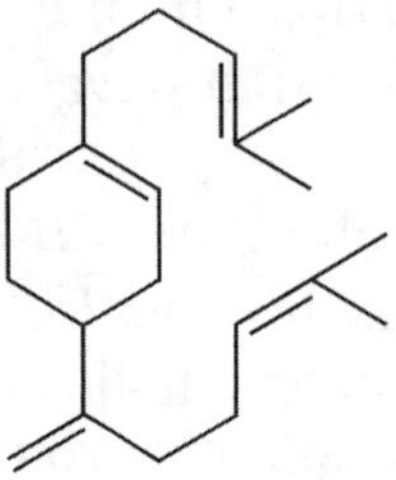

α–Camphorene
(Monocyclic)
$C_{20}H_{32}$

White Camphor Oil

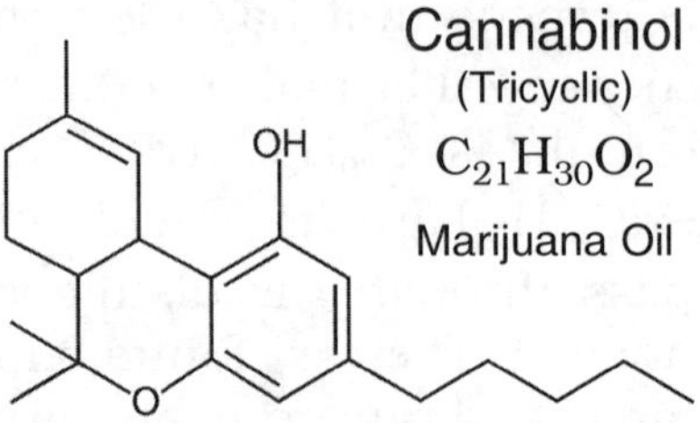

Cannabinol
(Tricyclic)
$C_{21}H_{30}O_2$

Marijuana Oil

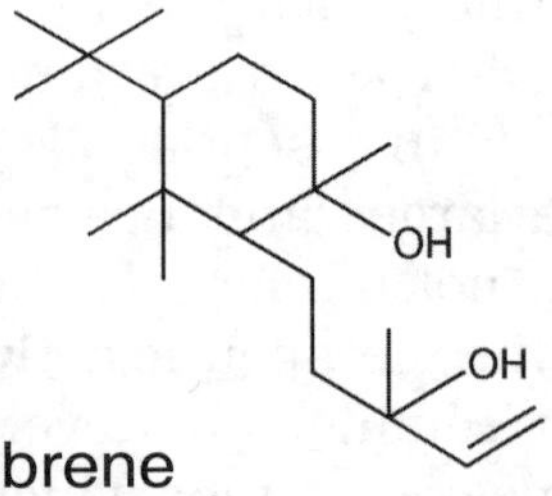

Sclareol
(Monocyclic)
$C_{19}H_{36}O_2$

Sage and
Clary Sage Oils

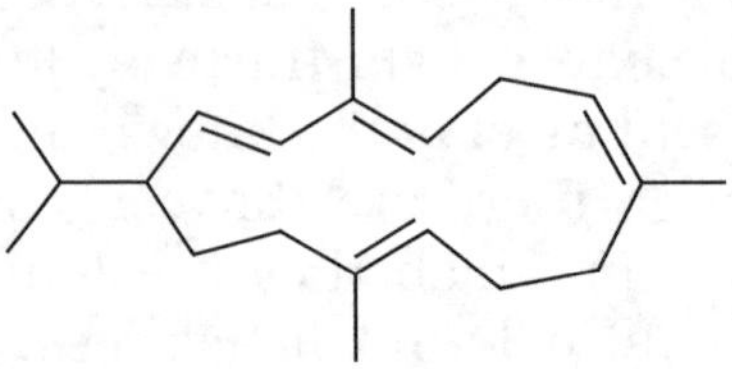

Cembrene
(Monocyclic)
$C_{20}H_{32}$

Pine Oil

There seems to be some confusion as to the genus of this plant. While we have given its scientific name as *Laurus camphora* in the table, it is also known as *Cinnamomum camphora* and *Cinnamomum officinalis*. When botanists work independently in different countries, sometimes the same plant gets two or more scientific names and several of them can become entrenched in the literature.

Therapeutically, diterpenes have some of the same properties as sesquiterpenes. Additionally, they are also considered to be expectorants and purgatives with some effectiveness against fungi and viruses.

Shown above are structural diagrams of four diterpenes as a sample of the great variety of shapes possible with bigger molecules (more Legos® to play with). While the strict formula for a diterpene should include the hydrocarbon, $C_{20}H_{32}$, liberties are taken in naming compounds when their formulas are close, as with cannabinol and sclareol above, which are oxygenated. When hydrocarbons are oxygenated, this can often add or subtract one or two carbons or hydrogens. Notice that the tricyclic cannabinol molecule has a heterogeneous ring (i.e. a ring not composed of all carbons). It is a Coumarin. (see p. 374-75)

Triterpenes

Examples of distilled oils containing triterpenes include birch (1%), marijuana (2%), and myrrh (6%). Myrrh is a very viscous oil, partially due to its triterpene content. As mentioned earlier, diterpenes, with a molecular weight of 272 amu, are about as heavy as as a compound can be and still pass through the distillation process in significant quantities. Triterpenes, that weigh in at a whopping 408 amu are just too fat to make it most of the time, but sometimes they come through. Among aromatic oils, the main place you find triterpenes is in oils extracted by expression (as in citrus oils) or by solvents (as in jasmine, onycha, and neroli). Technically, oils extracted by solvents should not be called "essential." Their proper designation would be "essences" or "absolutes." (See Table Forty.)

Squalene ($C_{30}H_{48}$) comprises 2–7% of jasmine absolute (*Jasminum officinale*). Jasmine cannot be extracted by distillation. The heat destroys the desired constituents. Therefore, it is extracted by solvents—usually with an alkane like hexane (C_6H_{14}). This is how and why such a large molecule as squalene can be present in the fragrant oil. If it were distilled, it would probably not be there except in traces.

Squalene is found in large amounts in shark liver oil as well as in olive oil (up to 1%). It is also found in wheat bran oil, rice bran oil, and yeast. It is employed in our bodies in the biosynthesis of cholesterol, an essential steroid. Squalene is also known as spinacene and supraene. It is found in sebum, a natural waxy secretion of our skin. Sebum protects us from hostile microbes and has been shown to be a shield from lethal high frequency radiation.

Extensive research is being done to document the immune enhancement, cholesterol controlling, and anticarcinogenic properties of squalene. It may some day be employed in the prevention and treatment of some cancers. Squalene capsules are available in most health food stores. As for essential oils, it is available in jasmine.

The molecular structure of squalene is shown in the illustration below, along with that of triacontane. As you can see, squalene ($C_{30}H_{48}$) is actually an acyclic terpene composed of six isoprene units. It is a long chain of thirty carbons. Triacontane ($C_{30}H_{62}$) is an alkane comparable to squalene in weight and formula. The molecular weight of squalene is 408 while that of triacontane is 422. Both are structured as acyclic chains of 30 carbons. But triacontane is different. It does not manifest the aromatic and biologically mobile characteristics of squalene. Triacontane, a form of paraffin, is not found in any essential oil but forms

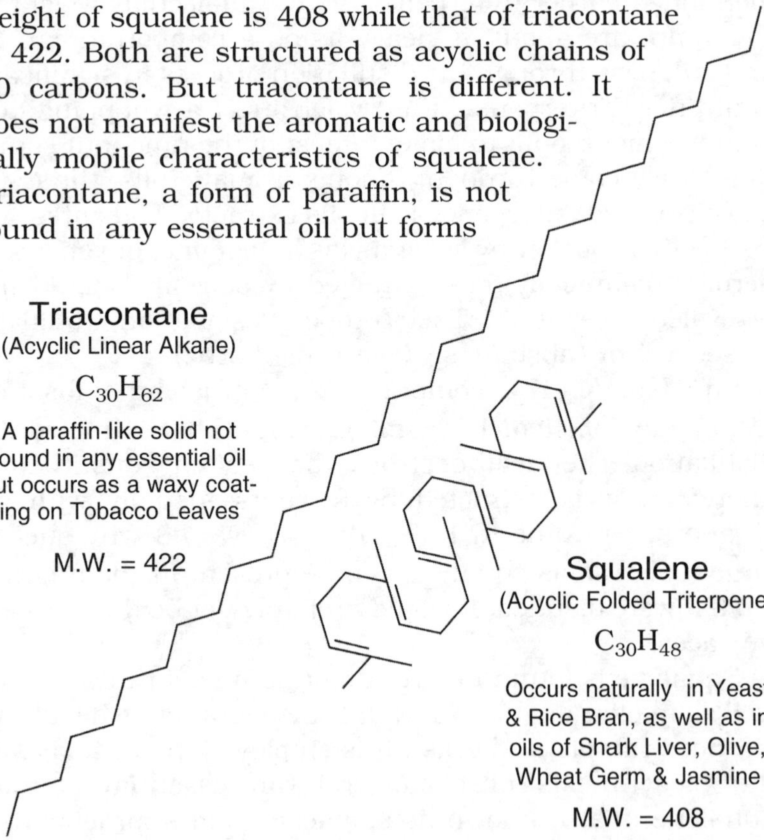

Triacontane
(Acyclic Linear Alkane)

$$C_{30}H_{62}$$

A paraffin-like solid not found in any essential oil but occurs as a waxy coating on Tobacco Leaves

M.W. = 422

Squalene
(Acyclic Folded Triterpene)

$$C_{30}H_{48}$$

Occurs naturally in Yeast & Rice Bran, as well as in oils of Shark Liver, Olive, Wheat Germ & Jasmine

M.W. = 408

Squalene and Triacontane Molecules Compared

the waxy coat on a tobacco leaf. The longest alkane in any essential oil is pentacosane ($C_{25}H_{52}$)—an ingredient of rose oil. Triacontane is of a greasy, waxy texture while squalene is not. The different properties between triacontane and squalene have to do with differences in shape. Their weights are about the same. Triacontane is linear, i.e. stretched out in a straight long line while squalene is an accordion-folded molecule following the template of five almost-complete hexagonal rings. A molecule of triacontane is almost three times the length of a molecule of squalene, as you can see in the figure. In fact, we had to slant it at a 45° angle just to fit it on the page. In contrast, because of its compact size, squalene can do things and go places triacontane can only dream of going.

This illustrates the fact that when it comes to volatility, viscosity, and other physical, chemical, molecular mobility, and other behavioral properties of oil compounds, molecular weight, size, and shape are all important factors. In fact, the difference in many nonaromatic vegetable oil compounds (like caprylic or lauric acid) and aromatic essential oil compounds isn't that they are heavier molecules, but that they are big, long and stretched out.

Caution Regarding Jasmine

Please do not take jasmine internally. Because it is an absolute, and not a true essential oil, it usually contains traces of petrochemical solvents, like hexane. Jasmine absolute is also one of the most commonly adulterated of fragrances.

It takes more than three million jasmine blossoms, plucked in the dark hours of early morning, before sunrise, to produce one pound of oil. A pound of true pure jasmine absolute can cost $1200 or more. A pound of synthetic jasmine can be produced for less than $5.

Unless you know and can trust your producer, you never know what you are getting in jasmine oil except that if its price is cheap, you can know without question that the oil is a fake or has been diluted. And even when you have the highest quality jasmine, it is still an absolute extracted with chemicals, so don't take it internally. If you want squalene as a nutritional supplement, get it from olive oil, wheat bran oil, or shark liver oil.

Compound Personalities Compared

The most active ingredients of an oil, the ones that capture our senses and attention, are the oxygenated hydrocarbons (including oxygenated terpenes). These are the alcohols, ethers, aldehydes, ketones, acids, esters, oxides, lactones, coumarins, and furanoids discussed in the next chapter. Phenols and phenylpropanoids are also a class of oxygenated hydrocarbons already discussed. It is the oxygenated molecules of an oil that usually provides its personality, character, zest, and sex appeal.

The most important group of hydrocarbons in oils is the terpene family, the topic of this chapter. While their therapeutic benefits are undisputed, terpene hydrocarbons don't usually dominate fragrance or flavor. They prefer to administer their benefits in quiet, unassuming ways—unlike the phenols, which are usually strong, brazen, and aggressive.

Among the personalities of various oil compounds, monoterpenes are like mothers. They are coordinators, quenchers, unifiers, and organizers—providing balance and coherence to the actions of the hundreds of participants in an essential oil. Monoterpenes are the ones that see that the healing objectives are not forgotten while supplying encouragement and support to everyone along the way. Monoterpenes don't mind if another constituent gets the credit for a job well done. They are content to be of support and to make good things happen behind the scenes, creating an environment of resonance and harmony. Monoterpenes are humble servants, working quietly and hard to make everyone else look good.

Sesquiterpenes are wise, responsible ones who will see a job through to the end, the ones who help pace everyone so that they all finish the race. They are the sensible big brothers watching over every one else and gently guiding them in ways of benefit and healing. Sesquiterpenes are the ones who do what no one else wants to do, like emptying the trash, clearing flawed files, and cleaning out cellular information that is no longer useful. They will also corral an unruly companion, kindly and firmly, taking it under its big brother wing, helping it to behave in a positive and beneficial way. Sesquiterpenes are chaperones of the more aggressive molecules, making sure their work in the body is productive and constructive and not destructive. They are the illumined ones who, like the monoterpenes, don't mind to work in service and humility, seeing that everyone else gets the best job done and not caring who gets the credit. Phenolics are the unruly little boys, full of energy, but needing guidance. They are fighters, the purgative ones. They are the ones who clean the receptor sites, clearing out any unwelcome guests that don't belong in those areas. They are warriors and policeman, looking for invaders such as viruses, bacteria, parasites, petrochemicals, heavy metals, pharmaceutical drugs, and other aliens. When they find them, they destroy them and/or usher them out of the body. Phenols and phenylpropanoids are initiators of healing processes, clearing the way for the many other types of healing compounds in an oil, to carry out their divinely designated assignments. In the absence of phenols, the ketones of an essential oil will take over and perform their purgative tasks. In Psalm 51, David cries out to God, "Purge me with hyssop and I shall be clean." Hyssop is about 50% ketones—compounds that purge us of toxins—material, emotional, and spiritual.

Thank God for PMS

Like a good football team, essential oils have a whole book of plays to be applied according to the needs and demands of the situation. Oils work in dozens of ways, mostly unknown and misunderstood, but their "PMS" battle plan is one of their best plays. It is the PMS Paradigm that explains how a single anointment or application of essential oils to bring about an instant and permanent healing. I know this happens first hand, having been healed instantly and permanently of 43 years of continuous back pain with a single application of raindrop oils. This was in the Fall of 1999, and I am still healed. Thanks to PMS, I now have the strong back of a young man. Here's how PMS theory works, where P = Phenol or Phenylpropanoid. M = Monoterpene. S = Sesquiterpene. When you receive a variety of oils by inhalation, orally, or through the skin, that includes these three classes of compounds, what happens is thought to be as follows:

P— First, the phenolics clean the receptor sites.

S— Second, sesquiterpenes delete bad info from cellular memory.

M—Lastly, monoterpenes restore or awaken the correct information in the cell's memory (DNA).

The PMS Paradigm is a useful working hypothesis that provides practical guidance for mixing and applying oils in an effective, therapeutic way. Let's express it another way: (1) When cellular intercommunication is restored in the body by clean, well-functioning receptor sites, (2) When garbled or miswritten information in the cellular job description has been erased, and (3) When God's image of perfection, that was always there in the field of the cell from our creation, has been revived and re-installed, then whatever our disease or condition had been, the conditions for its presence exist no more. Our disease or condition was the consequence of miscommunications between cells and erroneous information within the cells that caused them to malfunction. When these basic errors have been corrected, as is possible with PMS, the problem disappears. It can take time, like days, weeks, or months, but it can also be instantaneous.

Of the 73 mentions of healing in the New Testament, only 30 were miraculous or instantaneous. 55% of them took place over time with additional therapy and loving care. (See *Healing Oils of the Bible* pp. 91-92.) Regardless of how long it takes, once the exterior cellular miscommunication and interior cellular misinformation has been fixed, you are healed. Furthermore, it can be a permanent healing because the root conditions in cellular memory have been corrected. And what is even better, you don't need those oils any more because a true healing has taken place.

This is unlike pharmaceuticals that cover up symptoms, making you think you are well or getting better, when, in fact you are still sick and will need to continue taking drugs to the death. Once you are healed by the help of essential oils, you don't need the oils any more. No life-long dependencies develop, as they do, deliberately and by design, with drugs.

To understand how monoterpenes can restore proper programming after the phenols have cleansed the receptor sites and the sesquiterpenes have deleted cellular misinformation, you need to realize that essential oils act as channels between the physical body and the body's electromagnetic field, a fact that is recognized and applied in raindrop technique. There is more on this in Part Three. Suffice it to say here that our physical vehicles are secondary to and reflections of our subtle bodies composed of light and field energy. God's image is preserved there and can be downloaded from the subtle realm into the materially manifested realm by such agents as monoterpenes. This is how monoterpenes restore things to what they should be once the way has been cleared and the cells prepared by the other compounds. When the interferences to cellular communication have been removed the conditions for healing have been established and set into motion. If maintained by appropriate attitudes and life style changes, healing is assured and is only a matter of time—sometimes hours, sometimes days or weeks, and sometimes minutes or seconds. Such is the power of essential oils.

After a true healing, the disease or condition won't return unless we continue to engage in the life style, thought patterns, emotional state, bad habits, toxic environments, or other activities that brought that disease or condition upon us in the first place. Thus, it is within your control to prevent backsliding, to prevent a relapse. This commitment to a revised life style following a healing is called "repentance" in the *Bible*. Repentance is part of healing, as mentioned in Mark 6:12-13 and James 5:14-16. For more on this, read *Healing Oils of the Bible*.

Finding and Creating PMS Oils

The best way to create a PMS oil is to blend several oils to provide a proportion of all three classes of compounds. Also keep in mind that the receptor site cleansing function performed by phenols can also be accomplished by ketones and/or alcohols, although the alcohols are less aggressive in their cleansing actions as the phenols or ketones and it takes more of them to accomplish the same end. So we could also talk about KMS and/or AMS blends of oils as healing in the same ways as PMS combinations. Instead, we will continue to use the letter "P" where it is understood that it could be P, K or A. A therapeutically effective PMS proportion seems to lie in the range of:

> 10-50%   Phenols/Ketones/Alcohols,
> 10-60%   Monoterpenes, and
> 3-20%   Sesquiterpenes.

You don't need as much of the sesquiterpenes as you do of the phenols and monoterpenes. Table Sixty-Eight in

Part Two, p. 586, lists fourteen oils that contain these proportions as a single species. For example, tea tree oil is fairly well balanced as a PMS oil with 33% phenols, 52% monoterpenes, and 17% sesquiterpenes, which may be a reason for its popularity as an oil with universal applications. Marjoram is also reasonably well balanced with 37% phenols/alcohols, 44% monoterpenes, and 4% sesquiterpenes. Hyssop oil is about 50% ketones/phenols, 30% monoterpenes, and 8% sesquiterpenes and can also act alone as a balanced PMS oil. You can go to Table Sixty-Eight for a list of single PMS oils. However, for a good PMS anointment, blends are best.

Keep in mind that some compounds fit more than one class and can play dual roles. For example, methyl salicylate constitutes 85-90% of the oils of wintergreen and birch. Methyl salicylate is an ester, but it is also a phenol. (See Table Thirteen and the discussion on aspirin earlier in this chapter.) Likewise, you can have monoterpene alcohols and phenols, sesquiterpene ketones and aldehydes, and phenolic ethers and esters. In these cases, compounds can manifest qualities of more than one family of substances—like manifesting qualities of the two families represented by your mother and your father. Cedarwood, which is considered the highest of sesquiterpene bearing oils, is only about half sesquiterpene hydrocarbons, the rest of the oil being sesquiterpene alcohols (20-40%) and sesquiterpene ketones (14-25%). All three classes of these cedarwood compounds manifest their sesquiterpene qualities and their alcoholic and ketonic personalities as well.

Most blends of oils contain a balance of all three—PMS—which is one reason blends are often more effective than using single oils. By combining phenolic, monoterpene, and sesquiterpene oils, you automatically get your balance of the top, middle and base notes of a good blend.

There are 41 cross-referenced tables of oil compounds in Part Two of this book to facilitate the creation of custom blends for therapeutic purposes. The 113 oils whose chemical analyses are given in Table Thirty-Two are averaged together in Table Thirty-Two-A. This summary represents "An Average Essential Oil" which is 31% phenols/ketones/alcohols, 30% monoterpenes, and 12% sesquiterpenes. Thus, a blend of more than 100 of the most commonly used essential oils would be a perfect PMS balance. One company, Young Living Essential Oils, Inc., has a blend like that. It is called Legacy®.

Quick Reference Guide to PMS Content in Oils

To conclude this chapter, let's make some brief lists of oils that are predominantly one of the three: Phenols, monoterpenes or sesquiterpenes. Most essential oils have one or two of these classes of compounds and a few have some of all three, See Table Sixty-Eight, p. 586, for single oils with the PMS proportions. The following three lists will give you an idea of what oils could work together to make a PMS anointing blend. For more complete lists, see Tables 46, 48, and 49. The percents given here are averages only and can vary by 10% or more from batch to batch in the real world. To simplify things so you can easily scan these lists at a glance, we have used only the common plant names for the oils. You can get the botanical names from the cross-references in Part Two. Only a sample of phenolic, monoterpene, and sesquiterpene oils are listed here. For complete lists of alcoholic or ketonic oils, which can also cleanse receptor sites, see Tables Thirty-Five and Forty-Four respectively:

Examples of Phenolic Oils
(For a complete list see Table Forty-Eight, p. 571)

Wintergreen	97%
Birch	90%
Anise	89%
Clove	77%
Basil	76%
Tarragon	75%
Fennel	71%
Oregano	70%
Tea Tree	63%

Thyme	50%
Mountain Savory	49%
Peppermint	39%
Cinnamon	26%

Examples of Monoterpene Oils
(For a complete list see Table Forty-Six, p. 569)

Grapefruit	93%
Silver Fir	92%
Bitter Orange	90%
Mandarin	90%
Orange	90%
Tangerine	90%
Balsam Fir	83%
Lemon	80%
Angelica	80%
Frankincense	78%
Celery Seed	77%
Cypress	76%
Parsley	75%
Fleabane	73%
Galbanum	72%
Elemi	72%
Douglas Fir	70%
Nutmeg	68%
White Fir	65%
Lime	62%
Bergamot	55%
Juniper	54%
Cistus	53%
Marjoram	52%
Pine	51%
Black Pepper	50%
Blue Tansy	50%
Dill	50%
Spruce	50%
Caraway	48%
Yarrow	43%

Examples of Sesquiterpene Oils
(For a complete list see Table Forty-Nine, p. 572)

Cedarwood	95%
Patchouly	85%
Sandalwood	83%
Ginger	77%
Blue Cypress	73%
Myrrh	65%
Vetiver	59%
Vitex	58%
German Chamomile	54%
Black Pepper	53%
Spikenard	52%
Ylang Ylang	48%
Marijuana	46%

Peculiarities of the PMS Lists

You can see by a glance at the PMS lists that monoterpenes are, by far, the most common of the PMS compounds. As the main ingredient in an oil, monoterpenes do not necessarily dominate their therapeutic qualities since the various oils on the above list all act differently. Many of the monoterpene-dominant oils, like the citrus and fir oils, are virtually void of phenols and sesquiterpenes.

Notice how no single oil is listed on all three or even on two of the lists. No oil is strong in all three of the PMS compounds. Oils that are not strong in any one of these classes of compounds may offer a balance of all three, as was mentioned earlier with tea tree and marjoram oils. (See Table Sixty-Eight, p. 586)

Generally speaking, if you want a strong representation of all three PMS compounds, you need at least three oils—one to represent each class. This is why you need to use blends or sequential layering of several different oils to get the full benefit of the PMS healing process.

The Chemistry of Raindrop Technique

Raindrop technique is a protocol for applying oils to the feet and back in a sequence involving various techniques of massage, reflexology, and laying on of hands. It was developed over a period of years by D. Gary Young, N.D., a naturopathic physician and producer of essential oils.

Raindrop is a powerfully effective healing modality and anointing procedure that has benefited hundreds of thousands. For scientific research on the outcomes of raindrop technique, see *A Statistical Validation of Raindrop*, listed in the bibliography. Training seminars and video/DVDs on raindrop are provided by several educational agencies listed in the resource section at the end of this book.

The PMS Chemistry of Raindrop Oils

Oil	*P/K/A	M	S	Other
Valor®	8%	54%	4%	17% esters
Oregano	72%	18%	4%	
Thyme	58%	37%	3%	
Basil	77%	3%	0	
Wintergreen	97%	0	0	
Marjoram	37%	44%	4%	
Cypress	8%	76%	14%	
Peppermint	63%	10%	9%	
Weighted Means:	44%	35%	5%	

* P/K/A = % Phenols + %Ketones + %Alcohols. M = % Monoterpenes. S = % Sesquiterpenes.

Except for Marjoram, the essential oils used in raindrop are not PMS balanced individually, but applied and layered in sequence, as they are, they constitute a PMS anointment with amazing healing capabilities—physically, spiritually, and emotionally. The single oils used for raindrop technique (in the order they are applied) are oregano, thyme, basil, wintergreen (or birch), marjoram, cypress, and peppermint. All but cypress and wintergreen are members of Lamiaceae, the mint family. Valor® is a blend used at the beginning and end of the procedure. Valor contains 15 parts spruce, 7 parts frankincense, 6 parts blue tansy, 2 parts rosewood, and 1 part balsam fir in an almond oil base. This translates into the following aromatic composition for Valor: 0% phenols, 1% ketones, 7% alcohols, 54% monoterpenes, 4% sesquiterpenes, and 17% esters.

The weighted mean in the Chemistry of Raindrop Table on the previous page is what a combination of all of these oils would produce with Valor included three times since it is used in triple the quantity of any of the other oils administered during raindrop. This means that over the course of receiving a full raindrop the recipient will receive oils whose aggregate proportions are 44% phenols, ketones, and/or alcohols, 35% monoterpenes, and 5% sesquiterpenes along with 4% esters (from the Valor). Esters are soothing, calming, and can lead to emotional releasing. They also provide the fragrance of the Valor (viz. the bornyl acetate in the spruce). These percents, formed by the combination of these eight oils, fit the profile of a perfect PMS blend even though only marjoram, and possibly Valor, fits that profile individually. Hence, the combination of raindrop oils as delivered to the client in a full raindrop session is a PMS anointment.

Notice that although the weighted mean for raindrop oils falls within the parameters of a PMS blend, it is weighted toward the phenolic side. The strong phenolic bias of raindrop technique is the main reason British aromatherapists are afraid of it. According to British beliefs on essential oils, phenolic oils should never be applied undiluted to the skin (as in raindrop), should never be used in such quantities (as in raindrop), and should never be applied repeatedly over extended periods of time (like some people who receive raindrops monthly and even weekly).

All I can say is that those of the British school who have expressed those opinions to me have never seen, done, nor received a raindrop and refuse to do so. One personal raindrop experience would change their minds and dispel their fears. For scientific data on the safety and effectiveness of raindrop, see *A Statistical Validation of Raindrop* mentioned in the bibliography.

In discussing the chemistry of raindrop, cypress deserves special commentary. Cypress is dominant in monoterpenes—56-95%. However, it also contains up to 20% sesquiterpenes such as α–cedrene and δ–cadinene and the sesquiterpene alcohol, cedrol. The identifying odor of cypress is thought to be mainly due to an ester, iso-valerate, composing less than 2% of the oil. Synthetic iso-valerate is sometimes added to commercially produced cypress oils to reinforce the fragrance when it has been diluted to increase profit. Thus an unwary buyer can be fooled into thinking the oil is pure and full strength.

What makes pure unadulterated cypress chemically unique among essential oils is its diterpenoid content—up to 3%. From Tables Sixteen and Thirty-Two, you can see that cypress contains five diterpene alcohols and one diterpene acid. No other oil contains such a variety of diterpenes. In fact, the vast majority of oils contain no diterpenes at all. Diterpenes (272 amu) are double the weight and size of monoterpenes (136 amu) and seem to share many of the same qualities as sesquiterpenes (204 amu). They may even function inside cells as erasers of bad information in cellular memory, like sesquiterpenes. In any case, cypress oil stands out among the raindrop oils as being very different. In fact, cypress oil stands out among all essential oils as being very different.

Cleanliness is Next to Godliness

Seeing how the raindrop oils consist predominantly of cleansing compounds (47% phenols, ketones, and alcohols), one can understand why raindrop is such a powerful detoxifying technique—cleansing receptor sites and rid-ding the body of toxins at all levels in every organ and in every tissue. As your mother may have said to you when you were a child, "Cleanliness is next to Godliness." And so it is when it comes to achieving and maintaining the Godly state of health the Lord meant for us all to enjoy. Cleansing the bodily temple at a cellular level—that is what raindrop technique does.

Of course, the compounds of raindrop oils are not all phenolic. There is also a good dose of monoterpenes and a balanced quantity of sesquiterpenes. Regardless of the PMS proportions, the raindrop combination works well. This suggests that the most important part of health and wellness is keeping the body inwardly clean. Raindrop technique works effectively as a cleanser from the insides of the cells to the body surface. Whatever the chemico-electro dynamics may be, raindrop works wonders—both physically and emotionally, as hundreds of thousands who have experienced it will testify. Raindrop represents a balanced PMS anointing on the phenolic side. But then, the PMS Paradigm isn't everything.

PMS Isn't Everything

Note the absence of some important healing oils in the PMS lists—like geranium, helichrysum, jasmine, lemongrass, melissa, Roman chamomile, rosewood, rose, sage, and clary sage. These oils, and many others, have less than 5% of any of the PMS compounds, which is why they are not on these lists.

Remember, PMS is only one of many healing etiologies with essential oils. There are many processes by which aromatic oils work their wonders—some of which are not even chemical, but are electric, magnetic, and vibrational. The multiple manners by which aromatic oils work their healing magic is complex and is only beginning to be understood by scientists and aromatherapy practitioners. Anointing with PMS oils may not always bring about the healing we desire. Different oils may be required to meet the special needs of the person and the situation. If there are emotional or spiritual roots to a disease, the oils that address feeling and consciousness may be the most helpful. These include oils with esters, ethers, aldehydes, ketones, and oxides, as well as the unique combinations of specific compounds each individual oil provides. To state that phenols, monoterpenes, and sesquiterpenes behave in such and such ways individually or in combination to bring about healing in certain ways is a generalization that is not always true. Not all phenols are alike. Neither are all monoterpenes or sesquiterpenes. Each specific compound will manifest, not only its family characteristics (phenolic, monoterpenic, ketonic, or alcoholic, etc.), but has its own singular personality as well.

So please don't use the lists of PMS oils to restrict your therapeutic applications of essential oils in any way. They can be helpful when seeking the specific oils containing PMS compounds, but PMS compounds are only a portion of the therapeutic agents that give essential oils their powers. That is why we must also study and apply the oils that are principally composed of alcohols, ethers, aldehydes, ketones, esters, oxides, coumarins, and/or lactones. There is a vast armamentarium of effective healing oils that do not involve PMS. Learn to use them all. Essential oils are complex in their compositions and complex in their healing actions. The PMS paradigm explains a lot and provides a useful rationale for using oils in many situations, but far from all situations.

As for applying the PMS theory, you will have no problems locating suitable PMS oils with lists of this chapter and the tables in Part Two. May the PMS be with you.

PMS as a Spiritual Analogue

In one's individual search for God, there are three stages along the way:

(1) There is the **Purgative Stage** where one is cleansed in preparation for spiritual endeavor. This is analogous to the function of the phenols (or ketones/alcohols) that cleanse our receptor sites and prepare us for the release of our emotional and spiritual blockages.

(2) There is an **Illuminative Stage** where the darkness is dispelled and cleared from our consciousness. This is analogous to the function of the sesquiterpenes that erase erroneous data in our cells and eradicate the dark emotions and spiritual deficiencies that block our vision of God and our capability of manifesting his gifts.

(3) Then there is the **Unitive Stage** where we are ready and able to unite and commune directly with God, as well

as with his saints, angels, and other divine personages. This is analogous to the function of the monoterpenes that assist in re-establishing the divine image of God that was implaced within us at our creation—the manifestation of which is our purpose in being.

King David's Experiences PMS

An example of an oil that has PMS capabilities without phenols is hyssop (*Hyssopus officinalis*). Hyssop was used in Biblical times to cleanse one from bad habits and sinful tendencies by addressing these issues at the level of cellular memory. (Psalm 51) Hyssop oil contains 20-40% monoterpenes, 4-12% sesquiterpenes, and only 2-4% phenols, but is rich in ketones—over 50%.

While hyssop contains enough sesquiterpenes to fall within the parameters of a PMS oil, in Biblical times it was often combined with cedarwood oil (*Cedrus atlanticas*) which contains the highest known concentration of sesquiterpenes of all essential oils (95%). (See Leviticus 14:6, 10-12.) However, in PMS healing, sesquiterpenes seem to be needed in the least quantity with the need for cleansing agents (phenols or ketones) and/or coordinating/programming agents (monoterpenes) being required in the largest quantities. Experience indicates hyssop to be an effective healing oil with all the attributes of PMS.

It is instructive to analyze the 51st Psalm in this light. In this psalm, King David is repenting to God for committing adultery (with Bathsheba) and committing murder (by arranging for the death of her husband, Uriah). (See II Samuel, chap. 11.) Tendencies to commit compulsions and engage in wrongful actions are imbedded in the DNA of our cells. David did not want to be driven to commit such heinous acts ever again and in his begging for God's mercy, he applied the oil of hyssop to his body and inhaled its vapors with these words:

> "Purge me with hyssop and I shall be clean. Wash me and I shall be whiter than snow. . . Blot out all my iniquities. Create in me a clean heart, O God, and renew a right spirit within me."
>
> (Psalm 51: 7, 9-10)

All of the elements of PMS are in these verses. "Purge me with hyssop and I shall be clean" implies a cleansing of the receptor sites (P). "Blot out all my iniquities" suggests that unwanted tendencies be deleted from the DNA (S). "Create in me a clean heart" and "Renew a right spirit within me" suggests the reprogramming and restoration of God's perfect image (M). Whatever the reason, David's sincere supplication to God and his self-anointing with oil of hyssop must have worked. There is no Biblical record of David committing any such deeds ever again.

To make this discussion complete, it should be mentioned that some Biblical scholars have concluded that the hyssop plant of Biblical times was actually marjoram (*Origanum marjorana*). Insofar as PMS qualities are concerned, the above analysis of Psalm 51 still applies inasmuch as marjoram is also a PMS balanced oil. (See Table Sixty-Eight in Part Two.)

Key Points of Chapter Nine

1. The basic building block of thousands of essential compounds is the isoprene unit, C_5H_8.

2. Two isoprenes = 1 terpene unit, $C_{10}H_{16}$. Compounds composed of terpene units (or isoprenes) are called terpenes.

3. Compounds containing one terpene unit (two isoprenes), $C_{10}H_{16}$, are called monoterpenes.

4. Compounds containing of one-and-a-half terpene units (three isoprenes), $C_{15}H_{24}$, are called sesquiterpenes.

5. There are also compounds containing two, three, and four terpene units called diterpenes $C_{20}H_{32}$, triterpenes $C_{30}H_{48}$, and tetraterpenes, respectively.

6. Terpene units can be joined together without any apparent limit, even in the thousands, creating huge molecules like rubber. However, for distilled oils, a triterpene ($C_{30}H_{48}$) is the largest molecule you will find because larger ones cannot pass through the distillation process.

7. Tetraterpenes ($C_{40}H_{64}$) provide color to plants, insects, and animals. The two most famous tetraterpenes are carotene, the orange color of carrots, and lycopene, the red color of tomatoes. Tetraterpenes are found in pressed oils (like citrus) and solvent-extracted oils (like jasmine, neroli, and onycha).

8. Essential oils contain only the lightest and smallest of plant molecules, which are unique in that they can pass through skin, through the blood-brain barrier, and through cell membranes to bring healing at cellular levels.

9. Essential oils do not contain all of the healing capabilities of plant compounds. There's healing in the big molecules, too, which are accessed, not through essential oils, but by eating whole fresh plants and by applying dried herbs, where the large plant molecules are concentrated.

10. Phenols or phenolic compounds contain a phenol molecule (C_6H_6O), which is a benzene ring (C_6H_6) with a hydroxyl radical (OH) attached.

11. Phenylpropanoids are a type of phenolic compound with a propyl radical (C_3H_7 or C_3H_6) attached to the molecule.

12. Examples of phenolic compounds include methyl salicylate, cinnamaldehyde, p-cuminol, estragole, anethole, carvacrol, thymol, terpenenol, borneol, menthol, eugenol, and myristicin.

13. Examples of phenolic oils include wintergreen, birch, cinnamon, cumin, basil, fennel, oregano, thyme, tea tree, citronella, peppermint, clove, and nutmeg.

14. Methyl salicylate ($C_8H_8O_3$), which composes 85-90% of wintergreen and birch oils, has analgesic properties that have been compared to cortisone and aspirin ($C_9H_8O_4$).

15. Monoterpenes ($C_{10}H_{16}$) are found in every essential oil ranging from 1% to as much as 95% of the oil. Monoterpenes are volatile, but are usually mild in odor.

16. The most popular monoterpenes are α–pinene, β–pinene, d–limonene, l–limonene, sabinene, camphene, γ–terpinene, myrcene, and p-cymene.

17. The eight compounds just listed all have the formula ($C_{10}H_{16}$) except p-cymene which has the formula

($C_{10}H_{14}$), but is still considered a monoterpene. P-cymene has an extra double bond that gives it a higher resonance energy than most monoterpenes, thus giving it special healing powers. Many oils contain p-cymene.

18. Sesquiterpenes ($C_{15}H_{24}$) compose the largest group of naturally occurring terpenes in the world and occur in most, if not all, essential oils. Sesquiterpenes are not particularly volatile, but can range from odorless to strongly fragrant.

19. The sesquiterpene found in more oils than any other is β-caryophyllene. Other sesquiterpenes found in essential oils include α–bergamotene, bisabolene, δ–cadinene, α–copaene, α–curcumene, γ–curcumene, elemene, α–farnesene, β–farnesene, guaiene, humulene, α–selenene, and α-ylangene.

20. Chamazulene ($C_{14}H_{21}$) is considered a sesquiterpene, but is actually not a natural compound found in the living plant. It is an artifact of distillation which removes a methyl radical (CH_3) from naturally occurring matricene (a true sesquiterpene—$C_{15}H_{24}$) reducing the formula to that of chamazulene ($C_{14}H_{21}$).

21. Chamazulene, although an unnatural artifact, has special therapeutic properties and is, thus, a desirable artifact. The greater the concentration of chamazulene in the oils that contain it, the more valuable the oil.

22. Oils containing chamazulene include German chamomile, blue tansy, helichrysum, and yarrow.

23. Chamazulene is dark blue in color. Some dishonest oil dealers purchase the cheaper Moroccan chamomile, add synthetic chamazulene, and sell it at a high price as if it were German chamomile.

24. Diterpenes are found in only a few oils. Diterpene molecules, which weigh 272 amu, are among the heaviest that will pass through distillation into an essential oil.

25. Triterpenes are not found in most distilled oils, but mainly occur in oils that are expressed (such as citrus) and absolutes that are extracted by solvents (like jasmine, onycha, and neroli).

26. One of the most significant triterpenes found in aromatic oils is squalene which constitutes 2-7% of jasmine oil. Ongoing research suggests that squalene may have anticarcinogenic, cholesterol regulating, and immune boosting capabilities.

27. Phenolics, Monoterpenes, and Sesquiterpenes work together as the PMS trio, delivering a triple whammy to conditions of sickness and disease at the level of cellular intelligence (DNA). The PMS trio can sometimes result in an instantaneous healing.

28. Phenolics cleanse receptor sites. Sesquiterpenes delete faulty information in cellular memory. Monoterpenes restore or awaken the correct cellular information. By these three processes, the roots of a disease or condition can be eliminated at its cellular source and result in a permanent healing—sometimes instantaneously.

29. Ketones and alcohols can substitute for phenols in cleansing receptor sites. Hence, we can also talk about KMS and/or AMS combinations of oils.

30. Of the three PMS classes of compounds, monoterpenes are by far the most common.

31. Single oils generally contain significant amounts of only one of the three PMS compounds and many contain no significant amounts of either of the other two.

32. It usually takes at least three different oils, either layered or blended, to achieve a PMS anointing and receive the full benefit of the PMS healing process.

33. A therapeutically effective PMS proportion seems to lie in the range of: 10-50% Phenols/Ketones/Alcohols, 10-60% Monoterpenes, and 3-20% Sesquiterpenes.

34. The oils of raindrop technique consist of seven single oils and one blend layered on the feet and back, one after the other, that provide a perfect PMS anointment. Raindrop has demonstrated its therapeutic benefits on hundreds of thousands of clients since its introduction in the 1980s.

35. Besides their role in restoring God's image to our cells, monoterpenes are mitigators, quenchers, and coordinators. They keep compounds with strong personalities, (ketones and phenols), in line so that they do only good.

36. Sesquiterpenes help in keeping potentially unruly compounds (phenols and ketones) under control and focused on their appointed healing tasks until complete.

37. The PMS Paradigm isn't the only healing modality of essential oils, but it does explain a lot and provides a practical guide for healing applications. Oils containing other types of compounds also have their unique healing capabilities. All should be utilized in appropriate ways when applying essential oils for health and healing.

38. Tea tree, marjoram, and hyssop are all PMS balanced oils. (A complete list of such oils is given in Table Sixty-Eight, p. 586.)

39. Psalm 51 is a Biblical example of hyssop (or marjoram) oil being used in a PMS anointment to address emotional and spiritual issues at a cellular level.

♥ CHAPTER TEN
COMMON COMPOUNDS
IN ESSENTIAL OILS

Several times in previous chapters we have said that "The Chemistry of Essential Oils Made Simple" can be summarized in a single sentence, which was stated as follows:

"The chemistry of essential oils consists of simple hydrocarbons, oxygenated hydrocarbons, and their isomers."

To this point, you have read a great deal about hydrocarbons and their isomers, but the only oxygenated hydrocarbons we have discussed are phenols, phenylpropanoids, and certain alkane alcohols. Now we are ready to spend a whole chapter on oxygenated hydrocarbons. This is going to be exciting, because the oxygenated compounds of essential oils are the ones that give oils most of their pleasing, pungent, emotionally satisfying aromas and other outstanding qualities we enjoy so much. Oxygen is where the action is. It is the fuel of life and a source of the unique healing energies for essential oils as well.

Among other things, you will learn that monoterpenes and sesquiterpenes, which play key roles in the healing process as hydrocarbons, yet play an even greater variety of roles when oxygenated. Mono- and sesquiterpenes can both be oxygenated into a vast variety of therapeutically active substances. These include terpene alcohols, terpene ethers, terpene aldehydes, terpene ketones, terpene acids, terpene esters, terpene oxides, terpene coumarins, terpene furanoids, and terpene lactones. We will briefly study and discuss all of these.

Eighteen Categories of Oil Compounds

To this point we have studied three main types of compounds including five subtypes of one of them:

1. Alkanes (Chapter Five)
2. Phenols (Chapter Six)
3. Terpenes (Chapter Nine)
   a. Monoterpenes
   b. Sesquiterpenes
   c. Diterpenes
   d. Triterpenes
   e. Tetraterpenes

Let's add six more general classes of compounds:

4. Alcohols
5. Ethers
6. Aldehydes
7. Ketones
8. Carboxylic Acids
9. Esters

After we have discussed these, we will add four more:

10. Oxides
11. Lactones
12. Coumarins
13. Furanoids

Besides the hydrocarbons and oxygenated hydrocarbon listed above, in Chapter Four we also briefly mentioned two classes of sulfur (S) compounds found in essential oils (thiols and sulphides) as well as two classes of nitrogen (N) compounds (pyrroles and diazines). However, we will say no more about S and nitrogen N compounds in this book, since they are not major players in essential oils. When we get to furanoids near the end of this chapter, we'll quit considering new categories. Adding the S and N compounds of Chapter Four to the list above, we will have mentioned twenty-two types and subtypes of essential oil compounds in this book. Within these twenty-two categories of compounds are thousands of constituents that comprise essential oils. More than 600 different compounds, and the oils that contain them, are compiled in Part Two of this book.

In Table Seventeen, we use the symbol R to stand for a functional hydrocarbon group. Remember that a hydrocarbon is a compound or group composed of only two elements—H and C. R could be a benzene ring (C_6H_6), an isoprene unit (C_5H_8), a terpene unit ($C_{10}H_{16}$), a sesquiterpene ($C_{15}H_{24}$) or a radical like methyl (CH_3), ethyl (C_2H_5), propyl (C_3H_7), or butyl (C_4H_9). There are endless possibilities. We also use another symbol, R´, referred to as "R-prime," which represents an additional hydrocarbon functional group when there is more than one group in a molecule.

Compounds Behave Like People

It would be nice if you could take a list of the compounds or classes of compounds in an oil and predict, from that list, what the oil will do when applied on a person. That would make the applied chemistry of essential oils simple, like a cookbook. Unfortunately, that is impossible for three reasons:

(1) Part of the chemistry of an oil's reaction to a person has to do with that particular person's own chemistry. Hence, no two compounds or oils will consistently evoke the same response from everyone. Different people respond differently and receive different benefits.

(2) The behavior of a specific compound in an oil varies according to the influence of its companions in the oil. This is just like the behavior of people. Do we act the same around our spouse as with our children? When around our business associates as with our next door neighbors? In the company of our church brothers and sisters as when we deal with people at the bank or the grocery store? No. We are actually many different people with many personalities and many faces. What we manifest at any time or place depends on with whom we are present at the time. The components of oils are like that, too.

(3) Essential oils do not entirely act within the laws of chemistry, but also possess properties best described by quantum physics. In other words, essential oils exist as packets of probabilities until applied to a person at which time the intents of the anointer and the anointed deter-

mine which of the possibilities actually manifests. Hence, like people, the compounds in oils respond to the thoughts and wishes of those applying and receiving them at any given moment. See Part Three for more on this.

For example, as a class of compounds, ketones are used with caution by most aromatherapists because of their theoretical effects on hormonal balance and the central nervous system—based on data from animal and single component studies. However, ketones like fenchone, carvone, pinocamphone, and dozens of others are mild and harmless as members of a working team of compounds in an essential oil. Remember indole (Chapter Four, p. 127), a foul smelling misbehaving nitrogen compound by itself, but which becomes a sweet smelling well-behaved floral fragrance in the buffering presence of the other compounds in jasmine, neroli, and narcissus oils.

Hence, the generalizations given in Table Seventeen for the six classes of compounds listed there are not to be taken as always true. They aren't. But they can be valuable as guidelines.

Oils are Like a Chocolate Cake

Aromatic oil compounds do not act in isolation, which is why single compound studies are not a valid way to study the action of a whole, natural oil. To appreciate how the behavior of the individual ingredients in an oil cannot be understood when considered alone as isolates, consider a chocolate cake.

Its ingredients consist of flour, shortening, sugar, eggs, salt, bitter chocolate, baking powder, and vanilla extract. Could you appreciate the attributes of a piece of chocolate cake by studying flour alone? Or shortening? Or bitter chocolate? Of course not.

Would you be able to judge the taste of a piece of chocolate cake by eating half-a-cup of sugar, a couple of raw eggs, or a tablespoon of salt separately? Hardly.

If you swallowed a teaspoon of baking powder or an ounce of pure vanilla extract, would this give you any clue as to the experience of a piece of chocolate cake? I don't think so.

After a mouthful of baking power, you might even conclude that chocolate cake must be horrible and toxic to contain such a disagreeable ingredient.

None of these ingredients are good by themselves. In fact, most of them are distasteful or inedible and, perhaps, are actually hazardous when ingested alone. Yet, combined in proper proportions and baked in an oven, the result is a delectable dessert that has none of the attributes of any individual ingredient acting alone.

How is it that a group of disgusting, not-too-tasty, not-too-appetizing ingredients can combine to make something so wonderfully satisfying and so good? Romans 8:28 comes to mind. "All things work together for good for those who love God, who are called according to his purpose."

So it is with healing oils. The compounds of an essential oil work together for good when grown, harvested, distilled, and applied by those who love God, who are called according to his purpose. Essential oils amplify intent. When one's intent is born of prayer and spiritual desire, according to God's purpose, oils can only work in concord to do good.

Thus it was, in Biblical times, that the healers and essential oil producers were also priests and priestesses—persons of spiritual intent, dedicated to a godly life. These special people not only did the praying, the laying on of hands, and the anointing with oils, they were also the "perfumers, confectionaries, and apothecaries" mentioned in the *Bible* who grew, harvested, and distilled the oils.

General Formulas for Oxygenated Hydrocarbons

The general formulas given in Table Seventeen on the next page show how the oxygen atoms are attached to the molecule. For the compounds on the left (alcohols, aldehydes, and acids), there is a hydrocarbon group (R) attached on the left and an H atom attached on the right. For the compounds on the right (ethers, ketones, and esters) a hydrocarbon group (R) is also attached on the left, but on the right, instead of an H atom, is another hydrocarbon functional group (R').

Table Seventeen
Six Important Types of Oxygenated Hydrocarbons

ALCOHOLS (Tables 35, 51, 52)

General Formula: **ROH**

Suffix: -ol
Example: Linalol
Oil: Lavender
General Properties: energizing, stimulating, toning, cleansing, bactericidal, antiviral, antiseptic, sweet floral fragrances, gentle and mild

ETHERS (Tables 42, 67)

General Formula: **ROR'**

Suffixes: -ole, -cin, or -ether
Example: Anethole
Oil: Fennel
General Properties: soothing, balancing, calming, sedative, anesthetizing, emotionally releasing, antidepressant, (Some ethers are toxic)

ALDEHYDES (Tables 36, 53, 54)

General Formula:
$$\underset{\text{RCH}}{\overset{\text{O}}{\|}}$$

Suffixes: -al or -aldehyde
Example: Geranial
Oil: Geranium
General Properties: strong aromas, antimicrobial, antiviral, anti-inflammatory,

KETONES (Tables 44, 57, 58)

General Formula:
$$\underset{\text{RCR'}}{\overset{\text{O}}{\|}}$$

Suffix: -one
Example: Carvone
Oil: Spearmint
General Properties: strong odors, decongesting, analgesic, sedative, promote healing, cleanse receptor sites

---

CARBOXYLIC ACIDS (39, 67)

General Formula:
Also written as
RCOOH
$$\underset{\text{RCOH}}{\overset{\text{O}}{\|}}$$

Suffix: acid
Example: Cinnamic acid
Oil: Cinnamon
General Properties: stimulating, cleansing, chemically active, antimicrobial, react with alcohols to make esters

ESTERS (Tables 41, 55, 56)

General Formula:
$$\underset{\text{RCOR'}}{\overset{\text{O}}{\|}}$$

Suffixes: -yl & -ate, or -ester
Example: Methyl salicylate
Oil: Wintergreen
General Properties: soothing, balancing, emotionally releasing, antifungal, hormone-like, calming, fruity odors & flavors

Alcohols and Ethers are configured alike where ethers have an R', the alcohols have an H. Think of an alcohol as an O atom holding hands with a hydrocarbon (R) on the left and a hydrogen atom (H) on the right. Then think of an ether as an O atom holding hands with two hydrocarbon groups, one on each side—R and R'. They can be different hydrocarbon groups or two of the same. That's an ether.

Aldehydes and Ketones are configured alike where ketones have an R', the aldehydes have an H. Think of an aldehyde as a carbonyl group (C=O), C atom double bonded to an O, where the C is holding hands with a hydrocarbon (R) on the left and a hydrogen atom (H) on the right. Then think of a ketone as a carbonyl group holding hands with two hydrocarbon groups, one on each side—R and R'. That's a ketone.

Carboxylic Acids and Esters are configured alike where esters have an R', the acids have an H. Think of a carboxylic acid as a carbonyl group (C=O) where the C is holding hands with a hydrocarbon (R) on the left and an OH on the right. Then think of an ester as a C atom double bonded to an O above where the C is holding hands with a hydrocarbon on the left and an O atom on the right which is grasping onto another hydrocarbon group (R') on the right. That's an ester.

Notice that it takes two O atoms to make hydrocarbons into acids and esters while only one is needed to make hydrocarbons into alcohols, ethers, aldehydes and ketones. There can sometimes be more than one oxygen in these cases yielding double alcohols (called "diols"), double aldehydes (called "dials"), double ketones (called "diones"), etc. Some compounds are both alcohols and ketones.

You can see from the above descriptions that alcohols /ethers, aldehydes/ketones, carboxylic acids/esters, are three pairs of compounds that relate to one another by the similarities of their general formulas. Thus, you can see why we have listed the compounds in pairs in the manner which we have in Table Seventeen.

Alcohols

Oils composed mostly of alcohols include rosewood (83%), coriander (76%), garden thyme (74%), catnip (64%), geranium (60%), and rose (60%). (See Tables 18, 19, 35, 51, and 52.) The names of alcohols end in -ol. What defines an alcohol is an OH (hydroxyl radical) attached to a hydrocarbon group (R). (See Table Seventeen) There are hundreds of alcohols in essential oils.

We have already discussed phenols, which are a type of alcohol. However, phenols all include a six-carbon ring to which the OH radical is attached, which makes phenol (C_6H_6O) the defining functional group of a phenolic alcohol.

Table Eighteen
Monoterpene Alcohols Found in Essential Oils

Name	Formula*	Example of an Oil Where Found
Borneol	$C_{10}H_{18}O$	Lavandin (*Lavandula x hybrida*)
Carotol	$C_{10}H_{20}O$	Carrot Seed (*Daucus carota*)
Citronellol	$C_{10}H_{20}O$	Rose (*Rosa damascena*)
Geraniol	$C_{10}H_{18}O$	Geranium (*Pelargonium graveolens*)
Isopulegol	$C_{10}H_{20}O$	Lemon Eucalyptus (*E. citriodora*)
Lavandulol	$C_{10}H_{18}O$	Lavender (*Lavandula angustifolia*)
Linalol	$C_{10}H_{18}O$	Rosewood (*Aniba roseaodora*)
Myrtenol	$C_{10}H_{18}O$	Myrtle (*Myrtus communis*)
Nerol	$C_{10}H_{18}O$	Neroli (*Citrus aurantium*)
α–Terpineol	$C_{10}H_{18}O$	Ravensara (*Ravensara aromatica*)
Terpinen-4-ol	$C_{10}H_{18}O$	Tea Tree (*Melaleuca alternifolia*)
Thujanol	$C_{10}H_{18}O$	Mountain Savory (*Satureja montana*)

* For monoterpene alcohols, the chemical formula always contains 10 C atoms, but the number of hydrogens can vary. Their Molecular Weight is around 150–154 amu. Their volatility is high.

Table Nineteen
Sesquiterpene Alcohols Found in Essential Oils

Name	Formula*	Example of an Oil Where Found
α–Bisabolol	$C_{15}H_{26}O$	Lavandin (*Lavandula x hybrida*)
α–Santalol	$C_{15}H_{26}O$	Citronella (*Cymbopogon nardus*)
Cadinol	$C_{15}H_{26}O$	Cedarwood (*Cedrus atlantica*)
Caryophyllol	$C_{15}H_{26}O$	Vitex (*Vitex negundo*)
Elemol	$C_{15}H_{26}O$	Elemi (*Canarium luzonicum*)
Farnesol	$C_{15}H_{26}O$	Geranium (*Pelargonium graveolens*)
Guaiol	$C_{15}H_{26}O$	Blue Cypress (*Callitris intratropica*)
Ledol	$C_{15}H_{26}O$	Ledum (*Ledum groenlandicum*)
Nerolidol	$C_{15}H_{26}O$	Jasmine (*Jasminum officinale*)
Patchoulol	$C_{15}H_{26}O$	Patchouly (*Pogostemon cablin*)
Santalol	$C_{15}H_{26}O$	Sandalwood (*Santalum album*)
Viridiflorol	$C_{15}H_{26}O$	Niaouli (*Melaleuca quinquenervia*)

* A sesquiterpene hydrocarbon contains 15 C and 24 H atoms. A sesquiterpene alcohol usually has an additional 2 H atoms. Their Molecular Weight is usually 222 amu. Their volatility is low.

Thus, phenols are special alcohols built on a ring. They possess such unique and special properties that they are treated separately from the other alcohols found in essential oils. In this section we mainly want to discuss the other alcohols, but we will make some comparisons.

Non-phenolic alcohols are mild and gentle, possessing pleasant floral odors, and are generally regarded as being of low toxicity, non-skin irritating, and safe to use on children and the elderly. Non-phenolic alcohols are considered by some to be the most therapeutically beneficial of all essential oil components.

By contrast, phenolic alcohols are usually strong and aggressive, with sharp, powerful odors. They can be irri-

Examples of Monoterpene Alcohol Molecules

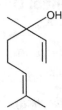

Linalol
$C_{10}H_{18}O$
Lavender, Coriander,
Basil, Bergamot,

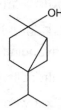

Thujanol
$C_{10}H_{18}O$
Thyme, Mountain Savory,
Rosemary, Marjoram

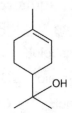

α–Terpineol
$C_{10}H_{18}O$
Bay Laurel, Ravensara,
Anise, Tea Tree, Juniper

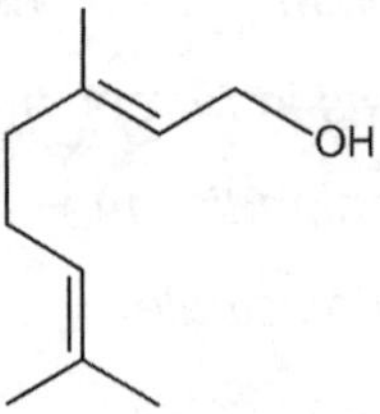

Geraniol
$C_{10}H_{18}O$
Geranium, Clary Sage,
Basil, Neroli,

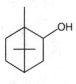

Borneol
$C_{10}H_{18}O$
Ginger, Sage, Rosemary,
Thyme, Frankincense,
Lavandin, Pine, Yarrow

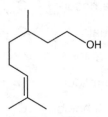

Citronellol
$C_{10}H_{20}O$
Citronella, Melissa, Rose,
Mandarin, Eucalyptus

Examples of Sesquiterpene Alcohol Molecules

Bisabolol
$C_{15}H_{26}O$
German
Chamomile
Oil

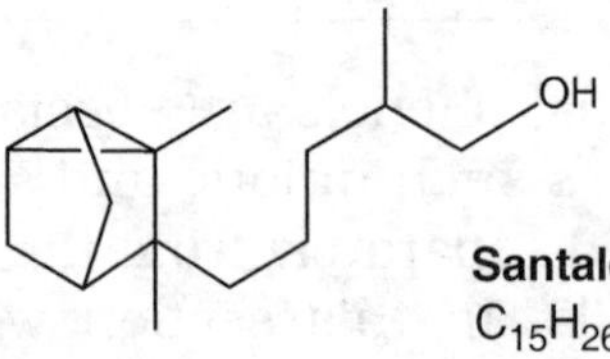

Santalol
$C_{15}H_{26}O$
Sandalwood Oil

Farnesol
$C_{15}H_{26}O$
Rose, Neroli,
Ylang Ylang,
German
and Roman
Chamomile Oils

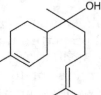

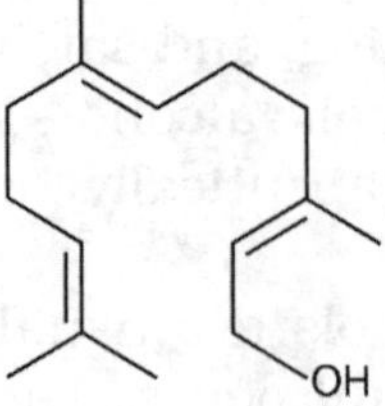

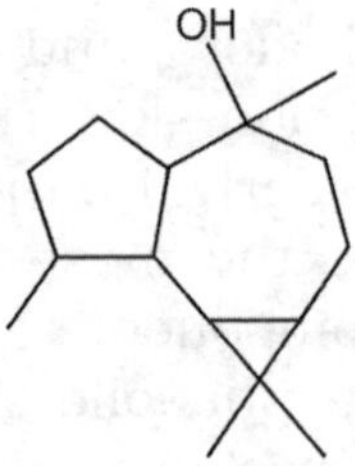

Viridiflorol
$C_{15}H_{26}O$
Peppermint,
Naiouli (MQV),
Sage,
and
Myrtle Oils

tating to the skin and should be used with some discretion. There is concern by some aromatherapists over possible liver toxicity from long-time usage of oils with phenolics, but the studies that suggest this are not for whole oils containing phenolics, but for isolated phenolic compounds. It appears in practice that the potential hepato–toxic properties of phenols are quenched by the other constituents when applied as an ingredient of a natural oil. Phenolic compounds have their own unique therapeutic qualities, especially the phenylpropanoids, but they act in different ways than the non-phenolic alcohols. Phenolic compounds in oils are effective antiseptics and are also cleansers of cellular receptor sites. (See PMS Paradigm discussed in Chapter Nine, pp. 291-304.)

Non-phenolic alcohols are also antiseptic and also can cleanse receptor sites, as mentioned in the PMS section of Chapter Nine. However, they are milder—not as strong as phenolics.

Some of the most common oil alcohols are actually oxygenated terpenes. Geraniol, linalol, citronellol, and terpineol are all monoterpene alcohols where their molecules all have the 10 C atoms and the two isoprene units of a monoterpene, but where the number of H atoms can vary from 16 to 20.

The compounds, α-bisabolol, α-santalol, guaiol, patchoulol, and farnesol, are all sesquiterpene alcohols where their molecules all have the 15 C atoms and the three isoprene units of a sesquiterpene, but where the number of H atoms can vary from 22 to 28.

Diterpene Alcohols

Table Fifteen in Chapter Eight lists several diterpene alcohols. One of them, cannabinol, a diterpene phenol, is discussed in the text following the table along with its structural formula. The molecular model for sclareol is also shown in the same figure.

Jasmine (*Jasminum officinale*) contains two isomers of phytol, a diterpene alcohol, comprising some 10-20% of the oil. Its large molecular size (about 290 amu) helps the characteristic fragrance of jasmine, which is composed of many smaller molecules, to last longer. Phytol may also have emotionally balancing benefits.

Sclareol is a diterpene alcohol that exhibits hormonal properties and is found in clary sage (*Salvia sclarea*). (See Chapter Eleven for a structural diagram.) Sclareol ($C_{19}H_{36}O_2$) is not only a double terpene, but a double alcohol—possessing two OH radicals. Sclareol has a molecular weight of 297. Double alcohols are called "diols." Estradiol ($C_{18}H_{22}O_2$) and androstenediol ($C_{19}H_{31}O_2$) are hormones produced in the human body by both men and women. These two sexual hormones are both double alcohols. Note the similarity in their formulas with that of sclareol. Sclareol is thought to mimic some of the properties of both estrogens and androgens as well as stimulating our bodies to secret these hormones, helping to restore hormonal balance to both men and women.

Alkane Alcohols

Some of the non-terpene alcohols in essential oils are derived from the alkane series such as butanol ($C_4H_{10}O$), hexanol ($C_6H_{14}O$), heptanol ($C_7H_{16}O$), octanol ($C_8H_{18}O$), nonanol ($C_9H_{20}O$), and decanol ($C_{10}H_{22}O$). All but the first one are found in lemon oil (*Citrus limon*) while butanol, heptanol, and nonanol are in ginger (*Zingiber officinale*). A trace of hexanol is found in Basil (*Ocimum basilicum*), lavender (*Lavandula angustifolia*), and clary sage (*Salvia sclarea*) and a trace of octanol in melissa (*Melissa officinalis*), peppermint (*Mentha piperita*) and Moroccan thyme (*Thymus satureioides*). None of these have rings in their structures. (See Chapter 4 for molecular models.)

Ethers

Oils composed mostly of ethers include anise (88%), tarragon (75%), fennel (66%), and basil (65%). (See Tables 20 and 42.) The names of ethers end in -ole (as in apiole), -cin (as in myristicin), or -ether (as in diethyl ether). What defines an ether is an O atom with a hydrocarbon group attached to each side—R and R'. (See Table Seventeen on page 314.) Ethers are not as common as alcohols, ketones, terpenes and other types of compounds in essential oils. In fact, they are rather uncommon among the most popularly used oils. Because of toxicity concerns, certain oils high in ether content are avoided in aromatherapy.

Table Twenty
Ethers Found in Essential Oils

Name	Example of an Oil Where Found
Anethole	Anise (*Pimpinella anisum*)
Apiole*	Parsley Seed (*Petroselinum sativum*)
Ascaridole*	Boldo (*Peumus boldus*)
Asarole*	Calamus (*Acorus calamus*)
Elemicin	Elemi (*Canarium luzonicum*)
Estragole	Tarragon (*Artemisia dracunculus*)
Myristicin	Nutmeg (*Myristica fragrans*)
Safrole*	Sassafras (*Sassafras albidum*)

* Because of concerns over the possible toxicity of these four compounds (apiole, ascaridole, asarole, and safrole), the oils in which they are found in significant amounts (viz, parsley seed, boldo, calamus, and sassafras) are avoided by many aromatherapists. Asarole and elemicin are isomers of the same formula, $C_{12}H_{16}O_3$.

Ethers do not often occur in essential oils as simple ethers. They almost always occur also as phenols. That means that one of the hydrocarbon units that make the ether includes a benzene ring (C_6H_6) with an attached hydroxyl radical (OH). These include anethole $(C_{10}H_{12}O)$ and estragole $(C_{10}H_{12}O)$, which we already discussed as examples of phenolic compounds in Chapter Seven. (Also see Table Thirteen in Chapter Nine.) While phenolic compounds are generally strong in odor and strong in action, phenolic ethers are regarded as being even stronger.

Safrole $(C_{10}H_{10}O_2)$, asarole $(C_{12}H_{16}O_3)$, ascaridole $(C_{10}H_{16}O_2)$, and apiole $(C_{12}H_{14}O_4)$ are also phenolic ethers found in oils. Most aromatherapists avoid oils containing

Examples of Ether Molecules

Elemicin
$C_{12}H_{16}O_3$
Elemi Oil

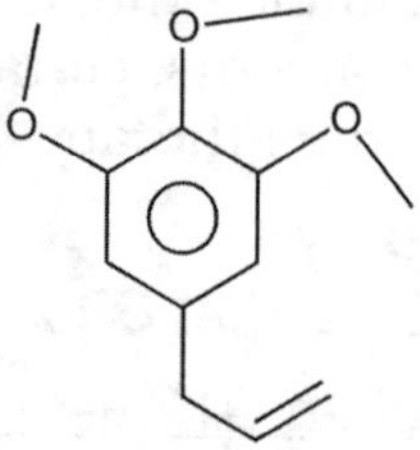

**Asarole
(Asarone)**
$C_{12}H_{16}O_3$
Calamus Oil

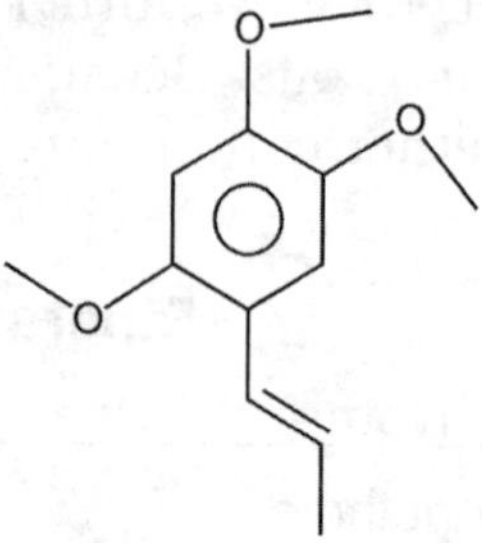

Myristicin
$C_{11}H_{12}O_3$
Nutmeg Oil
Parsley Seed Oil

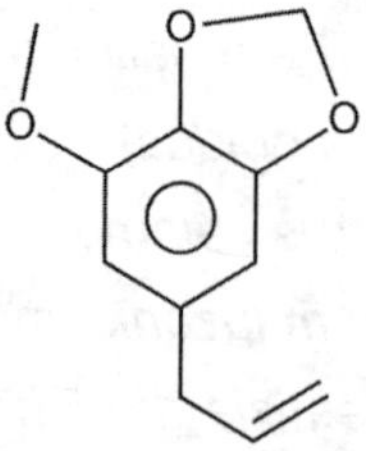

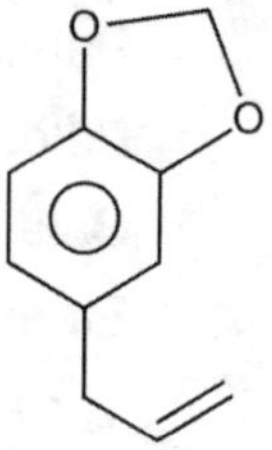

Safrole
$C_{10}H_{10}O_2$
Sassafras Oil

significant percents of any of these four compounds.

If you compare the structural formulas above with those of anethole and estragole given in Chapter Six, you will be struck by the similarities. In fact, the estragole molecule is incorporated in elemicin, myristicin, and safrole while the anethole molecule is incorporated in asarole. There isn't as much variety in the appearances of ether molecules found in essential oils in comparison to some other classes of oil compounds like the monoterpenes and sesquiterpenes. Notice that elemicin and asarole are isomers of $C_{12}H_{16}O_3$.

The shapes above may remind you of animals. To me, asarole looks like a little frog with its four legs spread out while elemicin looks like a turtle with flippers swimming. Myristicin looks like the same turtle, but with its hind legs tied together. Safrole can also be a turtle with its hind legs tied together, but with only one front flipper. Safrole could also be a frog with a missing leg. You decide. Consider this a chemical Rorschach test.

Asarole ($C_{12}H_{16}O_3$), as an isolated compound, has been shown to produce duodenal tumors in mice, but whether this translates into a risk to humans is not known. Asarole is found in calamus oil (*Acorus calamus*). Calamus (or cane) is mentioned in Exodus 30:22-25 as an ingredient in the holy anointing oil used daily in the temple. Although the evidence of its reputed toxicity is ambiguous, some aromatherapists avoid calamus for that reason even though it was a Biblical oil used for centuries by the Hebrews. The *Bible* does not mention tumors as being a problem among temple priests who were exposed to this oil on a daily basis. There is some confusion about the common name of asarole. It is also called "asarone," "α-asarone," and "β-asarone," which would imply that it is a ketone, which it is not. Asarole is its proper scientific name.

Safrole ($C_{10}H_{10}O_2$) is another compound of suspected carcinogenicity because tumors on the livers of rats have been produced when applying this isolated compound in concentrated form. However, safrole is the main ingredient in sassafras oil and clinical applications have shown it to be therapeutically beneficial and not harmful. Nevertheless, most aromatherapists are afraid to apply sassafras oil and don't.

Apiole ($C_{12}H_{14}O_4$) and ascaridole ($C_{10}H_{16}O_2$) are other ethers considered to be hazardous because of their aggressiveness toward the nervous system demonstrated in animal studies. Thus, parsley seed oil (*Petroselinum sativum*), which contains apiole, and boldo oil (*Peumus boldus*), which contains ascaridole, are generally avoided in aromatherapy.

While oral administration of large doses of boldo oil to rats has caused convulsions, the oil has been found useful as a remedy for gonorrhea and is used in gall bladder treatments. Boldo leaf extracts have also been approved as a flavor for alcoholic beverages by the U.S. Food and Drug Administration (FDA).

Myristicin ($C_{11}H_{12}O_3$), which constitutes 4% of natural nutmeg oil (*Myristica fragrans*), has no contraindications as a constituent of the whole oil. However, as a concentrated extract isolated from the oil, it is a hallucinogen when inhaled. When commercial laboratories, interested in its hallucinogenic properties, tried to make synthetic myristicin, they found that synthetic myristicin is not hallucinogenic at all. Apparently, the isomeric mix of the natural compound could not be duplicated in a laboratory. Myristicin is also found in parsley seed oil (*Petroselinum sativum*).

The good ethers (anethole, elemicin, estragole, and myristicin) and the oils in which they are found (anise, fennel, elemi, basil, tarragon, and nutmeg) are widely used and highly regarded in the practice of aromatherapy. Estragole also goes by the name of "methyl chavicol."

In summary, some ethers have been found toxic in laboratory conditions (apiole, ascaridole, asarone, and safrole) and the oils in which they are found (parsley seed, boldo, calamus, and sassafras) are usually avoided in aromatherapy. Whether this is a legitimate concern with regard to the safety of humans remains to be proven. When there is doubt, most aromatherapists prefer to err on the conservative side.

Aldehydes

Oils composed mostly of aldehydes include cassia (80%), cambava (75%), and lemongrass (67%). (See Tables 21, 36, 53, and 54.) The names of aldehydes end in -al or -aldehyde. What defines an aldehyde is a carbonyl group (C=O) with a hydrocarbon functional group (R) attached on the left and an H atom on the right. (See Table Seventeen on page 314.) There are hundreds of aldehydes in essential oils. They are responsible for some of the most delightful fragrances in the perfume and cologne industry. The popular perfume, Chanel No. 5®, is a blend of aldehydes—all synthetic.

Aldehydes are sometimes described as having properties in between those of alcohols and ketones—being stronger than alcohols and milder than ketones. The beneficial properties of aldehydes are that they are antiviral, anti-inflammatory, and calming to the nervous system. They are relievers of emotional stress, tend to reduce blood

Table Twenty-One
Aldehydes Found in Essential Oils

Name	Example of an Oil Where Found
Anisaldehyde	Anise (*Pimpinella anisum*)
Citronellal	Citronella (*Cymbopogon nardus*)
Benzoic aldehyde	Onycha (*Styrax benzoin*)
Cinnamaldehyde	Cassia *(Cinnamomum cassia)*
Citral	Lemongrass (*Cymbopogon flexuosus)*
Citronellal	Lemon Eucalyptus (*E. citriodora*)
Cuminal	Cumin (*Cuminum cyminum*)
Geranial	Lime (*Citrus aurantifolia*)
Myrtenal	Roman Chamomile (*Chamaemelum nobile*)
Neral	Melissa (*Melissa officinalis*)
Phellandral	Peppermint Eucalyptus (*E. dives*)
Valeranal*	Valerian (*Valeriana officinalis*)
Vanillin aldehyde*	Vanilla (*Vanilla planifolia*)

  * Aldehydes in essential oils are always strong contributors to the fragrance,usually in a pleasant way, but not always. Valeranal has a disgusting smell to many people. Vanillin aldehyde, however, is the flavor of the vanilla bean and vanilla ice cream, loved by almost everyone.

pressure, can dilate blood vessels, and may reduce fevers. Inappropriately used, aldehydes can cause skin irritation, but if a vegetable oil is applied promptly, there is no permanent problem. Sensitization of the skin can occur with synthetic aldehydes because they tend to remain in body tissues for long periods of time, but this is not a problem with natural aldehydes since they are metabolized quickly.

Some aldehydes are also aphrodisiac. This is one reason women (and men) have worn perfumes and colognes for thousands of years. This is why aldehydes are among the most prized of substances to those who compound perfumes and fragrances for body products like shampoos, soaps, lotions, and cosmetics.

Examples of Aldehyde Molecules

Geranial
$C_{10}H_{16}O$
Geranium
Lemon, Lime
Lemongrass
Ginger
Rosewood

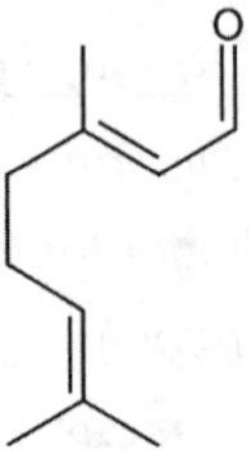

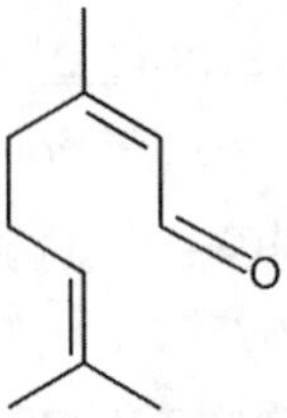

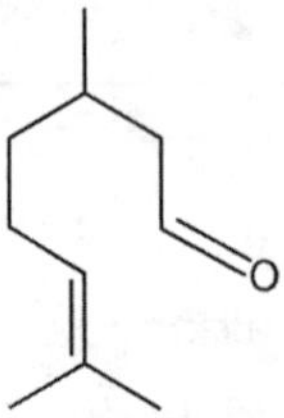

Citronellal
$C_{10}H_{18}O$
Citronella,
Melissa
Grapefruit
Pine, Lemon
Eucalyptus
citriodora

Neral
$C_{10}H_{16}O$
Neroli, Melissa
Ginger, Rose, Lemon
Rosewood, Bergamot,
Lemongrass

Cinnamic Aldehyde
C_9H_8O
Cassia
Cinnamon

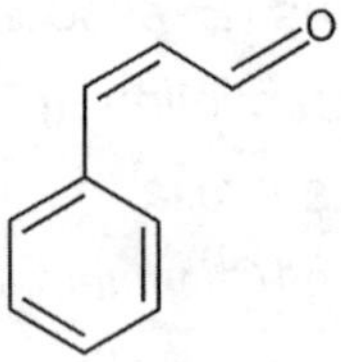

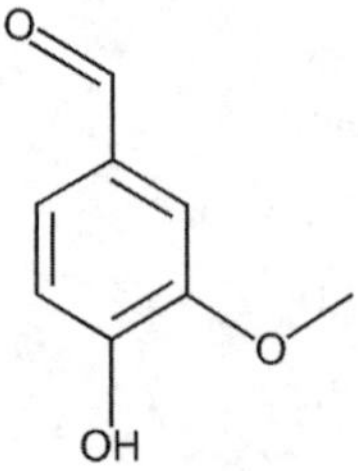

Vanillin Aldehyde
$C_8H_6O_3$
Onycha
Vanilla

The most common aldehydes in oils are geranial $(C_{10}H_{16}O)$, neral $(C_{10}H_{16}O)$, citronellal $(C_{10}H_{18}O)$, cuminal $(C_{10}H_{18}O)$, and cinnamic aldehyde (C_9H_8O). Several isomers of cinnamic aldehyde (also called cinnamal or cinnamaldehyde) are the compounds that provide the taste of cinnamon to chewing gum, breath mints, and red hot candies. Cassia oil contains about twice the cinnamal concentration of cinnamon bark oil and has a potent flavor like super-concentrated sweet cinnamon. Geranial and neral are monoterpene aldehydes as you can see by the $(C_{10}H_{16})$ in their formulas given above. Citronellal and cuminal are considered monoterpene aldehydes, too, even though they have a couple of extra hydrogens. Cuminal is the dominant fragrance of cumin oil and the taste of cumin seed. Cinnamic and vanillin aldehydes are considered to be phenols as well as aldehydes because of their unsaturated aromatic rings.

A Case of Quenching

Geranial, neral, and citronellal are powerful skin irritants when applied as isolated compounds. Together they comprise about 5% of lemon oil. Interestingly, when these compounds are applied in the whole lemon oil their abrasive personality is mellowed by the presence of monoter-penes (mostly d–limonene).

This is an example where terpenes play their role as coordinators, quenchers, buffers, and peacemakers among the other chemical personalities—providing balance and coherence to the actions of the hundreds of participants in an essential oil. Terpenes are the enforcers that keep all of the other constituents in line and on task so that healing takes place in the least time and without side effects.

Duplicate Names

Some of the names of aldehydes can be confusing inas-much as geranial is also called α–citral and neral is also called β-citral. If you see references to citral in other books, they are referring to either geranial, neral, or both mixed together. The way this confusion started was in the fact that researchers discovered these compounds independ-ently in different plants, at different times, and in different countries. When researchers first discovered these aldehy-des in the rinds of citrus fruit (orange, grapefruit, etc.), it was natural for them to call them "citrals." Meanwhile, when other researchers found certain aldehydes in gerani-um and neroli oils, it was natural to name them "geranial" and "neral." respectively. It was not until years later that it was realized that geranial and α-citral, as well as neral and β-citral, were pairs of identities, both chemically and structurally. Hence, two sets of names had already become entrenched in the literature.

Neroli is actually not an essential oil because it is extracted by chemical solvents, not by distillation or expression. Neroli absolute is actually of citrus origin being extracted from the blossoms of the bitter orange tree (*Citrus aurantium*).

The example of duplicate names for geranial, neral, and the citrals is not the only one. The more you study the chemistry literature of essential oils, the more apparent contradictions you find. Even the formulas, both chemical and structural, can vary from reference to reference, for what should be the same compound. Geranial, neral, and citral are actually the common or trivial names for these compounds. If one deals only with the scientific names assigned by International Union of Pure and Applied Chemistry (IUPAC) discussed in Chapter Four, then the confusion disappears. Compounds can have several common names, but theoretically, they have only one official scientific name.

There is also some confusion in the botanical naming of plants from which oils are derived. For example, *Chamaemelum nobile* and *Anthemis nobilis* are actually both the same plant whose common name is Roman chamomile. Like chemists working in different labs and different countries, when botanists in separate locations in the world find and name a new plant, they may be unaware for some time that the same species has already been identified and named otherwise by a different scientist elsewhere. Also, the naming of plants is less precise and objective than the naming of compounds whose formulas are fixed. Plants are named by visual appearance and what looks like one thing to one botanist may look different to another. Hence, Roman chamomile has been identified by different botanists as being in two different genera. *Chamaemelum nobile* has become the accepted name in current literature, but *Anthemis nobilis* can still be found in many texts.

I mention these things because you will encounter these apparent contradictions if you read a variety of books on aromatherapy. It's not that one book is right and another is wrong. It may be that they simply compiled their information from different sources with different origins and even different languages. Reconciling these differences is an international task requiring cooperation of scientists and aromatherapists throughout the world. Such endeavors are not easy. Perhaps, some day, there will be an International Union of Aromatherapy and Essential Oil Chemistry (IUAEOC) that will tackle these issues and clarify them for us all.

The Odor of Dirty Socks

While most aldehydes are pleasant smelling, some are not. Some say the odor of valerian oil (*Valeriana officinalis*) is "a bit cheesy." Others describe it as the "smell of dirty socks." That would be pretty close, in my opinion. The source of its rank odor is valerian aldehyde and valerinic acid. Where valerian grows wild, as in the Canadian Rocky Mountains, on warm fall days following an overnight frost, the roots of valerian exude a rotten stench that makes you think a garbage heap must be nearby. The therapeutic value of valerian lies not in its noxious fragrance, but in its sedative properties that stem from the sesquiterpenes present in the oil. In Germany, valerian oil is accepted by medical officials as a tranquilizer and as an effective treatment for restlessness and sleep disturbances. If you have a bottle of valerian oil, give it a sniff. Some people like it. You might also see if your cat likes it. Valerian oil contains two cat pheromones: actinidine and valerianine.

Alkane Aldehydes

Several alkane aldehydes are found in essential oils in small amounts—always less than 3% and usually less than 1%. They are as follows:

Hexanal	$(C_6H_{12}O)$	Clary Sage, Lavender, Myrtle
Octanal	$(C_8H_{16}O)$	Rose, Lemon, Mandarin
Nonanal	$(C_9H_{18}O)$	Lemon, Grapefruit, Orange
Decanal	$(C_{10}H_{20}O)$	Coriander, Lemongrass, Mandarin, Petitgrain
Undecanal	$(C_{11}H_{22}O)$	Lemon, Bitter Orange

Cream Soda and Vanilla Ice Cream

Onycha (*Styrax benzoin*) is an interesting oil mandated by God as an ingredient in the holy incense burned daily in the temples of the Israelites. (Exodus 30:34) Onycha has a variety of unusual molecules including some large diterpenes that make it a very viscous oil. It is actually not a true essential oil, but an absolute extracted by solvents. Onycha contains an interesting aldehyde which is a main contributor to its unique aroma—vanillin aldehyde.

Vanillin aldehyde is the compound in the vanilla bean (*Vanilla planifolia*) that gives us that rich aroma and flavor we love to taste in cream soda and vanilla ice cream. If you have a bottle of onycha oil, check it out. Most people can clearly detect the vanilla. Onycha also contains several acids, including benzoic and cinnamic acids, which also contribute to its distinctive smell, giving it a medicinal note. Onycha is a very healing oil, good for the skin, and excellent in massage. With onycha, your massage therapist can make you smell like a vanilla wafer with a medicinal touch. Onycha oil is also known as "friar's balm" and "Javanese frankincense." It comes from Indonesia.

Ketones

Oils composed mostly of ketones include cedar bark and cedar leaf (both 86%), as well as Idaho tansy (73%), and marigold (65%). (See Tables 22, 44, 57, and 58.) The names of ketones end in -one, like the name, "ketone," itself. What defines a ketone is a carbonyl group (C=O) with a hydrocarbon functional group attached on both sides—left (R) and right (R'). (See Table Seventeen on page 314.) While ketones are not as prevalent in essential oils as monoterpenes and alcohols, as you can see from Table Twenty-One and the figures of molecular models on the following page, lots of oils have ketones. Ketones come in countless variations and are responsible for some of the most powerful, unusual, and usually pleasant flavors and fragrances of all classes of compounds.

Like aldehydes, ketones have strong distinctive aromas. We have already experienced a couple of them in the taste and fragrance of dill and spearmint which are due to a chiral pair of ketone isomers called carvone. (See Chapter Seven.) While many essential oils contain little or no ketones, those that do are usually noteworthy in some special way.

Oils without ketones include all of the expressed citrus oils such as orange, lemon, lime, grapefruit, mandarin, tangerine, etc. Neither cypress, sandalwood, nor any of the melaleuca oils contain ketones either. However, most other oils do contain some ketones, at least traces. All it takes is a trace of a ketone to influence the fragrance and, perhaps, the therapeutic action as well.

Table Twenty-Two
Ketones Found in Essential Oils

Name	Example of an Oil where Found
Camphor	Rosemary (*Rosmarinus officinalis*)
d–Carvone	Caraway (*Carum carvi*)
l–Carvone	Spearmint (*Mentha spicata*)
Fenchone	Fennel (*Foeniculum vulgare*)
Jasmone	Jasmine (*Jasminum officinale*)
Khusimone	Vetiver (*Vetiveria zizanoides*)
Menthone	Corn Mint *(Mentha arvenis)*
Octanone	Lavender (*Lavandula angustifolia*)
Nootkatone	Vetiver (*Vetiveria zizanoides*)
Pentanone	Myrrh (*Commiphora myrrha*)
Pinocamphone	Hyssop (*Hyssopus officinalis*)
Pinocarvone	Roman Chamomile (*Chamaemelum nobile*)
Piperitone	Peppermint Eucalyptus (*E. dives*)
Pulegone	Peppermint *(Mentha piperita)*
n-Shyuobunone	Calamus (*Acorus calamus*)
Tagetone	Marigold (*Tagetes glandulifera*)
α–Thujone	Sage (*Salvia officinalis*)
β–Thujone	Western Red Cedar (*Thuja plicata*)
α–Vetivone	Vetiver (*Vetiveria zizanioides*)
Verbenone	Rosemary (*Rosemarinus officinalis*)

* Ketones in essential oils are strong contributors to fragrance. While ketones are not as common in essential oils as terpenes and alcohols, some oils are more than 50% ketone in composition—oils such as vetiver, wild tansy, hyssop, and western red cedar, for example.

Ketones in essential oils are thought to be calming and sedative, helpful as an expectorant or decongestant, can be analgesic, aid in digestion, and may encourage wound healing. In addition, they provide a variety of pleasant fragrances, some of which can be emotional releasing.

Rosemary is an oil with two chemotypes, each being a ketone. There is rosemary CT camphor (which is up to 30%

Examples of Ketone Molecules

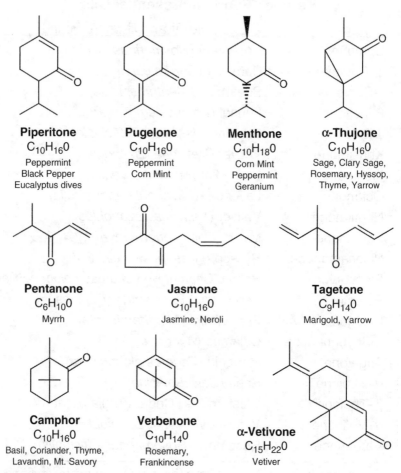

Piperitone
$C_{10}H_{16}O$
Peppermint
Black Pepper
Eucalyptus dives

Pugelone
$C_{10}H_{16}O$
Peppermint
Corn Mint

Menthone
$C_{10}H_{18}O$
Corn Mint
Peppermint
Geranium

α-Thujone
$C_{10}H_{16}O$
Sage, Clary Sage,
Rosemary, Hyssop,
Thyme, Yarrow

Pentanone
$C_6H_{10}O$
Myrrh

Jasmone
$C_{10}H_{16}O$
Jasmine, Neroli

Tagetone
$C_9H_{14}O$
Marigold, Yarrow

Camphor
$C_{10}H_{16}O$
Basil, Coriander, Thyme,
Lavandin, Mt. Savory

Verbenone
$C_{10}H_{14}O$
Rosemary,
Frankincense

α-Vetivone
$C_{15}H_{22}O$
Vetiver

camphor with only a trace of verbenone) and there is rosemary CT verbenon (which is up to 37% verbenone with only 1-10% camphor).

Camphor is a ketone that has been misnamed. It ends in -or instead of -one. Its proper common name should be more like "camphone." It's official scientific name is 1,7,7-trimethylbicyclo[2.2.1]heptan-2-one. The scientific name ends in -one, but who can say it? You'll never see it except in highly technical publications where the exact compound has to be precisely stated. I say, let's just stick with "camphor." The way it got misnamed is because camphor has been a popular compound extracted from natural sources for more than 200 years and was named before the nomenclature rules were established by IUPAC. (See Chapter Five, pp. 149-150.)

Properly named or not, camphor is a popular fellow invited to be a party to many essential oils. (They say he smells good and does fun things.) These oils include basil, coriander, lavandin, rosemary, mountain savory, lemon eucalyptus, thyme, wild tansy, blue tansy, sage, yarrow, ormenis, and white camphor,

The Secret of the Marigolds

Organic gardeners know about companion planting. They know that if you plant string beans and potatoes side by side, in alternating rows, that the fragrance of the bean plants will repel potato bugs and the fragrance of the potato plants will repel the bugs that attack beans. This way you can avoid using pesticides and keep the insects and caterpillars from destroying your produce. Companion planting is actually a practical application of essential oils, a form of aromatherapy, since the secret of repelling the insects is in the oil molecules released to the atmosphere by these plants.

Another companion planning trick is to plant rows of marigold flowers around your vegetable garden. Marigold flowers (*Tagetes glandulifera*) are a pleasure to see, but not to smell. The odor of marigold blooms is not pleasant to most people. If you have ever smelled a marigold you know what I mean, Well, guess what? Bugs and critters don't like the smell of marigolds either. If you have ever gardened, you know that it is not only the flying and crawling insects that eat your plants, it is the rabbits and gophers also. Many people simply put up a fence. However, encircling your garden with marigolds creates a protective barrier which rodents won't cross and insects try to avoid.

The key to marigold's repellent abilities is in a ketone called "tagetone." Marigold oil is composed of up to 60%

tagetone. That's enough to stop most furry mammals, as well as many bugs, from munching on your nearby vegetables. Tagetone takes the temptation away.

While we, as humans, can take advantage of the tagetone in marigolds for our own purposes, the marigold plant was probably not thinking of us when it formulated its fragrance, but of itself. It's bitter smelling oil saves it from being eaten by just about everything.

Among the therapeutic properties of marigold oil is that it will drive parasites out of your intestinal tract. So even the critters that can live inside of us will flee in the presence of marigold. Marigold oil is not only an effective general insect repellent, it is also an insecticide in some cases. It will kill mosquitoes and their larvae.

Alkane Ketones

In the figure showing examples of ketone molecules, you will see two that look a little different than most of the essential molecules seen throughout this book. The top four (piperitone, pugelone, menthone, and thujone) are all monoterpene ketones, as you can see by their shapes and formulas. Camphor and verbenone are also monoterpene ketones while vetivone is a sesquiterpene ketone. Jasmone is a strange looking creature, but it, too, is a sesquiterpene ketone which you can recognize from its formula. Pentanone and tagetone are something else. They are alkane ketones. To this point we have discussed alkane alcohols and alkane aldehydes. Now we will discuss alkane ketones.

You may remember from Chapter Five that alkanes are long chain molecules with no rings. From this chapter you have learned that ketones consist of a carbon atom double-bonded to an O atom with a hydrocarbon group on both sides. If you look at the molecular models for pentanone and tagetone, this is exactly what you have. The center carbon is double-bonded to an oxygen with a pair of hydrocarbons on each side like a pair of wings. These two molecules look like birds flying toward you. The following four alkane ketones are found in these four essential oils:

Hexanone	$(C_6H_{12}O)$	Ginger, Rosemary
Heptanone	$(C_7H_{14}O)$	Ginger, Rosemary, Rosewood
Octanone	$(C_8H_{16}O)$	Lavender, Melissa, Basil
Nonanone	$(C_9H_{18}O)$	Ginger

Ketones and Aldehydes as Pheromones

Pheromones are chemicals released by animals, particularly by insects, that carry information and invoke responses in others. Pheromones can be alcohols, oxides, acids, and esters. But most often they are aldehydes or ketones. There are sex pheromones, alarm pheromones, attack pheromones, and probably many other types of pheromones.

Sex pheromones can be released by either females and/or males when seeking a partner with whom to mate. Ethyl cinnamate $(C_{11}H_{12}O_2)$, an ester, is the sex pheromone of the male oriental fruit moth while tetradecenolide $(C_{14}H_{24}O_2)$, a lactone, is the female sex pheromone of the Japanese beetle. Hundreds of thousands of moths, butterflies, and various other insects seek and find their mates this way. Even mammals do it. Anyone owning a female cat or dog knows that if their pet goes into heat, males for miles will come to visit, having caught a whiff of their species' mating pheromone on the wind.

Not all pheromones are for the purpose of matching males and females. Sometimes, alarm pheromones are released when a colony of creatures are threatened. Hexanal $(C_6H_{12}O)$, an aldehyde, is an alarm pheromone released by certain species of ants when their anthills are approached by a human or other potentially threatening creature. Ants foraging for many meters around will sense the smell and head immediately for home to fight off any would-be invaders.

Interestingly, hexanal is a trace compound in both clary sage and lavender oils, both prized for their emotionally calming qualities. It would be interesting to see if a drop of clary sage or lavender oil on an anthill would have an alarming or a calming effect on its residents.

British Concerns About Ketones

British schooled aromatherapists are wary of oils containing ketones and have many warnings and precautions about them based on studies of isolated ketones administered in high doses to animals. While there may be some validity to their concern, for the most part their reluctance to use ketone-containing oils is unwarranted by actual experiences of people. Extreme dosages of any oil can be harmful. Extreme doses of any substance can be harmful, even lethal.

Common sense appears to provide a sufficient degree of protection from any toxic reactions to therapeutic grade oils, even those with ketones. As you can see from the foregoing figures, tables, and discussion, not to mention Tables 44, 57, and 58 in Part Two, there are a lot of oils containing significant percents of ketones—including harmless oils like spearmint, dill, and peppermint. To exclude every oil with a ketone would be to cripple the practice of aromatherapy for healing purposes.

Robert Tisserand is a leading British aromatherapist. In his book, *Essential Oil Safety*, he makes a categorical statement on page 75, "Thujone-rich and camphor-rich oils are all neurotoxic and potentially convulsant." If we take Tisserand seriously in this, we would be reluctant to use more than a dozen oils just named in this chapter.

Oils rich in thujone include sage (*Salvia officinalis*), wild tansy (*Tanacetum vulgare*), and western red cedar (*Thuja plicata*) which contain approximately 40%, 70%, and 85% thujone respectively.

Oils rich in camphor include juniper (*Juniperus communis*), sage (*Salvia officinalis*), rosemary CT cineole (*Rosmarinus officinalis*), blue tansy (*Tanacetum annum*), lavandin (*Lavandula x hybrida*), yarrow (*Achillea millefolium*), coriander (*Coriandrum sativum*), and rosemary CT verbenon which contain between 5% and 15% camphor in each.

Tisserand and many other British authors make the same precautionary statement for hyssop (*Hyssopus offic-*

inalis), warning of its neurotoxicity because it contains about 50% pinocamphone—a ketone.

Tisserand also implicates peppermint oil (*mentha piperita*) because of its menthone (16%) and pulegone (4%) content. Tisserand's concerns are because studies with high doses of peppermint oil have produced convulsions, loss of reflexes, and paralysis in rats. Tisserand does not say if the oil in the experiment was therapeutic or flavor grade oil—a key piece of missing information. There are no instances of these problems occurring when humans use therapeutic grade peppermint in reasonable amounts.

Thujone, camphor, pulegone, and menthone are all monoterpene ketones. The first three are mutual isomers with the same formula—$C_{10}H_{16}O$—while menthone is slightly modified with a formula of—$C_{10}H_{18}O$. To aromatherapists of the French school, when applied to the skin, oils with thujone have nerve and hormone balancing properties. Camphor is an ingredient in many popular over-the-counter medications. Vicks VapoRub®, for example, is a salve containing camphor (10%) used by millions of American mothers to rub on their children to help clear the congestion of a chest cold. Menthone is also an ingredient in many common medications to clear congestion. Peppermint oil, containing menthol ($C_{10}H_{20}O$), menthone ($C_{10}H_{18}O$), and pulegone ($C_{10}H_{16}O$), is one of the safest of all oils. It is applied neat to the skin in raindrop technique and is taken orally in drinking water and by other means by thousands of Americans without a single case of convulsions, paralysis, or other dire consequences that Tisserand would lead you to believe. As for tansy with its alleged toxicity from thujone, I have already commented on this in Chapter One by describing an oral dose I took during a public speech to make a point about its safety.

Pennyroyal (*Mentha pulegium*) is an oil which is 60-90% pulegone. It always seems to be on the forbidden lists of British aromatherapists. It has been used in attempted abortions where pregnant mothers have died. However, in these cases huge overdoses of more than 100 ml were taken orally. This is hardly representative of normal aromatherapy practice. According to the *PDR for Herbal Medicines*, "acute poisonings with oil of pennyroyal are not to be feared with proper administration." According to Daniel Penoel, M.D., pennyroyal has some therapeutic benefits in treating skin diseases, dysmenorrhea, and bronchitis. Even with these benefits, this oil is not used by most aromatherapists.

I mention these things because you may encounter alarmed responses from British trained aromatherapists if you say that you use oils containing ketones—especially the ones listed in the previous paragraphs. They will claim that if you do use such oils, they should be diluted down to a 1-2% maximum concentration in a neutral carrier oil, that they should never be taken orally, should never be used during pregnancy, and should never be used over prolonged periods of time as it will endanger your liver.

Tell them that when therapeutic grade oils are used in moderation, they can be safely utilized within the parameters of common sense. Anything can be toxic in a massive overdose, which is the way most animal studies are conducted. Ask them if there are any human studies with whole therapeutic grade oils that have indicated the risks of which they speak? If someone of this school tells you that ketone containing oils (especially those with thujone) can cause miscarriages when inhaled or applied during pregnancy, ask them if they can cite even one study involving humans that has shown this to be true. They won't be able to do it. There are no such studies.

Carboxylic Acids

Oils containing the highest concentrations of acids include onycha (19%), oregano (4%), and lemon eucalyptus (4%). (See Tables 23 and 39.) The names of acids incorporate the word, "acid," in their nomenclature, which makes them foolproof to identify. What defines a carboxylic acid is a carbonyl group (C=O) with a hydrocarbon functional group (R) attached on one side and an OH (hydroxyl radical) attached on the other. Lumped together, a carboxylic acid is a compound incorporating a carboxylic acid functional group of one C atom, two O atoms, and one H atom—COOH. Carboxylic acids can be written as a hydrocarbon group (R) attached to a COOH group. (See Table Seventeen.)

Carboxylic acids are also called "organic acids," and differ from inorganic acids in that they always contain carbon and oxygen. Inorganic acids do not contain carbon and are stronger than most organic acids. Inorganic acids are also called "mineral acids." Examples of mineral acids are sulfuric (H_2SO_4—battery acid) and hydrochloric (HCl—murietic acid. (HCl is a constituent of many prescription drugs). There are no mineral acids in essential oils.

The oxygenated hydrocarbons discussed so far (alcohols, ethers, aldehydes, and ketones) only require one O atom. Carboxylic acids require two O atoms, as will the next class of compounds we will discuss—esters. As we will see, acids and esters are related.

Carboxylic acids are never a main ingredient in essential oils and rarely comprise more than 1-2% of an oil. The main reason for this is that acids are chemically aggressive compounds that tend to react with other compounds. Since essential oils are mixtures of many compounds, it is difficult for an acid to be part of the mix because it will want to react with something. When an acid reacts with another compound, both the acid and the other compound are changed into something else. The acid is no longer an acid. The only acids that can survive as such in an essential oil are very weak ones and/or those that occur in low concentrations.

The most likely reaction an acid would have in a mix of essential oil compounds is to react with an alcohol. When a carboxylic acid reacts with an alcohol, the result is an ester. We will talk about esters next, but for now let's continue our discussion of acids.

What is pH?

What is pH? If you go to a chemistry book for an answer to this question it will tell you that pH is a measure of acidity in an aqueous solution. It will say that pure water has a pH of 7.0, which is neutral. It will say that a pH value below 7.0 indicates an acid solution and that a pH above 7.0 is basic or alkaline (which is the opposite of acidic). The book may even tell you that the number values of the pH scale are negative logarithms of the hydrogen ion concentration in the solution and that the pH values of most solutions run from 0 to 14, but could be less than 0 and more than 14, but what does that mean? Chances are, when you get through reading all of this in your chemistry book, you still won't know what pH really is, or why it is called "pH," or why 7.0 is neutral instead of some logical number like zero. And you probably won't know why the lower the pH value the higher the concentration and the stronger the acid. None of this makes logical sense to the majority of beginning chemistry students, so they just accept it, learn how to use it, and memorize what they need to know in order to get through the course with a passing grade. You can survive a lot of chemistry courses and do a lot of chemistry in the lab by blindly accepting these things on faith.

But I always wanted to know why pH = 7.0 means "zero acidity" when it would seem more logical to let the number 0.0 represent "zero acidity." And why does a lower pH number mean more acid instead of less? Why is any pH above 7.0 basic, while below 7.0 is acidic? And I wanted to know why it is called "pH," with a little "p" and a capital "H?" If you really want to understand pH, read on. By the end of this section, you will be able to explain pH better than most chemists.

First of all, "pH" means, literally, "potential Hydrogen." The little "p" is for 'potential" and the big "H" is the chemical symbol for hydrogen. Since the characteristic feature of an acid is its willingness to give up H^+ ions, "potential Hydrogen" is a well chosen name for a scale to measure acidity.

Second, pH has no meaning except for compounds or elements that will dissolve in water—H_2O. Since oils, in general, do not dissolve in water, pH is not a term usually applied to oils. There are some exceptions. Some oil compounds do dissolve in water, but only to a very limited extent. To dissolve in water, the molecules of a compound have to be willing and able to do one of two things: (1) Separate from those of its own kind and be surrounded entirely by water molecules; or (2) Break into a pair of partial molecules (called ions) and allow the ions to be surrounded entirely by water molecules.

Oil molecules don't like to do this. They have a strong preference for sticking together with other oil molecules and generally refuse to separate into parts (ionize), preferring to remain as intact molecules. Oils are particularly opinionated about giving up hydrogen atoms as ions, and generally refuse to do it.

What is an Ion?

To understand acids and bases, you need to understand ions. We learned in Chapter Three that elements and compounds are electrically neutral. Protons and electrons are the sources of all the electricity in this world. They constitute the fundamental units of electrical energy. Protons and electrons carry electric charges that are equal in size, but opposite in sign—protons (P^+) being positive, electrons (e^-) being negative. When protons and electrons are present in equal numbers in an element, compound, or mixture—the net charge is zero or neutral.

Since the atoms of elements all contain equal numbers of both particles, they are electrically neutral. Since the molecules of compounds are made of atoms, they are also electrically neutral. When an atom or a molecule loses or gains a proton or an electron, the result is a partial atom or molecule which is electrically unbalanced. These are called "ions." They are also called "free radicals."

Ions are either positively or negatively charged depending on whether there is a surplus of electrons or protons. Molecules are said to "ionize" when they dissociate into two parts with a surplus of electrons on one part and a surplus of protons on the other. One part will have become a positive ion while the other will have become a negative ion. An ion can be as simple as a single electron (e-) or a single proton (P+). In the case of acids, a single proton (P+) breaks away on its own leaving the rest of the molecule behind as a negative ion.

If you will recall from Chapter Three, a hydrogen atom is a single electron orbiting around a single proton. Hence, another way to look at a proton (p+) is to consider it as a hydrogen ion (H+)—i.e. a hydrogen atom missing its electron. Free hydrogen ions are what make acids acids. The greater the tendency for a compound to give up hydrogen ions when in solution, the greater the strength of the acid or the "more acid" it is. Hydrogen ions (protons–P+) are extremely aggressive, which is why acids are corrosive and have a bite. This is a bite we like in lemons and the tartness of fruits, orange juice, and the taste of blackberry pie.

Pure water is neither acid nor alkaline. It does not easily ionize, which is why it is a poor conductor of electricity. An electrical current requires electrically charged particles free to move in order to flow. This is why we add sulfuric acid to the water in a car battery, which turns water from a poor conductor into a very good conductor.

Because of its low ionization potential, water is a very stable compound. However, water does spontaneously and naturally ionize to a limited extent. The formula, H_2O is sometimes written as HOH to indicate that the O atom has an H atom on each side. (See the diagram of a water molecule in Chapter Four, p. 134.)

Now suppose one H atom broke away from a water molecule leaving its electron behind attached to the OH part. You would then have two ions. H+ and OH- (a hydrogen ion and a hydroxyl ion). Back in Chapter Five we talked about "OH" being a "hydroxyl radical." Don't be confused. They are the same thing, only here we are calling them ions instead of radicals.

The definition of an acid is a water solution with a surplus of H+ ions. The definition of an alkaline or base is a solution with a surplus of OH- ions. But when pure water ionizes there are always exactly the same number of H+ ions as OH- ions so there are no surpluses. Therefore, pure water is neither acidic nor basic. Even though some of its molecules are dissociated into H+ and OH- ions at all times, water is still neutral. To be otherwise, there has to be a surplus in the solution of one ion or the other.

Now here is the really important part of this discussion. So pay close attention. Natural pure water at room temperature (25° C or 77°F) will spontaneously ionize to the extent that one H_2O molecule per billion will dissociate into H+ and OH-. This is a constant property of water. This never changes. Any time you want to count the ionized molecules in a water sample, you will always find that only one in a billion, or one billionth of the H_2O molecules present, have ionized. In other words, for every billion water molecules you would find one H+ ion and one OH- ion. Expressed as a percent, that means one ten-millionth of a percent of the water molecules present have dissociated into ions.

Why a pH of 7.0 Means Neutral

Here is where a pH value of 7.0 being neutral comes from. Water is neutral, neither acid nor base, because it has equal numbers of H+ and OH- ions present at any given time. The portion of H_2O molecules ionized at any time is always one ten-millionth of a percent. Expressed as a fraction, this is 1/10,000,000%.

Notice that there are seven zeros in the denominator of this fraction. The pH scale counts these zeros as its numerical value. A pH of 7.0 means that 1/10,000,000% of molecules of water are ionized in any given instant. Since pure water ionizes in equal numbers of equally charged particles (H+ and OH-), the water has no surplus of H+ or OH- ions and is neutral. Therefore, a pH (potential Hydrogen) of 7.0 represents the situation where the water contains exactly the same number of H+ and OH- ions. Hence, pH = 7.0 means neutral, neither acid nor base. The numeral, "7" is the number of zeros in the fractional percent concentration of H+ ions, namely, 1/10,000,000%. Since both ions are present in equal numbers, one can also say, with equal validity, that the numeral, "7" is the number of zeros in the fractional percent concentration of OH- ions.

Therefore, the number 7.0 as the neutral value for pH is not an arbitrary value chosen by scientists. It is a number given to us by the nature of water, itself, a consequence of the mathematics applied to water's natural state of ionization which, according to Romans 1:20, should tell us something of the nature of God who created water. Throughout the *Old and New Testaments* of the *Bible*, the number seven represents completeness and perfection. God created the heavens and the earth in seven days (Genesis 1:1-2:4). Land is to lie fallow every seventh year (Leviticus 25:2-7). The finest quality silver is to be refined seven times (Psalm 12:6). There are seven churches mentioned in Revelation 2-3 and seven deacons in Acts 6:1-6. When Peter asked Jesus if forgiving someone seven times was enough, Jesus replied, "not seven times, but seventy times seven." (Matthew 18:21-22)

This is where and why a value of 7.0 for pH comes to mean "neutral." This is why the measure of a solution of "zero acidity" is 7.0 on the pH scale, and not 0.0. The idea of zero meaning "zero acidity" only seems to make more sense than 7.0 until you understand where the numbers are coming from. In fact, a pH of 0.0 actually implies an extreme acid which leads us to answer the next question of why lower pH numbers mean higher levels of acidity. But before we can do that, we need to cover some more background.

What Makes an Acid Acid?

Since pH means "potential Hydrogen" and pure water has no potential hydrogens that are available for chemical action because all the loose H^+ ions are matched by an OH^- ion, what would it take to turn water into an acid? In other words, where can H_2O get some surplus H^+ ions to make it acidic? The answer is to dissolve a hydrogen-containing compound in the water that is willing to release its H atoms as H^+ ions. Such compounds are called acids. There are thousands of them.

Hydrogen ions are protons. Since acids are defined to be

compounds that, when dissolved in water, are willing to release H^+ ions, chemists sometimes call acids "proton donors."

When a compound releases all or most of its "potential hydrogens" or H+ ions, we call that a "strong acid." Hydrochloric acid (HCl), sulfuric acid (H_2SO_4), and nitric acid (HNO_3) are strong because they dissociate completely from their H+ ions in water. We say such compounds become totally dissociated or 100% ionized. Highly ionized solutions readily conduct electricity, which is why the fluid in a wet cell (like a car battery) is a strong acid. Partially ionized solutions (like pure water) can conduct electricity, but not well. They are called poor conductors. A totally non-ionized substance conducts no electricity at all. These are called insulators.

Why pH Less than 7.0 is Acid

The numeral "7" as the indicator for a neutral pH comes from the natural ionization that occurs with water where the concentration of H+ ions is 1/10,000,000 of a percent. The numbers of the pH scale are the numbers of the zeros in the fraction that expresses the percent H+ ions present. Since water is neutral, 1/10,000,000% H+ ion concentration means neutral. There are seven zeros in this fraction, hence a pH value of 7.0.

Expressed in words, 1/10,000,000% means "one ten-millionth of a percent." Now let's add an acid compound, like HCl, which is naturally present in most fruit juices. Let's add enough HCl to the water that there are enough additional H+ ions to increase the concentration from one ten-millionth of a percent to one-millionth of a percent. Expressed as a fraction, that would be 1/1,000,000%. Now count the zeros. There are only six. This makes the pH of this solution 6.0. We definitely have an acid solution now with lots of surplus H+ ions and the pH value is now less than 7.0. By comparison, your saliva has a pH of 6.5, which is slightly acid.

Now let's add more HCl to the solution until there are enough H+ ions to increase the concentration from one millionth of a percent to one hundred-thousandth of a percent. Writing this in fractional form, we get 1/100,000%. Now count the zeros in the denominator. There are only five. This corresponds to a pH of 5.0. The pH of black coffee is 5.0, which is more acid than your saliva.

Getting back to the mathematics, a concentration of 1/100,000% (pH = 5) is ten times more than a concentration of 1/1,000,000% (pH = 6) which is ten times more than 1/10,000,000% (pH = 7). In other words, each difference of one unit on the pH scale represents a tenfold change in the concentration of H^+ ions. When each unit on a measuring scale represents factors of ten, we call that a "logarithmic scale."

Now you not only know that the pH scale is "logarithmic," but you know what "logarithmic" actually means. What's more is that you understand why lower and lower numbers of pH mean higher and higher levels of acidity.

If some more HCl is added to our solution such that the concentration of H^+ ions increases from one hundred-thousandth of a percent to one ten thousandth of a percent, that would be 1/10,000%. notice that here we have only four zeros in the denominator which would be a pH of 4.0. A pH of 4.0 represents a greater H+ surplus than pH = 5.0 or 6.0, and, thus, a greater level of acidity.

Tomatoes typically have a pH of 4.0. Vinegar and soda pop generally have a pH of 3.0. Lemon juice measures around 2.2 while the digestive juices of your stomach have a pH of 1.2. Hence, your stomach acids are 10 times stronger than lemon juice, 100 times more than vinegar, 1000 times more than tomato juice, 10,000 more than coffee, and more than 3 million times more than the digestive juices in your mouth. Now you know why aspirating vomit into your lungs can kill you.

If we take this process one step further, adding enough HCl to our acid solution to bring the concentration of H+ ions to 1% we will discover the meaning of pH = 0.0. A concentration of 1% would be a concentration of 1/1%. There are no zeros at all in this denominator. Thus, a pH of 0.0 would represent a powerfully strong acid, indeed! There are such things. You don't want to mess with them.

Everything About pH Summarized

1. "pH" is a scale by which chemists measure the acidity or alkalinity of a solution.

2. The terms, acidity and alkalinity, have no meaning except in regard to aqueous (H_2O) solutions.

3. Solutions with a surplus of H+ ions are acid. Solutions with a surplus of OH- ions are basic or alkaline. Solutions with equal numbers of H+ and OH- ions are neutral. Pure water is neutral.

4. "pH" means "potential H" in the form of hydrogen ions (H+). Hydrogen ions are protons.

5. The numerical values of pH come from the number of zeros in the denominator when H+ concentrations are expressed as fractions of a percent.

6. The reason a pH value of 7.0 represents "neutral," or "zero acidity or zero alkalinity," neither acid nor base, is because pH represents the concentration of H+ ions in pure water which are always exactly balanced by the concentration of OH- ions, resulting in a neutral solution.

7. The reason decreasing pH numbers stand for increasing levels of acidity is because larger and larger values of H+ concentration expressed as fractions have decreasing numbers of zeros in the denominators.

8. The pH scale is logarithmic, meaning that a change of one unit represents a ten-fold change in acidity.

Now that you have seen a full and detailed explanation of pH, you know why chemistry books normally just leave it out and let the student just accept pH by rote, teaching them to use the scale and make calculations with it without trying to explain, exactly, where these numbers come from or why.

Applying pH to Daily Living

Since most essential oil compounds don't ionize in water and, hence, manifest neither acidity nor alkalinity, what does pH have to do with essential oils? Here's an answer to that excellent question.

A proper pH for various body fluids is vital to life and health. Our stomach acids are supposed to be strongly acid for the purpose of digesting food. Our pH for gastric juice is around 1.2—the most acid substance in our bodies and is necessary to digest proteins. Our saliva is also a digestive juice, but much milder than stomach acid since it is contained in our mouth. Normal pH for saliva ranges from 6.0 to 6.8, which is the same for our urine. When either urine or saliva gets above 7.0 (alkaline), that is not good. Saliva needs to be slightly acid to begin the digestion process.

The urine is supposed to be slightly acid because eliminating acid is one of the functions that kidneys do. Urine becomes alkaline when kidneys are not doing their job or when we eat more protein that our bodies need and can process. Excess protein intake can result in urine of such high acidity as to damage the kidneys. To prevent this, our bodies dump ammonia (NH_3) into urine to raise its pH into safe alkaline levels above 7.0. High levels of ammonia in the urine is not a good sign. Our bodily pH is regulated by several mechanisms, but the most important is the action of alkali and alkaline earth elements in our bodies. These are sodium-Na, Potassium-K, Calcium-Ca, and Magnesium-Mg. (See p. 102) The effect of these elements in our bodies is to regulate acidity and maintain a healthy alkalinity. The sources of these alkalyzing minerals are fruits and vegetables. Too much protein and grain, which are acid producing, can use up our store of the alkali and alkaline minerals, forcing our bodies to add ammonia to our acid urine to prevent kidney damage.

Blood is a completely different story. The ideal pH of arterial blood is 7.45 and for venous blood 7.35. Any pH very much above 7.6 or below 7.3 is a serious problem.

If pH is too high, we can develop a chemical state called alkalosis. Too many OH^- ions circulating in your body is not good. Symptoms of alkalosis include sore muscles, creaking joints, bone spurs, protruding eyes, drowsiness, seizures, edema, night cramps, asthma, chronic indigestion, itching skin, and hard dry stools. People suffering from alkalosis are highly nervous, prone to hyperventilation, and can go into convulsions. A blood pH of 8.0 or above can be deadly in a matter of minutes.

If pH is too low, we can develop a chemical state called acidosis. Too many H^+ ions circulating in your body is not good. Symptoms of acidosis include frequent sighing, insomnia, water retention, recessed eyes, rheumatoid arthritis, migraine headaches, low blood pressure, foul-smelling stools accompanied by a burning sensation in the anus, difficulty swallowing, alternating constipation and diarrhea, and sensitivity of teeth to vinegar and acid fruits. When people die, their body immediately starts turning acid and the decomposition process begins. A blood pH of 7.0 or below can result in death in less than 15 minutes.

Our body regulates blood pH three ways: (1) By our diets, (2) By our respiration, and (3) Through our kidneys. What we eat can metabolize into acids or alkalines.

There are many published lists of acid-forming and alkaline-forming foods, often available at health food stores. You can't go by the acidity of the food, itself. Paradoxically, citrus fruits, which are high in acids all metabolize into alkalines in our bodies. Hence, eating citrus is a way to raise pH and increase alkalinity. White sugar, on the other hand, is one of the worst foods for increasing acidity. Other acid–forming foods include alcohol, coffee, eggs, meat, fish, mustard, catsup, flour products, soft drinks, pasta, pepper, cheese, butter, ice cream, and sauerkraut.

Alkaline–forming foods include apricots, avocados, corn, dates, grapefruit, grapes, lemons, millet, oranges, raisins, and vegetables in general. For alkaline–forming sweeteners, try honey, molasses, agave, or maple syrup.

Breath is another pH regulator. Breathing lowers blood acidity. Shallow breathing or holding one's breath raises it. When one's air supply is cut off, acidosis sets in. Excess breathing (i.e. hyperventilation), on the other hand, leads to blood pH levels that are too high. (i.e. alkalosis) This is where aerobic exercises can help.

As for your kidneys, they are designed to selectively secrete more acid than alkaline, but can go the other way if necessary. Thus, your kidneys, in conjunction with the liver, are a vital regulator of body pH.

Bacteria, yeast, and fungi love an acid environment. They can grow uncontrollably in our bodies when our blood pH is too low. When these microbes flourish, they secrete exotoxins and mycotoxins, which are poisonous to our systems and make us sick. Such organisms can hibernate in our bodies and so long as our pH is high enough, they sleep. When it drops too low, they awaken and attack. Hence, proper maintenance of blood pH is vital to staying well.

Applying pH to Essential Oils

Here is where essential oils come into the picture. Acids attack oils and destroy them. When the blood in your tissues is on the acid side, essential oils are compromised in what good they can do and it takes more of them to achieve the same effects.

One of the benefits of incorporating essential oils into one's daily life is that they increase the alkalinity of the body, not because oils are alkaline, but because of how they respond to acids. While an acidic condition in the body will destroy essential oil molecules, during the destruction process there are benefits gained by the person. The aggressive parts of an acid are the free hydrogen ions H^+ that cause bodily damage wherever they circulate. When a therapeutic grade oil enters the body, its molecules willingly sacrifice themselves to the acid, engulfing and neutralizing the H^+ ions so that you don't have to suffer their mischief any more. With a reduction of H^+ ions in the body, pH is raised toward a healthier alkaline state. In this way, even though essential oils are neither alkaline nor acid in and of themselves, their effect upon a person is to alkalize their bodies and move them toward a higher state of health and wellness.

Many people with unhealthy acid conditions in their systems will respond negatively to the scent of essential oils saying "That stinks," or "Get those things out of here. I can't stand them." This reaction is not because the oils, themselves, are unpleasant. What is unpleasant is the fact that the oils have stirred up toxins which need to be eliminated. It is the toxins that cause the unpleasantness. Detoxification is not always a pleasant experience, but a necessary one to maintain health and experience longevity. When a person's acidity and toxicity levels are reduced, they will find that they actually like and enjoy the very fragrances they formerly could not tolerate.

This statement is also true for people with "acidic" personalities. Negative and destructive emotions, such as hate, resentment, bitterness, anger, etc., act as spiritual acids that eat away at our peace and happiness and come between us and our relationships with others and with God. Spiritually acidic people may respond negatively to the scent of an essential oil, saying "Get that stuff away from me!" or "I can't stand that smell!" Such a reaction is an indication that unpleasant thoughts or feelings have been stirred up by the essential oils that the individual has been unwilling to deal with, preferring rather to shove them into their unconscious mind. This phenomenon is the basis for emotional release with oils where, by the use of essential oils people who are willing to better themselves allow the oils to bring their repressed emotions to the surface where they can release them.

Those that practice raindrop technique have usually observed that when essential oils are applied to the back, for some people they soak in rapidly and disappear, like water drops on a sponge, while in others the oils remain visibly on the surface and are absorbed only slowly and reluctantly through the skin. How this is related to bodily pH is somewhat of a mystery. Some that soak up the oils like sponges are healthy alkaline people whose bodies readily accept and utilize essential oils. Some less healthy acid people also readily absorb the oils as if their bodies were craving them. In eny case, to gain maximum benefits from a raindrop session, it is wise to avoid acid-forming foods for a day or so prior to receiving it. This, of course, includes most fast foods such as fried chicken, deep fried fish, burgers, french fries, sugar-containing beverages, ice cream, and other sweets.

To gain the optimal benefit of essential oils, keep your body pH levels in the normal ranges by right diet, right exercise, lowering the stress in your life, and avoiding the use of antibiotics and pharmaceuticals (which increase acidity). Breathing, ingesting, and rubbing essential oils on the skin raises body pH and helps to maintain proper pH balance. It also raises one's spiritual pH and helps to elevate and maintain one's peace and calmness, a joyful state of mind, and a loving heart.

Oils Containing Acids

As you learned in Chapter Two, fatty oils are composed almost completely of acidic compounds. That's why they are called "fatty acids." (See pp. 56-57.) However, they are all very weak acids. Nevertheless, this is why, given enough time, unrefrigerated vegetable oils (and butter) will start decomposing and go rancid. Essential oils, on the other hand, rarely contain acids in more than trace amounts. They never go rancid, having shelf lives measured in thousands of years. One

Table Twenty-Three
Carboxylic Acids Found in Essential Oils

Name	Example of an Oil Where Found
Aminobenzoic Acid	Mandarin (*Citrus reticulata*)
Angelic Acid	Angelica (*Angelica archangelica*)
Anisic Acid	Anise (*Pimpinella anisum*)
Benzoic Acid	Onycha (*Styrax benzoin*)
Cinnamic Acid	Cinnamon (*Cinnamomum verum*)
Citronellic Acid	Citronella (*Cymbopogon nardus*)
Geranic Acid	Geranium (*Pelargonium graveolens*)
Phenylacetic Acid	Neroli (*Citrus aurantium*)
Sedanolic Acid	Celery Seed (*Apium graveolens*)
Valerinic Acid	Valerian (*Valeriana officinalis*)
Vetiveric Acid	Vetiver (*Vetiveria zizanioides*)

* Carboxylic acids in essential oils are not common and never occur as major ingredients.(i.e. almost always less than 1% of the oil)

apparent exception to this is onycha oil (*Styrax benzoin*) which contains up to 30% carboxylic acids. However, onycha is not a true essential oil since it is extracted from the gum of a tree by solvents, not by distillation.

When vegetable oils are used as a base for massage oils containing essential oils, these can eventually spoil because of the activity of the fatty acids in the base. When an oil blend is mostly essential oil with only a little base oil, the shelf life is quite long, measured in years. When a massage oil is blended according to British standards (i.e. less than 5% essential), these can go rancid in months depending on storage conditions. Refrigeration retards spoilage.

Table Twenty-Three lists some essential oils containing small amounts of carboxylic acids followed by a few graphics of acid molecules on the next page. You will notice that the presence of acids is so rare and unusual in essential oils that many of them are virtually unique to a single oil and are named as such. For example, anisic acid is found only in anise oil, citronellic acid only in citronella oil, and vetiveric

Examples of Carboxylic Acid Molecules

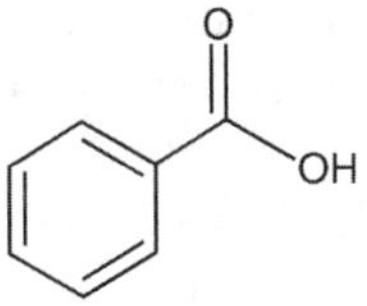

Benzoic Acid
$C_7H_6O_2$
Onycha, Peruvian
Balsam (Tolu)

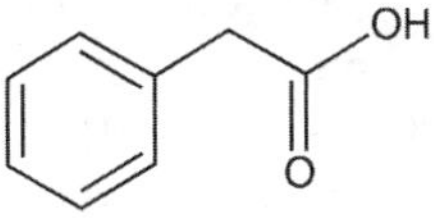

Phenylacetic Acid
$C_8H_8O_2$
Neroli

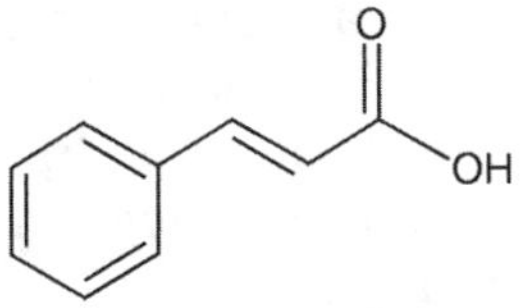

Cinnamic Acid
$C_9H_8O_2$
Cinnamon, Cassia,
Onycha, Tolu, Coca

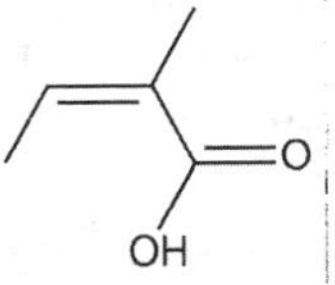

Angelic Acid
$C_5H_8O_2$
Roman Chamomile
Angelica

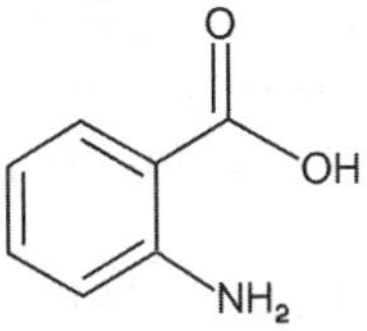

Aminobenzoic Acid
$C_7H_7O_2N$
Neroli, Mandarin
Orange, Lemon, Bergamot

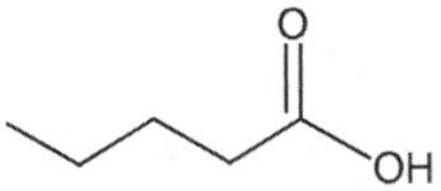

Valerinic Acid
$C_5H_{10}O_2$
Valerian

acid only in vetiver oil, etc. Phenylacetic acid, one of the fragrances of neroli oil, is formed by the combination of acetic acid and an aromatic ring (benzene).

All of the essential oil acids in the figure of examples shown above are light in molecular weight, ranging from 100 amu for angelic acid to 148 amu for cinnamic acid. This is why all of them are so volatile and strongly aromatic. Note that four of the displayed acids are monocyclic and phenolic in that they have a benzene ring while two of the acids are acyclic and non-phenolic. The molecules with benzene rings are of a higher resonance energy and assume the behavior of wave forms more than ensembles of atomic particles. They impart electromagnetic frequencies to oils.

Also note that the aminobenzoic acid molecule is unique in that it contains an amine radical—NH_2—which has a nitrogen atom. This acid is found in traces only as a transient ingredient because its role is to combine with various alcohols in the oil to form esters, which we will discuss in the next section. Aminobenzoic acid is not a true amino acid, but a by-product in the metabolism of tryptophan, which is a true and essential amino acid. Amino acids are virtually absent from essential oils. Aminobenzoic acid is widespread in nature occurring in such things as brewers yeast and plays a role in the biosynthesis of vitamins.

Valerinic acid in combination with the aldehyde, valerianal, is the source of the unpleasant smell of valerian oil as mentioned earlier in this chapter in the section entitled "The Odor of Dirty Socks," p. 328.

Cinnamic acid is found in a range of plants and their oils. Besides cinnamon (*Cinnamomum verum*), cassia (*Cinnamomum cassia*), and at least ten other species of *Cinnamomum*, it is found in onycha (*Styrax benzoin*), Peruvian balsam or tolu (*Myroxylon peiera*), and coca (*Erythroxylon coca*).

These last two are South American plants. Tolu absolute is used in the perfume and food industries because its chemistry offers a variety of tastes and fragrances including cinnamon, clove, vanilla, and chocolate. Tolu essential oil also has therapeutic applications. Tolu resin is mostly esters, but contains 12–15% cinnamic and benzoic acids.

The coca plant is the source of cocaine, which is present in the leaves which are chewed by natives for its narcotic and anesthetic effects. Extracts of the coca plant used to be an ingredient in Coca-Cola® when the company first started marketing its drink in the late eighteenth century. Coca is not to be confused with cacao, another South American plant (*Theobroma cacao*) whose seeds are the source of chocolate. "*Theobroma*," by the way, means "food of the gods," from the Greek where "*theos*" means god and "*broma*" means food.

Angelic acid is interesting. It is found in the oils of angelica (*Angelica archangelica*) and Roman chamomile (*Chamaemelum nobile*). Look closely at the molecular shape. It is an isoprene unit (a little horsey) with an acid radical attached to its front foot. (See Chapter Nine, p. 257.) Notice the isoprene formula (C_5H_8) buried in the formula for angelic acid ($C_5H_8O_2$).

The Taste of Berries and Smell of Hospitals

Benzoic acid (which contains a benzene ring—C_6H_6) is a powerful antimicrobial agent, as are many acids. It is found in concentrations of up to 20% in onycha oil (*Styrax benzoin*) along with cinnamic acid (up to 10%). Onycha contains more acid than any other aromatic oil. Its high acid content, in combination with its esters, aldehydes, and alcohols, makes it a powerful antiseptic, effective against most microbes and even fungi. For more than 200 years, oil of onycha was dissolved in ethyl alcohol as an antiseptic called "tincture of benzoin." It was used in hospitals and clinics throughout the world. Onycha oil has a unique fragrance emanating from its vanillin aldehyde content combined with benzoic and cinnamic acids and the esters created by these acids. It is the smell people used to associate with hospitals.

During the twentieth century, hospitals began to use synthetic antiseptics rather than the natural oil of onycha in alcoholic solution. The synthetics were less expensive and easier to obtain, but were eventually discovered to be less effective. Synthetic antiseptics also create resistent strains of bacteria against which they are no longer effective. Medical practitioners are now rediscovering that tincture of benzoin remains unequaled in the breadth of its antiseptic cleansing properties. Furthermore, natural substances like onycha oil do not create virulent resistant strains of bacteria and will always be effective into the future, unlike synthetics and unaturals whose days of effectiveness are numbered. What man creates is transient and temporary. What God creates is good forever. In fact, in Genesis 1:31, God says that his creations are "very good."

The fact that tincture of onycha oil addresses a broader spectrum of pathogens than any synthetic agent is due, not to a single ingredient, like benzoic acid, but to the synergy of all of its components. Synthetic benzoic acid can be made in a lab, but it does not have the properties of the whole oil of onycha. Not only is onycha more effective, it is also non-toxic to humans, which can be a problem with antiseptics artificially produced from petrochemicals.

Onycha oil is one of the ingredients in the holy incense whose formula was given to Moses by God to burn in the temple every day. (Exodus 30:34-36) Because of its highly antimicrobial properties, burning this incense would effectively fumigate the temple, keeping the atmosphere free of harmful germs, thus offering protection to the priests and other personnel, as well as to those of the public who came to offer their sacrifices and prayers to God.

Benzoic acid is also an acid in cherries and berries of many species that makes them tart. Benzoic acid is used as a preservative for various foods, fats, and fruit juices. It is also employed in the making of dyes for cloth and in the curing of tobacco. It has also been found useful for its antifungal properties. Benzoic acid is also found in vetiver oil (*Vetiveria zizanioides*).

Esters

Oils composed mostly of esters include birch and wintergreen (both over 90%), as well as onycha (70%) and clary sage (64%). Bornyl acetate (an ester) is the main ingredient in the smell of the evergreens such as pine, spruce, juniper, and fir. (See Tables 24, 41, 55, and 56.) What defines an ester is a carbonyl group (C=O) with a hydrocarbon functional group (R) attached on one side and an oxygen atom (O) on the other side to which is attached another hydrocarbon group (R'). (See Table Seventeen.)

The names of esters either incorporate the word "ester" in their nomenclature or consist of two parts, the first ending in "-yl" and the second in "-ate." To remember that the suffix, -ate, indicates an ester, just say to yourself "We want to know what Ester ate?" It is appropriate to associate esters with eating inasmuch as the flavors of most fruits are combinations of esters. What defines an ester is a C atom double-bonded to an O atom above and another O on one side with hydrocarbon groups (R and R') attached on both sides. (See Table Seventeen, page 314.)

Esters are oxygenated hydrocarbons requiring two O atoms per molecule, like carboxylic acids. Phenols, alcohols, ethers, aldehydes, ketones, and oxides require only one oxygen. When there is more than one oxygen in these compounds, we sometimes add the prefix "di" as in "diphenol," "diol," "dione," or "dioxide." From Table Seventeen (on page 314) you can see that esters and acids are a similarly constructed pair. Alcohols and ethers are another similar pair while aldehydes and ketones form yet another parallel twosome.

Esters are biosynthesized in oils by the reaction of a carboxylic acid with an alcohol. This is one reason only a few weak acids are found in essential oils. Because most volatile oils contain alcohols, the presence of an acid almost always results in the production of an ester and the disappearance of the acid. The chemical reaction is as follows:

a carboxylic acid + an alcohol $\rightarrow$ an ester + H_2O

In this equation, the arrow symbol translates as the word "yields." In a sentence, the equation reads like this: "A carboxylic acid combined with an alcohol yields an ester plus water." This example illustrates how all equations can be stated in plain English as a sentence. Mathematics is simply a language written in the form of a shorthand. Understanding math is learning how to translate formulas into the familiar tongue we normally speak. But we digress. This isn't a math book. It's a chemistry book.

Since ester is a child conceived and born by the marriage of an acid to an alcohol, its double name reflects both parents with the given name taken from the parent alcohol and the family name from the parent acid. In methyl salicylate, for example, the alcohol is methyl alcohol (methanol) while the acid is salicylic acid. Methyl salicylate was discussed in Chapter One regarding the *Merck Manual* and depicted in Chapter Nine in the discussion on aspirin, which it resembles chemically and structurally.

Esters are among the most pleasant of fragrances and often lend to an oil their characteristic personality even when present in minor quantities. The ester, linalyl acetate (the child of linalol and acetic acid), is the dominant fragrance of lavender oil. Esters compose some of the most highly prized perfumes and also provide many fruity flavors like grape, cherry, strawberry, and banana. There are thirty different esters that combine to make the taste of orange. One could say that "Ester has good taste."

Not all esters in essential oils existed in the living plant. Some are artifacts of distillation where weak acids present in the fluids of the plant are stimulated to react with the alcohol content in response to the heat. However, in all cases, the resulting esters are considered aromatically and therapeutically desirable. You can remember the acid-alcohol reaction given on the previous page by the following illustration.

Rum and Coke®

The idea of mixing acids with alcohols to produce esters brings to mind an interesting idea. Rum and Coke® is a popular drink among those who imbibe liquor, especially in certain Latin American countries. Considering that rum's main ingredient is ethyl alcohol (ethanol—C_2H_6O) and Coca-Cola® is principally an acid (carbonic acid—H_2CO_3), combining the two could create an ester that gives the mixed drink its appealing and unique taste and aroma. Bartenders are actually playing chemistry. The chemical reaction equation would look like this:

$$H_2CO_3 + C_2H_6O \rightarrow C_3H_6O_3 + H_2O$$

The equation reads, "one molecule of carbonic acid combined with one molecule of ethyl alcohol yields one molecule of an ester plus one molecule of water."

If we were to follow the conventions of naming esters in this drink, we could say that it is a combination of "rumol" (the alcohol) and "cokeic acid" (the acid). Using that as our basis, the name of the ester would be "rumyl cokate." If we used the scientific names "ethanol" and "carbonic acid." the name of the ester would be "ethyl carbonate." In the *Merck Index* it is identified as an ester called "dimethyl carbonate" since the ethyl radical (C_2H_6) splits into two methyl radicals ($CH_3 + CH_3$) in its structure. We will let you decide which is the better of the three choices.

Whether a mixture of rum and coke actually produces this particular ester depends on many factors such as temperature, pressure, concentration, and the presence or absence of certain catalysts or enzymes. Dimethyl carbonate has several isomers and is not the only ester that could result by this combination. The purpose of this presentation is to help you remember the way esters are named and the manner they are biosynthesized in living plants—by the reaction of a carboxylic acid with an alcohol.

Esters in Essential Oils

Oils containing esters usually contain the parent alcohols as well, but not the parent acids. For example, a major ingredient in lavender oil is the ester, linalyl acetate (about 35%) while another major compound in lavender is linalol (also about 35%). Linalol is the parent alcohol for linalyl acetate. As for the parent acid (acetic), lavender contains not even a trace. Cistus oil contains bornyl acetate and also borneol, its parent alcohol, but does not contain acetic acid, the parent acid. Another example is geranium oil which contains the esters, geranyl formate, geranyl acetate, geranyl butyrate, and geranyl tiglate. Geranium also contains the parent alcohol for all of these esters—viz. geraniol. But as for the acids (formic, acetic, butyric, and tiglic), not a trace of these is found in the oil.

Acetic acid ($C_2H_4O_2$), the acid of vinegar, is a major player in procreating esters for oils, yet this acid is rarely found in any oil. It is too strong. Myrrh is an exception to this. It contains a trace of it. acetic acid is too active to remain an acid but, instead, reacts with whatever alcohols are available to form esters. Apples contain a variety of esters, including ethyl acetate, that give the fruit its distinctive apple taste. When apple juice ferments, the esters can revert back to the parent alcohol (ethanol) to make hard cider and/or transform into the parent acid (acetic) to make vinegar.

While most oils are not primarily composed of esters, almost every essential oil has at least small amounts of one or more in their makeup. There may be more varieties of esters in aromatic oils than any other class of compounds. Oils with esters as main ingredients include wintergreen (97%), birch (90%), Roman chamomile (65%), petitgrain (57%), lavender (39%), bergamot (37%) and spruce (34%). If you are familiar with the fragrances of these oils or those in Table Twenty-Four, you will appreciate the tremendous variety of fragrances offered by esters.

In general, the natural esters occurring in plant oils are nontoxic, safe to use, and pleasant to the nose. Esters are

Table Twenty-Four
Esters Found in Essential Oils

Name	Example of an Oil Where Found	%
Methyl Salicylate	Birch (*Betula alleghaniensis*)	85%
Terpinyl Acetate	Cardamom (*Elettaria cardamomum*)	50%
Linalyl Acetate	Bergamot (*Citrus bergamia*)	40%
Isobutyl Angelate	Roman Chamomile (*Cham. nobile*)	40%
Neryl Acetate	Helichrysum *(Helichrysum italicum)*	30%
Benzyl Acetate	Jasmine (*Jasminum officinale*)	25%
Bornyl Acetate	Spruce (*Picea mariana*)	25%
Eugenyl Acetate	Clove (*Syzygium aromaticum*)	15%
Citronellyl Formate	Geranium (*Pelargonium graveolens*)	15%
Benzyl Benzoate	Ylang Ylang (*Cananga odorata*)	10%
Menthyl Acetate	Peppermint (*Mentha piperita*)	9%
Geranyl Acetate	Citronella (*Cymbopogon nardus*)	7%
Bornyl Valerate	Valerian (*Valeriana officinalis*)	5%
Cinnamyl Acetate	Cassia (*Cinnamomum cassia*)	3%
Methyl Anthranilate	Mandarin (*Citrus reticulata*)	2%

* Most essential oils have some esters present. A few, like some of those above, are composed principally of esters. Most esters are known for their mild and pleasant properties—highly prized by perfumers for their fragrances and valued by aromatherapists for their balancing,

among the most popular classes of compounds in the perfume industry. Esters also provide most of the tastes we enjoy in fresh fruits and fruit juices.

The essential oil with the most varieties of esters (more than a dozen) is Roman chamomile which can be up to 75% esters. Esters are known for their soothing, relaxing, and stress-releasing effects. Maybe that is why rum and Coke is so popular in some cultures. It is also interesting to note that the original recipe for Coca-Cola® contained flavorings of six essential oils: cinnamon, coriander, lemon, neroli, nutmeg and orange.

Examples of Ester Molecules

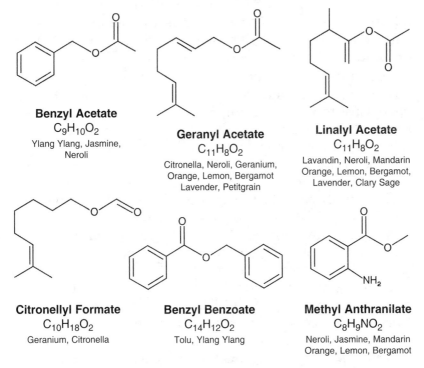

Benzyl Acetate
$C_9H_{10}O_2$
Ylang Ylang, Jasmine,
Neroli

Geranyl Acetate
$C_{11}H_8O_2$
Citronella, Neroli, Geranium,
Orange, Lemon, Bergamot
Lavender, Petitgrain

Linalyl Acetate
$C_{11}H_8O_2$
Lavandin, Neroli, Mandarin
Orange, Lemon, Bergamot,
Lavender, Clary Sage

Citronellyl Formate
$C_{10}H_{18}O_2$
Geranium, Citronella

Benzyl Benzoate
$C_{14}H_{12}O_2$
Tolu, Ylang Ylang

Methyl Anthranilate
$C_8H_9NO_2$
Neroli, Jasmine, Mandarin
Orange, Lemon, Bergamot

Table Twenty–Four, shown above, gives a sample of various esters with an example of an essential oil that contains each of them along with the percent of the oil that ester comprises. See if you can figure out which alcohol and which carboxylic acid paired up to produce the ester offspring in each listing.

The figure above gives six examples of ester molecules. Three are acyclic, two are monocyclic, and one is bicyclic. The top three are from reactions of acetic acid with benzyl alcohol, geranol, and linalol, respectively. Benzyl benzoate is formed from benzyl alcohol and benzoic acid—both of which contain a benzene ring—which is why the resulting ester, benzyl benzoate, has two benzene rings. Benzyl benzoate is used commercially as a fixative in perfumes. Its natural occurrence in ylang ylang increases the half-life of that oil. It is also used to extend the taste of candies and chewing gum.

Fear and Formic Acid

Citronellyl formate is from a reaction between citronellol and formic acid. Formic acid is the simplest possible carboxylic acid and the smallest in molecular size (M.W. = 46 amu). Formic acid contains only one carbon—CH_2O_2. Except as a passing participant in the making of esters, formic acid is usually not found in essential oils. It is too aggressive to remain in an oil intact as an acid. That is a good thing. Formic acid is the burning toxin in some ant bites and wasp stings as well as the sting in stinging nettles. As for its fragrance, it is pungent to say the least. One whiff of formic acid and your eyes will water, your nose will run, your throat will burn, you will start coughing, and you'll probably get sick to your stomach.

You may have noticed that people who are afraid of bees and hornets are more likely to be stung than those who are not. This is because formic acid acts like an alarm pheromone to certain stinging insects and drives them into an attack frenzy to protect their territory. Since you secrete traces of formic acid in your sweat when you feel scared, fear of stinging insects can actually draw them to attack you. At the same time, a calm and fearless person standing nearby may not be stung at all.

Formic acid is considered a hazardous chemical. This is not an ingredient you want to experience in an essential oil or in any other context. But its ester, citronellyl formate, is fruity and floral like a rose.

There is one notable exception to the absence of formic acid in essential oils. Paradoxically, oil of myrrh, which is one of the mildest and gentlest of all the aromatic oils, contains a trace of formic acid.

Methyl anthranilate is an unusual ester in that it incorporates a nitrogen atom. It is found in neroli, ylang ylang, bergamot, jasmine, lemon, mandarin, orange, and other essential oils. It has a fragrance we would identify as orange or orange blossom. Found naturally in cherries and grape juice, synthetic anthranilate is used as an imitation for cherry or grape. Since methyl anthranilate is produced by nature, companies can use the synthetic version for artificial flavorings and still put "natural flavorings" on their label. (See Chapter Four for more on this.)

Oxides

Oils composed mostly of oxides include cajuput (60%), ravensara (55%), blue mallee (90%), and eucalyptus (68%). (See Tables 25, 26, 47, 61, and 62.) Oxides are usually derived from other compounds such as terpenes, alcohols, or ketones which have been oxidized. The names of oxides usually identify the parent molecule to which the word "oxide" is merely added. Thus we have names like "α-pinene oxide" (where α-pinene, a monoterpene, has been oxidized), "linalol oxide" (where linalol, an alcohol, has been oxidized), and "bisabolone oxide" (where bisabolone, a ketone, has been oxidized).

Organic oxides are another example of oxygenated hydrocarbons. However, in oxides an O atom is attached to the hydrocarbon in a special way, like no other. In the oxy-

Examples of Oxide Molecules

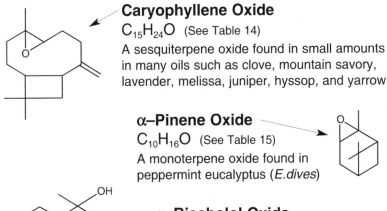

Caryophyllene Oxide
$C_{15}H_{24}O$ (See Table 14)
A sesquiterpene oxide found in small amounts in many oils such as clove, mountain savory, lavender, melissa, juniper, hyssop, and yarrow

α–Pinene Oxide
$C_{10}H_{16}O$ (See Table 15)
A monoterpene oxide found in peppermint eucalyptus (*E.dives*)

α–Bisabolol Oxide
$C_{15}H_{24}O_2$ (See figure following Table 18)
An oxide derived from a sesquiterpene alcohol comprising 32-42% of German chamomile oil

genated molecules mentioned thus far, an oxygen atom was placed between a hydrocarbon (R) and a hydrogen atom (H)—(as in phenolics, alcohols, and acids), or double bonded to a single carbon (C)—(as in aldehydes, ketones, acids, and esters), or placed between two hydrocarbons (R and R')—(as in ethers and esters). (See Table Seventeen.)

Oxides are different. In oxides, the oxygen is bonded to two different carbon atoms of the same molecule forming a triangular ring. In the three examples given on the previous page, see how the oxygen atom reaches out in two directions to grab the hands of two different carbons. This is what defines an oxide and sets it apart from all other types of oxygenated hydrocarbons.

Table Twenty-Five (shown below) lists a number of oxides found in essential oils. See if you can identify the parent compound that was oxidized in each one. There are four terpenes, three alcohols, and two ketones. Manool oxide is an oxidized diterpene alcohol called manool. As for

Table Twenty-Five
Oxides (Other than Cineole) in Essential Oils

Name	Example of an Oil Where Found	%
Bisabolol Oxide-A	German Chamomile (*Matricaria Recutita*)	28%
Bisabolone Oxide	German Chamomile (*Matricaria Recutita*)	12%
Caryophyllene Oxide	Carrot Seed (*Daucus carota*)	4%
Piperitone Oxide	Peppermint (*Mentha piperita*)	3%
Manool Oxide	Cypress (*Cupressus sempervirens*)	0.5%
Linalol Oxide	Hyssop (*Hyssopus officinalis*)	0.4%
Rose Oxide	Rose (*Rosa damascena*)	0.3%
α-Pinene Oxide	Peppermint Eucalyptus (*E. Dives*)	0.2%
Sclareol Oxide	Clary Sage (*Salvia sclarea*)	0.1%
Humulene Oxide	Clove (*Syzygium aromaticum*)	0.1%

* Oxides are not common in essential oils, except for 1,8 cineole, which is very common. Except for those containing cineole, German Chamomile contains more oxides than any other essential oil.

rose oxide, who knows? Rose oxide does not reveal its parent compound in its name. It is found, however, not only in rose oil, but geranium oil as well.

Favorite Oxide of the Plant Kingdom

As you can see from Table Twenty-Five, except for the high level of oxides in German Chamomile, the presence of oxides in essential oils other than 1,8 cineole is not only uncommon, but when they do occur, they usually exist as minor or trace constituents only. However, there is one oxide whose recipe has evidently been passed on ("through the grapevine" perhaps) to hundreds of plants, becoming a favorite for many species. Most aromatic oils contain at least traces of this popular compound. In a number of essential oils, it constitutes more than half of their makeup. It is, by far, the leading oxide in all of aromatherapy. That oxide is 1,8 cineole—also called "eucalyptol" or "cajuputol."

For reasons unknown to humans, hundreds of plants know how to make 1,8 cineole. Whether they all went to the same school where its biosynthesis was taught or if they all discovered its formula independently on their own by coincidence, we don't know. (We suspect they all had the same teacher.) One thing we do know, hundreds of plants love it and produce it for their own purposes and enjoyment. If there were a popularity contest for the favorite oxide among plants, 1,8 cineole would definitely be voted as "King of the Oxides."

Notice that none of the three common names for this compound follow the nomenclature convention for oxides. "Cineole" makes it sound like an ether while "eucalyptol" and "cajuputol" make it sound like an alcohol when, in fact, it is neither an ether nor an alcohol. It is a true oxide. The misnaming of this compound has to do with its long 200 year history of familiarity in the fields of medicine and aromatherapy. It was labeled long before the rules for naming organic compounds were established.

The molecular shape of 1,8 cineole is given in the figure on the next page, along with that of 1,4 cineole, another

The Cineole Sisters

$C_{10}H_{18}O$ $C_{10}H_{18}O$

1,8 Cineole   Molecular   1,4 Cineole
Eucalyptus   Numbering   Melaleuca
Oils   System   Oils

oxide of the same family. These two oxides are isomers. Also shown is the conventional numbering system for this molecular structure, which was first mentioned in Chapter Seven. Browsing through this book you will see that numerous essential oil molecules use this particular model as a template for their structures. In order to identify the specific carbons to which various radicals and atoms are attached, the numbering system shown on the template has been adopted by scientists. From this you can see how the numbers in the names of the two types of cineole identify where the oxygen atom is grabbing on with its two arms and hands.

Table Twenty-Six (on the next page) is a partial list of essential oils containing 1,8 cineole. It gives you a sample of the many species of plants who have figured out how to manufacture this compound. You can also see from the table why two alternate names for 1,8 cineole are "cajuputol" and "eucalyptol," since these oils contain such high percents of the compound. Also notice that German chamomile, which is top of the list in Table Twenty-Five, with a 47% oxide content, is devoid of cineole.

While many oils contain 1,8 cineole, some exhibit a considerable range of concentrations. For example, the possible concentration of 1,8 cineole in tea tree oil can range

Table Twenty-Six
Essential Oils Containing 1,8 Cineole

Common Name	Botanical Name	% 1,8 Cineole
Blue Mallee	(*Eucalyptus polybractea*)	90%
Gully Gum	(*Eucalyptus smithii*)	75%
Black Peppermint	(*Eucalyptus radiata*)	67%
Eucalyptus	(*Eucalyptus globulus*)	67%
Cajuput	(*Melaleuca cajuputi*)	60%
Spanish Marjoram	(*Thymus mastichina*)	58%
Ravensara	(*Ravensara aromatica*)	55%
Niaouli (MQV)	(*Melaleuca quinquenervia*)	50%
Rosemary CT cineole	(*Rosmarinus officinalis*)	47%
Bay Laurel	(*Laurus nobilis*)	42%
Myrtle	(*Myrtus communis*)	38%
Cardamom	(*Elettaria cardamomum*)	32%
White Camphor	(*Laurus camphora*)	30%
Rosalina	(*Melaleuca ericifolia*)	15%
Lemon Eucalyptus	(*Eucalyptus citriodora*)	10%
Thyme	(*Thymus vulgaris*)	10%
Sage	(*Salvia officinalis*)	9%
Tea Tree	(*Melaleuca alternifolia*)	9%
Lavandin	(*Lavandula x hybrida*)	6%
Yarrow	(*Achillea millefolium*)	6%
Basil	(*Ocimum basilicum*)	5%
Peppermint	(*Mentha piperita*)	4%
Nutmeg	(*Myristica fragrans*)	3%
Fennel	(*Foeniculum vulgare*)	3%
Rosewood	(*Aniba roseodora*)	2%

NOTE: Oils containing significant amounts of 1,8 cineole are noted for their respiratory decongesting and sinus clearing attributes. Such oils are used commercially in many products such as VicksVapoRub®, for example.

from zero to 18%. Roman chamomile can contain from zero to 25% while ravensara can range from 20% to 60%. These differences reflect the nature of the growing conditions in different locations around the world which produce chemotypes with more 1,8 cineole or less.

The Safety of Cineole

1,8 cineole has been lab tested in isolation with mixed conclusions. Some reports suggest that it might be neurotoxic to an unborn child and a potential abortive agent, but no actual incidents have been reported to confirm these concerns. Tisserand (*Essential Oil Safety*) reports that "1,8 cineole can cause serious poisoning when accidentally instilled through the nose." The only cases of lethal poisoning attributed to cineole seem to be cases of extreme amounts—5-30 ml of eucalyptus (*globulus*) oil taken orally in a single dose by children. This oil can be up to 80% 1,8 cineole. Cineole has also been described as "a skin irritant" with precautions against using it in massage unless diluted to "a maximum of 2%." (Tisserand) These reports, anecdotes, and cautions are all found in British publications.

By contrast, the U.S. Food and Drug Administration (FDA) has classified *Eucalyptus globulus* (Blue Gum) oil as "GRAS," meaning "generally regarded as safe for internal use." Other oils listed in Table Twenty-Five also classified as GRAS by the FDA include basil, Roman chamomile, fennel, ginger, bay laurel, lavender, tea tree, nutmeg, peppermint, sage, and thyme. When an oil has been given GRAS status for internal use, it goes without saying that such an oil may also be considered safe for inhalation and transdermal applications.

Gold Bond® medicated cream is a topical remedy that has been on the market for over 100 years in the U.S. and is still popular today, It is sold everywhere over the counter in pharmacies and grocery stores. Second on its list of active ingredients is 1,8 cineole. The first active ingredient in Gold Bond® ointment is methyl salicylate, discussed in Chapter One and elsewhere in this book. Its third active ingredient is thymol. If 1,8 cineole or methyl salicylate posed a serious toxicity problem Gold Bond® salve would have been taken off the market decades ago.

As for the possibility of any buildup of 1,8 cineole to toxic levels when used repeatedly over extended periods of time, research indicates that the half-life of 1,8 cineole in the human body is of the order of only 10–20 minutes.

Any data on cineole (or any other essential oil compound) tested as an isolate in concentrated doses cannot be validly applied to the effects of using the whole oil. Furthermore, abuse of any substance by ingesting extreme doses, including an essential oil, is not a valid test of its safety or utility under common sense conditions and normal usage. While it is possible that cineole could pose a risk as a single compound, when applied as one ingredient among many in a whole, natural, pure oil, its risks (if any) are quenched and controlled by the company of the other compounds. The chemistry of essential oils can only be understood in the whole, not by separation of its constituents and analysis of its parts. The aerodynamics of an airplane can only be understood by flying the craft, not by disassembly and analysis of its separate parts.

Lactones

Oils containing the highest percents of lactones include catnip (13%) and celery seed (11%). (See Tables 27, 45, and 70.) Lactones are a special kind of ester.

Referring back to Table Seventeen (page 314), or the section on esters a few pages back, you will see that esters are characterized by having a C atom with two O atoms attached: One double–bonded O and one single–bonded O with hydrocarbon groups (R & R') on two sides.

The difference between a lactone and any other kind of ester is that the single-bonded O atom is part of a hydrocarbon ring whereas in a regular ester, it is not.

Hermaphroditic Molecules

Referring back to the section on esters, you see that it takes two molecules to make an ester—an acid and an alcohol, a mommy and a daddy. Lactones are created from

Table Twenty-Seven
Lactones in Essential Oils

Name	Example of an Oil Where Found
Achillin	Yarrow (*Achillea millefolium*)
Aesculetine	Peppermint (*Mentha piperita*)
Alantolactone	Sweet Inule (*Inula graveolens*)
Bergaptene	Fennel (*Foeniculum vulgare*)
Bergamottin	Lemon (*Citrus limon*)
Butanolide	Lavender (*Lavandula angustifolia*)
Citropten	Petitgrain (*Citrus aurantium*)
Coumarin	Lavandin (*Lavandula x hybrida*)
Furanogermacrene	Myrrh (*Commiphora myrrha*)
Herniarin	German Chamomile (*Matricaria recutita*)
Limettine	Lime (*Citrus aurantifolia*)
Nepetalactone	Catnip (*Nepeta cataria*)
Psoralen	Bergamot (*Citrus bergamia*)
Scopoletin	Roman Chamomile (*Chamaemelum nobile*)
Umbelliferone	Anise (*Pimpinella anisum*)

* Lactones never compose the principal portion of any oil, but their strong ketone-like qualities can influence an oil's therapeutic actions even when present only in small quantities. Lactones containing a furan ring are phototoxic. Furanogermacrene is a sesquiterpene lactone.

a single molecule that is both an acid and an alcohol—a hermaphrodite—like an earthworm that is male on one end and female on the other. These strange molecules are called "hydroxy acids." Hydroxy acids have an acid radical (COOH) at one end and a hydroxyl radical (OH), an alcohol, at the other. It is a creature with an acid head and an alcoholic tail. If the acidic end bends around and reacts with the alcoholic end a ring is formed and you get a lactone. In other words, the snake (hydroxy acid) bites its own tail forming a heterogeneous ring. During the process a water molecule is also given off, just as in the normal alco-

Examples of Lactone Molecules

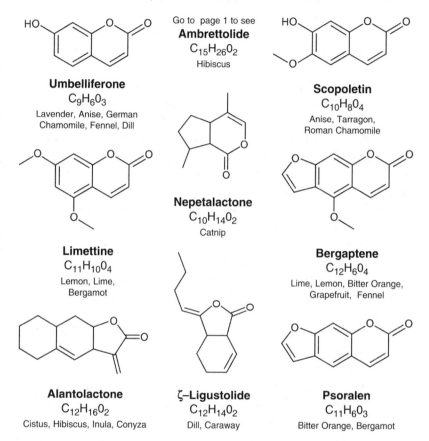

Umbelliferone
$C_9H_6O_3$
Lavender, Anise, German
Chamomile, Fennel, Dill

Go to page 1 to see
Ambrettolide
$C_{15}H_{26}O_2$
Hibiscus

Scopoletin
$C_{10}H_8O_4$
Anise, Tarragon,
Roman Chamomile

Limettine
$C_{11}H_{10}O_4$
Lemon, Lime,
Bergamot

Nepetalactone
$C_{10}H_{14}O_2$
Catnip

Bergaptene
$C_{12}H_6O_4$
Lime, Lemon, Bitter Orange,
Grapefruit, Fennel

Alantolactone
$C_{12}H_{16}O_2$
Cistus, Hibiscus, Inula, Conyza

ζ–Ligustolide
$C_{12}H_{14}O_2$
Dill, Caraway

Psoralen
$C_{11}H_6O_3$
Bitter Orange, Bergamot

hol/acid reaction that creates an ester.

Lactones get their name from lactic acid $(C_3H_6O_3)$—the simplest of the hydroxy acids. (See Williams, pp. 71-72.) Lactic acid is an extremely common compound in nature. You will find it in molasses, apples and most fruits, tomato juice, beer, wine, and sour milk. It gets its name from "*lactis*" the Latin word for milk. Lactic acid is also present in most of our body organs. Lactic acid levels increase in our blood and muscles during vigorous exercise. However, except as a transient participant in the process of forming lactones, lactic acid is not found in essential oils.

The names of lactones are not as consistent and easy to recognize as in other classes of compounds. Properly named, they should end in –olide or –lactone, but more often they end with –ine, –ene, –in, –en, or –one. The -ine ending is misleading since it is normally reserved for peptides and amino acids which are all nitrogen-containing compounds not found in essential oils. The –ene ending is confusing in that it erroneously implies a terpene. The –one ending can also be confusing since this is customarily used to identify ketones. However, since lactones manifest some of the same properties as ketones, perhaps this is not altogether misleading. Like ketones, lactones are generally decongesting and expectorant. Sweet inule oil (*Inula graveolens*) and other oils containing lactones have been used to treat bronchial congestion.

Another difference in naming lactones (compared to naming other esters) is that most esters have double common names whereby the parent acid and parent alcohol can be identified. Not so with lactones. They are children of a single parent.

In the figure on the previous page there are eight examples of lactone molecules. The top two are actually phenolic lactones with a benzene ring (C_6H_6) and an attached hydroxyl radical (OH). They are well behaved phenolics however. Umbelliferone is used in many suntan lotions as a protector from sunburn.

Nepetalactone has a five-sided, homogeneous ring of carbons and is a sex pheromone of the female cat. It is the ingredient in catnip that felines of both sexes love so much. Because of this lactone, the oil of catnip is a sedative to mice, rats, cats (and people, too). Nepetalactone has also been found to be an effective deterrent against roaches and other insects. Actinidine and valerianine are lactones in valerian oil (*Valeriana officinalis*) which are also cat pheromones.

Bergaptene, alantolactone, ζ-ligustolide, and psoralen all have a five-sided, heterogeneous ring with four carbons and one oxygen. This pentagonal ring is a functional group called "furan." Compounds containing furan are called furanoids. Furanoids respond in a special way to sunlight. We will discuss them later in this chapter.

Lactones are often mild in aroma, but some have strong fragrances and fruity flavors. Such lactones are found in apricots, oranges, raspberries, peaches, and strawberries. Lactones are found in expressed oils (like citrus) and in absolutes (like jasmine)—usually in low concentrations of 1-3%. However, lactones exist in minor and trace quantities in a lot of oils.

Some large-molecular-weight lactones (like achillin or furanogermacrene) contain a sesqiterpene unit $(C_{15}H_{24})$ and may have special healing qualities. Ambrettolide, a large sesquiterpene lactone molecule with a strong musky odor, is found in hibiscus seed oil (Turn to page 1 to see a molecular diagram). While many lactones do not have strong odors, they do tend to have strong actions. Even a small percent of lactones in an essential oil can produce noticeable effects.

Dr. Penoel reports that lactones seem to possess antiseptic, antiparasitic, antitumoral, antispasmodic and antiinflammatory properties as well as being supportive of the liver and immune system.

Oils with traces of lactones include caraway, cassia, cinnamon, cistus, clove, clary sage, conyza, cumin, German chamomile, fennel, hibiscus, inule, juniper berry, lavandin, lavender, melissa, myrrh, onycha, peppermint, Roman chamomile, rosemary CT verbenon, spikenard, and yarrow. In most of these oils, the lactones include some coumarins, a special kind of lactone we will discuss next.

Coumarins

Oils containing the highest concentrations of coumarins include fleabane (8%) and bitter orange (6%). (See Tables 38 and 70.) Coumarins are a subgroup of lactones and are widely distributed in nature. They are lactones with a benzene ring. One of this group is actually called coumarin $(C_9H_6O_2)$. (See the figure two pages ahead.) It has the fragrance of newly mown hay. In fact, coumarin, dicoumarol, and other coumarins are exactly what you smell when you cut clover or alfalfa or when you mow your lawn. Cutting grass and harvesting green cover crops releases coumarins into the air. Coumarins are found in most green vegetables, like broccoli, spinach, cabbage, lettuce, collard greens, and string beans, contributing a flavor to vegetables we characterize as the "taste of green." Green vegetables are also rich sources of natural vitamin K which is a blood coagulant. Coumarins also provide the flavor and aroma to coconut.

The name, "coumarin" comes from the Caribbean word "coumarou" for the tonka tree (*Dipteryx odorata*). Tonka bean extracts were formerly used as flavoring agents. In 1954 the U.S. FDA prohibited coumarin as a flavoring in food because of animal studies indicating possible toxicities. However, these studies are now considered of questionable validity and coumarin continues to be used as a flavoring in Europe and Great Britain. In addition to tonka beans, the coumarin compound ($C_9H_6O_2$) and other natural coumarin derivatives have been found in sweet vernal grass (*Anthoxanthum odoratum*), sweet clover (*Melilotus albus*), and red clover (*Trifolium pratense*).

Coumarins, like most lactones, are powerful. Even when present in an oil in small amounts, they can have strong therapeutic actions. Coumarins are thought to be antispasmodic, as are many other esters. Coumarin containing oils, such as khella (*Ammi visnaga*), have been used for their bronchiodilating properties to treat asthma.

Compounds incorporating the coumarin molecule as part of its structure are called "coumarins." If you look back at the previous figure showing lactone molecules, you will see that all but nepetalactone, ζ-ligustolide, and alantolactone are coumarins. According to Franchomme and Penoel, coumarins manifest anticonvulsant, antispasmodic, antiviral, antibacterial, and antifungal properties. Bergaptene and psoralen are furanocoumarins, which we will discuss later in this chapter.

Coumarin, Coumadin and Warfarin Molecules Compared

Coumarin
$C_9H_6O_2$

Clary sage, Rosemary, Spikenard, Onycha,
Lavandin, Lavender, Cinnamon, Cassia, Tonka
Bean, Red Clover, Sweet Vernal Grass

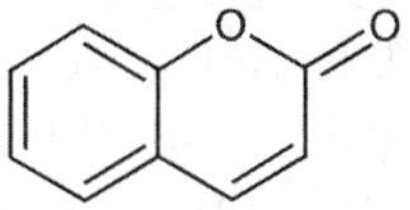

Warfarin
$C_{19}H_{16}O_4$

Anticoagulant and Rodenticide.
Causes rats to
hemorrhage to death internally

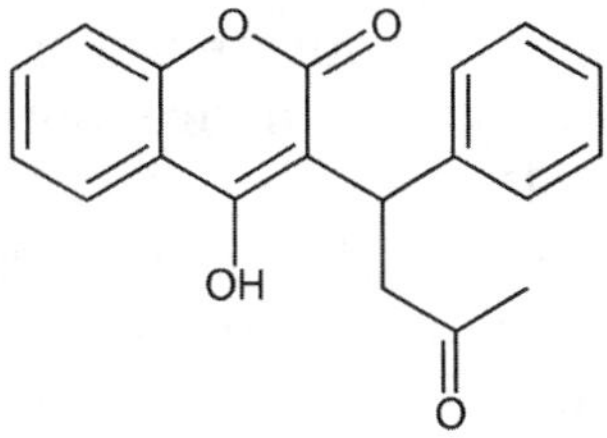

Coumadin®
$C_{19}H_{15}NaO_4$

Anticoagulant and Patented Drug
(Bristol-Myers-Squibb) A blood thinner
to prevent unwanted blood clots

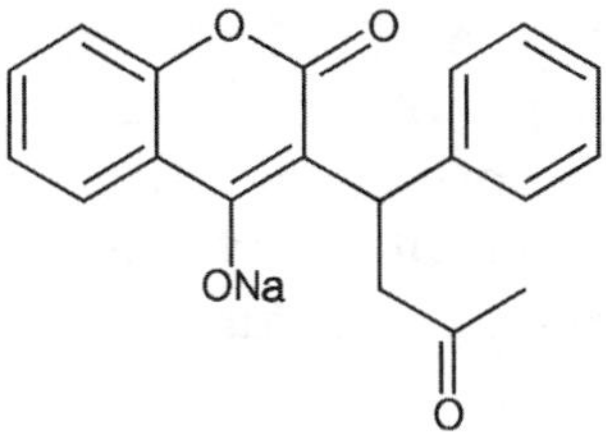

Coumarin vs. Coumadin®

There is some confusion and concern about coumarins and coumadins and their effects on human blood. The similarity of the two words causes many people to mistakenly think they are compounds with similar pharmaco-biological actions in our bodies. They are not similar. Here is why.

Coumadin® is a drug manufactured by Bristol-Myers-Squibb (BMS) for thinning the blood to prevent unwanted blood clots in blood vessels that can lead to strokes. Its formula is ($C_{19}H_{15}NaO_4$) while that of coumarin is ($C_9H_6O_2$). Coumarin is biosynthesized by plants in nature while Coumadin® is synthesized by technicians in laboratories. So the first thing is to realize is that one is natural, the other artificial, and that they have significantly different chemical formulas.

Structurally, you can see in the figure above that Coumadin® incorporates a coumarin molecule in its structure. Even so, the two molecules are quite different in overall shape, size, and biochemical properties. Warfarin ($C_{19}H_{16}O_4$) is another artificially manufactured drug containing a coumarin functional group. Warfarin is generic, meaning it is not patented or owned by anyone. Because warfarin and Coumadin® have a coumarin molecule (functional group) as part of their structure, they are both technically classified as "coumarins." But this does not mean they are similar in action. As we learned in Chapter Six, benzene (C_6H_6) by itself is a highly toxic ring compound, but as a functional group it is incorporated in every protein in our bodies as well as in the molecules of most foods we eat and essential oils that we apply without any of the toxicity of benzene. Coumadin® and warfarin are both blood anticoagulants. Coumarin is not.

According to Tisserand and Balacs (*Essential Oil Safety*), "Although coumarin derivatives are used as anticoagulant drugs (such as warfarin, dicoumarin, etc.) coumarin itself is not anticoagulant." They go on to say that coumarin is used in the treatment of lymphedema (swelling and puffiness of the lower limbs) as well as various cancers. Natural coumarin, as found in essential oils, is also reported to be a stimulant and supporter of the immune system.

While coumarin ($C_9H_6O_2$) resembles neither warfarin nor Coumadin®, the two latter compounds resemble each other so much, you have to look closely to see the difference. Coumadin® is actually a clever chemical modification of warfarin.

Warfarin's name has nothing to do with warfare. It was coined from "Wisconsin Alumni Research Foundation (WARF) plus the last four letters of coumarin." WARF was instrumental in developing warfarin as a rodenticide. Warfarin is a generic compound which could be used to thin blood and prevent blood clots like Coumadin®. However, since its formula is public property, anyone can make and sell warfarin. Drug companies like monopolies. Bristol-Myers-Squibb (BMS) figured out how to modify warfarin so that it was still an anticoagulant, but would be in a form they alone could own and distribute. They accomplished this by simply replacing one of the hydrogens in warfarin with a sodium atom (Na). (See the molecular models.) Thus, they created a patentable product for which they have a monopoly. Doctors prescribe Coumadin® millions of times a year, making a fortune for BMS.

Examples of Applied Chemistry

If you want to know how BMS scientists discovered that replacing an H atom with an Na atom would work, go back to Chapter Three and the Periodic Table. You may recall that any element in the same vertical column can replace any other element in that column in a compound. This is because all elements in the same vertical column have the same valence. Sodium (Na) is in the same vertical column as hydrogen (H) which makes this simple substitution chemically possible, turning warfarin into Coumadin®.

Other elements in the hydrogen column include lithium (Li), potassium (K), and rubidium (Rb) which may have also worked. What BMS chemists did was to take these elements and substitute them one by one in the various hydrogen locations of the warfarin molecule until, by trial and error, they found the one that worked best. It turned out to be a sodium atom (Na) at the location of the hydrogen (H) in the hydroxyl radical (OH) of the warfarin molecule. The generic name of Coumadin® is "sodium warfarin." Coumadin® is a brand name chosen for its marketing appeal that just happens to sound a lot like "coumarin." And therein lies the source of the confusion.

The point is this: the concerns over natural coumarins in essential oils being potential blood thinners that could exaggerate or interfere with Coumadin® drug therapy have no basis in scientific fact or medical experience. Coumarin is not an anticoagulant. Coumadin® is. As you can see at a glance, the molecular formulas and structures of the two are not at all alike, even though Coumadin® contains coumarin in its structure. This fact does not imply they have similar properties. Countless recipes call for flour and salt, but that does not make them all taste alike.

Vitamin K
$C_{11}H_{11}NO$

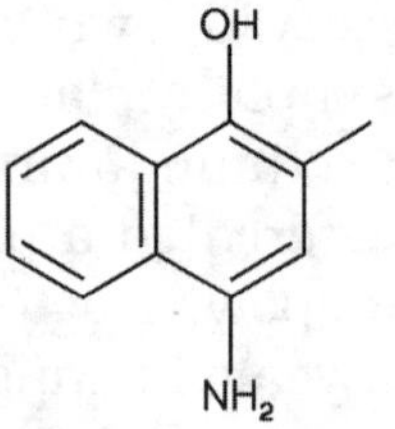

OH

NH$_2$

Compare with
Size and Shape
of Coumarin
(on p. 375)

There are a number of lactones in oils that incorporate a coumarin molecule and none of them are anticoagulants. Coumadin® is not synthetic coumarin, as the names suggest. The main similarity between the two is in the superficial similarity of their names, not their chemistry.

In fact, in size and shape, the molecular structure of coumarin is more like Vitamin K than it is like Coumadin®. (See the figure above) Vitamin K is a term for several related compounds that are natural blood coagulants found in green vegetables. Vitamin K is also manufactured by the friendly flora (bacteria, yeast, and fungi) that live in our bodies. Vitamin K is necessary to form blood clots to seal off wounds and prevent hemorrhage when we are cut. In the Danish and German languages it is called "koagulatingvitamin," which is where the "K" comes from. Although similar in structure, coumarin compounds in essential oils do not have the blood clotting properties of Vitamin K. Vitamin K is the antidote for warfarin or Coumadin® poisoning. Coumarins in oils are neither coagulants nor anticoagulants.

Coumarins in oils do not act alone. They act in concert with all of the other constituents. It has been suggested that if coumarins in oils do have any effect upon the blood, it would be as an adaptigen. That is, if the blood needs thinning, it would thin, if it needs thickening, it would thicken, but if the blood is just right, coumarin-containing oils would have no effect. The natural coumarins in essential oils would only act toward restoring a healthy balance, leading to neither unwanted clotting nor hazardous hemorrhaging and would have no effect if the blood is of normal viscosity.

Such is the nature of essential oils in that the same oil can regulate bodily functions in opposite directions, or not at all, depending on the need. This is called homeostatic intelligence—a sense of which way the body needs to be nudged to attain a healthy balance. Such intelligence, present in essential oils, is absent from pharmaceutical drugs which operate in one direction only whether the body needs it or not, leading to potentially dangerous bodily imbalances.

Heparin is another class of natural anticoagulants found in the lungs of cows, the intestines of pigs, and in many other places. Heparins are huge molecules consisting of a string of saccharides (sugars) and functional groups containing sulfur and nitrogen. Their molecular weights vary from 6,000 to 30,000 amu. However, natural heparin is not sold by drug companies. Aventis, Inc., markets a synthetic suite of heparin molecules called Lovenox® whose technical name is heparin sodium or enoxaparin sodium. Lovenox is also called "low weight heparin" since its molecular weights range from 2,000 to 8,000 amu—much lighter than natural heparin.

Lovenox® is used with the administration of certain anesthetics with surgical procedures to prevent unwanted blood clots. There are five pages of fine print in the *PDR* concerning the contraindications, warnings, precautions, and adverse reactions of Lovenox. Lovenox is another example of where a natural compound has been modified by making use of the Periodic Table to replace hydrogen atoms (H) with sodium atoms (Na) to create a synthetic drug with serious side effects, but one that is patentable and profitable.

Furanoids and Phototoxicity

Furanoids (or furans) are compounds containing a heterogeneous, five-sided ring called "furan" with the formula of C_4H_4O. (See the figure on the next page.) It can be either a stand–alone molecule or a functional group. The furanoid compounds of essential oils are usually lactones or coumarins whose names may start with furano- or furo-

The Furan Molecule
(or Functional Group)
C_4H_4O

or end with -furan, but not always. Names of furanoid compounds that are neither lactones nor coumarins may start with furfur- or fur-. There are several essential oils containing furans, mostly expressed oils of certain citrus fruits. They are not found in distilled citrus oils. (See Chapter Two for definitions of "expressed" oils versus "distilled" oils.)

Oils with the highest concentrations of furanoids include myrrh (23%), fleabane (8%), and peppermint (5%) which are not phototoxic, as well as bitter orange (4%), bergamot (3%), and lemon (2%) which are phototoxic. (See Tables 43 & 70, pp. 567 & 592.)

A class of furanoids in oils are furanocoumarins whose molecules each have three rings—the two six-sided rings of coumarin plus the five-sided ring of furan. Bergaptene and psoralen are furanocoumarins. Alantolactone and ζ-ligustolide are furanoid lactones, but are not coumarins. Furfural, in myrtle oil, is a furanoaldehyde while menthofuran, in peppermint oil, is a furanoxide.

The five-sided furan ring can make a compound phototoxic if there are no compounds in the oil to quench it. The furan pentagon acts like a molecular prism, or magnifying glass, that favors the frequencies and wavelengths of ultraviolet (UV) light. In other words, the dimensional lengths of a furan ring can resonate with the wavelengths of UV light and amplify that portion of the spectrum. What that means is that you apply oils with furanoid compounds to your skin and then go out into sunlight or lie in a tanning booth, it is possible that you could experience severe sunburn, dermal discoloration, and other skin disorders—some permanent. Therefore, it is important to know what oils contain furanoids, especially furanocoumarins.

Oils containing photoactive furanoid compounds suffi-cient to cause concern about their phototoxicity are listed below. Some authorities would also include fennel (*Foeniculum vulgare*), anise (*Pimpinella anisum*), and cumin (*Cuminum cyminum*) on this list. Notice that the list does not include all of the citrus oils, only some of them. According to Tisserand and Balacs (*Essential Oil Safety*), the expressed oils of Mandarin (*Citrus reticulata*), Sweet Orange (*Citrus sinensis*), Tangelo (*Citrus x hybrida*), and Tangerine (*Citrus nobilis*) are not phototoxic. Neither are the distilled oils of lemon, lime, and grapefruit, even though their expressed oils are. However, distilled citrus oils are seldom used in aromatherapy since their aromas are considerably reduced by distillation. Distilled citrus oils are mostly used for flavorings. Neroli absolute (*Citrus aurantium*), extracted from bitter orange blossoms, is also non-phototoxic, containing not even a trace of any lactone, coumarin, or furanoid.

Essential Oils Considered Phototoxic

Angelica	(*Angelica archangelica*)
Bergamot	(*Citrus bergamia*)
Bitter Orange	(*Citrus aurantium*) rind
Grapefruit	(*Citrus paradisi*)
Lemon	(*Citrus limon*)
Lime	(*Citrus aurantifolia*)
Petitgrain	(*Citrus aurantium*) leaves
Rue	(*Ruta graveolens*)

The Mystery of Myrrh

Myrrh (*Commiphora myrrha*) is a puzzle. It contains at least ten types of furanoid compounds (20-27%), more than any other oil—yet it is not phototoxic. Many ancient Egyptians, who lived under the intense tropical desert sun, applied myrrh oil on their skin daily without sunburn reactions. In fact, the cones seen on the heads of figures in Egyptian heiroglyphics were fat saturated with myrrh allowed to melt slowly and run down over their bodies as a protection from the sun and as a repellent to biting insects, as well.

Queen Esther of the *Old Testament* (Esther 2:12) was massaged daily with liquid myrrh for six months prior to her marriage to the king and apparently suffered no ill skin effects from sunlight. In fact, myrrh seems to act more like a sunscreen, protecting the skin from ultraviolet light instead of increasing its sensitivity to burn. Yet it contains major quantities of furanoids.

Evidently, there are compounds in myrrh (perhaps the sesquiterpenes) that mitigate or quench the solar amplifying properties of the furans. In fact, the quenchers in myrrh cause the furanoids to resonate in such a way as to dissipate UV energy in harmless forms (like heat), thus offering sunscreen protection—the opposite of phototoxicity.

In terms of physics, furanoids can resonate with UV light in two opposing ways, depending on their configuration: One reinforces the UV radiation resulting in wave magnification while the other results in destructive interference with the UV radiation resulting in wave cancellation.

Here again, we have an example of how compounds change their behavior according to their company—hazardous and toxic in one setting yet safe and therapeutic in another. (See pp. 23-24 for more on myrrh.)

When is One Safe from Phototoxicity?

Phototoxic oils pose problems only if applied to the skin followed by exposure to a source of ultraviolet light. This is true even when the essential oil is diluted in a neutral carrier oil. There is no risk of phototoxic reactions unless oils have been applied directly to the skin.

Using phototoxic oils for flavorings in food and drink poses no hazard. It is only on the skin that there is a problem. So don't worry if you like a few drops of bergamot or orange in your drinking water while you sunbathe. Just keep it off of your exposed skin.

Most authorities recommend waiting twelve hours following an application of phototoxic oils to the skin before exposure to sunlight or the UV radiation of a tanning booth. This would be true even if one tried to wash them off since they would have already penetrated deep into the skin, beyond the touch of soap and water. Applying oils with furanocoumarins after sundown, before going to bed, poses no problems then or the next day, provided one is not retiring to a tanning bed that evening.

It is wrong to think that the phototoxic effects of an applied oil diminish immediately with time following their application. Experiments with bergamot have shown that one's phototoxic response can actually be worse an hour or two after the oil has been applied then if you were to be exposed to sunlight immediately after the application.

One can go out into sunlight after applying phototoxic oils if the parts of the body receiving the oils are well covered with clothing. That would be sufficient protection.

People with fair skins are more susceptible to phototoxic reactions than those of color. In fact, experiments have shown that with a person of brown or black skin it takes up to seven times more oil with furanocoumarins to elicit a phototoxic response than with a Caucasian. A suntan gives a white person some increased protection.

Bergamot can be purchased "FCF," which means "furanocoumarin free." What they do is to remove the bergaptene. This is sometimes called "deterpenizing" the oil, even though bergapten is not a terpene. It just has a name that makes it sound like a terpene. FCF bergamot is not phototoxic. It can be safely applied in sunlight. However, you want to be sure you can trust the label and that the oil is truly furanocoumarin free. Aromatherapists generally prefer unrefined bergamot containing bergapten because the fragrance of deterpenized bergamot is not as appealing. Its therapeutic actions are also altered and diminished by removal of some of its natural compounds.

The table of Essential Oils Considered Phototoxic is a list of single oils. If any of these are included in a blend of oils, the blends will also be phototoxic. Popular commercial blends containing phototoxic components (usually citrus) include Gentle Baby®, Joy®, White Angelica®, Citrus Fresh®, Thieves®, RC®, and many others. Read the labels.

The Chemistry of Essential Oils Made Simple

This chapter abundantly illustrates what we stated near the beginning of this book in Chapter Three, which is restated in the box that follows:

> The chemistry of essential oils consists of simple hydrocarbons, oxygenated hydrocarbons, and their isomers.

This statement refers specifically to the following:

• Hydrocarbons (two types): Terpenes and Alkanes

• Oxygenated Hydrocarbons (eleven types): Phenols, Alcohols, Ethers, Aldehydes, Ketones, Carboxylic Acids, Esters, Oxides, Lactones, Coumarins, and Furanoids

• And Isomers Without End . . . Millions and Millions

In a sentence, that is the chemistry of essential oils made simple. In the process of reading this far, we hope you have also seen the handiwork and love of God in the molecules of therapeutically active oils.

Key Points of Chapter Ten

1. This book has covered the following classes and subclasses of compounds: 1. Alkanes, 2. Phenols, 3. Terpenes—(Monoterpenes, Sesquiterpenes, Diterpenes, Triterpenes, Tetraterpenes), 4. Alcohols, 5. Ethers, 6. Aldehydes, 7. Ketones, 8. Carboxylic Acids, 9. Esters, 10. Oxides, and 11. Lactones—(Coumarins and Furanoids), as well as brief mention of thiols, sulphides, pyrroles, and diazines (in Chapter Four).

2. Specific compounds behave differently depending on the other compounds in the oil mix. The same compound won't necessarily act the same in one oil as in another.

3. When some compounds in an oil influence others to perform gently and safely, when in isolation they would be harsh and unsafe, this is called "quenching" by aromatherapists. In chemistry it would be called a form of "buffering."

4. You cannot determine the behavior of an oil by analyzing its components isolated from the oil. Oils can only be studied as a whole. Essential oils are more than the sum of their parts.

5. Alcohols and ethers, aldehydes and ketones, carboxylic acids and esters, are chemically related pairs of classes of essential oil compounds.

6. Alcohol names end in –ol and are defined as a hydrocarbon group with an OH radical attached.

7. Ether names end in –ole, –cin, or –ether and are defined as an oxygen atom with two hydrocarbon groups, one on each side.

8. Aldehyde names end in –al or –aldehyde and are defined as a carbonyl group (C=O) with a hydrocarbon group (R) on one side and a hydrogen atom on the other.

9. Ketone names end in –one and are defined as a carbonyl group (C=O) with two hydrocarbon groups R & R'), one on either side.

10. Carboxylic Acid names end in "acid." They are defined as a carbonyl group (C=O) with a hydrocarbon on one side and an OH on the other.

11. Esters are the product of a chemical reaction between an alcohol and an acid. Esters have double names. The first name identifies its parent alcohol and ends in -yl. The second name ends in –ate and identifies its parent acid.

12. Esters are defined as a carbonyl group (C=O) with a hydrocarbon (R) on one side and an oxygen atom (O) on the other to which is attached another hydrocarbon (R').

13. pH means "potential Hydrogen," which refers to the availability of hydrogen ions H+ in a water solution. H+ ions are protons, which are very aggressive and are what gives acids their bite.

14. The pH scale is a logarithmic scale that assigns numbers to levels of free H+ ions in a solution. A pH of 7.0 means there are the same number of H+ ions as OH– ions, which exactly cancel each other. Pure water has a pH of 7.0, meaning that 1/10,000,000% of the water molecules are dissociated into H+ and OH– ions. The number 7.0 refers to the number of zeros in this fraction of a percent.

15. A pH level less than 7.0 means there are more H+ ions than there are OH– ions, which is an acidic solution. A pH level more than 7.0 means there are more OH- ions than H+ ions and the solution is basic or alkaline.

16. The pH scale can be thought of as running from 0 to 14 where the values correspond to the number of zeros in the fractional percent that expresses the H+ concentration.

17. To be healthy is to have a blood pH from 7.35–7.45, which is on the alkaline side. When our bodies become less alkaline (acid) and pH falls, we become prone to getting sick.

18. Acids destroy oils. An acid person requires more oils to get the same results as a healthy alkaline person. Inhaling, ingesting, and applying oils to the surface of the body raises pH and helps maintain a healthy alkaline balance.

19. Oxides are created in oils when other compounds in the oils are oxidized. Oxide names consist of the name of the parent compound followed by "oxide."

20. There are many types of oxygenated hydrocarbons in essential oils, but the oxygen in an oxide is attached, not to one carbon, but to two.

21. The most popular oxide is 1,8 cineole which is contained in dozens of oils, some of which are over 50% 1,8 cineole.

22. Lactones are esters where the single-bonded oxygen is part of a heterogeneous ring. Lactones are formed by the reaction of a hydroxyl acid molecule with itself, which is acid on one end and alcoholic on the other.

23. Lactone names can end in –one, –ine, –in, –en, or –ene. If named properly, they would all end in either –lactone or –olide, but most don't.

24. Coumarins are lactones that have a benzene ring as part of their structure.

25. Coumarins in essential oils are neither coagulants nor anticoagulants and do not act independently of the other compounds in the oil. With respect to blood thinning, seem to act as hemostats or adaptigens with the homeostatic intelligence to regulate blood viscosity toward to a healthy balance, having no effect when the blood is normal.

26. Furanoids are compounds with a furan functional group—a five-sided heterogeneous carbon ring with an O atom. Their names may begin with furano-, furo-, furfur-, or fur- or may end with -furan," but not always. The most common furanoids in essential oils are furanocoumarins—i.e. coumarins with a furanic functional group.

27. Oils containing furanoid compounds can be phototoxic unless the oil contains other compounds to quench their ability to magnify UV light.

28. The most common phototoxic oils are expressed citrus oils of bergamot, bitter orange, grapefruit, lemon, and lime. The distilled oils of these same sources are not phototoxic.

29. The expressed oils of some other citrus fruits, such as mandarin, sweet orange, tangelo, and tangerine, are not phototoxic.

30. Alphabetical listings of hundreds of compounds and the oils that contain them are given in Tables 69 and 70 in Part Two of this book.

31. This chapter abundantly illustrates a statement we have stated several times throughout this book:

> "The chemistry of essential oils consists of simple hydrocarbons, oxygenated hydrocarbons, and their isomers."

♥ CHAPTER ELEVEN
ESSENTIAL OILS
VERSUS DRUGS

In this chapter we will review what is in the literature, mention possible interactions between pharmaceuticals and essential oils, discuss the effects of oils with homeopathic remedies, how oils can take the place of some drugs without undesirable side effects, how some oils can imitate or stimulate hormones, how prescription drugs work, how drug companies manipulate molecules for profit, and why oils heal and drugs don't.

Oil/Drug Interactions

A frequently asked question concerning the therapeutic use of essential oils is whether they might react with a prescription drug or other allopathic medication. The question is usually framed as "Can a person take prescription drugs and use essential oils at the same time without ill effect?" or "Will oils cancel the benefits of drugs (or vice versa)?" or "Could there be a dangerous interaction between a drug and an essential oil?"

Hazardous interactions between different essential oils applied together are unheard of. By contrast, interactions between different prescription drugs taken together are very likely to result in an unpleasant, if not dangerous, outcome. In fact, one in seven patients in a hospital will suffer an adverse drug interaction while there, sometimes fatal. When a pharmaceutical interaction occurs, the solution most often prescribed to control the situation and save the patient is another drug. Often the additional drug only makes matters worse. Doctors have such faith in their pharmacological training they will usually continue to prescribe drugs even when, before their very eyes, they can see that they aren't working.

As mentioned in Chapter Three, medical doctors are conditioned to believe the body functions almost entirely by chemistry. Hence, they believe that virtually any problem, condition, or sickness manifested in the body has a chemical solution. Even emotional, psychological, and spiritual problems are treated by allopathic doctors as if they are of chemical origin and have a chemical solution. That is why their first mode of attack is almost always a pharmaceutical one. As for subtle electricities, energies, vibrations, consciousness, prayer, and the will of the patient—such concepts are alien to allopathic education and practice. It is a rare physician that even acknowledges nutrition as important and if they do, they had to acquire their appreciation and knowledge on their own, outside of medical school.

What the Authorities Say?

A medical definition of an interacting drug combination is "a clinically significant change in the pharmacologic response to a drug, documented in humans, that is more or less than it would have been had that drug been used alone." In other words, when a drug's usual effects upon a patient are reduced, increased, or altered when taken with another drug, that is a drug interaction. Some interactions are okay. Some even desirable. But many are adverse. Some can be fatal.

The problem is that drug interactions are mostly unpredictable, there being only limited data or information available by which physicians can know in advance whether or not there will be a problem. The research is not there to any great extent because to test every drug in combination with every other drug to see what interactions are possible is an impossible task since such combinations and permutations would number in the trillions. Hence, there is little interest and little funding for such research, except for the studies drug companies feel they must do to protect themselves from lawsuits for negligence.

This brings us to the topic of interest in this chapter, viz. possible interactions between allopathic drugs and essential oils. In searching for answers to this, I consulted the following twenty-nine references:

1. **Advanced Aromatherapy: Science of Essential Oil Therapy**
   by Kurt Schnaubelt

2. **Aromatherapy for Health Professionals**
   by Shirley and Len Price

3. **The Aromatherapy Practitioner Reference Manual**
   by Sylla Sheppard-Hanger

4. **Aromatherapy Scent and Psyche**
   by Peter and Kate Damian

5. **Chemistry of Essential Oils: Introduction for Aromatherapists, Beauticians, Retailers, & Students.**
   by David G. Williams

6. **Clinical Aromatherapy: Essential Oils in Practice**
   by Jane Buckle

7. **Clinical Aromatherapy for Pregnancy and Childbirth**
   by Denise Tiran

8. **Complete Book of Essential Oils & Aromatherapy**
   by Valerie Ann Worwood

9. **Essential Chemistry for Safe Aromatherapy**
   by Sue Clarke

10. **Essential Oil Safety**
    by Robert Tisserand and Tony Balacs

11. **Essential Oils Desk Reference**
    edited by Brian Manwaring

12. **Essential Oils Integrative Medical Guide**
    by D. Gary Young

13. **Freedom Through Health**
    by Terry Shepherd Friedmann

14. **Illustrated Encyclopedia of Essential Oils**
    by Julie Lawless

15. **Integrated Aromatic Medicine 1998**
    English version edited by Brian Manwaring

16. **Integrated Aromatic Medicine 2000**
    English version edited by Brian Manwaring

17. **Integrated Aromatic Medicine 2001**
    English version edited by Brian Manwaring

18. **L'Aromatherapie Exactement**
    by Pierre Franchomme and Daniel Penoel

In nineteen of these twenty-nine references, I could find no information on drug/oil interactions whatsoever. The ones apparently devoid of such information are as follows (identified by number): 1, 3, 5, 9, 11, 12, 13, 14, 15, 16, 17, 19, 20, 21, 22, 23, 25, and 29. Three of the 29 books are authored by two medical doctors—Terry Friedmann, MD (13) and Daniel Penoel, MD (18 and 21). Friedmann and Penoel are probably the world's leading medical authorities on therapeutic applications of essential oils alive today. If drug/oil interactions were a problem, why wouldn't they mention it? Also, references 15, 16, and 17 contain more than fifty technical articles on essential oils by pharmacists, biologists, biochemists, and more than a dozen medical doctors—none of which mention any adverse drug/oil interactions.

Worwood (8) and Higley (28) have information on using essential oils to overcome drug addictions and dealing with withdrawal symptoms. These oils include basil, bergamot, birch, eucalyptus (*globulus*), fennel, grapefruit, lavender, marjoram, nutmeg, orange, parsley, peppermint, Roman chamomile, rose, sandalwood, and wintergreen.

Higley (28) also lists oils that can help repair brain damage caused by antidepressant drugs. These include elemi, frankincense, lavender, onycha, and rose, as well as several trademarked blends such as Brain Power®, Clarity®, Joy®, and Valor®.

Damian (4) and Schnaubelt (19) have excellent discussions of how pharmaceuticals work versus oils, but do not discuss interactions between the two.

The only references I could find that attempt to deal with the issue of essential oil/drug interactions are Buckle (6), Price (2), Tiran (7), Tisserand (10), Valnet (27), and the *PDR for Nutritional Supplements* (24).

In the case of the PDRs, the famous one on pharmaceutical drugs (25), has thousands of pages and millions of words on drugs and their descriptions, indications, contraindications, adverse reactions, and warnings, including information on drug/drug interactions, but there is nothing in that book about essential oils and how they might interact with drugs.

The *PDR for Herbal Medicine* (23), specifically written for medical doctors who prescribe drugs, contains information on some 200 essential oils, but no data on possible interactions with pharmaceutical drugs.

The *PDR for Nutritional Supplements* (24) contains quite a bit of information on possible interactions between various nutritional oils and other herbs and supplements, but contains no information on essential oils and drugs. The oils mentioned with their possible interactions include borage, evening primrose, fish, flaxseed, perilla, hempseed, vitamin E, and mineral oils—all of which are fatty oils, not essential. In most cases, the potential interaction involved blood thinning potential and possible hemorrhage when these oils were used with aspirin, warfarin, heparin, garlic oil, and other anticoagulating substances. The interactions mentioned were postulated as theories, as yet unsubstantiated by actual data on humans.

In the case of Buckle (6), Tiran (7), and Tisserand-Balacs (10), they express many concerns and cite numerous animal studies, some with whole essential oils and some with isolated components of oils. In the whole oil studies, it was not specified if these were therapeutic grade oils or if they were adulterated, modified, or synthetic oils intended for flavors and perfumes. Hence, any interactions observed in these studies could as well be due to the adulterants in the oils as to their natural constituents, which Buckle acknowledges.

All of these authors (Buckle, Tiran, Tisserand, and Balacs) are of the British school of aromatherapy, which tends to present essential oils as potentially hazardous and not to be used undiluted (neat) on the skin or taken orally unless prescribed by a medical doctor or other suitably trained professional. They all concede that adverse drug reactions with oils are extremely unlikely (or nonexistent) when inhaled or applied transcutaneously in massage. Their serious concerns are expressed only for oral administrations of essential oils. While they speculate on various theoretical risks in great biochemical detail, they do not present a single study using a whole therapeutic grade oil on a human being that would substantiate their concerns. Their point of view is to err on the side of being conservative, cautioning against the use of certain oils with certain types of drugs. They provide no scientific evidence to justify their conservative course and candidly admit that definitive data do not exist.

Unfortunately, to follow their advice would be to deny many benefits of many oils to many people. Buckle acknowledges that the French attitude toward essential oils, including possible drug interactions, is more liberal and less restricted than the British viewpoint, and allows that there is merit in both ways of thinking.

Oils and Allergic Sensitizations

British authors often talk about "sensitizations to essential oils," as if they could be potential allergens causing allergies. They are confused. It is impossible for an essential oil to cause an allergy. Essential oils can cause nonallergenic detoxification reactions, which are often confused with allergies. But they cannot sensitize and cause allergies. (See Chapter Twelve for a thorough discussion of these points.)

A common discussion seen in British books is that one can determine allergic sensitizations to oils by a patch test. That is where you apply an oil to the skin, cover it with a bandage, and wait 24 hours to see if there is a reaction on the skin in the form of a rash or other dermal malmanifestation. If a reaction occurs, they consider that proof of sensitization (i.e. an allergic reaction).

Buckle (6), a practicing nurse, states on page 86, "I have found that patients taking several medications at the same time are more likely to be sensitive to essential oils than patients who are not taking several medications." She seems to be suggesting that one's proness to allergic reactions to oils is increased as one takes larger numbers of prescriptions.

What is actually happening here is a detox reaction. Pharmaceuticals are toxins to the body. Essential oils are cleansers of foreign substances. They can take substances that are not necessarily soluble in water and make them soluble, like soap does to grease, thus making it possible for them to be flushed out via the blood and lymph and, eventually, through the bowels, kidneys, and sweat glands.

Essential oils are one way to cleanse the body from a buildup of medications. The more medications one takes, the greater the buildup and the more likely oils will bring them to the surface in a reaction. This is the phenomenon that Nurse Buckle has observed, which she seems to interpret as an allergy.

Buckle's observation is a good one. It suggests that essential oils do react with drugs in some ways, helping to metabolize them out of the system, which is good. Chances are, the metabolism of the drugs via the agency of the oils takes place after the drugs have done their work and have had their desired effects. Hence, the oils would not be interfering with the drug's intended actions, but are only facilitating and accelerating the necessary clean up after their work is done.

What Do Aromatherapy Doctors Say?

One resource that actually presents observations on humans of an interaction between drugs and oils is the book by Jean Valnet, MD (27). On page 39 he mentions that "some essences have been found to complement the action of antibiotics." He gives niaouli (*Melaleuca quinquenervia*) as an example of an oil that "will increase the activity of streptomycin and penicillin." Valnet also mentions that some oils containing aldehydes and ketones can "inactivate antibiotics." Other than these examples, Valnet does not discuss any other essential oil/drug interactions.

The fact that Valnet only briefly mentions them while Penoel and Friedmann, two other medical doctors, do not mention them at all in their books, suggests that adverse interactions between drugs and oils is not a serious problem—hardly worth mentioning.

Essential oils as agents for transdermal transfer of drugs is mentioned in several of the references. Pharmaceutical patches for nicotine addiction or hormone replacement therapy (HRT) have been shown to be more effectively absorbed when essential oils are applied to the skin where the patches are applied. This would be a form of drug-oil interaction that is considered useful and beneficial in the minds of allopaths.

We also discussed in Chapter Ten how coumarin compounds in essential oils are confused with Coumadin®, a synthetic anticoagulant drug whose generic name is sodium warfarin. Many practicing aromatherapists have thought that oils containing coumarins could be contraindicated when a person is taking anticoagulant drugs on the theory that coumarins are also anticoagulants and might cause too much thinning of the blood that could result in hemorrhages. However, coumarins in essential oils are not anticoagulants and pose no such hazards.

Wintergreen and birch oils might pose a risk of excessive blood thinning in combination with anticoagulant drugs, since they are both mainly composed of methyl salicylate, which has aspirin-like properties. However, such an occurrence would only be possible with large oral doses of these oils. They pose no such hazards when inhaled or applied to the skin.

To conclude our discussion on possible adverse interactions between essential oils and pharmaceutical medicines, we quote from page 82 in Price (2):

> "Essential oils are composed of chemicals which are known to be active, gain access to cells by virtue of being fat soluble, and are metabolized by the body. It has been found by experience that some oils are relaxing, some sedative, some sharpen the memory, some promote the circulation, and so on. Therefore it may be assumed that, as active agents, they may react with other drugs present in the body. However, there has been no evidence so far which would imply any adverse significant reaction between essential oils and allopathic drugs, and they have been used together successfully in hospitals."

While there is scientific evidence that oils can and do sometimes interact with drugs, modifying their effects, there are no human studies with whole therapeutic grade oils that have ever demonstrated a negative reaction that should be cause for concern. These are the facts.

Oils and Homeopathy

Homeopathy is based on the principle of "like cures like." The idea is that a substance that can cause a healthy person to manifest symptoms of a particular disease can cure a sick person actually suffering from that disease. Homeopathic remedies take such substances and dilute them in a special way so that the remaining solution (usually water) contains not even one molecule of the substance, but only the "vibrational essence." Such an idea is incomprehensible to an allopathically trained physician schooled in classical chemistry. Nevertheless, success stories of homeopathic cures abound. Many credible healers employ homeopathic remedies and thousands swear by their efficacy. Many, finding no cure in allopathy, find healing in homeopathy.

The question arises as to whether or not homeopathic remedies and essential oils might contradict and interact with one another in undesirable ways. Since it is generally agreed that stimulating substances such as coffee will negate a homeopathic remedy, it is reasonable to wonder if some therapeutically active oils might do the same.

Homeopaths, themselves, cover the spectrum of opinions on this. Some prohibit the simultaneous use of essential oils altogether while others use both modalities together with little reservation. Terry Friedmann, MD, has applied homeopathic and essential oil therapies together for years in his practice and does not mention any antagonism between the two modalities in his book (13).

Since essential oils follow one's intent, perhaps the different experiences of different homeopaths is a reflection of their attitudes towards the oils. If they believe the two types of remedies will work together in mutual support, that is what they observe in their practice. If they believe essential oils will negate homeopathic remedies, then that is what they find in their practice. Their attitudes become self-fulfilling prophecies through the responsiveness of the oils. (See *Quantum Physics, Essential Oils, & the Mind-Body Connection* by Stewart listed in the bibliography.)

We will not resolve the controversy in this book since the range of opinions of practicing homeopaths extends from total prohibition to unreserved use. That is the fact of the matter. There may be some ground for compromise, however. Many homeopathic practitioners do agree that peppermint oil (*Mentha piperita*) should be avoided, and possibly eucalyptus (*Eucalyptus globulus*) and camphor (*Laurus camphora*) as well. Others say that floral oils such as rose (*Rosa damascena*), lavender (*Lavandula angustifolia*), geranium (*Pelargonium graveolens*), and the chamomiles (*Chamaemelum nobile* and *Matricaria recutita*) are okay, as are the absolutes of neroli (*Citrus aurantium*) and jasmine (*Jasminum officinale*).

If this is a personal decision you need to make as to

whether to use both homeopathy and aromatherapy concurrently or separately, you can always find a definitive answer for yourself in any given instance. Simply pray about it and ask God, the master and author of both healing modalities. He will answer and guide you. There may not be a general answer applicable in all situations, but there is always a specific answer applicable for the here and now, which is all you need. Such answers are not available through secular science. They are available only by your receptivity to and attunement with God.

When you are acutely sick and suffering and no health care provider seems to have an answer to your particular malady, you can't wait for science to find a solution. But God is always available and he always has an answer if we are ready to receive it and surrender to it.

Big Consequences from Small Things

We have seen in Chapter Seven on Biochemistry how minor differences in an oil molecule, even between isomers of the same formula, can make profound differences in how we perceive and respond to an oil. To illustrate this point further, let's consider a class of natural human ligands known as steroids.

Steroids are a type of hormone made by the human body that are all derived from cholesterol, as shown in the figure on the next page. Cholesterol is an integral part of every living cell and is the precursor for the synthesis of our essential steroids. All steroids are built on a set of four rings, three hexagons (six-sided) and one pentagon (five-sided) as seen in the pictures on pages 399 and 401.

As you can see in the figure on the next page, there is not much difference between these three molecules. Cholesterol is the largest with a molecular weight of 386 amu. Pregnenolone and progesterone weigh 316 and 314 amu respectively. These are all larger than most aromatic oil molecules whose weights usually fall between 50 and 250 amu. The weights of steroids fall between that of a diterpene ($C_{20}H_{32}$ M.W. = 272) and a triterpene ($C_{30}H_{48}$ M.W. = 408). They are very close to the weights and sizes

Cholesterol: The Mother of Steroids

Cholesterol
$C_{27}H_{46}O$

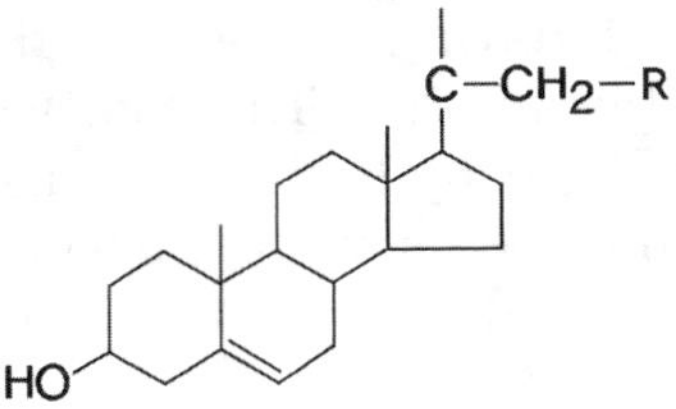

$R = C_5H_{11}$
(A pentyl radical)

Pregnenolone
$C_{21}H_{32}O_2$

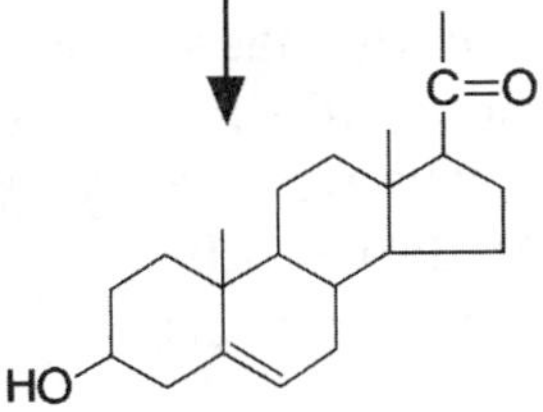

DHEA
and other
Steroids

Progesterone
$C_{21}H_{30}O_2$

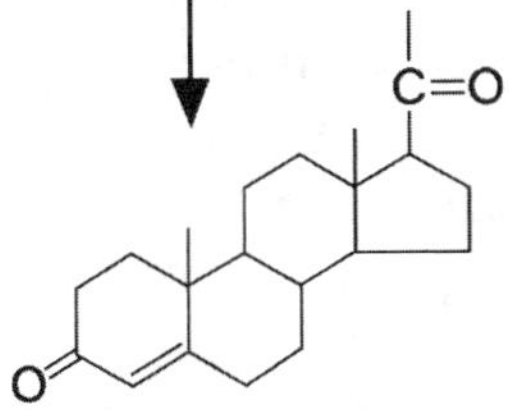

Various
Androgens &
Estrogens

Cortisol, Cortisone,
and other Steroids

of some diterpene alcohols and ketones ($C_{20}H_{32}O_2$ M.W. = 304) found in oils.

As classes of compounds, steroids are either alcohols (having one or more OH radicals attached and names ending in -ol) or ketones (having one or more double bonded O atoms attached and names ending in -one). Thus, cholesterol is an alcohol while progesterone is a double ketone with two double-bonded O atoms. Pregnenolone has both an OH and a double-bonded O, so it is actually a ketone–

alcohol, but its name is that of a ketone.

Notice in the figure on the next page that the -diols are all double alcohols having two OH radicals while the -diones are all double ketones. There is even one triple alcohol, estriol, with three hydroxyl radicals. The little lines extending up from the tops of the molecules have invisible methyl radicals (CH_3) at their ends. We call these "methyl spikes."

Steroids are essential to living and do many things for us—including control of body mass. This is why some body builders use them to stimulate muscle growth. However, what athletes and weight lifters use are synthetic steroids, which have potentially dangerous side effects, some of which can even result in death. The steroids our bodies produce pose no such hazards.

Neither pregnenolone nor progesterone produce any sexual characteristics in our bodies. They are sexually neutral. They are equally important in both men and women. However, the hormones that make us male or female are created from these two. Our sexual hormones are shown on the next page where the arrows on the left are coming from pregnenolone (upper left arrow) and progesterone (lower left arrow). There are four male hormones and three female hormones. Male hormones (androgens) range from 287–291 amu while female hormones (estrogens) are slightly lighter, ranging from 270–288 amu. This is because the male steroid molecules each have 19 carbons while the female steroids each have only 18.

Men and women both need all seven of these hormones. Whether a person manifests male or female characteristics depends on the balance. Men are predominantly androgenic in hormonal balance while women are mostly estrogenic. When these get out of balance, men can become effeminate and women can become masculine.

What I want you to notice is that there is not much difference between male and female hormones. In fact, the estrogens are actually made of slightly altered androgens. For example, compare androstenediol (upper right corner) with estradiol below. Change a couple of double bonds and

The Difference Between Man and Woman
(Just a Few Atoms in the Right Places)

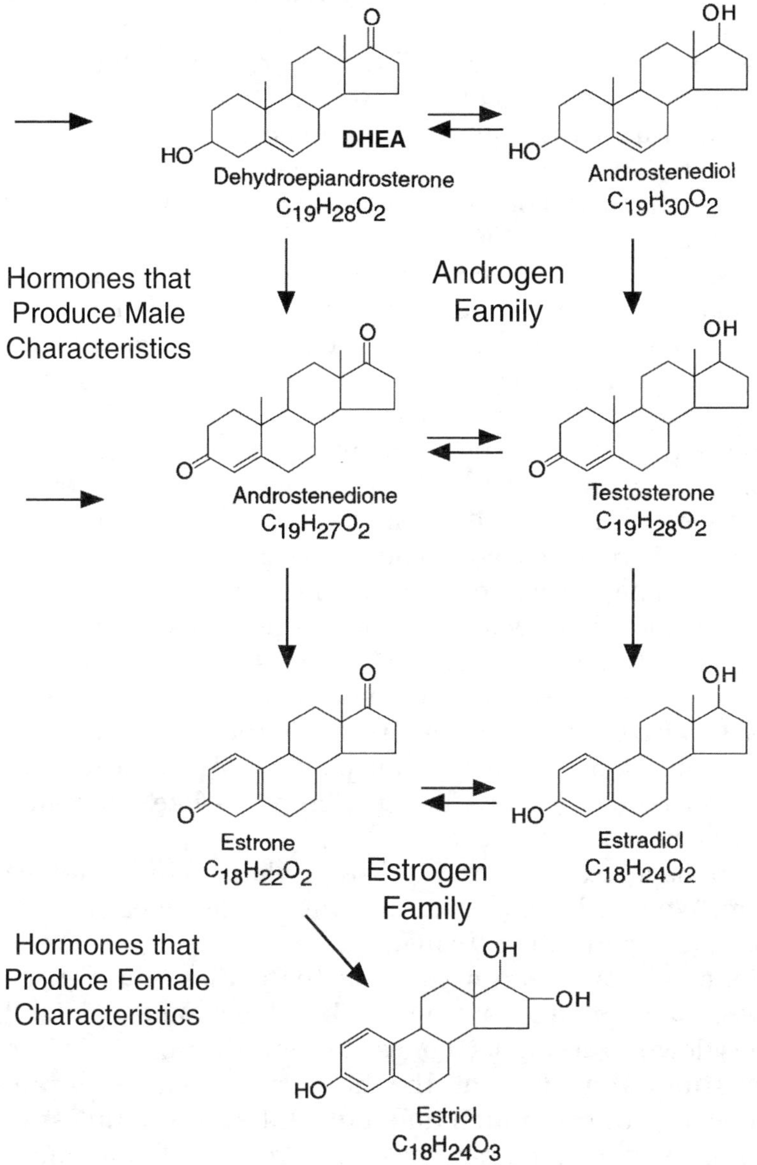

DHEA
Dehydroepiandrosterone
$C_{19}H_{28}O_2$

Androstenediol
$C_{19}H_{30}O_2$

Hormones that
Produce Male
Characteristics

Androgen
Family

Androstenedione
$C_{19}H_{27}O_2$

Testosterone
$C_{19}H_{28}O_2$

Estrone
$C_{18}H_{22}O_2$

Estrogen
Family

Estradiol
$C_{18}H_{24}O_2$

Hormones that
Produce Female
Characteristics

Estriol
$C_{18}H_{24}O_3$

remove one methyl spike and you can make an androgenic diol into an estrogenic diol.

Compare androstenedione (left middle) with estrone (directly below) and again, simply rearrange a few double bonds, remove a methyl spike and you make a male hormone into female. In fact, all of the androgens have two methyl spikes while all of the estrogens have only one. The removal of a methyl spike from a male steriod to make a female steroid is analogous to the removal of Adam's rib. "The rib that the Lord God had taken from the man he made into a woman." (Genesis 2:22) The point is that a small change in a molecule, from an androgen to an estrogen, makes a profound difference in the manifested results.

Androgens cause men to have beards, broad shoulders, narrow hips, hairy bodies, tenor and bass voices, strong arms, hard muscular chests, and to function primarily from their left brains—not to mention that androgens play a role in dozens of peculiarly masculine personality traits and preferences—like sitting in a tree from sunup to sundown in the freezing cold to shoot a deer or refusing to consult a roadmap or ask directions when driving.

Estrogens cause women to have smooth faces, narrow shoulders, broad hips, nearly hairless bodies, alto and soprano voices, weaker arms, soft skin, strong legs, soft breasts, and to function primarily from their right brains—not to mention that estrogens play a role in dozens of female personality traits and preferences—like shopping, which men usually detest.

Men have testicles and prostate glands and produce sperm. Women have ovaries and uteri, release eggs, have babies, and can nurse them.

Volumes have been written on the endless differences between a man and a woman, but biochemically it all comes down to seven hormones and how they balance. The interesting thing is that the hormones themselves are chemically not that much different. But even the tiniest of differences in a ligand can make the greatest of differences in a result—even to such extremes as male and female, life and death.

This brings us to a discussion of the differences between pharmaceutical drugs (which are all synthetic) and therapeutic grade essential oils (which are all natural).

Estrogens, Estrogens Everywhere

Gynecologists and drug companies have promoted birth control pills for decades, ever since they became available in the 1960s. They still promote them. Hormone replacement therapy (HRT) is a more recent medical product and is being marketed to the extreme by physicians and pharmaceutical companies who want every woman in menopause to be on these drugs for life. The pill and HRT are both synthetic estrogens. They aren't true estrogens, like estrone, estradiol, and estriol, the three estrogens made by the human body.

"Estrogen" is not a specific compound. It is a class of compounds. Their name is from the Greek word, *estrus*, meaning "heat" or "ovulation." An estrogenic substance is one that stimulates a woman in ways that prepare her body for fertilization and pregnancy. estrogenic substances can also cause a man to manifest feminine characteristics, both psychologically and physically.

There are only three true human estrogens—estrone, estradiol, and estriol—which were shown in the figure on page 401. There are also "phytoestrogens," which come from plant sources and can be used by women (and men) who need additional estrogen or seek a hormonal balance. Phytoestrogens are found in some essential oils. *Phyto* is a Greek word meaning "plant." There are also estrogenic substances that originate from petrochemicals. These include many plastics (especially when heated in a microwave oven), pesticides, herbicides, and industrial by-products such as dioxin. These are called "xenoestrogens." *Xeno* is a Greek word meaning "strange." And then there are the "synthetic estrogens" created and patented by drug companies. These are the ones that doctors prescribe.

So we have human estrogens produced by humans, phytoestrogens produced by plants (that can be used beneficially by people), xenoestrogens that result from accidental properties of petrochemical products (which aren't good for people), and synthetic estrogens produced by drug companies and prescribed by doctors (which universally carry negative side effects). Since estrogens are growth stimulators, the beef and pork industry feeds them to livestock to accelerate weight gain and produce more meat more profitably.

As a result, those who live in industrialized countries, like the U.S., live in an estrogenic environment. All of the estrogenic substances used, eaten, and prescribed end up in our soils, atmosphere, groundwater, and streams which ultimately re-enter our food supplies. Hence, everyone is being dosed with estrogens in America, whether they know it or not.

The problem is with the artificial estrogens. Human and phytoestrogens are biodegradable. God makes these and the earth's natural environment, which he also made, is capable of handling them. Xeno- and synthetic estrogens are not readily biodegradable. They can hang around in our environment for many years, accumulating and recycling over and over. What effect this is having on the physical, mental, and psychological health of the general population is not known. It can't be good.

Why Not Prescribe Natural Hormones?

Phytoestrogens are milder than a woman's own estrogens and are easily utilized and metabolized by our bodies. Xeno and synthetic estrogens are considerably more powerful than human estrogens and are not easily eliminated from the body. Thus, their effects last a long time.

Doctors could recommend phytoestrogens and drug companies could synthesize exact copies of the estrone, estradiol, and estriol that the human body makes, but they don't and they won't. They can't patent a natural substance, create a monopoly, and make large amounts of money. It is as simple as that.

The problem is that synthetic estrogens are harmful, even potentially fatal. When drug companies say they are spending millions of dollars to "find cures" or "better drugs," etc., they are not really trying to find any cures or any drugs that are better for you, they are trying to find a patentable product from which they can make a fortune. They want drugs that patients must take regularly for the rest of their lives, because it is in marketing a drug habit that the largest revenues are derived. If they sell you a cure, there is no repeat business, no steady income from your usage. If they sell you a drug that merely manages your illness, but keep you perpetually unhealed and dependent, they will have arranged to extract a lifetime of regular payments from you.

And what's more, negative side effects from a drug actually work in their favor. If they sell you a drug that is harmful, then they can increase their income even more by then selling you another drug or procedure to treat the problems they created for you with the first prescription, thus netting them additional income. If there are no adverse side effects associated with their product, their income is reduced.

Everything I am saying here is well known and understood by every doctor and every drug company. It is not that they just don't realize what they are doing. They know full well. As mentioned earlier in this book, in Galatians 5:19-21, St. Paul writes a list of works not pleasing to God. Included on the list is "sorcery" or "witchcraft," as translated into English. but the Greek word is "*pharmakeia*," meaning literally "drugs from a pharmacy."

Manipulating Molecules

The illustration on the next page shows two of our natural estrogens (estrone and estradiol) and two examples each of synthetic counterparts sold by drug companies as substitutes for estrone and estradiol. You can see right away that "hormone replacement" is an ambiguous statement. They want you to believe that they are replacing your hormones with real estrogens. In reality, they are replacing them with phony imitations. You can see that what they have done is to take a real estrogen and alter it just enough to be able to patent it. All they did was bend a few bonds into or out of the page while deleting or adding

Natural Estrogens vs. Synthetic Estrogens

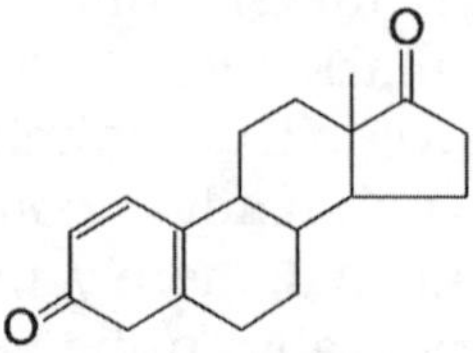

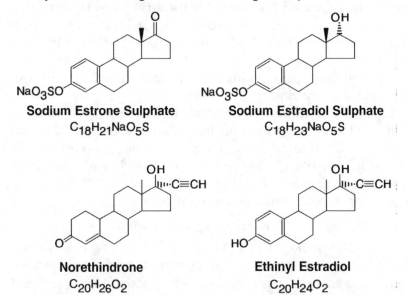

Estrone
$C_{18}H_{22}O_2$

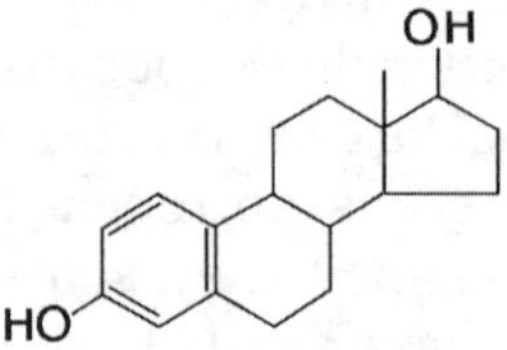

Estradiol
$C_{18}H_{24}O_2$

①Natural Estrogens • The Ones Our Bodies Make①

---

②Synthetic Estrogens • Ones Drug Companies Make②

Sodium Estrone Sulphate
$C_{18}H_{21}NaO_5S$

Sodium Estradiol Sulphate
$C_{18}H_{23}NaO_5S$

Norethindrone
$C_{20}H_{26}O_2$

Ethinyl Estradiol
$C_{20}H_{24}O_2$

a few things. The molecular sizes of our own estrogens run from 270-288. The sodium sulphate versions are larger, weighing in at 372-374 amu. The two bottom versions are 295-298 amu. The larger molecular size means that they stay in your body longer and are more difficult to eliminate, not to mention that they confuse our receptor sites and cause other mischief.

Notice that the elements chosen to modify the natural

estrogens are sodium (Na) and Sulfur (S). Checking back in the Periodic Table, you will see that sodium is in the same vertical column as hydrogen and sulfur is in the same vertical column as oxygen. All elements in the same column have the same valence and can be substituted for one another in a compound. Thus, companies can create new compounds with properties similar to the natural versions that can be patented into a profitable monopoly. Natural hormones do not produce the adverse effects as do the synthetic ones. However, this fact does not deter drug companies from their aggressive campaigns to market their inferior and potentially harmful products, while lobbying to inhibit the sale of natural products.

The sodium sulphate estrogens are for HRT (hormone replacement therapy) and are sold by two companies. One of them is Cenestin®, by Duramed Inc., and the other is Premarin®, by Wyeth Inc.

Norethindrone and ethinyl estradiol are for birth control and are sold by a dozen different companies under 18 different brand names. Some of them you may know: Brevicon®, Demulen®, Desogen®, Levlen®, Loestrin®, Lo/Ovral®, Modicon®, Neolova®, Nordette®, Norinyl®, Ortho Cyclen®, Ortho-Cept®, Ortho-Novum®, Ovcon®, Ovral®, Tri-Levlen®, Tri-Normyl®, and Triphasil®.

The problem with any synthetic estrogen is that it will always have side effects that neither plant estrogens nor our own estrogens possess. According to John R. Lee, M.D., in his book *What Your Doctor May Not Tell You About Menopause*, the following symptoms can be caused or made worse by these estrogens: acceleration of the aging process, allergies, breast tenderness, decreased sex drive, depression, fatigue, fibrocystic breasts, foggy thinking, headaches, hypoglycemia, increased risk of strokes, infertility, irritability, memory loss, miscarriage, osteoporosis, premenopausal bone loss, PMS, thyroid dysfunction, uterine cancer, uterine fibroids, water retention, weight gain, gall bladder disease, and a variety of autoimmune disorders such as lupus.

The scandal of doctors urging women to go on HRT is

not just that they are prescribing dangerous substitutes for the real hormones a woman needs. The scandal is that post menopausal women are not estrogen deficient, as they would lead you to believe. Most women in menopause have enough estrogen, which is about half what it was during their childbearing years. But half enough is enough. The problem is a progesterone deficiency.

As to why women in industrialized countries past the age of 40 or 50 suffer a progesterone imbalance, read John Lee's excellent book mentioned above. It is a preventable deficiency, but the preventive measures call for major changes in Western lifestyles which result in adrenal exhaustion in middle-aged women. Women in simple, primitive cultures never experience menopausal problems.

Progesterone is the hormone a woman must have in dominance during pregnancy to retain the pregnancy. That is why it is called the "pro-gestation" hormone. It supports gestation. But progesterone has other benefits for both men and women. In women, it quenches or mitigates the harmful consequences of having too much estrogen. "Too much estrogen" means "out of balance with progesterone." Realizing this early on, the drug companies now include a synthetic progesterone in the pills they compound for HRT. But, again, it is a synthetic compound, not real progesterone. What is sold for HRT today is called a "conjugated estrogen." This is a mixture of some nine variations of synthetic estrogen like the sodium sulphate versions, shown earlier, blended with a synthetic progesterone.

Horse Urine

You might like to know where drug companies get their raw materials from which to create synthetic estrogens. Notice in the list of birth control pills one called "Loestrin." It is sold by Parke-Davis. When drug chemists create and name their compounds, they sometimes hide their origin in the name, unknown to the public. The "-rin" part is in reference to "uRINe." That's right. Horse urine.

The chemists at Wyeth Laboratories were even more clever. Their product name, "Premarin," was fashioned out of the words PREgnant MAres uRINe. They confine preg-

Natural Progesterone vs. Synthetic Progesterone

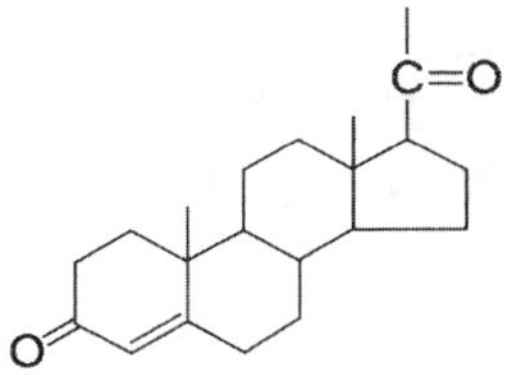

Progesterone
$C_{21}H_{30}O_2$

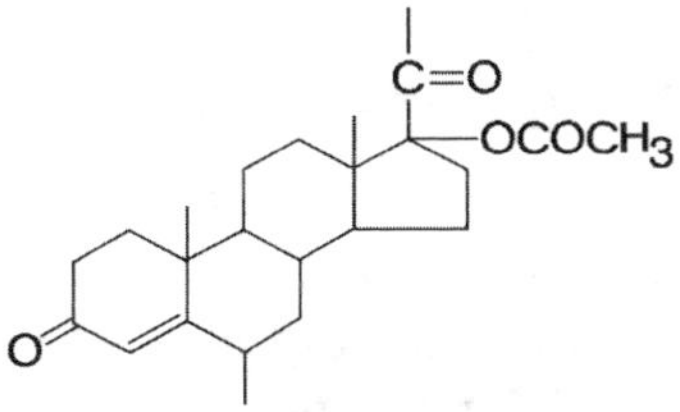

Medroxyprogesterone
$C_{23}H_{36}O_4$

nant mares attached to various devices to capture their urine from which they manufacture Premarin®. If women knew the misery and abuse such horses suffer, they would think twice about patronizing these products.

The truth is, despite what doctors say, few women really need them. Post menopausal women rarely need more estrogen. They need more progesterone, the real stuff, not fake progesterone. Synthetic progesterone is called "progestin." Its technical name is "medroxyprogesterone," as seen above. Here again, the drug companies have only changed a few parts of the molecule to make something they can own and sell. They could make and sell you a synthesized version of the natural hormone, but they won't. When companies dealing in natural products try to sell natural hormones, they often get into trouble with the U.S. Food and Drug Administration (FDA) and their products can be taken off the market. Meanwhile, the FDA approves of the fake versions. Your body benefits from real progesterone while it is harmed by progestin, the false version. Table Twenty-Eight, on the next page, shows the benefits and risks from both kinds of progesterone taken from Lee's book on menopause.

The only thing progestin can claim as a possible benefit is possible protection from endometrial cancer. All other aspects of progestin are negative. Natural progesterone also protects from endometrial cancer as well as breast cancer. What most women do not realize is that endometrial cancer is purely an iatrogenic (doctor-caused) disease. You can't get endometrial cancer unless you have taken

Table Twenty-Eight
Natural & Synthetic Progesterone Compared

Conditions	Natural Progesterone	Synthetic Progestin
Sodium and water into body cells		X
Loss of mineral electrolytes		X
Intracellular edema		X
Depression		X
Risks of Birth Defects		X
More body hair, thinner scalp hair		X
Thrombophlebitis, embolism risk		X
Decreased glucose tolerance		X
Allergic reactions		X
Risk of cholestatic jaundice		X
Acne, skin rashes		X
Protects from endometrial cancer	X	X
Protects against breast cancer	X	
Normalizes libido	X	
Less hirsutism, regrowth of scalp hair	X	
Improves lipid profile	X	
Improves new bone formation	X	
Improves sleep patterns	X	

Adapted from *What Your Doctor May Not Tell You About Menopause*
by John R. Lee, MD, Warner Books, 1996.

synthetic estrogens—either birth control pills or HRT.

HRT is also sometimes promoted as a preventive from bone loss and osteoporosis. But osteoporosis is not due to an estrogen deficiency. Neither is it due to a calcium deficiency. Your bones have two types of cells: osteoblasts and osteoclasts. The blasts build new bone and the clasts tear out old bone. The blasts are builders. The clasts are wreckers. Osteoporosis happens when the clasts get ahead of the blasts. Taking calcium won't fix the problem. Calcium is like bricks and mortar. It is a building material. You can pile all the bricks you want at the work site, but unless you have masons to put them in place, no construction takes place. The osteoclasts get ahead of the osteoblasts when there is a hormonal imbalance, like too much estrogen and not enough progesterone. Here is another myth the medical community has foisted upon the unwary public trying to justify its all out promotion of the pill and HRT.

The point of this discussion on our male and female hormones is to demonstrate to you that our bodies are operated by molecules. When the right molecules are in place and allowed to operate, we are well. The right molecules come from nature, provided by God. When the wrong molecules enter our bodies, those made by pharmaceutical companies, we can never be completely well. Tiny changes in a good molecule can turn it into a bad molecule. It just isn't nice to fool with Mother Nature. She has it right. Our task is to understand what God has done and live in harmony with it. Not to try to supplant his good molecules with artificial ones that may have some benefits, but always, without exception, have untoward side effects. For more detail in this area I strongly recommend Dr. John Lee's excellent book, *What Your Doctor May Not Tell You About Menopause.* (See bibliography.)

Fennel, Anise, and DES

Besides its antiseptic, analgesic, and antiparasitic properties, fennel is estrogenic as an herb and as an oil. Dating from Egyptian papyri of 1600 BC, it has been used for thousands of years as a regulator of menstrual cycles and for the treatment of premenstrual syndrome. Fennel is 60% anethole ($C_{10}H_{12}O$), a phenolic ether, which is also the dominant constituent in anise oil (87%). While each of these two oils has its unique therapeutic characteristics that make them different, both manifest hormonal qualities—but not necessarily from anethole, their major constituent.

Another constituent common to both fennel oil and anise oil is p-anol—a natural phenylpropanoid ($C_9H_{10}O$). P-anol is a minor constituent in both oils, comprising no more than 1-2%. DES (diethylstilbesterol) is a synthetic, nonsteroidal estrogen. The p-anol molecule is exactly like half of a DES molecule ($C_{18}H_{20}O_2$). Chemists only have to link a pair of p-anol molecules together tail to tail to make DES. Administered as a natural ingredient in an essential oil, p-anol has no known negative side effects, has a mild fragrance of cloves, and is thought to be one of the sources of the hormonal benefits provided by fennel and anise. By contrast, DES, which joins a pair of p-anol molecules into a single unnatural one has serious side effects.

P-anol has been used by drug companies to synthesize DES as a prescription drug. Originally extracted from fennel and anise, p-anol was synthetically produced for drug manufacturing purposes. The figure below shows how DES can be created by the marriage of two p-anol molecules. This is not a marriage made in heaven (by God), but one made only in a laboratory (by man). For decades, DES was widely prescribed to pregnant women until it became clear, after accumulating more than forty years of data, that the drug causes delayed cancers in offspring daughters manifesting in their late teens and early twenties.

After this fact was established in the 1970s, it soon became illegal to administer DES to expectant mothers, but prescriptions of DES were still approved for many years thereafter to dry up a mother's milk when she did

Synthesizing the Unnatural from the Natural

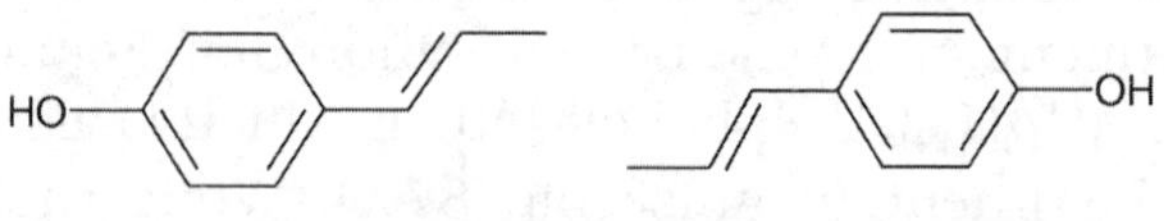

p-Anol
$C_9H_{10}O$

Two p-Anol Molecules as Found in Fennel and Anise Oils
(p-anol is a natural essential oil compound with estrogenic properties)

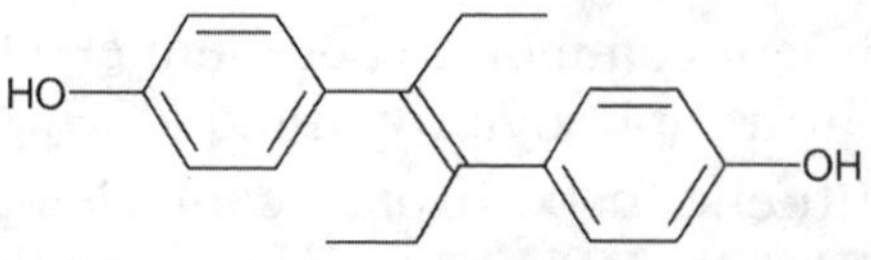

DES
$C_{18}H_{20}O_2$

One DES Molecule Synthesized from Two p-Anol Molecules
(Diethylstilbesterol (DES) is a synthetic estrogenic drug)

not wish to breastfeed. One of the actions of DES is to block the receptor sites for prolactin. Prolactin is a natural maternal hormone stimulated by the baby's suckling at the breast that stimulates the flow of mother's milk.

Besides the suppression of human milk production, another negative side effect of prescribing DES to lactating women was the loss of the benefits of prolactin. This hormone, designed by God, has an emotional impact. It stimulates motherly feelings and instincts, thus enabling women to be better parents—more sensitive, patient, loving, and responsive to their newborn baby's needs. When it was eventually found that DES is carcinogenic, not only to the female children of expectant mothers, but to the adult mothers, themselves, the drug was finally banned altogether. But not until thousands of women were diagnosed with cancer from the drug, many of whom died.

Hormones, Estrogens, and Essential Oils

There are several oils besides anise and fennel that have hormonal benefits. Sage, clary sage, blue tansy, tarragon, niaouli, cypress, myrtle, and wild tansy are among them. Chamazulene, found in blue tansy, helichrysum, and German chamomile oils, is a large sesquiterpene molecule that also appears to have hormone-regulating abilities.

Dr. Jean Valnet found that cypress oil seems to serve as a homologue to a woman's natural ovarian hormones. The exact compounds contained in cypress that are responsible for this have not been identified. Dr. Valnet also considers viridiflorol to be estrogenic and can be obtained through oils such as Niaouli (*Melaleuca quinquenervia*), myrtle (*Myrtus communis*), and sage (*Salvia officinalis*).

In Dr. Daniel Penoel's practice, anise oil has been used to increase breastmilk production. This oil apparently stimulates the release of prolactin, the lactation hormone. This fact is especially ironic in that p-anol, found in anise, is used to synthesize DES, a drug used to suppress lactation, as was just discussed. Dr. Penoel has also found that if a woman is experiencing menstrual irregularity tarragon oil can help restore regular menstrual periods. Other oils that have helped with this problem include sage, clary sage, German chamomile, and fennel.

While the hormonally active constituents of anise, fennel, and tarragon oils probably involve their main ingredients, anethole and estragole—both isomers of the formula, $C_{10}H_{12}O$—it is probably the minor ingredients, like p-anol ($C_9H_{10}O$), that give them their hormonally balancing qualities. But who can say if it is actually one or two particular constituents responsible for these beneficial effects when, in fact, compounds in an oil act in concert with all of their companions to produce results no single component could do alone?

Sclareol is a diterpenol found in sage (*Salvia officinalis*) and clary sage (*Salvia sclarea*) that is considered to have estrogenic qualities. That is to say, its presence in our bodies tends to stimulate the same receptor sites that estrogens do and help balance our hormones. Notice in the figure on the next page that the sclareol molecule has 19 carbon atoms, the same as natural androgens. (Natural human estrogens have only 18 carbons—see figure on p. 401.) While primarily considered for their estrogenic properties, the oils in which sclareol are found offer hormone balancing benefits to both men and women, demonstrating their androgenic properties as well.

It is interesting to note that the dried herb of clary sage is added to cigar tobacco. Compare the smell of a cigar with the oil of clary sage and you will recognize the aroma. Does this mean that cigars have hormonal attributes?

Sclareol and viridiflorol look like neither estrogen nor androgen molecules. Sclareol's molecular weight is 296 amu, which is slightly heavier than our natural estrogens and androgens which range from 270 to 291. Viridiflorol's molecular weight of 221 amu is less. Even though their physical shapes and sizes are not the same, sclareol and viridiflorol can apparently communicate with many of the same receptor sites as our sexual steroids evoking bodily responses as if they were hormones. These compounds may also stimulate our bodies to produce their own natural estrogens and androgens—which can explain why they have beneficial steroidal effects without being steroids.

Estrogenic Oil Molecules

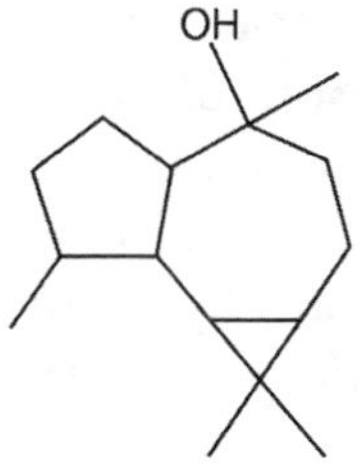

Viridiflorol
$C_{15}H_{25}O$ M.W. = 221
Niaouli, Myrtle, & Sage Oils

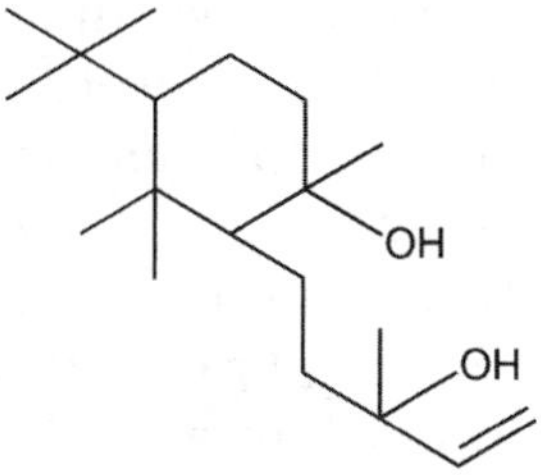

Sclareol
$C_{19}H_{36}O_2$ M.W. = 296
Sage & Clary Sage Oils

In Chapter Seven we pointed out that when molecules approach cellular receptor sites to gain access to the intelligence within, it really isn't like a mechanical key inserted into a mechanical key hole, as we sometimes visualize. Message-carrying molecules vibrate and sing to receptor sites such that if they strike the right resonance, the receptor site opens. Mechanical, molecular shape may not always be the key to what songs a molecule can sing. If you think about it, neither is the size and shape of a singer an index to the songs they can sing. Sclareol and viridiflorol are essential oil molecules that can sing estrogen and androgen songs that can help balance our bodies in beneficial ways—without adverse side effects.

Exactly how essential oil molecules invoke hormonal responses in our bodies is not well defined by science at this time. Aromatherapists just know, by experience and observation, that such responses really do occur, bringing many benefits. *L'Aromatherapie Exactement* by Franchomme and Penoel contains considerable material on the shapes of essential oil molecules and their abilities to mimic hormones, stimulate hormonal receptor sites, and even act as raw materials from which our human bodies can build hormone molecules.

There are a variety of sources for estrogens in plants. Several species of willow (*Salix sp.*) and genera of palm trees (Palmaceae) are reported to contain both estrone and estriol corresponding exactly to the steriodal hormones of the human body. (See figure on p. 401.) There does not appear to be any essential oils available from either of these plants, but if there were, they would probably be hormonally balancing in their therapeutic properties.

For actual applications of specific essential oils for hormonal balancing purposes, see the books by Higley, Manwaring, Young, Price, Franchomme, Penoel and Friedmann, reviewed in Chapter One and/or listed in the bibliography.

Why Oils Heal and Drugs Don't

If you tell most medical doctors that essential oils can bring about healing with no negative side effects, they won't believe you. This is because in medical school, students are repeatedly told by their professors that all effective medicines have negative side effects, and if they don't, then they can't be effective.

When I was in medical school one professor emphasized this point in a colorful, graphic manner with specially prepared slides. In each slide specific drugs were depicted as evil looking demons or goblins. As he presented each picture, he explained, "Although ugly and capable of doing harm, these 'demons' are also the bearers of some good. So long as the benefits outweigh the risks, we use them," he summarized. "We have no choice," he continued, "because if a drug has no dangers, then it can have no benefits. That's just the way it is. And that's why it is essential that only qualified physicians be allowed to prescribe medicines," he concluded.

Actually, the professor was telling the truth. Within the restricted practice of allopathy (MDs) the only real medicines are physician prescribed pharmaceuticals. Such medicines always do have negative side effects. All of them. No exceptions. Hence, doctors are trained to accept the bad with the good as the price of effective medicine.

The Danger is in the Drug

The principal dangers of prescription drugs are intrinsic to the drugs, themselves, not in how they are administered. No matter how careful the physician may be in prescribing and how compliant the patient may be in following doctor's orders, even then deaths and damages occur. In fact, according to the U.S. Centers for Disease Control, more than 100,000 Americans die every year, not from illegal drugs, not from drug overdoses, not from over-the-counter drugs, and not from drug abuses, but from properly prescribed, properly taken prescriptions. In the United States, more people die from doctor's prescriptions every ten days than were killed in the 9/11 terrorist attacks on the Pentagon and World Trade Center Towers in 2001.

Why is this so? Why do allopathic drugs always have undesirable effects (along with their apparent benefits) while one can find healing with natural products, such as essential oils, with no undesirable effects? The answer to this is biochemical.

Why Companies Sell Dangerous Products

It is illegal to patent any natural product. The way to big profits in the medicine industry is to create an unnatural substance that never before existed in nature, then patent it, and obtain a monopoly. Hence, the molecules of pharmaceutical drugs are all strange to the human body. In all the history of humankind, such molecules were never encountered or taken into any human body. Hence, the body does not easily metabolize them. God never made your body to accept and deal with these chemicals and antibiotics.

Non-toxic natural organic substances are usually easily eliminated by the body when their usefulness has run their course. Up to a point, your body can even deal with and eliminate natural toxic substances. But when your body receives a synthetic substance, even one that may seem benign or inert (like plastic), your body does not know how to metabolize and eliminate it. If sent to the liver to break it down into disposable compounds, the liver says, "Hey. What is this? I don't know what to do with it. Here, kidneys, you take it." Then the kidneys react saying, "Hey liver, don't send it to us. We don't know what it is either. Send it to the pancreas. Maybe it will have an enzyme that can deal with it." Then the pancreas objects,

"Hey guys, what do you think you are doing? I don't want this stuff. Dump it in the blood or the lymph or try the spleen. Maybe the spleen can filter this thing out or something." Finally, the substance ends up in a long term waste holding area of the body (usually fat tissue, including the brain) where it can remain for years and even for a lifetime, perturbing normal body functions as long as it remains. That's why you can find traces of prescription drugs in your body taken in childhood, decades ago.

On the other hand, natural molecules, such as those found in essential oils, are easily metabolized by the body. In fact, your body was created to handle them. When an essential oil molecule finds the receptor sites it was designed to fit and conveys its information to the cell, or participates in other therapeutic functions, it moves on to to the liver, kidneys, and bowels and leaves the body. It's benefits have been conveyed and its job is complete.

By contrast, the unnatural molecules of man-made drugs attach themselves to various tissues, disrupting normal function for years while the body tries to figure out what to do with them. Meanwhile, they wreak mischief with our bodily functions and even our minds. Pharmaceuticals are biochemical nightmares that disturb bodily functions and block true healing.

Who is in Control?

Another reason commercial drug companies don't want to sell natural products is that they are not in complete control of their production. When you synthesize everything in a laboratory, you are in control. You can produce your medicines at will in any quantity whenever you choose. This way you can meet market demands as they materialize.

When you depend on nature to grow your product, God is in control. You are at the mercy of the seasons. You can only grow so much with a given year's crop. If a year's supply runs out before the next crop is ready for harvest, then you and your customers just have to wait. Meanwhile, you lose potential sales and profits.

Drug companies want to be totally in charge of producing their products. They don't want God to be in charge. By omitting God from the manufacture of their medicines, they have omitted his healing power.

Drugs Versus Oils

Drugs and oils work in opposite ways. Drugs toxify. Oils detoxify. Drugs clog and confuse receptor sites. Oils clean receptor sites.

Drugs depress the immune system. Oils strengthen the immune system. Antibiotics attack bacteria indiscriminantly, killing both the good and the bad. Oils attack only the harmful bacteria, allowing our body's friendly flora to flourish.

Drugs are one-dimensional, programmed like robots to carry out certain actions in the body, whether the body can benefit from them or not. When body conditions change, drugs keep on doing what they were doing even when their actions are no longer beneficial.

Essential oils are multi-dimensional, filled with homeostatic intelligence to restore the body to a state of healthy balance. When body conditions change, oils adapt, raising or lowering blood pressure as needed, stimulating or repressing enzyme activity as needed, energizing or relaxing as needed. Oils are smart. Drugs are dumb.

Drugs are designed to send misinformation to cells or to block certain receptor sites in order to trick the body into giving up symptoms. But drugs never deal with the actual causes of disease. They aren't designed for that purpose. While they may give prompt relief for certain uncomfortable symptoms, because of their strange, unnatural design, they will always disrupt certain other bodily functions. Thus you always have some side effects.

Oil molecules deliver helpful information to cells and cleanse receptor sites so that they bring your body back to natural function. Oils are balancing to the body. Drugs are unbalancing to the body. Oils address the causes of disease at a cellular level by deleting misinformation and reprogramming correct information so that cells function properly and in harmony with one another. With drugs,

Table Twenty-Nine
Essential Oils and Pharmaceuticals Compared

Essential Oils	Pharmaceuticals
Properties	**Properties**
1. Natural, wildcrafted or grown organically	1. Unnatural, synthetic, chemically or gentically engineered
2. Hundreds of constituents, not all known	2. One or two active ingredients, all of which are known
3. Never two batches the same.	3. Every batch the same (purity)
4. Not patentable (God made)	4. Patentable (man made)
Effects and Consequences	**Effects and Consequences**
5. Restores natural function	5. Inhibits natural function
6. No adverse interactions	6. Many adverse interactions
7. Antiviral	7. Usually not antiviral
8. Improves intercellular communication	8. Disrupts intercellular communication
9. Corrects and restores proper cellular memory (DNA)	9. Garbles and confuses cellular memory (DNA)
10. Cleanses receptor sites	10. Blocks receptor sites
11. Builds the immune system	11. Depresses immune system
12. Emotionally balancing	12. Emotionally unbalancing
13. Side effects beneficial	13. Side effects harmful
14. Leads toward independence and wellness	14. Leads toward dependence and chronic disease
Philosophy/Paradigm	**Philosophy/Paradigm**
15. Assumes wellness as natural state, invulnerable to illness	15. Assumes natural state prone and vulnerable to illness
16. Assumes body and mind capable of self-healing	16. Assumes body and mind need external assistance to heal
17. Integrated wholistically, body, mind, and soul as a unit	17. Fragmented, treats body parts, mind and emotions separate
18. Build natural defenses and let body deal with disease	18. Supplant natural defenses and attack disease itself
19. Treats internally at level of cellular intelligence	19. Treats externally at level of gross symptoms
20. Theistic, historic roots in religion when healers were priests	20. Secular, historic roots in materialism motivated by money

misinformation is fed into the cells so that some temporary relief may be obtained, but there is seldom any true healing. Drugs usually only trade one kind of disease condition for another.

Because essential oils, properly applied, always work toward the restoration of proper bodily function, they do not cause undesirable side effects. They are feeding the body with truth. Drugs feed the body with lies. While no amount of truth can contradict itself, it doesn't take many lies before contradictions occur and the body suffers ill effects.

Eighteen Doctors Speak Out

Not all physicians are caught up in the idea that the only good medicines are ones that can also be harmful. Here are some comments by physicians themselves on the practice of medicine. Most of these quotes were downloaded from the the Global Institute for Alternative Medicine (GIFAM) website: www.gifam.org.

"Every educated physician knows that most diseases are not appreciably helped by medicine."

Richard C. Cabot, M.D. Professor Harvard School of Medicine; Author of *Differential Diagnosis*, *The Art of Ministering to the Sick*, and other books.

"Every drug increases and complicates the patient's condition."

Robert Henderson, M.D.

"The cause of most disease is in the poisonous drugs physicians superstitiously give in order to effect a cure."

Charles E. Page, M.D., Silver Springs, Maryland

"The person who takes medicine must recover twice, once from the disease and once from the medicine."

William Osler, M.D. Canadian physician; President, American Association of Physicians; author of *The Principles and Practice of Medicine*.

"If all the medicine in the world were thrown into the sea, it would be bad for the fish and good for humanity."

Oliver W. Holmes, M.D. American poet, novelist, and physician.
Professor of Medicine, Dartmouth College and Harvard University.

"Medicine is only palliative, for back of disease lies the cause, and this cause no drug can reach."

Wier Mitchel, M.D.

"Our figures show approximately four and one half million hospital admissions annually due to the adverse reactions to drugs. Further, the average hospital patient has as much as a 30% chance, depending how long he is in, of doubling his stay due to adverse drug reactions."

Milton Silverman, M.D. Professor of Pharmacology, Univ. of California Author, *The Drugging of America*, *Prescriptions for Death*, and other books

"Drug medications consist in employing, as remedies for disease, those things which produce disease in well persons. Its *Materia Medica* is simply a lot of drugs or chemicals or dyestuffs—in a word poisons. All are incompatible with vital matter. All produce disease when brought in contact in any manner with the living. All are poisons."

R.T. Trall, M.D., Author of *The True Healing Art* and other books. Quote from a lecture to members of the U.S. Congress, Washington D.C.

"Medical practice has neither philosophy nor common sense to recommend it. In sickness the body is already loaded with impurities. By taking drug–medicines more impurities are added, thereby the case is further embarrassed and harder to cure."

Elmer Lee, M.D., Vice President, American Academy of Medicine.

"There are over 10 million adverse reactions yearly from FDA-approved over-the-counter and prescription drugs. We are not talking about mild nausea or headaches. Between 60,000 and 140,000 people die each year from adverse drug reactions. Each year, more Americans die after taking prescription drugs than died in the entire Vietnam war. Over half the drugs approved by the FDA since 1976 were later found to be much more toxic than previously thought. Several had to be removed from the market."

Julian Whitaker, M.D., Author of *Reversing Heart Disease, Guide to Natural Healing, The Heart Surgery Trap,* and other books.

"What hope is there for medical science to ever become a true science when the entire structure of medical knowledge is built around the idea that there is an entity called disease which can be expelled when the right drug is found?"

John H. Tilden, M.D. Author of *Impaired Health, Etiology, Hygienic, and Dietetic Treatment of Appendicitis*, and other books and articles.

"The greatest part of all chronic disease is created by the suppression of acute disease by drug poisoning."

Henry Lindlahr, M.D. Author of *Diagnostic Methods, Nature Cure: Philosophy and Practice, Natural Therapeutics,* and other books.

"Drugs never cure disease. They merely hush the voice of nature's protest, and pull down the danger signals she erects along the pathway of transgression. Any poison taken into the system has to be reckoned with later on even though it palliates present symptoms. Pain may disappear, but the patient is left in a worse condition, though unconscious of it at the time."

Daniel H. Kress, M.D. Author of *The Cost to Society of Cigarettes: A Century of Analysis, Ulcers and Smoking*, and other books.

"Why would a patient swallow a poison because he is ill, or take that which would make a well man sick?"

L.F. Kebler, M.D. Author of *Technical Drug Studies*, *Medicated Soft Drinks*, and other works.

"We are prone to thinking of drug abuse in terms of illicit drugs such as heroin, cocaine, and marijuana. It may surprise you to learn that a greater problem exists with millions dependent on legal prescription drugs."

Robert Mendelsohn, M.D. Chairman, Illinois State Medical Licensing Board; Author of *Confessions of a Medical Heretic*, *How to Raise a Healthy Child in Spite of Your Doctor,* and other books.

"In the field of medicine today, there are many ancient therapeutic modalities that are becoming available to us. Among them are acupuncture, homeopathy, nutritional concepts, and massage. Also available is aromatherapy, in which the use of essential oils works at a deep cellular but also vibratory level."

Gladys Taylor McGarey, M.D. Former President of the Arizona Board of Homeopathic Medical Examiners and former President of the American Holistic Medical Association.

"There are significant efforts by insurance companies to exclude preventive health care and education and the use of natural, inexpensive remedies, while ignoring the benefits of nutrition. At the same time they pay huge medical claims to hospitals for surgery and pharmaceutical products. There is an unwritten agreement between hospitals and insurance providers to reimburse the hospitals for services performed in hospitals—to scratch each other's backs—so to speak. There is a hidden agenda in this. If insurance providers pay hospitals for patients' medical claims, then at the end of the year the insurance companies can go to the state insurance commissions with their track records and request a premium increase. A premium increase translates into more profit for the insurance carriers as well as the hospitals."

Terry S. Friedmann, M.D. Author of *Freedom Through Health* and other publications. Cofounder and Board Member, American Holistic Medical Association

"The necessity of teaching mankind not to take drugs and medicines, is a duty incumbent upon all who know their uncertainty and injurious effects; and the time is not far distant when the drug system will be abandoned."

Charles Armbruster, M. D.

So there you have it, why oils heal and drugs don't. It's all in the biochemistry of how they affect the body. Let's hope Dr. Armbruster is right, that "the time is not far distant when the drug system will be abandoned." Pharmaceutical companies and their army of drug dealing doctors could market and sell natural products with genuine healing capabilities, but most won't. There isn't any money in it.

Emergency Medicine is the Best of Medicine

In Dr. Robert Mendelsohn's book, *Confessions of a Medical Heretic*, he describes medicine as a practice of religion rather than a practice of science. Doctors practice what they believe, not what they can substantiate by valid science. According to Mendelsohn, in the religion of medicine, physicians are the high priests and their ecclesiastical robes are their white coats. Hospitals are the temples where many holy waters are dispensed in the form of drugs, antibiotics, and vaccines. People tithe to the church of medicine by dutifully paying their insurance premiums. The word, "prescription" is very close to the term, "pre-scriptural," thus implying a scriptural basis for their use. The *Holy Bible* containing the scriptures of medicine is the *Pharmaceutical PDR*. For millions of people, their faith and confidence in the religion of medicine is far greater than their belief in the institutions of worship they may attend. In a crisis, they would sooner call 911 than call upon God in prayer.

Dr. Mendelsohn was a practicing pediatrician at the Michael Reese Medical Center in Chicago, a professor at the University of Illinois School of Medicine, Chairman of the Illinois State Licensing Board, and appeared on national television many times. He is author of another book entitled, *How to Raise a Healthy Child in Spite of Your Doctor*, where he states, "When it comes to treating a sick child, one grandmother is worth two pediatricians." He also often said, "If you always assume your doctor is wrong, most of the time you will be right." In Dr. Mendelsohn's opinion, "The best of medicine is emergency medicine." I agree. When it comes to chronic disease, they have little or nothing to offer—no cures, only treatments and disease management.

I don't want to imply that there is no use for medical care as we have it today. If I were in a serious accident with a massive head injury, damage to my internal organs, or a broken limb I would want to go to the nearest emergency room as fast as possible with the best physicians and nurses on staff. Allopathic medicine is wonderful in a cri-sis and saves many lives. Emergency medicine is what they do best. In a traumatic situation where you could die unless immediate action is taken, allopathy with all of its drugs, surgeries, equipment, and other paraphernalia can be just what you need to get you through the crisis.

But as for healing, allopathic medicine doesn't offer much. After you have been rescued by allopathic measures from imminent death in an emergency situation, the healing is still up to you by seeking other modalities. And when it comes to a chronic illness like cancer, arthritis, diabetes, or cardiovascular disease, allopathy has no cures and usually makes matters worse.

One reason medical practitioners do best in a crisis is because that is the emphasis in their training. In fact, in America, 85% of medical expenditures are for crisis applications—responding to accidents, acute life-threatening conditions, or patching up the body when seriously advanced disease has occurred and death may be imminent. Meanwhile, less than 6% of health care expenditures are for prevention and wellness education.

True healing can only take place with the participation of the patient on all levels—mental, spiritual, emotional, and physical. The idea of "leaving it to the doctor," leads to unending sickness and poor health. Health care and health maintenance is something you do for yourself, with the help of God. Not something for which you pay your money and continue to do as you please without altering your life style.

Health care is your responsibility—not the government's, not the insurance company's, not the health care system's, and not the doctor's.

Can the Present Health Care System Change?

In my opinion, changing the medical system toward natural and spiritual forms of healing that encourage more individual responsibility is impossible. The system can't change. It won't change. It must be replaced. There was a time for horses and buggies, but when automobiles came along people gave up their former ways of transportation. There is also a time to repair your car and keep it, and a time to discard it for a new one. The medical profession is a sophisticated machine but it rests on a fallacious foundation. Its philosophical basis is like a Model-T Ford stuck in the mud that can't move and won't change.

There is a time to repair the old car and a time to replace it. The current medical system is an old car, beyond repair, parked on a false foundation. It survives, not because it serves the good of humanity, but because it has become politically entrenched in our society. The time has come to remove its legal franchise and replace it by allowing alternative modalities to flourish free of the shackles placed upon them by allopathy's monopolistic intent.

Terry Friedmann, MD, in his book, *Freedom Through Health*, envisions a new holistic system to replace the current one that emphasizes personal responsibility and fosters cooperative relationships among many modalities with allopathy playing only a minor role. Dr. Friedmann's new health care model would include nutrition, exercise, stress management, and aromatherapy, to address the whole person—mentally, physically, emotionally, and spiritually. In their books, Robert Mendelsohn, MD, and Richard Gerber, MD, also foresee a new holistic medical paradigm— one not dependent on allopathic drugs and procedures as its primary focus.

The time has come to move on to paradigms and modalities based on different premises than those that underlie modern allopathy. Those of you who have opted out of the system in favor of essential oils and their physical, mental, emotional, and spiritual benefits are among the pioneers who are replacing the system.

As for those of you who have taken over-the-counter or prescriptions drugs over long periods of time, essential oils are your best friend because they can cleanse the residues of these toxins from your system once and for all and help restore your body back to its natural healthy state.

Key Points of Chapter Eleven

1. When a pharmaceutical drug's usual effects upon a patient are reduced, increased, or altered when taken with another drug, that is defined as a "drug interaction."

2. Adverse drug interactions are common and a major cause of sickness and death in the United States.

3. Adverse essential oil interactions are virtually unheard of and pose no threats to human wellbeing.

4. Since essential oils are biochemically active, the question arises as to whether there are adverse interactions between essential oils and pharmaceutical drugs when taken together.

5. In reviewing 29 references related to drugs and/or oils, 19 were found to be devoid of information on the topic of drug/oil interactions.

6. Most of those that did attempt to deal with the issue only offered speculations of theoretical interactions, mostly based on animal studies, perfume grade oil studies, or single component studies, without any hard data on human subjects to substantiate their concerns.

7. In references by the world's leading medical aromatherapists—Jean Valnet, MD, Daniel Penoel, MD, and Terry Friedmann, MD—only Valnet mentioned a possible drug/oil reaction. Valnet's only comment was that some oils can increase the effectiveness of antibiotics while others can inactivate them.

8. Some aromatherapists believe (erroneously) that essential oils can cause allergies, and mistake a detoxification reaction for an allergic one.

9. Insofar as drug/oil interactions happen or could possibly happen, there is no evidence so far to imply any significant adverse reactions between essential oils and allopathic drugs, which have been used together successfully without incident in some hospitals for many years.

10. As for essential oils interfering with or negating homeopathic remedies, the opinions of homeopaths at this time range from total prohibition of mixing the two modalities to unreserved applications of both.

11. As to whether to engage in homeopathy and aromatherapy simultaneously or separately is a choice individuals must make on their own. We recommend consulting God in the matter through prayer since he is the originator of both modalities.

12. The difference in male and female characteristics in humans lies in the balance among seven steroidal hormones—four androgens and three estrogens—all of which are present in both men and women. The structural and chemical differences in these compounds are only slight, but the differences in how they manifest is profound.

13. Synthetic estrogens, the ones marketed by drug companies and prescribed by doctors, all have adverse side effects.

14. Drug companies are not interested in marketing natural hormones because there is little profit in them. Natural hormones cannot be patented and do not create monopolies from which fortunes can be made.

15. Synthetic estrogens are often made from pregnant horse urine where the unfortunate mares are confined in inhumane conditions to collect their urine.

16. Many oils manifest hormonal properties in humans by imitating hormones, by stimulating hormonal receptor sites, and by stimulating our bodies to manufacture their own hormones, even using molecules of essential oils as raw materials.

17. The reason oils can heal and drugs don't is because our bodies were created to receive and make beneficial use of essential oils molecules, while synthetic drug molecules are strange and alien, and our bodies were not created to accept, metabolize, or make beneficial use of them.

18. The practice of medicine is more like a religion than it is like an applied science, but it is a false religion with a non-theistic foundation. Medical practice is based more on belief than on scientific fact, and the beliefs are more self-serving to the system rather than beneficial to the patient.

19. Emergency medicine is the best of allopathic medicine. It can save your life in a crisis, but as for healing, you need to find modalities other than allopathy for that.

20. The current health care system is an old car beyond repair. It cannot be fixed. It must be replaced. The time has come to disenfranchise the narrow monocular medical system we have, that offers few cures but mostly symptomatic treatments or disease management, and replace it with a pluralistic one of many modalities within which one can find true healing. The new system must be spiritually based, acknowledging and tapping into the only source of true healing, which is God.

21. Those who are using and learning about essential oils today are among the brave pioneers who are already replacing the old allopathic system with a better one.

♥ CHAPTER TWELVE
PRACTICAL ANSWERS TO
FREQUENTLY ASKED QUESTIONS

During the many times I have taught seminars on the chemistry of essential oils, certain questions seem to recur from class to class that need to be answered in this book. Rather than try to weave the answers into the general text of this book where they could be lost, I decided to just deal with them all right here, in the last chapter, just like I do in my classes. Customarily, I conclude all of my oil chemistry classes with a list of sixteen unrelated, miscellaneous topics, to wit. We will deal with each of these in the order given below.

1. Heat & Cold
2. Light
3. Air
4. Water
5. Adulteration
6. Shelf Life
7. BB Barrier
8. Skin
9. Allergies
10. X-rays
11. Plastic
12. Clockwise
13. Carrier Oils
14. Right Oils
15. More or Less
16. Oil Safety

1. Heat and Cold

To preserve an oil's chemical integrity, it only makes sense to store them in relatively cool places, like indoors away from sunlight and other sources of heat. The higher the temperature, the faster a chemical change can occur, if one is going to occur. It is a simple law of chemistry. Applying this idea to essential oils, one must distinguish between four kinds of oils that are called "essential."

(1) True essential oils are distilled and can either be a single species or a blend of species, all distilled. (2) Citrus oils are cold pressed or expressed from the rinds of the fruits and are called "essential oils," but technically they are not. They should be called "expressed oils." The properties and chemistry of expressed oils are not quite the

same as those that have been distilled. (3) Oils extracted by chemical solvents (not distilled or expressed) are called absolutes. These include jasmine, neroli, and onycha oils. Absolutes have physical and chemical properties of their own, different from expressed or distilled oils. (4) There are many blends that consist mostly of essential oils (70-90%), but also contain a fatty base like olive, almond, jojoba, coconut, wheat germ, grape seed, etc. We can call this category "carrier oil blends." The carrier oil blends formulated by British standards are 95-98% fatty base oil, but in North America such blends are usually mostly essential in content. Fatty oils are all expressed from seeds, never distilled.

True essential oils, expressed oils, absolutes, and carrier oil blends each have different responses to heat. Let me answer the question of heat separately for each of these four categories:

True Essential Oils and Heat

When it comes to pure distilled essential oils, either single species or blends of species, don't worry if such oils are temporarily exposed to hotter than normal temperatures. People often worry if their essential oils may have been damaged when they leave them in their car or van on a hot day and it gets to 110-140° F (45-60° C) inside the vehicle. They wonder whether the oils still have their therapeutic abilities or not. They don't know if they should still use them or throw them away for fear that they have been ruined.

My first response to such a query is to say, "If you have any oils that got hot in your car and you want to throw them away, please don't. Send them to me and I will pay you the postage." In other words, what I am saying is that unless you opened the bottles while they were hot, they are still as good as ever. Here's why.

The first thing to realize is this: True essential oils are the product of distillation at temperatures well above the boiling point of water (212°F or 100°C). In fact, they can come out of the still at temperatures of 240-260°F (115-125°C) and sometimes even higher. Hence, by the nature of the means of their separation from the plant, essential oils are high temperature substances. They are actually at home at high temperatures, more or less. In other words, the compounds of the oil are stable at those temperatures or else they would not have been able to survive the hot steam that lifted them from the plant.

While it is true that some plant oil compounds are altered by the heat of distillation, the resultant artifacts are also stable at those temperatures which is why they survive and remain in the finished oil. An example of this is the colorless sesquiterpene, matricene, found in the living plants of German chamomile, blue tansy, helichrysum, and yarrow. During the heat of distillation matricene is transformed into a transparent blue compound called chamazulene found in the extracted oils of these plants. (See Chapter Eight.)

It is also true that the flash points of some oils are between 100° and 140° F (38-60°C), which are temperatures that can be reached inside a closed vehicle on a hot day. Flash points are determined by slowly heating up an oil one degree at a time until a temperature is reached where a flash of fire results when a wand with a tiny flame at the tip is waved over the surface of the heated oil. What this procedure determines is the temperature of vaporization of the most volatile compounds of the oil.

When distilled aromatic oils are heated to the flash point in your car and confined to a tightly sealed bottle, the lightest oil components may temporarily separate, vaporizing within the bottle. However, as soon as the bottle is cooled down, these components condense, become liquid again, and remix with the rest of the oil, just as before, their chemical makeup unaltered,

Putting this bit of information into practice, means that if your oil bottles do get too warm, don't open them until they have cooled. Otherwise the lightest compounds may escape and upset the balance of your oil. Therefore, if your oils are left in a hot car, take them inside the house, and let them cool without removing any of the caps. Your oils will be just a good as new. Heat, up to a point, does not spoil the oil if its truly essential.

One can actually enjoy and benefit from essential oils by steam inhalation. Pour boiling water into a bowl. Add a few drops of your favorite oil or oils. Cover your head and the bowl with a towel, like a little tent, and breathe deeply.

Storing distilled essential oils at normal room temperatures is quite sufficient to preserve their quality indefinitely. Keeping them cooler than temperatures comfortable to you is not necessary, offers no advantages, and does not increase shelf life.

Expressed Oils and Heat

Expressed oils include all the citrus oils: bergamot, grapefruit. lemon, lime, mandarin, orange, and tangerine. Unlike true essential oils, expressed oils can be damaged by temperatures in excess of 100° F (38° C). Hence, they need to be kept in a cool place or at least stored at no higher than normal room temperatures. This includes blends of essential oils containing citrus components. While every compound in a true essential oil has passed through a high temperature process during its extraction, the compounds in an expressed oil have not been submitted to such temperatures and many of them will start breaking down with excessive heat.

To a great extent, this has to do with molecular size. The molecules in distilled oils are limited in size by the distillation process. A weight of 300 amu is about as heavy as they get. Among the terpenes, a diterpene or diterpenol (MW less than 300 amu) is usually the largest terpene you have in distilled oils. However, in expressed oils, you can get triterpenes and tetraterpenes, with molecular weights (MW) between 400 and 500 amu. Neither are there any proteins, amino acids, or polypeptides in essential oils, but in expressed oils there are traces of all of these. While the small volatile molecules of essential oils are not particularly bothered by temperatures under 200° F, the larger non-aromatic molecules in expressed oils are. They can start decomposing. As large molecules, they have little or no fragrance. When they break down into smaller molecules, due to the heat, they take on a variety of smells, most of which are unpleasant. We say "the oil has gone bad" or "has become rancid." Not only has their fragrance changed, but their therapeutic value has been reduced or destroyed. Refrigerating expressed oils can extend their shelf life for several years, but if you normally use up your oils within a year, you don't need refrigeration. Room temperature will do.

So keep your citrus oils, and any blends that contain them, in a reasonably cool place. Any temperature comfortable to you will be comfortable to them. Any temperature too hot for you will be too hot for them. A few of the popular blends of oil available commercially that contain citrus oils include: Citrus Fresh®, Joy®, Peace and Calming®, Inner Child®, Harmony®, Christmas Spirit®, and many others. Read your labels.

Absolutes and Heat

Aromatic oils extracted by chemical solvents are called absolutes. They include neroli, jasmine, and onycha. The reason these are not extracted by distillation is because their fragrant and therapeutic compounds are destroyed by heat. Unlike true essential oils, absolutes can be damaged by temperatures in excess of 90° F and are slightly more sensitive to high temperatures than expressed oils. Hence, they need to be kept in a cool place or at least stored at no higher than normal room temperatures. This includes blends of essential oils containing absolutes. While every compound in a true essential oil has passed through a high temperature process during its extraction, the compounds in an absolute oil have been obtained at relatively cool temperatures to maintain their delicate chemistry, which is easily destroyed by heat.

In expressed oils, this has to do with the large molecular sizes found in such oils, molecules that can break down to smaller, unpleasant smelling molecules. Absolutes also contain large molecules, since they have not passed through a distillation process that limits the molecular size of their components. Hence, they can degrade and decompose into undesirable fragrances with heat, like expressed oils. But the small molecules of absolutes are also degraded or destroyed by heat. So both the largest and the smallest molecules in an absolute can be deleteriously affected by heat, their aromas unfavorably altered and their therapeutic abilities compromised.

So keep your absolute oils, and any blends that contain them, in a reasonably cool place. In general, any temperature comfortable to you will be comfortable to them. Any temperature too hot for you will be too hot for them. If you are going to store them for more than a year, you can refrigerate them to be on the safe side. A few of the popular blends of oil available commercially that contain absolutes include: Awaken®, Chivalry®, Clarity®, Gentle Baby, ®, Forgiveness®, and Humility®. There are many others. Read your labels.

Carrier Blend Oils and Heat

Carrier blend oils contain true essential oils mixed with a fatty oil base. Popular base oils include almond, sesame seed, and olive. Carrier blend oils can be damaged by temperatures in excess of 100–130° F, depending on the type of fatty oil used as its base. This susceptibility to damage from heat is because of their fatty oil content, not because of their essential oil content. The fatty oils of a carrier blend are cold expressed from seed while the essential oil of a carrier bland are heat produced by steam distillation. Carrier blend oils need to be kept in a cool place or at least stored at no higher than normal room temperatures. Many compounds in a base oil will start breaking down with excessive heat.

This is mainly due to molecular size. The molecules of base oils are all larger than those of essential oils. Oils pressed from seed also contain proteins, polypeptides, and amino acids. Unless refrigerated, most of the molecules in a carrier oil will gradually decompose in time even without excessive heat. It is their nature to do so. Heat only accelerates the process. When fatty oil molecules break down into simpler compounds, they acquire undesirable tastes and odors. We say, "The oil has become rancid."

So keep your carrier blend oils in a reasonably cool place. Any temperature comfortable to you will be comfortable to them, although they will last longer if refrigerated.

Any temperature too hot for you will be too hot for them. A few of the popular blends of oil available commercially that contain carrier oils include: Acceptance®, Hope®, 3 Wise Men®, Exodus II®, SARA®, Valor®, and OrthoEase® There are many others. Read your labels.

Flames and Candles

While the temperatures inside of a car on a hot day won't damage a true essential oil, the heat of a candle will damage any oil. Here we are talking about 300-400°F (150-200°C). These temperatures are well above distillation temperatures and can cause much of the oil to decompose and even burn completely. Diffusers that operate by putting oils on a ceramic or metal tray with a candle flame or other heat source underneath will vaporize some of the oil intact, but will destroy most of it, including its therapeutic value. You may get aroma from such a device, but you won't get much therapy. Consider candles and flames as recreational aromatherapy, not a means for serious healing. If you are a candle maker and want to scent them with essential oils, buy cheap non-therapeutic oils. Save the good oils for healing. If you want to fill a room with an aroma with candle light, burn scentless candles while diffusing a good grade oil with a nebulizing diffuser.

Another thing about using heat to vaporize oils is that the most volatile compounds disperse into the air first with the heavier molecules coming later. Thus, you never receive the whole oil at one time in its natural balance.

In Biblical times, oils were diffused by means of censers (called incense burners). Censers are mentioned twenty times in the *Bible*. (cf. Numbers 16:46 or Revelation 8:3-5) Unlike candles, censers do not contain flames. They were metal or ceramic containers in which hot coals were placed in the bottom while the aromatic resins and oils were on a shelf several inches above where they were heated, vaporized, and dispersed. The oils and resins were not actually burned, even though the term "burning incense" was used.

The incenses of India, however, are actually burned. Such incenses are usually formed in sticks or tablets containing aromatic compounds mixed with solid materials that will smolder and glow like charcoal as it burns slowly, releasing the aroma in the smoke. This form of incense actually destroys much of the oil, but enough is vaporized to provide the desired scent.

While burning incense is not an ideal way to vaporize oils, it is not as destructive as a candle flame, and was an effective way to diffuse oils in ancient times before better technology was available, as we have today. (See the book, *Healing Oils of the Bible* for more on this.)

When it comes to fire, one must also keep in mind that essential oils are all inflammable. All oils will burn—essential and otherwise. Essential oils are neither explosive nor highly flammable, but in the presence of a flame, they can catch fire. They become dangerously flammable only if diluted with an alcohol, like methanol, ethanol, or propanol, as is done in some countries such as Taiwan.

Oils in Your Favorite Hot Beverages

Some people like to put a few drops of their favorite oil in their drinks—both cold and hot. Peppermint and cinnamon oils are favorites. Some routinely put a drop or two of an antiseptic oils (like clove or lemon) in their regular morning beverage as an immune system booster to stave off colds and flu.

Remember that one drop of an essential oil can represent the concentrated essence of a large volume of leaves or plant matter. So use sparingly. It has been said that a drop of peppermint equals the flavoring potency of more than twenty peppermint tea bags.

The question arises as to whether the heat in your drink could destroy some of the qualities of the oil. The answer is "No." The rule is this: If it is not too hot for you to drink, then it is not too hot for the oil either. However, when adding oils to a beverage in a pot heating over a stove, don't let it come to a boil. Otherwise you will lose some of the more volatile compounds in the oil and upset its balance. But don't worry if you forget and let it boil. Drink it anyway. No harm will be done.

Taking oils orally in hot drinks is good applied aromatherapy. You receive the benefits of the therapeutic molecules through the digestive tract, but you also enjoy the flavor and aroma, absorbing them directly through the sensitive tissues that line the mouth as well as through the nose, going straight to the lungs and brain. Try a drop of cinnamon or cassia in hot apple cider some time. You'll love it.

Before selecting an oil for flavoring your drinks, be sure they are pure therapeutic grade oils. Also check to see if they are rated by the U.S. Food and Drug Administration as

GRAS—"generally regarded as safe." Read the bottle labels or consult a book such as the *Essential Oil Desk Reference* or *Reference Guide to Essential Oils* for a list of GRAS oils. Always in aromatherapy, moderation and common sense should be exercised at all times.

Frozen Oils

We have talked about heat. What about cold? If your oils are delivered in cold weather and have been outside in the back of an unheated truck all day, some could arrive in a congealed, waxy, semi-solid state.

Not to worry. Even in the extreme, cold never hurt any oil—regardless of whether it is essential, expressed, absolute, or a carrier blend. If your oils are ever chilled to the freezing point, don't apply any heat to thaw them out. Keep the lids on and just let them warm up gradually to room temperature and they will be fine.

2. Light

Essential oils should always be kept in opaque containers or dark colored transparent bottles. In ancient Egypt and during Biblical times, essential oils were kept in alabaster boxes or jars of limestone, marble, and fired ceramics. They were usually sealed with a translucent or opaque layer of wax. Today most properly packaged essential oils are in dark amber (brown) or dark blue glass bottles. If you see an oil for sale advertised as "essential" in a clear white bottle, it is either a fraud (not a true essential oil) or the packager did not know any better and whatever essential oil may have been there has been long since destroyed by light.

The aroma and therapeutic value of an essential oil is made possible only because of the tiny size of the molecules. These are generally all less than 300 amu. Tiny molecules are aromatic because they are light enough to evaporate, get into the air, and enter our noses so we can smell them. Small molecules are therapeutic because they can penetrate skin and muscle tissue, pass through the blood-brain barrier, and even through cell membranes, addressing our ills at cellular levels right down to the DNA.

Polymerized Oils

Here is what happens to essential oils with long exposures to light. Light causes essential oil molecules to polymerize. Polymerization is a process by which small molecules join together to make larger molecules. Large molecules do not easily evaporate and have no aroma at room temperatures. Neither can they penetrate bodily tissues nor enter into cells. Large molecules have no therapeutic value like the small molecules of essential oils.

In other words, light will eventually destroy an essential oil, chemically altering it into a substance that is no longer of any value aromatically or therapeutically.

Now don't worry if your bottle tops are off for a while as you are doing a raindrop technique or if you blend one oil with another, temporarily exposing them to light. A few minutes, or even a few hours, of exposure to light won't substantially change the composition of your oils. We are talking about exposure to light over days, weeks, and months. That is what will destroy an essential oil.

3. Air

Extended exposure to air will cause an essential oil to oxidize. In other words, the molecules of the oil will take on extra oxygen atoms, which will change their chemistry and their therapeutic actions, perhaps destroying it altogether. For example, the main ingredient in all citrus oils (orange, grapefruit, lemon, etc.) is d-limonene—a monoterpene with a very faint fragrance of "citrus." Some say like orange. Some say like lime. In any case, it is not strong. When limonene is exposed to air for a long period of time, the most common thing it does is to evaporate. However, what does not evaporate can oxidize into another compound called limonene oxide which smells like turpentine.

You can readily see from the figure on the next page that as keys to open receptor sites and trigger cellular responses, d-limonene and limonene oxide would definitely fit different locks and cause different responses. Also note that a double bond in the ring has been lost, thus reducing the resonance energy of the molecule and, there-

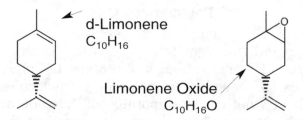

d-Limonene
$C_{10}H_{16}$

Limonene Oxide
$C_{10}H_{16}O$

by, its frequency. (See Chapter Six.) While d-limonene is thought to be a cancer fighter, the benefits of limonene oxide are dubious and unknown and certainly not the same as d-limonene.

How long does it take for a citrus oil to oxidize? I tried an experiment. I took a bottle with a little orange oil in the bottom, removed the lid, and removed the dropper cap. I let it sit for several months. It was at least a month before I could detect the turpentine-like scent of limonene oxide, and even then it was not very strong. It got stronger after two or three months. Meanwhile, the oil level in the bottle was going down as the volatile compounds evaporated. This illustrates a couple of points.

First of all, it takes a long exposure to air to chemically alter an oil. Secondly, the most damaging thing that happens to an oil exposed to air is not oxidation, but the loss of the most volatile components. This upsets the therapeutic balance of the oil and may result in the loss of the key ingredients.

You needn't be concerned about keeping your lids off too long under normal usage. First of all, most essential oil bottles not only have airtight caps, but they also have non-reactive plastic or Teflon® dropper caps that make it extremely difficult for any air to circulate into and out of the bottle even when the caps are off—even for extended periods of time, like overnight.

So don't worry about having your lids off for several minutes, or even for several hours, at a time. You aren't going to lose much by evaporation and as for oxidation, it isn't going to happen to any noticeable extent.

4. Water

The hydrocarbon components of an oil will not mix with water at all. Some float and some sink, but they don't mix. The hydrocarbons include alkanes, monoterpenes, sesquiterpenes, diterpenes, and triterpenes.

Some of the oxygenated hydrocarbons will mix with water to a limited extent, but generally do not react chemically (or very little) so that their compositional nature remains intact. Oxygenated hydrocarbons include phenols, phenylpropanoids, alcohols, ethers, aldehydes, ketones, carboxylic acids, esters, oxides, coumarins, lactones, and furanoids.

The only essential oil compounds that react chemically with water are acids, phenols, and esters. Acids will dissociate in water producing electrically charged hydrogen ions (H+), which carry a positive charge. Phenolic compounds can also dissociate in water like a weak acid, but only to a very minor extent. As for esters, we will discuss that in more detail later in this section.

Translated into simple terms, we are saying that if essential oils containing acidic or phenolic compounds are mixed with water, you may ionize some of the acids and phenols, changing the chemistry and, thus, the therapeutic action of the oil, but only slightly and undetectably.

As for acid reactions in water from acidic oil components, this will not be very important with most oils since carboxylic acids are not found in many oils beyond trace amounts. Furthermore, the ionization potential of the acids found in oils is low. In other words, they are always weak acids. Therefore, the therapeutic value of an oil containing carboxylic acids will not substantially change in contact with water.

Many oils contain phenolic compounds, but fortunately, the ionization of phenols in water is only slight, so not much is going to change when phenolic oils are in contact with water, but there will be some changes. Such changes will probably not materially alter the therapeutic value in the oil.

Let's Talk About Ester

When it comes to water, esters are something else. Esters are compounds that are the product of a chemical reaction between an alcohol and a carboxylic acid. (See Chapter Nine.) Stating it in the form of a chemical equation, the reaction is as follows:

a carboxylic acid + an alcohol $\rightarrow$ an ester + water

In the shorthand of chemistry, the arrow stands for the word "yields." Stated in a sentence, the above equation simply says that when you combine a carboxylic acid with an alcohol the blend can yield an ester with some water. This reaction can go both ways, depending on the thermodynamic parameters of the situation. Thus, we can also write the following equation:

an ester + water $\rightarrow$ a carboxylic acid + an alcohol

Reworded into a sentence, the equation just stated simply says that when you combine an ester with water the result can yield an acid and an alcohol.

Translating this into essential oil practice, it means that oils containing esters may be altered by contact with water, but not necessarily and not necessarily very much.

Most oils are not high in ester content and many contain only traces or no esters at all. However, a few oils are very high in esters. These include wintergreen (97%), birch (90%), Roman chamomile (65%), clary sage (64%), petitgrain (57%), lavandin (44%), helichrysum (43%), valerian (42%), lavender (39%), bergamot (37%), spruce (34%), and tsuga (33%). See Table Forty-One for a complete list.

I would not worry about any ester transformations in essential oils upon contact with water unless you are considering one of the oils high in esters, such as those listed above. The question of how water affects essential oils comes up in several contexts which we shall discuss next.

Bath Tubs and Drinking Water

People like to add drops of essential oils to their drinking water. This is generally no problem. Only the acids, phenols, and esters are potentially affected, but only in minor ways. Go right ahead. Any chemical changes that may occur won't significantly alter the benefits you will receive. Just be sure you are drinking from a non-reactive vessel like glass, ceramic, or stainless steel. Some oils dissolve plastic and styrofoam, as we will discuss later.

Some people like to add oils to their showers or bath tubs. There is really no problem here with water altering the chemistry of the oil, which would only be slight within the time you are bathing. The challenge is to add the oils to a bath in a way that concentrated droplets do not come into contact with sensitive areas of your body and cause unpleasant burning. It is best to combine the oil with a gel or with a solution of Epsom salts and pour the mixture under the running faucet so that the oil is dispersed throughout the bath, and not floating around in concentrated forms. Mixing aloe vera or a liquid bath soap in the tub before adding the oil also works to emulsify and disperse it harmlessly throughout the bath water. Instructions for adding oils to baths are given in the *Essential Oils Desk Reference* and in the *Reference Guide to Essential Oils*, listed in the bibliography.

When adding to a hot tub or bath, choose your oils carefully. Hot oils like peppermint, oregano, or cinnamon could result in an unpleasant experience. Use common sense.

Using oils in a hot bath or whirlpool allows your body to absorb them through the skin as well as through their fragrance. Soaking in a hot tub with a few drops of eucalyptus, or one of the other oils high in 1,8 cineole, is a good way to get relief from the aches and congestion of a cold, sinusitis, bronchitis, or the flu. (See Tables 26 or 62.)

Diffusers

Another context of bringing essential oils in contact with water has to do with diffusers. Some inexpensive aromatic oil diffusers operate by floating the oils on a water surface in a tray with a fan that blows through to disperse the oils into the air. While some chemical alterations in your acids, phenols, and esters may take place with such a diffuser, that won't be the most serious problem. The problem with a fan-powered evaporation type diffuser is that the lightest compounds blow off before the heavier ones. You never get the whole oil into the air at the same time. Thus, the balance of ingredients contained in the oil in its liquid form is never maintained in the vapor that results from a water-type diffuser. You should also know that some essential oils are denser than water and do not float. Cinnamon and cassia oils are examples of this.

The best diffusers are called "nebulizing diffusers" and employ unheated air at room temperature. This type of diffuser operates on the principle of "atomization." When oils are forced through a pinhole by a high pressure stream of air, when it bursts through the opening into the atmosphere, the oil explodes into billions of droplets so tiny that they consist of only a few molecules each. The resulting oil vapor contains all of the ingredients of the oil in the same balance as it was in liquid form, before it was atomized. Thus, you get all of the oil components in a highly vaporized form that maximizes its effectiveness and benefits. Since nebulizing diffusers use neither heat nor water, none of the potential problems associated with heat and water exist for this form of diffusion.

There is another beneficial aspect of atomizing type diffusers that other types of diffusers do not offer. Spraying of the oil at high velocity through the nebulizing nozzle actually energizes the oil, raises the levels of oxygen carried by the molecules, and increases its frequency. Thus, the healing potential of the oil is increased and raised to a higher level. Nebulizing diffusers are normally more expensive than some other types, but the difference in cost is well worth it for what you receive.

5. Adulteration

Exodus 20:14 says, "Thou shalt not commit adultery." Of course, neither God nor Moses were thinking of essential oils when these words were committed to writing. But the commandment does bear a meaning for essential oils. The composition of a true therapeutic grade essential oil is not an act of humankind. It is an act of God. We do not control it. God controls it through the plants. All we can do is to distill it as gently as we can, without chemical solvents, at minimum temperatures, and at atmospheric pressures in order to preserve the oil as closely as it was contained in the living plant.

Essential oils contain more than chemistry. They contain life force, which is preserved when extracted properly. The therapeutic value of the oils depends on this life force which depends on maintaining the balance of ingredients that were there in the plant and which pass through distillation. When you add anything but a neutral carrier or another essential oil to a therapeutic grade essential oil, you rarely improve its therapeutic value. You usually degrade it to one extent or another. If you add natural ingredients in order to increase the percent of a desirable compound, you upset the natural balance and reduce the healing properties. If you add a synthetic ingredient, you poison the oil and damage or kill its life force. Adding anything to an essential oil other than a neutral base oil or another essential oil is called "adulteration," and you know what the *Bible* says about adultery.

On the other hand, you need to know what the U.S. Food & Drug Administration (FDA) says about adultery. FDA regulations allow a company to label its oils as "100% pure" so long as they contain at least 5% of the actual oil alleged to be in the bottle. Think about that the next time you see a Brand X oil with 100% pure on its label. Some 100% brands really are pure. Others are not. You can smell the difference.

6. Shelf Life

People who use adulterated or synthetic oils worry about shelf life. Some British references on aromatherapy say one should throw away their oils every six months and purchase a fresh quantity. Such advice may be valid for certain carrier blend oils, but is not valid for pure unadulterated aromatic oils that are the products of distillation.

In order to discuss shelf life, you need to distinguish among various classes of scented oils. In Section 1 (*Heat and Cold*) of this chapter, we describe four types of fragrant oils: (1) Essential (distilled). (2) Expressed (usually citrus); (2) Absolutes (solvent extractions); and (4) Carrier Blend Oils (essential oils in a fatty base). The shelf lives of these classes of aromatic oils are different. While expressed, absolute, and carrier blend oils contain large molecules along with their small aromatic ones, pure essential oils obtained entirely by distillation contain only small molecules.

Large molecules tend to be less stable than small ones. Shelf life addresses the question of chemical stability. Aromatic oils are mixtures of many compounds. If a mixture of compounds remains stable, that is, if it does not decompose or change its chemistry over a long period of time in storage, we say it has a long shelf life.

If you are using pure distilled therapeutic grade essential oils, as described in Chapter Two of this book, then you don't have to worry about shelf life. Essential oils have been found in Egyptian tombs that were still aromatic and effective—their therapeutic properties intact— even after thousands of years. These oils were in moderately cool, dark places tightly sealed from exposure to air and the elements. That is all they required to maintain their potency. No one knows what their true shelf life may be. All we know is that it is measured in millennia, not months.

As for the British oils, there is a so called "aromatherapy grade" of oil that is actually only 1-5% essential oil dissolved in a fatty base oil. The large molecules of fatty vegetable oils are not as stable as the tiny ones that comprise essential oils. Fatty oils also contain proteins, polypeptides, and amino acids—unstable compounds not found in essential oils. Fatty oils can naturally break down into smaller molecules over time at normal room temperatures. We call this "going rancid." While large molecules have no smell, the smaller molecules resulting from the decomposition of fatty hydrocarbons do have a smell—an unpleasant one. Hence, an aromatherapy grade oil that is mostly vegetable oil does have a shelf life. Thus, the British texts that recommend pitching your oils every six months have a valid point in reference to "aromatherapy grade" oils.

A number of blends containing pure essential oils used in North America also contain some fatty oil such as olive, sesame seed, or almond. However, these blends consist of 80% or more of essential oils. These are not the same as the aromatherapy grade massage oils of England which are mostly fatty, but they do have a shelf life.

Expressed oils, absolutes, and carrier blend oils are sensitive to heat, such as in a car on a hot day. Heat accelerates any chemical reaction and if the large molecules in these oils are prone to gradual decomposition even at normal temperatures, this process will be hastened by heat. You can tell if any damage has been done to your oils by heat by testing the fragrance. If it still smells the same as when you bought it, it is still okay. If not, then damage has occurred. Exposure to heat in excess of 90-130° F can shorten the shelf life of expressed, absolute, and carrier blend oils, but does not shorten the shelf life of true essential oils. (See section on *Heat and Cold* at the beginning of this chapter for a more thorough discussion on the effects of temperature on oils.)

Absolutes, expressed oils, and oil blends that are mostly essential and only partly fatty all have a shelf life. Experience has shown that their shelf lives can be measured in years, unless the oil has been exposed to excessive heat. So if you have any such oils, your nose will know if they go bad. If you want to extend their shelf life, refrigerate them. However, if you are using such oils over periods of less than a few months, you don't need to go to the trouble of storing them in your refrigerator.

You don't have to refrigerate pure essential oils that are the products of distillation. Refrigeration does not extend their shelf life. A cool environment won't hurt them or help them. They will last indefinitely at normal living temperatures and will remain unaffected and intact even when occasionally exposed to the heat of a hot day in a car.

If anyone asks you about the shelf life of a pure therapeutic grade essential oil, just say, "5,000 years at least." If they ask you about the shelf life of an oil that has been expressed, solvent extracted, or mixed with a fatty base, just say, "It depends."

7. Blood-Brain Barrier

The "blood-brain barrier" is somewhat of a misnomer. It is more like a sieve than a barrier. Any molecule less than 500 amu in weight and relatively compact in size and shape can get through, provided it is lipid soluble. All hydrocarbons and most oxygenated hydrocarbons are lipid soluble. "Lipid soluble" means that the substance will dissolve in oil. Essential oils will always dissolve in another oil and are, hence, lipid soluble.

As for size, some fatty oil molecules are light in weight, like caprylic acid (M.W. = 144 amu) and lauric acid (M.W. = 200 amu), which are comparable to the weights of monoterpenes (136 amu) and sesquiterpenes (204 amu). Yet these fatty oil molecules do not pass through the blood-brain barrier while monoterpenes and sesquiterpenes do. The difference is in their structural shapes. Compare the shapes of monoterpenes and sesquiterpenes depicted in Tables Fourteen and Fifteen in Chapter Nine with the shapes of fatty molecules shown in the Table entitled "Shapes of Fatty Molecules" in Chapter Two. Essential oil molecules are compact in shape, almost always containing rings while fatty molecules come in long chains with no rings. Even the acyclic essential oil molecules (i.e. those without rings) come in bent chains that conform to the outlines of rings. Thus, essential oil molecules are condensed in size while fatty molecules are strung out and long. All oil molecules (fatty or essential) are lipid soluble but even when fatty molecules are relatively light weight (of the order of essential molecules), they are still not volatile and aromatic and do not penetrate the blood-brain barrier because of their long structure. (See pp. 56 & 288.)

The human skin possesses similar screening capabilities as our brain. The skin is a barrier also, but a barrier like a sieve that passes only molecules less than a certain weight and size and are soluble in oils. All essential oils pass easily through the skin and can penetrate into deep tissues all the way into the cells, themselves. Fatty oils do not because of their long shapes, even when their weights are not great. (See p. 56.)

The screening mechanisms of the brain and the skin are not exactly alike. Those of the brain involve osmotic potentials across cell membranes which, in some cases, can actually allow controlled numbers of water molecules (which are not lipid soluble) to pass through. By contrast, the skin has a layer of flattened, dead cells impregnated with oily-waxy compounds that repel water. Brain cells can also regulate the passage of various molecules by their receptor sites. But this is getting beyond where we want to go in this book where we want to keep things simple.

Basically, you can just say "If it will pass through skin,

it will pass through the blood-brain barrier and if it will not pass through the skin, neither can it enter the brain."

It is a good thing that the skin and brain pose protective barriers that are selective in the size, shape, and chemical nature of the molecules they will pass. For example, water (H_2O) is an extremely tiny molecule—only 18 amu in size. By comparison, even the smallest oil molecules are usually at least 100 amu in weight. So what keeps water from penetrating our brains and soaking into our bodies through the skin as easily as essential oils? Water molecules are certainly small enough in weight and size. The answer is in water's lack of lipid solubility.

Water does not mix with oil and will not dissolve in it. This is a fortunate fact. If molecular size were all there were to our brain and skin barriers, then every time we took a shower or soaked in a bath tub, we'd swell up like a sponge. We could get soaked in a rain and look like a blimp. And every time we took a breath of damp air, water molecules would pass through our nasal passages and accumulate in our brains. Too much water on the brain is not a good thing.

The beauty of essential oils being able to pass through the blood-brain barrier is in the benefits they provide physically, mentally, emotionally, hormonally, and spiritually. The fact that they pass through skin is also a wonderful attribute that provides them access to any part of the body by mere massage and anointment.

It must be remembered, however, that many harmful substances can also penetrate through the skin and into the brain. The two-fold criteria for passage are molecular size and lipid solubility. There are hundreds of toxic substances that qualify—including gasoline and many cleaning solvents, pesticides, or herbicides. These are all various forms of hydrocarbons (usually petrochemicals). Many of them are composed of molecules small enough in size and weight to penetrate skin and brain tissue.

Remember that essential oils can be helpful in detoxifying us from such substances should we come into contact with them and absorb some of their malicious molecules.

Essential oil molecules can penetrate into the tissues of our bodies that store such toxins and remove them, allowing them to leave the body through the kidneys, colon, respiration, and sweat.

8. Skin

In the application of essential oils to the skin, the chemistry of the oils is altered by the chemistry of the person. Women know that you can't tell what a perfume is going to smell like on a body when simply sniffed from a bottle. One must apply it to their own particular skin and then sample the fragrance. The resultant odor will be a chemical combination of the perfume and its reaction to the substances in and on your skin. A perfume that smells great on one person may smell yucky on another, depending on their individual chemistry.

Here is one reason why. The sweat glands of our bodies bring waste products to the surface which are eventually washed away when we bathe or shower. These are usually proteins or decompositional byproducts of proteins. The compounds of essential oils can react with these substances, changing the fragrance. These chemical reactions can also alter some of the constituents that pass through the skin into the body. Since no two people have identical bodies or identical chemistry, essential oils may not have the same effects on different people.

The therapeutic effects of an essential oil are a combination of the chemistry of the oil and the chemistry of the person receiving the oil. This is one reason different oils work (or don't work) for different people. This is why the intelligent application of essential oils require some experimentation on the part of the individual applying the oil.

Whereas experimentation on your own with pharmaceutical drugs would be dangerous, fortunately, experimentation with essential oils is safe enough for anyone who simply applies a little common sense and goes to no extreme. While skin effects can unpredictably alter some oil compounds as they pass through into the body or evaporate as aromas in the air, the ultimate test of efficacy is whether the oil's application caused a discernable therapeutic benefit or resulted in a pleasant perfume.

9. Allergies

Occasionally, a person receiving essential oils claims to have had an allergic reaction to them, but this is almost never the case. Such claims are most often based on a faulty understanding of what constitutes an allergy. It is common for people to jump to the conclusion that any untoward reaction to a substance, like an oil, is an allergy, when most of the time the reaction is something else. While some people occasionally react in an unpleasant manner to the application of an essential oil, usually in the form of a burning sensation or a skin rash, such a reaction is almost always one of three other things: 1. A detoxification response, 2. Inflammation from chemical irritation to tender skin, or 3. Manifestation of an emotional issue. Allergies can manifest with the same symptoms as any these three, but are of a different origen and etiology. Allergies tend to be permanent, even for a lifetime, while three non-allergenic reactions mentiioned above are temporary. In fact, they are usually therapeutic (e.g. a detox), indicating the initiation of a cleansing, healing process.

First, let's talk about what an allergy actually is. *Mosby's Medical Dictionary*, 6th edition, (2002) defines an allergic reaction as "an unfavorable physiological response to a substance (called an allergen) to which a person has previously been exposed and to which the person has developed antibodies." An allergen is defined as "a substance, which may not be intrinsically harmful, that can produce a hypersensitive reaction in the body."

Therefore, there are three requirements for an oil to cause an allergic reaction: (1) The person must have been previously exposed to that oil; (2) That person must have developed antibodies for certain compounds contained in that particular oil; and (3) there must be a hypersensitive reaction upon subsequent exposures to that oil. Is this possible? We shall see.

Substances that cause allergies are called "allergens," and are said to be "allergenic." Allergens to one person may not be allergens to another. Some people are allergic to many things while others seem to be allergic to nothing. Almost all allergens are proteins or polypeptides, both of which are large molecules composed of amino acids. All organisms, living or dead, are built from proteins and polypeptides. Thus, any life form could become an allergenic source to you—including your pet, a favorite food, certain fabrics, and/or even your own spouse or children.

Essential oils, however, contain no proteins or polypeptides and, thus, are virtually free of potential allergens. In fact, one can be allergic to an oil-yielding plant, like fennel, geranium, or goldenrod, but have no allergy to the essential oil distilled from that plant, since volatile oils contains none of the plant proteins, peptides, or amino acids that are the principle sources of allergic reactions in the plant. The molecules of proteins and polypeptides are too large to pass through the distillation process of a pure essential oil.

However, an oil pressed from seeds (vegetable oils), or one cold expressed from rinds (citrus oils), or absolutes, which are oils obtained by solvents (like jasmine, onycha, or neroli), can be allergenic. Unlike distilled essential oils, pressed, expressed, or solvent-obtained oils can contain traces of proteins and polypeptides. For example, some people are allergic to an oil blend called Valor® which contains oils of spruce, rosewood, blue tansy, and frankincense in an almond oil base. Their allergy is not to the essential oil content of that blend, but to the almond seed carrier, which is a fatty oil.

We used to say that allergies to a distillled essential oil are impossible, but in this edition of the book, we have had to modify that statement somewhat. Read on.

The Most Common Allergens

The most common allergens come from pollen, animal dander, feathers, vaccines, insect bites, bee or wasp venom, antibiotics, pharmaceuticals, and various foods—almost all of which involve proteins and/or polypeptides. Vaccines are particularly prone to cause allergies since they are usually composed of several alien proteins and are designed to produce an antibody reaction in the body. House dust is also a common allergen because of the proteins and amino acids of mites, microbes, pollen, viruses, fungi, mold, insects, mice droppings, and other biological substances in the dust.

Most allergens are harmless substances to most people and some may be toxic to one degree or another (like insect venom). However, it is not toxicity that makes an allergen. Allergic reactions are entirely different than and independent of toxic reactions. A substance can be both toxic and allergenic, to which the body will have two responses, both different and both originating from different mechanisms in the body. Most allergies are in response to good, wholesome things like bread, milk, blueberries, chocolate, pizza, seafood, kittens, puppies, and apple pie which have no inherent toxicities. Exposure to an allergen may be by inhalation, skin contact, hypodermic injection, stings, bites, ingestion of food or drink, or by intake of certain medicines or prescription drugs. Skin contact can be something as seemingly harmless as the use of latex rubber products which contain proteins. This includes some condoms and many hospital items such as latex gloves, catheters, tubing for respiratory equipment, and enema tips.

Allergic reactions can range from mild to deadly. Mild reactions include sneezing, runny noses, sinus congestion, watery eyes, headaches, skin rashes, itching, and hives. More severe reactions include asthma, profuse sweating, weakness, shortness of breath, diarrhea, nausea, acute dermatitis (with skin lesions and blistering), irregular heartbeat (arrhythmia), inflammation of the tissues around the eyes (conjuctivitis), swelling of the face and neck (angioedema), and bronchial spasms. Anaphylactic shock is a potentially fatal reaction, which is preceded by many of the foregoing symptoms, It can end by complete respiratory failure, suffocation, and death.

Allergies are among the most misunderstood of maladies, not only by the public in general, but among medical professionals as well. This is because the symptoms of an allergy can be so easily mistaken for something else, while something else can be mistaken for an allergy.

It is not God's plan that allergies should happen. Allergies are malfunctions of the immune system for which allopathic medicine has no cures. The current medical approach is to identify the allergens and prescribe a regimen of avoidance, and/or prescribe drugs that suppress the symptoms, without addressing the actual problem. Solving the problem involves getting at the root cause and making corrections at that level, which, for allergies, requires a psychosomatic approach.

The Spiritual Roots of Allergies

Most of the time, there are emotional or spiritual roots underlying a person's hypersensitivities to particular substances that manifest as true allergies or allergic-like reactions. In Chapter Seven we talked about interleukin 2. Interleukin 2 is a cytokine, a special type of ligand—a molecule that carries information between cells. Interleukin 2 enables the immune system to distinguish good proteins from bad ones. Without adequate secretions of interleukin 2, the immune system will mistake harmless substances for harmful ones resulting in allergy-like reactions. Interleukin 2 levels rise or fall depending on one's emotional state. A chronically negative emotional state, such as fear, anxiety, or unresolved grief, depresses interleukin 2 production and, thus, compromises immune function. This leads to mistakes on the part of the immune system, at cellular levels, that manifest as allergy-like symptoms. This is expressed in the *Old Testament* as follows:

> A merry heart does good like a medicine: but a broken spirit dries up the bones.   Proverbs 17:22

A habitually negative mental state damages your immune system and can lead to a host of different autoimmune diseases including allergies and other types of environmental sensitivities. In Biblical language, it says "a broken spirit dries up the bones." The marrow of your bones is where the white corpuscles and antibodies of your immune system are produced. For example, intense unresolved grief can cause extreme sensitivity to everything, turning a person into a "universal responder" or someone afflicted with "environmental illness syndrome" (EIS) or "Extreme Chemical Sensitivity" (ECS). Such people can become so sick that they react to nearly everything. Such people may not be able to wear clothes, touch a pet or another human being, eat most foods, or even come into contact with pure therapeutic grade essential oils. What they suffer is not a true allergy, but is an immune dysfuction mimicking an allergy. It is a case where the person is emotionally, mentally, and physically rejecting the world and everything in it over one's grief.

The solution is to recognize the problem, accept responsibility for creating it, resolve the grief, correct the depressed state, replace it with "a merry heart," and accept God's world as being good. Many essential oils are emotionally releasing and, accompanied with spiritual counsel, can help get to the roots and resolve the problem. Many oils are mood elevating, promoting a peaceful, happy state of mind. The Bible refers to "oils of joy," "oils of gladness," and "oils that make the heart glad," in Psalm 45:7-8; Proverbs 27:9; Isaiah 61:3; and Hebrews 1:9. Biblical oils known to "rejoice the heart" are frankincense, myrrh, cedarwood, cassia, and aloes (sandalwood).

Since essential oils can address issues at both emotional and cellular levels, you can understand why many people testify that their allergies or sensitivities have disappeared after they began using oils on a regular basis. Thus, rather than essential oils being a cause of allergies, they can actually help to resolve allergic sensitivities, at both their physical and emotional roots, and make them go away.

How the Immune System Works

There are hundreds of autoimmune diseases. Allergies are just one of them. No one inherits an allergy and no one is born with an allergy unless it was acquired in the womb late in pregnancy. Allergies are all acquired. An allergy is the immune system gone wrong. To know how we acquire allergies, you need a basic idea of how the immune system works.

One function of our immune system is to distinguish entities within our bodies that are "us" or "not us" and to recognize agents that are "friendly" or "unfriendly." Once an alien or hostile entity is identified, the immune system kills it, neutralizes it, and/or removes it from the body.

For living entities to be recognized as "not us" would include certain bacteria, viruses, fungi, parasites, tumors, and cancer cells. There are also good bacteria that our bodies need to function properly. It is crucial that the immune system be able to tell the good guys from the bad guys.

For non-living agents to be recognized as unfriendly would include foreign proteins and polypeptides, as well as some toxins and certain types of phenols, including some found in essential oils. Since we take in proteins, polypeptides, and phenols every day in our food and drink, it is vital that the immune system be able to accurately distinguish friends from foes.

We have two kinds of immunity: (1) Innate or nonspecific immunity; and (2) Acquired or specific immunity. We are born with certain innate immune capabilities which consist of two kinds of cells: (1) Phagocytes; and (2) Natural Killers. There are a variety of phagocytes, all of which are programmed to recognize alien or hostile entities. Their job is to eat them—like a little PAC-MAN®. Macrophages, a type of phagocyte, can be seen under a microscope as big blobs drifting around. They wrap around and engulf enemy agents and toxic particles when they find them—digesting or smothering them to death. Natural killer (NK) cells are programmed to destroy tumors, cancer cells, some microorganisms, and cells infected with viruses. Phagocytes and NK cells are generic fighters whose programming, skills, and techniques do not change over a lifetime. They are effective only up to a point. Here is where the other kind of immunity becomes necessary.

Specific immunity comes from the white blood corpuscles (lymphocytes) where cells learn to recognize specific alien or hostile entities for which they create special fighter cells specifically designed to attack and destroy that entity with a uniquely designed protein, called an antibody. These special cells are called "antibody producers." They can replicate themselves, along with their specialized antibody weapons, any time the body is invaded by the specific alien for which they are designed.

There are two types of lymphocytes (antibody producers): (1) B-cells; and (2) T-cells. B-cells are produced and educated in the bone marrow from which they are dispatched to roam throughout the body in search of enemy agents. B-cells also congregate in the nodes of the lymphatic system, The "B" in "B-cell" comes from "Bone." T-cells are also produced in the bone marrow, but are sent to the thymus gland where they complete their education and training. When necessary, they are deployed from the thymus gland to fight invaders. The "T" in "T-cell" comes from "Thymus."

Some essential oils, such as cypress (*Cupressus sempervirens*) and lemon (*Citrus limon*) may stimulate lymphocyte production and thereby boost our immune systems. While white corpuscles circulate with the red corpuscles of the blood, they reside principally in the lymphatic fluid which is where they get their first name, "Lympho." (Their last name, "Cyte," just means "cell.")

Unlike phagocytes and NK cells, B-cells, and T-cells can learn, adapt, and remember. All four of these are called "immune cells," but they don't all perform in the same ways. The phagocytes and NK cells are like security guards and policemen with restricted training and limited functions. They are on the prowl 24-hours a day, guarding us, protecting us, taking unruly and criminal entities into custody, and ushering them out of our bodies—dead or alive. B and T-cells comprise the military troops and leaders of our immune systems. They gather intelligence, prepare battle plans for present and future activation, and execute them.

Antibodies vs. Antibiotics

Don't confuse the term "antibody" with "antibiotic." To clarify this, a point for point comparison is given below:

(1) **Antibiotics** are produced outside of our bodies by laboratories and drug companies. (2) Antibiotics are antimicrobial agents that can destroy or interfere with the development of a living organism, but are not specific to a particular entity. (3) Antibiotics deal with living microorganisms only. (4) Each antibiotic is designed to deal with a spectrum of microbes, not just one. (5) Antibiotics are not living entities and have no reproductive capability.

(1) **Antibodies** are produced within our bodies by our own immune systems. (2) Antibodies are designer proteins on the surfaces of lymphocytes precisely tailored to combat specific entities (called antigens) identified as potentially harmful. (3) Antibodies deal with both living microbes and non-living substances (usually alien proteins). (4) Each antibody is designed to deal with only one antigen, not a spectrum. (5) Antibodies are produced by living cells with reproductive capability.

How White Corpuscles Work

When alien entities find their way into our bodies, they first encounter the phagocytes and natural killer (NK) cells. These two can control the situation most of the time. When the things get too much for them, they call in the elite troops, the Green Berets (viz. B-cells and T-cells).

The way lymphocytes (white corpuscles) work is this. When a foreigner is spotted, they sit him, her, or it down and obtain a complete history—including fingerprints, ID photos, genetic identity codes, and the works. In the language of lymphocytes, the general term they use for a foreigner is "antigen."

When an antigen enters the body, the lymphocytes quickly check their records to see if they already have a profile of this character on file. If they do, they pull out the battle plan already developed to deal with this foreigner, execute the plan, and get rid of the invader. The preformulated plan on file for a specific antigen is stored in the form of an "antibody" containing all the information on that specific alien, including how to kill it and eliminate it by attacking and disabling its software in its genetic code.

Antibodies are specialized proteins or polypeptide chains on the surfaces of white corpuscles, created as specialized weapons to destroy or neutralize specific antigens. When an army of foreigners (like a brigade of measles viruses, for example) invades your body, once identified, the antibody producing cells assigned to that specific antigen begin to multiply rapidly and proliferate copies of themselves in numbers sufficient to meet the size of the invading force. Thus, the army of trespassers is confronted with an opposing army of lymphocytic clones armed with antibody weapons that know all about them in detail, including their genetic weaknesses, which they will use to defeat them.

When a new antigen enters the body and the lymphocytes find no previous record of it, they arrest the stranger, interrogate it, and use the information obtained to design and create an antibody they can use to recognize and destroy it the next time one of its kind appears. Lymphocytic copies of that antibody then remain permanently on file, with the memory of this encounter.

Antibody-carrying B- and T-cells remain on standby duty, like National Guard or Reserve Units, until needed. The next time an antigen of that type comes to town, the specific B- or T-cell assigned to deal with it is instantly reactivated to deploy an effective defense of cloned soldiers (white cells) armed with tools (antibodies) designed to defeat the enemy. The battle between an antigen and an antibody is called an "antigen–antibody reaction." The process in which an antibody is first created for a specific antigen is called "sensitization." In the case of bacterial or viral antigens, the process of sensitization is also called "immunization," which may be natural or by vaccination.

We acquire natural immunities throughout all of our lives by this process. It is awesome to recognize the presence of so many well trained battalions of vigilant, intelligent soldier-protectors God has provided within our own bodies to preserve our health. So long as our immune system functions as God intended, we remain well. God's benevolent consciousness and intelligence is in our lymphocytes. When it fails, we become sick. Our immune systems fail when our contact with God has been compromised and the flow of his intelligent direction has been interrupted. Herein lies the spiritual roots of physical disease, including allergies.

How Allergies are Acquired

Allergies are acquired, not inherited. They do not transmit through the genes. Allergies are due to a malfunction of the immune system at the point of sensitization and, later, at the point of an antigen-antibody reaction. Almost all allergies have to do with proteins and/or polypeptides, but in some instances can be phenollic compounds. tThe immune system selects some of these to be labeled as antigens—"foreign" and/or "hostile." In the case of allergies, most of the time, the protein, polypeptide, or phenol is actually harmless, even beneficial, and should never have been identified as an enemy antigen. Hence, the immune system has made a mistake in labeling it as something to attack. When the immune system creates an antibody specific for that particular substance, we say that person has been "sensitized" to it for a future allergic reaction.

Because a person carries no antibodies for any newly contacted substance, there can be no antigen-antibody reaction with the first encounter. That comes later with the second and subsequent encounters. A person does not know they have acquired an allergy until the second or third time they make contact because, until then, they will have had no discernable reactions. However, inside of their bodies, ever since sensitization with their first exposure, they are carrying specific antibodies for the sensitizing substance. It could be years before they encounter that substance again. It doesn't matter how long. When the substance enters the body a second time, the ever vigilant antibodies, whose sole purpose for existence is to deal with that specific substance, will see it, remember it, recognize it, and mobilize their battle plan against it.

A normal antigen-antibody reaction would be no problem, if that is what would happen. The antibody cells would simply seek out the foreign protein molecules, neutralize them, and eliminate them. But an allergic reaction is not normal. An allergic reaction is when the antigen-antibody reaction is inappropriately intense, causing the person to suffer. A hypersensitive, inappropriately extreme reaction is an immune system gone out of control.

Therefore, an allergy consists of two mistakes on the part of our immune systems: (1) Misidentification of a harmless substance as an enemy; and (2) Overreaction upon subsequent contacts with that substance. If the immune system had been operating properly, it would have simply let the digestive system or the phagocytes take care of the foreign substance. With an allergy, there was never a true need to call in the military superbrains (lymphocytes) to create a customized weapon. Furthermore, there is never any justification for pulling out the computerized smart bombs (antibodies) and high powered artillery to unleash maximum force in an extreme response.

When the immune system misidentifies a substance as an antigen, that substance is called an "allergen." When an immune response to an allergen goes beyond a normal antigen-antibody reaction, becoming hypersensitive and extreme. it is called an "allergic reaction."

That is how allergies are acquired. Allergens are not the cause of allergies. Allergens are only the triggers. The cause is a problem in the immune system which usually has its origins in ones mind, emotions, and/or spirit which can only be corrected emotionally and spiritually. For many people, just being around essential oils on a daily basis, breathing them and applying them topically, has caused their allergies to permanently disappear.

There are some allopathic physicians who are beginning to recognize the connection between feelings and physical maladies such as allergies. They are developing a new science called psycho-neuro-immunology. Since essential oils are such excellent facilitators of emotional releasing and spiritual healing, we suggest that doctors could hasten their research and dramatically increase their understanding of psycho-neuro-immunology if they experimented with essential oils.

There is a book entitled, *A More Excellent Way,* by Henry Wright, that elaborates on the spiritual roots of allergies and relates everything to scripture. Pastor Wright's ministry from a church in Thomaston, Georgia, has brought about the healing of many people of their allergies and chemical sensitivities. You can contact them via email at info@beinhealth.com or via phone at 706-646-2074 or 800-453-5775. Their web site is www.beinhealth.com.

At this time, Pastor Wright does not use essential oils in his healing ministry, but he does understand the spiritual roots of disease and how to apply that understanding to bring about healing. If he were to include anointing with essential oils into his mission, he could experience even greater success in his ministry.

The Nature of Allergens

The original question we have been leading up to is whether or not one can have an allergic reaction to an essential oil. The question boils down to whether or not an essential oil can be an allergen.

Many essential oils contain phenolic compounds, and phenols can sometimes be allergens. The vast majority of allergens are proteins and/or polypeptides, both of which are composed of amino acids which all contain nitrogen as an essential element. Phenols contain no nitrogen. Protein and polypeptide molecules are also quite large compared to essential oil molecules. In fact, they are typically 100 to 1,000 times larger in both weight and size.

When nitrogen-free molecules are allergens, such as some phenols, they are larger than the average molecules found in essential oils. The molecular weights of 99% of the compounds in aromatic oils range from 100 to 300 amu. They are also structured in compact shapes and sizes, usually involving one or more rings. Allergens that do not contain nitrogen often incorporate large carbon chains, much longer than any found in essential oils.

The nature of allergens can be summarized as follows: (1) Allergens are almost always proteins or polypeptides which are large nitrogenous molecules. (2) In rare cases allergens contain no nitrogen, such as some phenols, but they are usually comprised of molecules that are heavier and larger than those found in essential oils, like toxicodendrol an allergenic phenol found in poison ivy. (see pp. 466-469.)

Potentially allergenic phenols in essential oils would be the heavier phenols ($\geq$ 250 amu), such as some phenolic ethers, phenolic sesquiterpenes, and phenolic diterpenes, which are in oils such as Anise, Clove, Fennel, Calamus, Tarragon, Basil, Nutmeg, Sasssafras, Cypress, or Clary Sage. Although allergic reactions to these, or any other essential oil, is extremely rare we felt like we should mention the possibility

Are Essential Oils Allergens?

Aromatherapists of the British school often warn about "sensitizations" from using essential oils undiluted on the skin or taken orally. They customarily dilute their essential oils with 95-98% neutral, fatty vegetable oils and oppose taking them orally. So their warnings apply more to carrier oils than essential oils, since most of what they use are not essential. They are alarmed by such practices as raindrop technique where many essential oils are applied neat (undiluted) to bare feet and back. Some opponents of raindrop technique actually claim that allergic reactions to raindrop applied neat to the skin can have serious consequences, including anaphylactic shock and respiratory failure. None of these allegations are true and no verifiable facts or studies are ever cited to support them. The research publication entitled, *A Statistical Validation of Raindrop Technique*, soundly refutes such allegations with data from thousands of actual raindrop sessions.

Back to the question: Are essential oils potential allergens? Consider the following facts:

(1) 90%+ of allergenic substances are composed of proteins or polypeptides, which are relatively large nitrogenous molecules. There are no proteins or polypeptides in essential oils. In fact, nitrogen-containing compounds are virtually non-existent in essential oils except in occasional trace amounts. (See Chapter Four.)

(2) Allergens are composed of large molecules. There are no large molecules in volatile or aromatic oils, otherwise they would be neither volatile nor aromatic. The relatively small size of essential oil molecules and their natural plant origins

makes them easily metabolized and eliminated, within minutes or hours. This is usually not enough time for an allergenic sensitivity to develop. It usually takes a large molecule that stays in the body well beyond its welcome before sensitization can occur. Unless sensitization occurs and antibodies produced and stored in the body, there can be no allergic reaction. There may be detox and other types of allergy-type reactions, but not true allergic ones.

(3) Some phenolic compounds can also be allergenic. There are some phenols in nature, such as in poison ivy, that are truly allergenic. Hence we must allow that some phenols in essential oils could also be allergens for some people. (See pp. 466-457 for a discussion of poison ivy.) See pp. 295, 571 & 582 for lists of oils containing phenols, but don't think that all phenols can provoke an allergy. Only some phenols with larger molecules can do this, such as phenolic ethers, phenolic sesquiterpenes, or phenolic diterpenes.)

The truth is that phenols in essential oils are very beneficial and are some of the most therapeutic compounds, both physically and emotionally. They cleanse receptor sites, clear toxins from tissues, and release associated emotional patterns. They pave the way for all types of healing. They are the main key constituents of essential oils that make raindrop technique so powerful. (See p. 470 and Chapter Nine)

Nonallergenic Reactions to Essential Oils

While allergenic reactions from pure therapeutic grade essential oils are rarely known happen, this is not true for perfume, massage, or food grade oils, depending on what synthetic substances and fatty oils are used to alter and dilute them. However, even in cases of reactions to non-therapeutic grade oils, resultant reactions, may be, but are not likely to be, true allergies.

To be an allergic reaction, there must be antibodies in the system of the person having the reaction, antibodies designed for that particular substance. There must also be a period of prior sensitization before an allergic reaction can occur. If a person has a reaction to an oil the first time they receive it, it cannot be an allergy because there was no prior exposure whereby sensitization and development of antibodies could have taken place. Such a reaction is nonallergenic. It is either emotional, a detox, or a chemical irritation.

Therapeutic grade essential oils are detoxifying to the body, which is a good thing. When the detoxification takes place at a rate greater than can be eliminated through our kidneys, colon, sweat glands, and respiration, then allergy-like symptoms can occur. Here is where aromatherapists of the British school make their mistake in interpreting allergy-like symptoms as allergies when, in fact, they are usually not. Allergic and the other types of reactions are quite different, even opposite in some ways.

According to data reported in *A Statistical Validation of Raindrop Technique*, (see bibliography) the most frequently reported negative results of applying undiluted oils was a burning sensation on the skin, skin rashes, nausea, headaches, and tiredness (in that order). Among the outcomes of thousands of raindrop sessions included in the report, no negative experiences more severe than these five items were reported. Not one case of a true allergic reaction was discovered by this study even though an honest effort was made to find and report such reactions if they existed.

In fact, none of the dire prognostications or potential sensitizations alleged by aromatherapists of the British school were seen in this study. This is true in spite of the fact that in gathering the data the research questionnaire was submitted to the antagonists of raindrop, soliciting their inputs and encouraging them to submit negative outcomes if they could document them.

In all the reports of negative outcomes with undiluted oils in that study, the experiences were temporary and interpreted as detox reactions. Given enough time, accompanied by a cleansing regimen, detox reactions to oils will cease and the oils that had caused a reaction initially will no longer do so. This is an indication that the cleansing is complete and proof that the reaction was no allergy.

When a detox reaction happens, stop using the oils for a while or reduce their quantity in order to slow down the release of toxins. Don't do another raindrop procedure for a while. Focus on cleansing procedures with lots of water, fiber, and fresh foods and, perhaps, some fasting, to flush out the toxins. Gradually use the oils again and eventually the toxins will be gone and you won't have unpleasant reactions to the oils any more. Many have had this experience. This proves that such reactions are not allergies, otherwise continued use of the oils would never result in cessation of the symptoms, but it would only increase the symptoms. So don't confuse a detox reaction with an allergic one. Detox reactions may be unpleasant, but are temporary and beneficial. They are the beginning of healing in a body full of toxins that would have eventually resulted in a serious chronic disease.

As a practical tip, persons with acidic conditions (low pH) in their bodies are more prone to untoward detox reactions, such as skin rashes, than those with a more alkaline (and healthy) body chemistry. Taking a teaspoon of any alkalyzing product, such as Alkalime®, before and/or after a raindrop session can prevent such experiences even with toxic clients.

The toxins most often found in our bodies today are usually the result of "modern living" where we breathe polluted air, drink polluted water, and eat foods contaminated with pesticides, preservatives, herbicides, and synthetic hormones. We also bathe our bodies in synthetic compounds and petrochemicals through all the personal care products we use such as hand creams, mouthwashes, shampoos, perfumes, hair-care products, antiperspirants, after-shave lotions, toothpastes, and deodorants. Many common household cleaners are also sources of hazardous substances. Vaccines and prescription drugs are another source of toxins that can accumulate in our bodies.

We may not be able to eliminate all toxic substances from our living environments, but we can apply essential oils to help cleanse us from foreign materials as much as possible and to flush out what has been stored in our bodies from previous exposures. In this way we may be able to improve our health and extend our longevity.

In summary, we can state the following: True allergies to essential oils are rare and have only to do with certain phenols. Allergy-like reactions to pure therapeutic grade essential oils are usually detox reactions, which, if handled with care and common sense, are usually a good thing and can represent a healing process that leads to recovery from many ills and a ticket to longer, healthier living. Besides detoxification, one must realize that there are also spiritual roots to allergies and allergic type sensitivities. (See pp. 453-454.) Also, for some people essential oils can also be a chemical irritant, causing inflammatory symptoms.

Allergic Reactions to Fatty Oils

While allergic reactions to an essential oil are generally not possible, allergies to fatty oils are. This is because fatty oils are not distilled. They are cold-pressed from the fruit and seed. Hence, they contain many large molecules that would not survive distillation but do come through a pressing. Among these large molecules are traces of proteins, amino acids, and polypeptides—all potential allergens.

For massage purposes, essential oils are often added to fatty oils and sometimes fatty oils are added to essential oils to increase their half-lives for fragrance and/or therapeutic reasons. When this is done, the possibility of an allergic reaction exists, not to the molecules of essential oil, but to the proteins and amino acids in the fatty oil. The fact that British aromatherapists routinely apply essential oils diluted in a fatty base may be why they are concerned about allergic sensitizations.

Fatty oils implicated as potential allergens include walnut, almond, olive, peanut, safflower, and virtually any vegetable oil. Although this is an uncommon occurrence, it is one you need to remember if someone you know has a genuine allergic reaction to what appears to be an essential oil when, in fact, the problem is in the carrier oil with which the aromatic oils have been blended.

We should also comment that allergic reactions are also possible with expressed oils (citrus) and aromatic oils obtained by solvents (such as jasmine, onycha, or neroli). These two types of oils are not true essential oils since they are not obtained by distillation. Pure distilled oils rarely contain allergens. Absolutes, expressed oils, and fatty oils (because of their larger molecules) can contain allergens, including carrier oil blends that are mostly essential.

Poison Ivy

We have stated that almost all allergens are proteins or polypeptides—both of which are composed of amino acids whose essential element is nitrogen. The most notable exception to this are the phenols in poison ivy and related species.

The most infamous and common non-nitrogenous allergens are the toxins found in poison ivy (*Rhus toxicoden-*

dron), poison oak (Rhus diversiloba), and poison sumac (Rhus venenata)—three plants of the same genus that are all native to North America. These three species share a common mixture of allergenic compounds, a family of diphenols, called "toxicodendrols" or "urushiols," for which the human body can produce antibodies. No one gets a poison ivy, oak, or sumac rash the first time they touch the plant. Before an allergic reactions can occur, sensitization has to take place followed by the production of the specific antibodies for toxicodendrol (or urushiol).

Some people produce antibodies for toxicodendrol and have a normal antigen-antibody reaction upon repeated exposures to the plants with no untoward effects. Such fortunate people have acquired an immunity to poison ivy, poison oak, or poison sumac.

Other people's bodies produce toxicodendrol antibodies and have a hypersensitive allergic reaction upon subsequent exposures. Such unfortunate people have acquired an allergy to one or more of these plants. The allergic symptom is a contact dermatitis or rash upon each exposure, sometimes increasing in severety each time.

Since toxicodendrol is not a single compound, but a mixture of five compounds that occur in different proportions in each of the three species of Rhus, an acquired immunity to one species (eg. poison ivy) may not mean one is immune to either of the other two (viz. poison oak or poison sumac).

Sometimes the reaction can be severe with red bumps, blisters, open lesions, swelling, and fluids weeping from the skin accompanied with intense itching. It is a case where the offending lymphocytes are on a rampage, having multiplied way beyond reasonable limits. Because they can circulate throughout the body, these antibodies can actually carry these unpleasant symptoms to places that never came into contact with the plant. They can also be transferred by one's own hand by first scratching an infected place on the body and then an uninfected place.

A poison ivy, oak, or sumac rash is a true allergic reaction, preceded by an initial contact with no symptoms from which

The Five Diphenols of Poison Ivy Oil

Toxicodendrol
(or Urushiol)
$C_{21}H_NO_2$

T–I	N = 33	$C_{21}H_{33}O_2$
T–II	N = 31	$C_{21}H_{31}O_2$
T–III	N = 29	$C_{21}H_{29}O_2$
T–IV	N = 27	$C_{21}H_{27}O_2$
T–V	N = 27	$C_{21}H_{27}O_2$

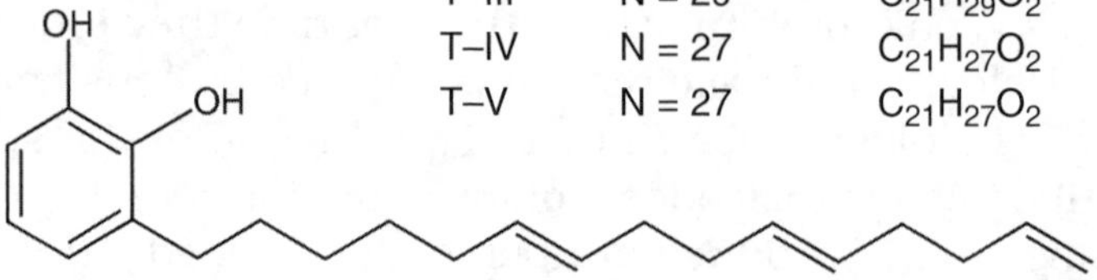

the body produces the antibodies that go berserk with subsequent exposures. In extreme cases a poison ivy, oak, or sumac allergy can internalize and become a life-threatening emergency requiring hospitalization. Thus, our own immune systems, created to protect us, can malfunction to the point of causing discomfort, pain, suffering, bodily harm, and even a threat of death.

Toxicodendrol is actually a relatively non-volatile compound. Its molecules are too big to evaporate at normal temperatures, which is a good thing. Otherwise, all you would have to do is get near one of these plants and you would come in skin contact with the vapors and would be breathing them into your lungs. However, when these plants are burned, the smoke is quite dangerous when inhaled and even when the smoke comes into contact with the skin.

The allergens of poison ivy oil (toxicodendrol or urushiol) are actually mixtures of five similar compounds, as shown above. They are all oxygenated hydrocarbons. They all contain a benzene ring of high resonance energy. They all have two OH radicals attached to the ring, which make them all diphenols. They all have a very long side chain of 15 carbons, which makes them very large in molecular size due to the long chain—much larger than any essential oil molecule. And they are all allergens. The only difference in these five kinds of toxicodendrol is in the number (N) of hydrogens (H) in the side chain which varies from 25 to 31. Note that T–IV and T–V have the same formula. They are isomers. The differences are where the double bonds are located in the side chain. The toxicodendrol molecule shown is T–V.

In molecular weight, they range from 311-317 amu, which is heavier than a diterpene (272 amu) and lighter than a triterpene (408 amu), but because of their structure, are a lot bigger in size than either of these. In fact, toxicodendrol resembles a fatty acid molecule more than an essential oil molecule. (See diagrams of fatty acid molecules in Chapter Two, p. 56.) Diterpenes are usually the largest molecules found in essential oils with the exception of trace quantities of a few triterpenes. Essential oil diterpenes and triterpenes are both compact in shape, not strung out in a chain like toxicodendrol, which may have something to do with why the former are therapeutic and nonallergenic while the latter is a toxic allergen. It's the long shape and size that really sets toxicodendrol molecules apart from essential oil molecules. Check out the numerous figures of essential oil molecules in this book and you won't find a single molecule that resembles toxicodendrol in appearance. All five varieties of toxicodendrol molecules have a side chain 15 carbons long. No essential oil molecule has a carbon chain that long. In fact, essential oil molecules typically have side chains of only 2 carbons (ethyl) or 3 carbons (propyl) with a maximum of 4 (butyl).

It is interesting to note that the formulas for T–I and T–II ($C_{21}H_{33}O_2$ and $C_{21}H_{31}O_2$) are within one H atom of the formula for pregnenolone ($C_{21}H_{32}O_2$), a vital steroid manufactured by our bodies and the precursor to all of the sexual hormones from the estrogens to testosterone. Furthermore, T–II and T–III are within one H atom of the formula of progesterone ($C_{21}H_{30}O_2$)—another steroidal hormone manufactured by our bodies which, among other things, is essential during gestation to retain pregnancy. Hence, two vitally important hormones in our bodies are very close to being isomers of poison ivy toxin. However, while their formulas are almost the same, their structures are entirely different. Steroids are shaped more like the compact molecules of diterpenes in aromatic oils while toxicodendron is shaped more like the long chain molecules of fatty acids.

This illustrates once again why the shape of a molecule is as important a determinant of its biochemical behavior as its chemical weight and composition. All of the variations of toxicodendrol have single rings (i.e. monocyclic) with long side chains. By contrast, pregnenolone and progesterone are both compact in size—consisting of four connected rings (i.e., tetracyclic) and no side chains.

Poison ivy, oak, and sumac—all species of the genus, *Rhus*—are the only plants with oil molecules known to be allergens. Toxicodendrol molecules are nonaromatic and do not resemble any essential oil molecule in size or shape and do not offer the beneficial properties of essential oils.

A Word About Phenols and Allergies

Since the allergens in poison ivy are phenols and since phenols are common and important compounds in essential oils (see pp. 295-296, 571 & 582), is it not possible that there could be occassional true allergic reactions to some oils? The answer is, "yes."

When a phenolic oil like oregano or thyme causes reddness or a rash, they are acting as a detox agent almost always, although although they can also act as a simple chemical irritants producing temporary inflammation. But a true allergy can also sometimes occur from exposure to the phenols in essential oils, like with some foods. For example, allergies to many fruits and vegetables (like strawberries or peanuts) are attributed to phenols. So in general, whereas essential oils are virtually non-allergenic, for some rare individuals, the phenols in essential oils can be truly allergenic. (For more information, Google "allergies & phenols" on the internet.)

10. X-Rays

People who carry their essential oils onto airplanes want to know if the x-rays at the security gates will damage them. The answer is probably yes, but only to a very minor extent and what damage occurs is repairable.

When a high frequency photon of electromagnetic energy (like an x-ray) makes a direct hit on a molecule, it can splinter it into pieces. Fragments of a molecule are free radicals, electrically unbalanced ions or groups of atoms looking for their missing parts. In some cases, a complete benzene ring (C_6H_6) can be broken from a larger molecule by radiation where, as free benzene, it is highly toxic, but as a functional group incorporated in another molecule is harmless or beneficial. (See Chapter Six.)

How X-Rays Can Damage Oil Molecules

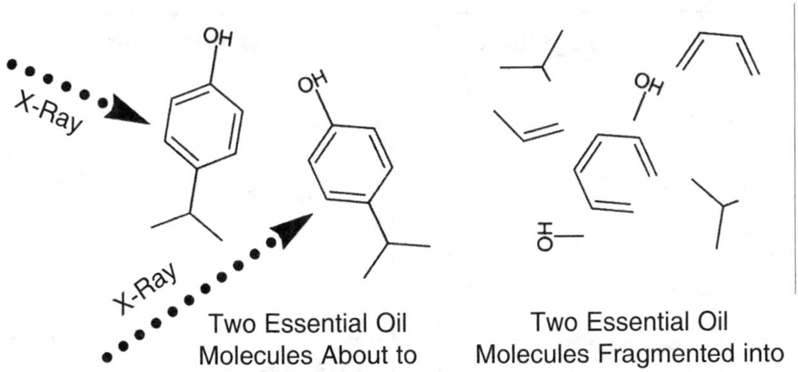

| Two Essential Oil Molecules About to be Hit by a Couple of X-Ray Photons | Two Essential Oil Molecules Fragmented into Free Radicals After being Hit by a Couple of X-Rays |

Free radicals are not nice to have floating around in your body because they will grab electrons and atoms from your tissues, accelerating the aging process, damaging organs and tissues, and, in some cases, causing cellular mutations that can become cancer. That is why when we are exposed to high doses of x-rays, gamma rays, nuclear radiation, microwaves, or other high frequency electromagnetic energies we can suffer various symptoms of radiation sickness.

Being irradiated by x-rays and other high frequency electromagnetic energy is not such a problem for essential oils as for people because oils contain no living cells that can be damaged and result in sickness. All that can happen in an oil is that a few molecules may be fractured into pieces. Percentwise it won't be many, say one in 10,000. That is because molecules and compounds are mostly space through which x-rays can pass harmlessly. It is only with a direct hit that a molecule is fractured.

Shown above are two p-cuminol molecules about to receive a dead hit from a pair of x-ray photons. (Notice how a benzene ring is incorporated into each of these molecules.) When a quantum of x-ray energy makes a direct hit on an oil molecule you get a bunch of partial molecules. Partial molecules are free radicals. In this figure, you see a couple of OH radicals on the loose looking for something to which to attach themselves. You also see a couple of propyl radicals (which

Table Thirty
Comparison of Antioxidant Capacities by ORAC Scores

Fruits and Vegetables		Essential Oils	
Carrots	210	Lemon	660
Lime Juice	305	Orange	1,890
Eggplant	390	Eucalyptus globulus	2,410
Yellow Corn	400	Cinnamon Bark	10,340
Cherries	670	Oregano	15,300
Red Bell Peppers	710	Hyssop	20,900
Red Grapes	739	Lime	26,200
Oranges	750	Celery Seed	30,300
Beets	840	Peppermint	37,300
Broccoli	890	Basil	54,000
Plums	949	Douglas Fir	69,000
Brussel Sprouts	980	Cumin	82,400
Raspberries	1,220	Geranium	101,000
Spinach	1,260	Marjoram	130,900
Strawberries	1,540	Cedarwood	169,000
Kale	1,770	Clary Sage	221,000
Blueberries	2,400	Myrrh	379,800
Wolfberries	25,300	Clove	1,078,700

Excerpted from the *Essential Oils Desk Reference*, Third Edition, Brian Manwaring, Editor, 2004 Essential Science Publishing Co., Orem, Utah, pp. 437-438.

look like little coat hangers). Meanwhile, there are two broken benzene rings that are quite unhappy, looking for some way to pull themselves together.

Interestingly, one of the healing properties of essential oils is that they can remove free radicals from our bodies, including benzene. This is because they are powerful antioxidants. Antioxidants are substances that can neutralize the damaging effects of free radicals and remove them from our bodies.

Fresh fruits and vegetables are high in antioxidants, but no food is as high in antioxidants as are most essential oils, which are many times more concentrated than undistilled produce. Table Thirty (above) lists eighteen representative essential oils and an equal number of fruits and vegetables with their ORAC scores. ORAC (Oxygen Radical Absorbance Capacity) is a scale developed by the U.S. Department of Agriculture in cooperation with scientists at Tufts University,

Boston, Massachusetts. The scale measures the antioxidant potential of various foods and substances.

You can see at a glance that essential oils, in general, are far more potent antioxidants than fruits and vegetables. In fact, two drops of essential oil of clove taken orally have the antioxidant power of . . .

5 pounds of carrots or 2.5 quarts of carrot juice
10 oranges or 20 ounces of orange juice
2.5 pounds of beets or 1 pint of beet juice
2.5 cups of raspberries or 1.3 cups of blueberries

Getting back to the subject of how to deal with x-rays, here is what you do when you go through an airport security gate and your oils have been irradiated. Don't worry about it. The oils have the capability of fixing themselves. However, a little prayer won't hurt. In research conducted by the Human Dimensions Institute in New York, it was found that enzymes damaged by UV radiation would repair themselves in response to healing prayers. If you want to minimize x-ray damages and help fractured oil molecules to reassemble themselves, then just say a little prayer over your oils before entering the security zone and again after you have passed through.

That's all you need to do. Give them a little love and your oils will pull themselves back together and be just fine. They will appreciate your attention and concern and, in gratitude, will serve you well in your next anointing or application.

11. Plastic

Some essential oils will dissolve some plastics. If you have ever put drops of lemon, cinnamon, wintergreen, peppermint, or other essential oil in a plastic bottle of purchased tea or drinking water, you can actually taste the plastic in your beverage. If you have ever put a few drops of oil in juice or water in a styrofoam cup, you will soon find that the cup springs leaks. If the oil floats (like peppermint), it will eat around the rim at the level of the contents. If the oil sinks (like cinnamon), it will eat right through the bottom of the cup. Plastic molecules are not something you want in your body.

What this demonstrates is the fact that if you do have petrochemicals in your body (such as molecules of plastic), essential oils have the capability of dissolving them and cleaning them out of your system.

Essential oils won't dissolve Teflon®, which is often used for stopper caps on essential oil bottles, but they can dissolve the plastics normally used to contain commercial drinking water and other beverages like tea, juice, and soda pop. If you want to add oils to your drinks, they should be in glass, stainless steel, or ceramic containers.

12. Clockwise

In applying essential oils, healing aromatherapists teach us to "energize" the oil with a "clockwise" spin. This is often done by placing the desired number of oil drops in the palm of our non-dominant hand (usually the left) and then stirring the oil in small clockwise circles with one or more fingers of the other hand. It can also be done directly on the site where oils are applied. Why is this done? And is there a scientific basis for it?

The reason it is done is because it has been observed, empirically, that the therapeutic effectiveness of the oil is increased by this procedure. Thus, we say "the oil has been energized." This is something you can verify yourself.

The concept dates back thousands of years to Chinese medicine where the yin and yang principles are said to rotate in opposite directions, both clockwise and counterclockwise. According to Chinese cooking principles, if one stirs food clockwise it corresponds to balancing conditions within the human body that may be unbalanced if stirred counterclockwise.

The science behind this practice is as follows: Back in Chapter Seven we discussed chiral molecules. These are isomers that come in pairs, each the mirror image of the other, like a right and a left-handed pair of gloves. The word, "chiral," comes from the Greek, *cheiro*, meaning "hand." Chiral pairs are designated as being d-isomers where d = *dexter* (meaning "right" in Latin) or l-isomers where l = *laevus* (meaning "left" in Latin).

For reasons known only to God, the major molecules that make up living systems on earth are all chiral in the same way. This is true for all terrestrial plants, animals and microorganisms. Amino acids are the basic molecular building material of living matter. All amino acids are l-isomers (left-handed). Right-handed amino acids can be made in a lab, but they are all dead and not found in living organisms. Proteins are macromolecules built of amino acids present in all living cells. About 50% of your body's dry weight is protein. Proteins are major structural components in all of our bodily tissues. They also catalyze our chemical processes as enzymes, transport oxygen, serve as hormones, regulate bodily functions, and make life possible as we know it. Whatever their role, each protein molecule is built from the levo-chiral molecules of amino acids. Levo-chiral molecules, and all substances built from them, possess a natural twist in a clockwise direction.

To remember this, take your left hand, stick up your thumb, and look directly at your thumb aimed at your face. Now slowly bend your fingers to make a fist with your left thumb pointing toward your face and notice which way your fingers curl. As you make the fist, your fingers move clockwise. Thus, levoratary (left-handed) molecules have a clockwise spin.

From dinosaurs to the tiniest protozoans and viruses. the proteins of this planet are all helical with a clockwise twist. This includes the molecules of DNA. Counterclockwise proteins and strands of DNA do not exist on planet earth as normal substances. Simple counterclockwise proteins have been synthesized in a lab, but they are dead, having no place in the life forms of this world.

The insistence of nature on just one chiral form in the molecules of terrestrial organisms is called "homochirality" by scientists. It is possible that the proteins of extraterrestrial creatures could be counterclockwise. We only know that on earth, at a microscopic level, all life turns in a clockwise direction. The universal existence of clockwise protein chirality on earth may have to do with the nature and orientation of the earth's magnetic field into which all earthly life is born. If an organism or living entity was discovered on earth whose genes and proteins were all counter-clockwise, you could know for a certainty that they were aliens from another planet. This fact could be the basis for a good science fiction movie.

Geopathology

There are some exceptions to the homochirality of proteins. The earth possesses a global magnetic field with a north-south polarity due to ferric minerals and movements in the core of the earth. However, at the earth's surface one experiences significant variations in the measurable field due to latitude and the magnetism of local rocks, ores, and crystalline mineral deposits. There are also dynamic electric fields (called Telluric currents) that move and change continually over the earth's surface that move differently from place to place.

This gives rise to a phenomena called "geopathology." In other words, some places on the earth are more in electromagnetic harmony with human function than others. Living in some locations support health, wellness, and strength while others promote sickness and weakness. The unhealthy places are said to produce "geopathic stress." People living in such geographically unfavorable places have higher rates of cancer and other diseases. What is interesting is that measurements of the blood of people living under geopathic stress find reverse polarized proteins. They rotate counterclockwise. When these people move to a different place, their blood cells return to the normal clockwise twist and their health improves. Cancer patients, in general, are found to have reverse twisted proteins in their blood. If the cancer goes away, the proteins return to their normal clockwiseness.

These examples of counterclockwise rotation do not change the fact that all proteins created on earth have a clockwise twist. It is just that in certain situations, the surrounding electromagnetic fields or other forces can actually unwind some proteins, including our DNA, and turn them backwards. When this happens, we have an abnormal situation. If not corrected, physical, mental, and/or emotional sicknesses will inevitably ensue.

There are times when counterclockwise motions are used in healing. For example, in getting access to repressed emotions or forgotten memories of traumatic experiences, those who do emotional release work with oils sometimes make small counterclockwise circles on the temples of the client to "unwind the DNA" to gain access to these subconscious memories. However, before the close of the session, clockwise circles are made to restore the DNA back to its normal helical twist.

Getting back to essential oils, when we make clockwise circles before applying them, we are placing a spin on the molecules that enables them to more easily engage with the proteins in every cell of our bodies as well as the strands of DNA that form our cellular intelligence. Thus energized, essential oil molecules can enter our bodies turning in synchrony and harmony, spinning in the same direction as our body parts on a microscopic level. In this way the oils can more effectively administer their therapeutic powers. For cancer patients or persons living in geopathic stress or who work in man-made electromagnetic environments that have reversed some of their proteins and set them up for sickness—properly polarized and energized essential oils can restore these twisted proteins back to their normal clockwise configuration, thus setting the person back on the path to wellness.

For more practical information on the consequences of geopathology and electromagnetic fields in general, and what you can do about them, see the excellent book, *Electromagnetic Pollution*, by DeVita available from CARE.

What is Clockwise?

When instructed to energize essential oils with clockwise circles, some people ask: Which way is clockwise? This is a very good question since clockwiseness depends on your point of reference. As you will see, the answer to this seemingly innocent and simple question goes beyond chemistry and the physical sciences.

If you make circles on the palm of your left hand that are clockwise from your viewpoint, the base of your fingers would be 12 o'clock and 3 o'clock would be to your right under the little finger. If you held the palm of your hand away from you and someone facing you made clockwise circles on your palm from their point of reference, your view, from the back of your hand, would see them going in a counterclockwise direction. The same circles would be clockwise to them but counterclockwise to you. It is like a ceiling fan that appears to turn clockwise when you view if from the floor but counterclockwise when viewed from above by a fly on the ceiling.

As another example, during the hurricane season (August thru November in the Northern hemisphere) you have probably seen satellite photos of spirally tropical storms on the television news as viewed looking down from space above the earth. They normally turn counterclockwise from this perspective. But if you could see it spiraling from below standing on the ground looking up, the turning direction would appear to be clockwise. Hence, the same set of storm clouds that appear to turn clockwise from above, would appear counterclockwise from below. To demonstrate this, make counterclockwise circles with your fingers looking down on them from above. Now slowly raise your hand with the fingers still pointing down until they are above your head with you looking up. Notice that now they turn clockwise even though you didn't change the direction you were circling .

The whole idea of making clockwise circles with essential oils is to match the clockwise twist of our proteins and DNA. The problem is that a clockwise circle in two dimensions on a surface (like your palm or a weather satallite image) and a clockwise twist in three dimensions in a protein are not the same thing. In actual proteins and DNA molecules, we are not talking about making a simple circle in a plane or surface. We are talking about a three-dimensional twisted helix which is clockwise on both ends, —whether you view it from top or bottom, from above or from below. Unlike the ceiling fan or tropical storm whose apparent direction of turning depends on the side from which you view it, the twist of proteins is the same regardless of your point of perspective. The difference comes from an added dimension—the third dimension.

By making clockwise circles on the oils with our fingers, it is our intent to prepare the molecules to rotate in the same direction as our proteins and, thus, make them more readily absorbable. But this is only partly accomplished by the physical act of making circles in a plane. It is also in response to our intent to energize the oils in a direction that synchronizes with our cells. The process works whether one understands it or not and regardless of one's point of reference in choosing which way is clockwise.

In making clockwise circles, we are not able to actually mimic or duplicate the three-dimensional nature of the clockwise twist of our cellular proteins, but our intent is to do so and the oils have a consciousness that understands that and responds accordingly. Oils follow our heart's intent, even when our left-brain understanding is faulty or incomplete and our physical motions (making clockwise circles) is an imperfect representative of how the cellular proteins are actually configured.

For a practical answer of what is clockwise, simply visualize yourself standing in front of or looking down on the hand with which you make the circles and make that motion clockwise from that viewpoint. Don't worry about anyone else's viewpoint. The intelligence of the oils will know what you want them to do. Making the circles is a means of your communicating with the oils by a sign language they understand. But this is beyond chemistry and beyond science as we know it. (See Part Three.)

I hope this answer makes things clear to you as to what clockwise is all about and how and why going through the motions of clockwise circles can improve the therapeutic efficacy of essential oils. Think about it.

13. Carrier Oils

A carrier oil is a fatty oil mixed with an essential oil. In British aromatherapy the blends used are mostly carrier oils with only 1-5% essential oil. However, many blends are be mostly essential (80-90%) with a proportionately smaller amount of carrier or base oil. There are, of course, many blends that are 100% essential.

The question often arises as to whether mixing a carrier oil with an essential "dilutes" the essential oil, reduces its effectiveness, or prevents the essential oil molecules from penetrating into tissues down to cellular levels, as we would like for them to do in therapeutic aromatherapy. The answer is "no." The addition of a carrier only slows down the rate of absorption. Your body will still receive all of the essential oil molecules, but stretched out over a longer period of time.

Of course, if you dilute essential oils to an extreme as the British recommend (only 2-5% essential oil in a fatty base), you are significantly reducing the total amount of essential oil available to the client and, thus, you are reducing the potential for healing. When a massage oil diluted to British standards is applied, the client will receive the small amount of essential oils present over an extended period of time, but not much therapeutic benefit is likely to result from such applications.

In raindrop technique, sometimes oils, such as oregano and thyme, can create a burning sensation when applied undiluted (neat) to the skin. To quickly stop the discomfort, a layer of fatty vegetable oil is applied to the skin. All of the oregano and thyme that has been applied will still completely enter the body through the skin, but at a slower rate. Meanwhile, the larger fatty molecules remain on the skin surface, unable to penetrate beyond a few millimeters into the skin.

Similarly, at the end of a raindrop session, after more than eight oils have been applied neat to the back over a period of time, a hot damp towel is placed on the back. Whereas there may be no discomfort from the applied oils before the hot compress is applied, it can subsequently produce a heating sensation that occasionally becomes quite uncomfortable. The solution is to apply some carrier oil to the skin where the unpleasant sensation is too much. The "burning" experienced is actually not thermal. It is chemical. It has to do with the rate at which the oils are being absorbed, a rate that is accelerated by the hot, damp towel. A little vegetable oil retards the rate and the receiver experiences a cooling sensation because of the slower manner in which the oils are being absorbed. The client still absorbs all of the molecules of essential oil they have received, but just over a longer period of time and without any sensations of excess heat.

14. Right Oils

Sometimes it happens that you have a situation that calls for a specific oil and you don't have it. What do you do then? The answer is, use what you've got.

The molecules of specific oils are specially suited to stimulate certain receptors in the body. Some administer best to the digestive tract, others to the cardiovascular system, others to the muscles, some to the pancreas, some to the nervous system, and so forth. They are like employees in a company trained for certain tasks, but not particularly trained in others. Some do secretarial work, others ship goods, some operate machinery, while others may meet customers and work in sales. When a company gets into a crunch in one department, they will call on those of other departments to provide temporary assistance, even though they were not trained in the job at hand. When the crisis has passed and the urgent task accomplished, the workers return to their usual jobs.

Oils can do that, too. A particular oil may not be the oil of choice for a particular task, but in a pinch, it will still get the job done. Oils follow intent. They respond to directions, delivered verbally, mentally, or by prayer. Just tell the oil what you want it to do, visualizing its molecules traveling to the desired locations in the body, performing the desired tasks, and it will happen. Essential oils are not ordinary medicines. They were not created by ordinary means. They are God's agents for healing that he provided for us to use, in his name, and with his guidance.

> There will grow all kinds of trees . . . Their fruit will be for food, and their leaves for healing. Ezekiel 47:12

> And the leaves of the tree are for the healing of the nations. Revelation 22:2

Part Two of this book has numerous tables that have cross-indexed the chemical components of more than one-hundred essential oils. By using these tables, you may be able to find oils with similar chemical constituencies that can be substituted one for the other. Thus, you may be able to find an equivalent oil that you have and can use when your first choice is not available.

Also realize that essential oils are not all chemistry. In quantum physics you would consider them as packets of possibilities, but in any given application they will only manifest what you intend them to manifest. What they do is up to you. That's how and why they work with prayer, following your intent. (See Part Three, p. 716.)

But most of all, just remember that if you don't have exactly the right oil, use what you've got. Let God take care of the rest. He is used to working with imperfect instruments and can still achieve the desired results in spite of a handicap.

15. More or Less

It has been said, with regard to using essential oils, which are highly concentrated, that "less is better." Sometimes this is so and sometimes not. How do you know when less is better and when more would be best?

The answer lies in the purpose of the application. If you are fighting an army of bacteria, viruses, fungi, or parasites, or if you are dealing with bee toxin, snake venom, spider poison, or cancer cells, then more is better. You need an army to fight an army. More is also better when you want to oxygenate brain tissue (e.g. applying frankincense. cedarwood, or sandalwood to a massive head injury to keep the brain tissues oxygenated).

However, if all you need to do is trip a few receptor sites to awaken your bodys organs and natural functions, less is better. You don't need to batter a switch with a baseball bat to get the lights to go on. A simple flick of the finger will do. One molecule is all it takes to trip a receptor site. In these cases, too much oil will actually produce a reduced response or, perhaps, no response at all. Here is why.

Every living cell has thousands of receptor sites, portals of entry for communication between itself and the other cells of your body. We have likened them to mechanical or magnetic locks to be opened by the proper keys. Actually, most receptor sites are more complicated than a simple lock. Many are like miniature computer keyboards. When the message-carrying ligand approaches the site with the right key, it unlocks the keyboard and types in a message to the DNA inside the cell.

Think about it. When you use a computer terminal, you touch one key at a time most of the time. What happens when you press many keys at once, like leaning on the console with your arm. The computer freezes up. Either something happens you don't want to happen or nothing happens until you clear the gibberish you have just made by pressing too many keys at once. In situations where all you want to do is send a message to the DNA via the molecules of essential oils, it only takes a few to get the message across. Too many molecules engulfing the surface of a cell creates "receptor site overload." When this happens, little or no useful information is conveyed to the inner cell.

I learned this by experience. In the early days when I first started using essential oils, I had heard that peppermint oil would keep you awake if you became drowsy while driving. One late evening, I decided to try it. I was pretty tired. Naturally, I thought using a lot of peppermint would be in order. I doused it on my head, on the back of my neck, put it on my hands, rubbed it on the steering wheel, and inhaled it deeply. I figured that would keep anyone awake. But it didn't. I nearly fell asleep at the wheel. I was puzzled. As I thought it over in the ensuing days, I realized I had committed "receptor site overload." When all I needed to do was trip a few receptors, I had laid down on the keyboard and jammed the computer. Hence, the peppermint failed to switch on my alertness buttons.

The next time I was driving late at night, I tried peppermint in a different way. This time, I merely opened the bottle and passed it under my nose with a sniff. That was enough. The receptors tripped and I was wide awake. Every now and then I would refresh the commands to my brain and body with another light pass of the bottle. That worked. That was a case where "less was better."

Remember this. A single drop of essential oil contains 40 quintillion molecules, Written out, that is a 4 with 19 zeros after it, viz. 40,000,000,000,000,000,000. You have 100 trillion cells in your body. Hence, one drop of oil is enough to cover every cell in your body with 400,000 molecules. Now you can see why a little essential oil can often get the job done and address every cell in your body.

There is also an approach to using essential oils called "subtle aromatherapy." This is similar to homeopathy where none (or very few) of the actual molecules of a substance are applied as therapeutic agents. Instead their vibrational essence is employed, which has been transferred to water or some other medium. In the case of essential oils, their energetic essence can be transferred to water or to a fatty base oil, which is applied to the various chakras, acupressure points, or electromagnetic centers of our bodies from where healing currents are directed to specific organs or body parts. Homeopathic aromatherapy is a field that extends well beyond the science of chemistry as currently understood. (See pp. 396-398 & Part Three.)

16. Oil Safety

Aromatherapy books from the British point of view are full of warnings, prohibitions, contraindications, and detailed discussions of safety issues based on numerous scientific papers. The data they cite is from animal studies, single-component studies, non-therapeutic grade oils, and anecdotes of children accidentally drinking large quantities of essential oil or women attempting to induce an abortion by large overdoses of strong oils generally considered unwise to take orally in any quantity. The data for such alarms also comes from oils meant only for fragrance or flavorings, where only trace amounts are used in various products. None of the concerns, none of the data, and none of the studies cited in these books applies to pure, unadulterated therapeutic grade essential oils applied with simple common sense.

In the first chapter of this book, we discussed these points and identified books that were British in their viewpoint. However, since the previous paragraph is predicated upon using only therapeutic grade essential oils, one must be cautious in choosing brands. While the quality of essential oils is regulated in Europe and in some other countries, it is not in the United States or Canada. Find a company contientious enough to regularly submits samples of its oils for independent testing outside of and ain addition to their own labs. If you see the letters, AFNOR, on the label, that means they comply with the French standard. (See pp. 7-9.) Definitions of a therapeutic-grade essential oil are discussed in Chapters One and Two. So the first rule of safety in using essential oils is to use safe oils purchased from a trustworthy source. Oils that have been diluted, modified, standardized, adulterated, or extended with synthetic compounds do present hazards. The best course is to avoid them.

This is not to say pure therapeutic grade oils are totally devoid of potential for harm. They are biologically active. They do penetrate to cellular levels and can gain access to all of the tissues in our bodies. As active agents, inappropriate or over-use of an essential oil could result in a problem. That is why the more you know and understand about the chemistry and biological actions of essential oils, the less likely it becomes that there will ever be a problem.

British oriented authors like to quote "lethal dose" (LD_{50}) statistics. LD_{50} is a term that designates the dosage of a substance that results in killing 50% of the rats, mice, guinea pigs, or other types of animals in a scientific study. Every substance has an LD_{50} number. Anything can be harmful or deadly if the dosage is sufficient.

Philippus Aureolus Paracelsus, a Swiss alchemist and physician of the sixteenth century (1493-1541) stated the following: "What is there that is not poison? All things are poison and there is nothing that cannot be poison. The dose alone makes it poisonous." As pointed out in Chapter Three on basic chemistry, numerous elements (like iron) essential to normal body function are toxic, even fatal, in large doses, yet we need them to exist in our physical forms. Paracelsus was right. Every essential oil has its therapeutic dosages and every essential oil has its LD_{50}.

Even water has its LD_{50}. Too much water imbibed too rapidly can upset the balances of ions inside and outside of our bodily cells and result in death. This has actually happened several years ago when a Kansas radio station held a contest to see who could drink the most water in the shortest time. One contestant died.

British aromatherapists err on the side of the conserva-tive, refusing to use aromatic oils undiluted in therapeutic doses, refusing to take them orally, and refusing to use many therapeutic oils at all on the basis of theoretical pos-sibilities of what might happen, even though they can cite no valid studies on humans to support their concerns. In the process of their fears and reluctance, they deny them-selves and their clients many opportunities for true heal-ing through the unique powers of essential oils. Hence, there is harm in becoming too cautious in one's approach to aromatherapy. Just because a substance carries the potential for harm does not mean a problem actually exists. It only means that caution is to be exercised.

Safety in the use of essential oils is different for the different pathways of application. It would be difficult, if not impossible, to inhale a lethal dosage of any essential oil or absorb that much through the skin. Only in oral applications are serious overdoses possible. In such cases where oral overdoses have occurred with serious consequences, it was deliberate on the part of the person or an accident with a child. Such occurrences never happen in the normal course of aromatherapy practice. This is unlike the normal experiences with drugs where harmful overdoses happen all the time even with the most careful of medical monitoring and precaution in prescription.

Books on the therapeutic application of essential oils all contain safety information. My advice is to ignore the ones with a British bias. They will talk you out of using most of the oils that could benefit you and cause you to dilute the oils they approve to levels that have little or no therapeutic value. The references by Higley, Manwaring, Young, Friedmann, Schnaubelt, Valnet, Franchomme, Penoel, and Price discussed in Chapter One or listed in the bibliography are sensible in their recommendations. Take their advice. Given below is a list of common sense precautions for you to consider in using essential oils:

Twelve Rules for Safety with Essential Oils

1. Keep them out of the reach of children. Consider them as you would any therapeutic product in your home.

2. Keep a bottle of vegetable oil handy. It will dilute an essential oil and slow down its rate of absorption if there should be any discomfort or skin irritation.

3. People with sensitive skin can use a patch test to determine if they would react to a particular oil. It is generally safe to apply essential oils to the soles of the feet even for people with sensitive skin.

4. Pregnant women should consult their health care professional before using essential oils. Those oils with hormonal qualities discussed in Chapter Eleven should

probably be avoided during pregnancy.

5. Essential oils rich in phenols should be used with caution when applying to the skin. Sensitive areas such as the throat and face should be avoided, as well as the tender skin of young children. (See Table Forty-Eight.)

6. Keep essential oils away from the eye area where even the vapors can cause irritation. Do not handle contact lenses or rub the eyes with essential oils on your fingers. Oils with high phenol content can damage lenses and irritate eyes. If essential oils accidentally get in the eyes, pour vegetable oil in the eyes to stop the burning. Don't use water. Water will drive the oils in faster, increasing the burning sensation.

7. Essential oils may be applied on or around the ears, but don't pour essential oils directly into the ears.

8. People with epilepsy, high blood pressure, or who are prone to convulsions should consult a health care professional before using essential oils. Hyssop, fennel, and wild tansy oils should probably be avoided in these cases.

9. Most commonly used essential oils have been designated by the FDA as being "Generally Regarded as Safe" for oral usage. This designation is abbreviated as "GRAS." Before ingesting them, GRAS oils, may be diluted with honey, milk, rice milk, olive oil, or other lipid dissolving liquid.

10. In using essential oils in bathwater, first add a dispersant, like a gel or liquid soap, to avoid concentrated droplets that can sometimes gravitate to sensitive areas of the body. There are ways to safely disperse oils in a bath given in most books on applied aromatherapy as well as in the section 4. of this chapter entitled, "Water."

11. Some oils are phototoxic. (See list near the end of Chapter Ten.) When applied to the skin, avoid direct sunlight or the rays of tanning lamps for at least twelve hours afterwards.

12. Keep essential oils in tightly closed glass bottles away from light in cool places. (Normal room temperatures are cool enough.) In this way, they will maintain their bal-

anced chemical composition and potency indefinitely.

Death or serious injury from proper use of essential oils is unheard of and non-existent. Balance this with deaths or serious injuries from proper use of prescription drugs, and there is no comparison. While not even one person dies from essential oils in a given year, thousands die every month in every year from properly applied pharmaceuticals. This is the yardstick by which the safety of essential oils should be measured. The differences are so extreme, there is really no comparison.

All things considered, essential oils are among the safest of all therapeutic modalities and one that is safe enough for even amateurs and untrained users to apply with only a remote possibility of harm. Nevertheless, the more you know and understand about essential oils, the better and safer your results will be.

Conclusion

This is the end of Part One of this book. Part One contains the material presented in the chemistry course offered by the Center for Aromatherapy Research and Education (CARE)—plus a lot more. The rest of the book consists of supplementary materials. Part Two consists of numerous tables that cross-index the chemistry of essential oils from every angle. Part Three is a discussion of essential oils that goes beyond chemistry. Part Four includes a glossary, an annotated bibliography, and a course outline for the CARE chemistry class.

Reading this book won't make you a chemist, although it will definitely increase your understanding of the science of essential oils and, perhaps, fill in some gaps in your education if you have been a student of chemistry. Our hope is that your experience with this book has accomplished the themes in the title and subtitle: That you have found the chemistry of essential oils to be simpler and more interesting than you had ever thought and that the chemistry of essential oils is truly God's love manifest in molecules.

Key Points of Chapter Twelve

1. Regarding heat, essential oils (products of distillation) should be kept sealed and in a reasonably cool place to preserve their chemical balance. Room temperature is sufficient. If you leave pure essential oils in your car on a hot summer day and it gets up to 140° F (60° C) inside, don't worry. Just don't open them when they are hot. Let them cool to normal temperatures and they will be just fine. No damage.

2. Oils that are not true or pure essential oils, such as expressed oils (citrus), absolutes (neroli, jasmine, onycha), or carrier blend oils (containing fatty oils, such as Valor®, Exodus II®, etc.), are subject to deterioration when exposed to temperatures over 90-140° F (32-60° C). If damaged, you can tell by their smell. If they smell different than when they were fresh, then damage has occurred and their therapeutic value reduced.

3. Candles and flames produce excessive heat that destroys the therapeutic properties of essential oils.

4. If your oils happen to be left out in below-freezing temperatures and solidify, don't worry. Just let them thaw out at room temperature and they will be fine. Cold never hurt any oil.

5. Regarding light, essential oils will polymerize when exposed to light for extended periods of time. Polymerization changes small, therapeutic, aromatic molecules into large, non-therapeutic, non-aromatic molecules, thus destroying their healing qualities. Keep them in dark colored glass or opaque containers.

6. Exposed to air for extended periods of time, essential oils can oxidize, thus changing their chemistry. However, it takes many days or weeks for oxidation to take place to any significant extent. When aromatic oils are exposed to air the most volatile components evaporate first, thus changing the proportions and balance of the oil. Keeping your bottle caps off for minutes or even hours does not expose oils to sufficient air circulation to make any discernable difference.

7. When essential oils come into contact with water, the only chemical compounds that can be affected are the acids, phenols, and esters. However, this is not a significant problem if you wish to put oils in your drinking water or bath water. The main thing is to diffuse your oils with a nebulizing diffuser and not one that floats oils on a water bath.

8. Adulteration, modifying, or extending essential oils with synthetic compounds poisons them and reduces or destroys their therapeutic capabilities.

9. Pure therapeutic grade essential oils properly stored and sealed have shelf lives measured in centuries, at least.

10. Expressed, absolute, or carrier blend oils have a shelf life measured in years if kept in reasonably cool places. These types of oils may be refrigerated to extend shelf life, but if you consume them in a matter of months or less than a year, room temperature is sufficient.

11. Any lipid soluble substance with a molecular weight less than 500 amu and a compact molecular shape will pass through the blood-brain barrier. It will pass through human skin as well. The molecules of essential oils will all pass through skin and the blood-brain barrier.

12. Essential oils pass through skin and in so doing are chemically altered to a small degree by the chemistry of the individual. This is one reason essential oils have slightly different fragrances and effects on different people.

13. It is impossible for the molecules of an essential oil to cause an allergy. Almost all allergies are in response to proteins or polypeptides which are never found in essential oils. When reactions to oils do occur, they are detox reactions, not allergic ones. When the affected person undergoes an effective cleanse, the reaction to a particular oil will no longer occur.

14. While it is not possible to develop allergies to the tiny molecules of essential oils produced by distillation, it is possible to develop an allergy to fatty oils. Since fatty oils are pressed from fruit and seed, they contain traces of proteins, peptides, and amino acids not found in essential oils. Allergies are possible from these large nitrogenous molecules. When essential oils are mixed with a fatty massage oil base, such allergic reactions become possible, not to the essential oils, but to the fatty base.

15. Poison ivy, poison oak, and poison sumac are botanically related plants that carry a non-aromatic oil that can stimulate a true allergic reaction. The allergens in this plant are a set of five similar compounds jointly referred to as toxicodendrol,

16. X-rays can fragment oil molecules, creating free radicals. However, essential oils are, themselves, one of the most effective free-radical scavengers known. Hence, after passing through the x-ray units in an airport security zone, don't worry about your oils. Pray for them and they will fix themselves.

17. Plastic bottles in which commercial beverages are sold can be dissolved by essential oils. So can styrofoam cups. If you want to add a few drops of an essential oil to your water, juice, or tea, you need to use a glass, stainless steel, or ceramic drinking container.

18. To increase the therapeutic effectiveness of an essential oil, you may stir the drops in the palm of your hand with the fingers of your other hand in a clockwise motion. The intent is to place a spin on the molecules of the oil that is in the same direction as the spin on all of our proteins, including our DNA, which is also clockwise. In this way, the molecules of oil can enter our bodies in synchrony and harmony with our body parts on a microscopic level, thus increasing their healing potential.

19. Adding a carrier oil to an essential oil only slows down the rate of absorption. All of the molecules of the essential oil will still enter your body, only at a slower rate than they would have without the fatty oil.

20. When you don't have the right oil, use what you have and ask the oil to do what you want it to do.

21. More oil is better when you are fighting an army of bacteria, viruses, fungi, parasites, insect bite poisons, snake venom, or cancer cells or when oxygenating brain tissue following a stroke or severe head injury. Less oil is better when what you want to do is trip a few receptor sites. Too much oil in the latter situation can cause receptor site overload and result in no response.

22. Essential oils are intrinsically safe, provided you are using genuine pure therapeutic grade oils. Common sense and moderation are usually sufficient to protect one from any possible adverse responses. Chances of a serious problem from inhalation or skin contact are almost non-existent. The few serious reactions that have been reported were all from oral overdoses, either adults deliberately consuming large quantities or by accidents with unsupervised children. Keep your essential oils out of the reach of children the same as you would the various medications you may keep in your house.

23. Reading this book won't make you a chemist, but it should show you that chemistry can be interesting, even fun, and can give you insight into how oils work. Besides a lot of practical tips for applying essential oils, what we hope you have gained from this book is an appreciation for God's presence in the oils he has created especially for us. With such appreciation, your intuitive application of the oils will increase as will your sensitivity to God's will in their uses. Essential oils are God's grace in fluid form.

END OF PART ONE

493

PART TWO

CATALOGS
AND INDEXES
OF COMPOUNDS
IN ESSENTIAL OILS

♥ Analytic Tables ♥

♥ COMMON AND SCIENTIFIC NAMES OF PLANTS

Table Thirty-One, beginning below, is in two parts: (1) Common Names First, followed by (2) Scientific Names First. The next section in this book is a tabulation (Table Thirty-Two, pp. 509-558) of representative analyses of 113 essential oils listed alphabetically by both common and botanical names.

All known common names of these oils have been inserted in the Table Thirty-Two list so that no matter what name you look up, you will find the oil you are looking for. For example, it won't matter if you look up coriander oil as "coriander," or by one of its other common names ("cilantro" or "Chinese parsley)" or if you search by its scientific Latin name ("*Coriandrum sativum*"), you can't help but find it since it is listed under all of these names.

There are species in Table Thirty-One (pp. 496-501) not listed in Table-Thirty Two and vice versa. Table-Thirty Two (p. 509) is designed such that by using it, you will find yourself learning botanical names without even trying to memorize them.

Table Thirty-One
Cross-Index of Botanical and Common Names

Common Names First

Alfalfa	*Medicago sativa*
Almond	*Prunus dulcis*
Aloes	*Santalum album*
Aloe Vera	*Aloe vera*
Ambrette Seed	*Abelmoschus moschatus*
Angelica	*Angelica archangelica*
Anise	*Pimpinella anisum*
Avocado	*Persea americana*

Balsam Fir	*Abies balsamea*
Barberry	*Beberis vulgaris*
Barley	*Hordeum vulgare*
Basil	*Ocimum basilicum*
Bayberry	*Myrica pensylvanica*
Bay Laurel	*Laurus nobilis*
Beet	*Beta vulgaris*

Bergamot	*Citrus bergamia*
Birch	*Betula lenta*
Birch	*Betula alleghaniensis*
Bitter Orange	*Citrus aurantium*
Black Cumin	*Cuminum cyminum*
Black Current	*Ribes nigrum*
Black Pepper	*Piper nigrum*
Black Peppermint	*Eucalyptus radiata*
Black Walnut	*Juglans nigra*
Blue Chamomile	*Matricaria recutita*
Blue Cypress	*Callitris intratropica*
Blue Gum	*Eucalyptus globulus*
Blue Mallee	*Eucalyptus polybractea*
Blue Tansy	*Tanacetum annuum*
Boldo	*Peumus boldo*
Borage	*Borago officinalis*
Burdock	*Arctium lappa*

Cabbage	*Brassica oleracea*
Cacao	*Theobroma cacao*
Cajuput	*Melaleuca cajuputi*
Calamus	*Acorus calamus*
Camphor, White	*Laurus camphora*
Canadian Hemlock	*Tsuga canadensis*
Canadian Red Cedar	*Thuja plicata*
Caraway	*Carum carvi*
Cardamom	*Elletaria cardamomum*
Carrot	*Daucus carota*
Cassia	*Cinnamomum cassia*
Castor	*Ricinus communis*
Catnip	*Nepeta cataria*
Cayenne	*Capsicum annuum*
Cedarwood	*Cedrus atlantica*
Celery Seed	*Apium graveolens*
Chamomile, German	*Matricaria recutita*
Chamomile, Roman	*Chamaemelum nobile*
Chaparral	*Larrea tridentata*
Chocolate	*Theobroma cacao*
Cinnamon	*Cinnamomum verum*
Cistus	*Cistus ladanifer*
Citronella	*Cymbopogon nardus*
Clary Sage	*Salvia sclarea*
Clove	*Syzygium aromaticum*
Clover, Red	*Trifolium pratense*
Coconut	*Cocos nucifera*
Combava	*Citrus hystrix*
Conyza	*Conyza canadensis*
Coriander	*Coriandrum sativum*
Corn	*Zea mays*
Corn Flower	*Centaurea cyanus*
Corn Mint	*Mentha arvenis*
Cumin, Black	*Cuminum cyminum*
Cypress	*Cupressus sempervirens*
Cypress, Blue	*Callitris intratropica*

Dandelion	*Taraxacum officinale*
Davana	*Artemisia pallens*
Dill	*Anethum graveolens*
Douglas Fir	*Pseudotsuga menziesii*

Echinacea	*Echinacea angustifolia*
Echinacea	*Echinacea pallida*

Echinacea	*Echinacea purpurea*
Elemi	*Canarium luzonicum*
Eucalyptus	*Eucalyptus dives*
Eucalyptus	*Eucalyptus globulus*
Eucalyptus	*Eucalyptus polybractea*
Eucalyptus	*Eucalyptus radiata*
Evening Primrose	*Oenothera biennis*
Everlasting	*Helichrysum italicum*

Fennel	*Foeniculum vulgare*
Fir, Balsam	*Abies balsamea*
Fir, Douglas	*Pseudotsuga menziesii*
Fir, Silver	*Abies alba*
Fir, White	*Abies grandis*
Flax Seed	*Linum usitatissimum*
Fleabane	*Conyza canadensis*
Frankincense	*Boswellia carteri*
French Marigold	*Tagetes glandulifera*

Galbanum	*Ferula gummosa*
Garlic	*Allium sativum*
Geranium	*Pelargonium graveolens*
German Chamomile	*Matricaria recutita*
Ginger	*Zingiber officinale*
Goldenrod	*Solidago canadensis*
Grand Fir	*Abies grandis*
Grapefruit	*Citrus paradisi*
Green Tea	*Camellia sinensis*
Gully Gum	*Eucalyptus Smithii*

Helichrysum	*Helichrysum italicum*
Hemlock Canadian	*Tsuga canadensis*
Hibiscus Seed	*Abelmoschus moschatus*
Hops	*Humulus lupulus*
Horehound	*Marrubium vulgare*
Horseradish	*Armoracia rusticana*
Ho Wood	*Cinnamomum camphora*
Hyacinth	*Hyacinthus orientalis*
Hydrangia	*Hydrangea arborescens*
Hyssop	*Hyssopus officinalis*

Idaho Balsam	*Abies balsamea*
Idaho Tansy	*Tanacetum vulgare*
Immortelle	*Helichrysum italicum*
Indian Rhubarb	*Rheum palmatum*
Inule, Sweet	*Inula graveolens*

Jasmine	*Jasminum officinale*
Juniper, Common	*Juniperus communis*
Juniper Rocky Mt.	*Juniperus scopulorum*
Juniper, Utah	*Juniperus osteosperma*

Khella	*Ammi visnaga*

Labdanum	*Cistus ladanifer*
Laurel, Bay	*Laurus nobilis*
Lavandin	*Lavandula x hybrida*
Lavender	*Lavandula angustifolia*
Lavender, Spike	*Lavandula latifolia*
Ledum	*Ledum groenlandicum*
Lemon	*Citrus limon*
Lemon Eucalyptus	*Eucalyptus citriodora*
Lemongrass	*Cymbopogon flexuosus*
Licorice	*Glycyrrhiza glabra*
Lime	*Citrus aurantifolia*
Linseed	*Linum usitatissimum*
Lobelia	*Lobelia inflata*
Lotus, White	*Nymphaea lotus*

Magnolia	*Magnolia glauca*
Mandarin	*Citrus reticulata*
Marigold	*Calendula officinalis*
Marigold, French	*Tagetes glandulifera*
Marijuana	*Cannabis sativa*
Marjoram	*Origanum majrorana*
Melaleuca	*Melaleuca alternifolia*
Melaleuca	*Melaleuca ericifolia*
Melaleuca	*Melaleuca leucadendron*
Melaleuca	*Melaleuca quinquenervia*
Melissa	*Melissa officinalis*
Morrocan Chamomile	*Ormenis multicaulis*
Mountain Savory	*Satureja montana*
Mugwort	*Artemisia vulgaris*
Mustard Seed	*Brasica nigra*
Myrrh	*Commiphora myrrha*
Myrtle	*Myrtus communis*
MQV	*Melaleuca quinquenervia*

Neroli	*Citrus aurantium*
Nettle	*Urtica dioica*
Niaouli	*Melaleuca quinquenervia*
Nutmeg	*Myristica fragrans*

Olive	*Olea europea*
Onion	*Allium cepa*
Onycha	*Styrax benzoin*
Orange	*Citrus sinensis*
Orange, Bitter	*Citrus aurantium*
Oregano	*Oreganum compactum*
Ormenis	*Ormenis multicaulis*

Palm	*Elaeis guineensis*
Palmarosa	*Cymbopogon martinii*
Parsley	*Petroselinum crispum*
Patchouly	*Pogostemon cablin*
Peanut	*Arachis hypogaea*
Pennyroyal	*Mentha pulegium*
Peony	*Paeonia officinalis*
Pepper, Black	*Piper nigrum*
Peppermint	*Mentha piperita*
Peppermint Eucalyptus	*Eucalyptus dives*
Petitgrain	*Citrus aurantium*
Pimento	*Pimenta racemosa*
Pine	*Pinus sylvestris*
Poison Ivy	*Rhus toxicodendron*
Poison Oak	*Rhus diversiloba*
Poison Sumac	*Rhus venenata*
Pumpkin	*Cucurbita pepo*
Purple Coneflower	*Echinacea purpurea*

Ravensara	*Ravensara aromatica*
Red Cedar	*Thuja plicata*
Red Clover	*Trifolium pratense*
Rhododendron	*Rhododendron caucasicum*
Roman Chamomile	*Chamaemelum nobile*
Rosalina	*Melaleuca ericifolia*
Rose	*Rosa damascena*
Rosemary	*Rosmarinus officinalis*
Rosewood	*Aniba roseaodora*
Rose of Sharon	*Cistus ladanifer*
Rue	*Ruta graveolens*

Safflower	*Carthamus tinctorius*
Saffron	*Crocus sativus*
Sage	*Salvia officinalis*
Sandalwood	*Santalum album*
Sassafras	*Sassafras albidum*
Savory, Mt.	*Satureja montana*
Sesame	*Sesamum indicum*

Sheep Sorrel	*Rumex acetosella*
Silver Fir	*Abies alba*
Slippery Elm	*Ulmus fulva*
Snake Oil	*Melaleuca alternifolia*
Spanish Marjoram	*Thymus mastichina*
Spearmint	*Mentha spicata*
Spike Lavender	*Lavandula latifolia*
Spruce	*Picea mariana*
St. Johns Wort	*Hypericum perforatum*
Sunflower	*Helianthus annuus*
Sweet Inule	*Inula graveolens*
Sweet Violet	*Viola odorata*

Tamanu	*Calophyllum inophyllum*
Tangerine	*Citrus nobilis*
Tansy	*Tanacetum vulgare*
Tansy, Blue	*Tanacetum annuum*
Tansy, Idaho	*Tanacetum vulgare*
Tansy, Wild	*Tanacetum vulgare*
Tarragon	*Artemisia dracunculus*
Tea Tree	*Melaleuca alternifolia*
Thyme	*Thymus vulgaris*
Tsuga	*Tsuga canadensis*

Valerian	*Valeriana officinalis*
Vanilla	*Vanilla planifolia*
Vetiver	*Vetiveria zizanioides*
Violet, Sweet	*Viola odorata*
Vitex	*Vitex negundo*

Walnut, English	*Juglans regia*
Walnut, Black	*Juglans nigra*
Western Red Cedar	*Thuja plicata*
White Camphor	*Laurus camphora*
White Fir	*Abies grandis*
White Lotus	*Nymphaea lotus*
Wild Carrot	*Daucus carota*
Wild Tansy	*Tanacetum vulgare*
Wild Yam	*Dioscorea villosa*
Wintergreen	*Gaultheria procumbens*
Witch Hazel	*Hamamelis virginiana*
Wolfberry	*Lycium barbarum*

Yam, Wild	*Dioscorea villosa*
Yarrow	*Achillea millefolium*
Ylang Ylang	*Cananga odorata*

Scientific Names First

Abelmoschus moschatus	Hibiscus Seed
Abies alba	Silver Fir
Abies balsamea	Balsam Fir
Abies balsamea	Idaho Balsam
Abies grandis	Grand Fir
Abies grandis	White Fir
Achillea millefolium	Yarrow
Acorus calamus	Calamus
Allium cepa	Onion
Allium sativum	Garlic
Aloe vera	Aloe Vera
Ammi visnaga	Khella
Anthemis mixta	Morrocan Chamomile
Anethum graveolens	Dill
Angelica archangelica	Angelica
Aniba roseaodora	Rosewood
Apium graveolens	Celery Seed
Arachis hypogaea	Peanut
Arctium lappa	Burdock
Artemisia dracunculus	Tarragon
Artemisia pallens	Davana
Artemisia vulgaris	Mugwort

Berberis vulgaris	Barberry
Betula alleghaniensis	Birch
Betula lenta	Birch
Borago officinalis	Borage
Boswellia carteri	Frankincense
Brassica oleracea	Cabbage

Calendula officinalis	Marigold
Callitris intratropica	Blue Cypress
Calophyllum inophyllum	Tamanu
Camellia sinensis	Green Tea
Cananga odorata	Ylang Ylang
Canarium luzonicum	Elemi
Cannabis sativa	Marijuana
Carthamus tinctorius	Safflower
Capsicum annuum	Cayenne
Cedrus atlantica	Cedarwood
Centaurea cyanus	Corn Flower
Chamaemelum nobile	Roman Chamomile
Cinnamomum cassia	Cassia

Cinnamomum camphora	Ho Wood
Cinnamomum verum	Cinnamon
Cistus ladanifer	Cistus
Cistus ladanifer	Labdanum
Cistus ladanifer	Rose of Sharon
Citrus aurantifolia	Lime
Citrus aurantium	Bitter Orange
Citrus aurantium	Neroli
Citrus aurantium	Petitgrain
Citrus bergamia	Bergamot
Citrus hystrix	Combava
Citrus limon	Lemon
Citrus nobilis	Tangerine
Citrus paradisi	Grapefruit
Citrus reticulata	Mandarin
Citrus sinensis	Orange
Cocos nucifera	Coconut
Commiphora myrrha	Myrrh
Conyza canadensis	Conyza
Conyza canadensis	Fleabane
Coriandrum sativum	Coriander
Crocus sativus	Saffron
Cuminum cyminum	Black Cumin
Cupressus sempervirens	Cypress
Cucurbita pepo	Pumpkin
Cymbopogon flexuosus	Lemongrass
Cymbopogon martinii	Palmarosa
Cymbopogon nardus	Citronella

Daucus carota	Carrot
Dioscorea villosa	Wild Yam

Echinacea angustifolia	Echinacea
Echinacea pallida	Echinacea
Echinacea purpurea	Echinacea
Echinacea purpurea	Purple Coneflower
Elaeis guineensis	Palm
Elettaria cardamomum	Cardamom
Eucalyptus citriodora	Lemon Eucalyptus
Eucalyptus dives	Peppermint Eucalyptus
Eucalyptus globulus	Blue Gum
Eucalyptus globulus	Eucalyptus
Eucalyptus radiata	Black Peppermint
Eucalyptus polybractea	Blue Mallee
Eucalyptus Smithii	Gully Gum

Ferula gummosa	Galbanum
Foeniculum vulgare	Fennel

Gaultheria procumbens	Wintergreen
Glycyrrhiza glabra	Licorice

Hamamelis virginiana	Witch Hazel
Helianthus annuus	Sunflower
Helichrysum italicum	Everlasting
Helichrysum italicum	Helichrysum
Helichrysum italicum	Immortelle
Hordeum vulgare	Barley
Humulus lupulus	Hops
Hydrangea arborescens	Hydrangia
Hypericum perforatum	St. Johns Wort
Hyssopus officinalis	Hyssop

Inula graveolens	Sweet Inule

Jasminum officinale	Jasmine
Juglans regia	English Walnut
Juglans nigra	Black Walnut
Juniperus communis	Common Juniper
Juniperus scopulorum	Rocky Mt. Juniper
Juniperus osteosperma	Utah Juniper

Larrea tridentata	Chaparral
Laurus camphora	Camphor
Laurus camphora	White Camphor
Laurus nobilis	Bay Laurel
Lavandula angustifolia	Lavender
Lavandula x hybrida	Lavandin
Lavandula latifolia	Spike Lavender
Lobelia inflata	Lobelia
Linum usitatissimum	Flax Seed
Linum usitatissimum	Linseed
Lycium barbarum	Wolfberry

Magnolia glauca	Magnolia
Marrubium vulgare	Horehound
Matricaria recutita	Blue Chamomile
Matricaria recutita	German Chamomile
Medicago sativa	Alfalfa
Melaleuca alternifolia	Melaleuca
Melaleuca alternifolia	Snake Oil
Melaleuca alternifolia	Tea Tree

Melaleuca ericifolia	Rosalina
Melaleuca cajuputi	Cajuput
Melaleuca quinquenervia	MQV
Melaleuca quinquenervia	Naiouli
Melissa officinalis	Melissa
Mentha piperita	Peppermint
Mentha pulegium	Pennyroyal
Mentha spicata	Spearmint
Myrica pensylvanica	Bayberry
Myristica fragrans	Nutmeg
Myrtus communis	Myrtle

Nepeta cataria	Catnip
Nymphaea lotus	White Lotus

Ocimum basilicum	Basil
Olea europea	Olive
Origanum marjorana	Marjoram
Origanum compactum	Oregano
Ormenis mixta	Morrocan Chamomile
Ormenis multicaulis	Morrocan Chamomile

Paeonia officinalis	Peony
Persea americana	Avocado
Pelargonium graveolens	Geranium
Peumus boldo	Boldo
Petroselinum crispum	Parsley
Picea mariana	Spruce
Pimenta racemosa	Pimento
Pimpinella anisum	Anise
Pinus sylvestris	Pine
Piper nigrum	Black Pepper
Pogostemon cablin	Patchouly
Prunus dulcis	Almond
Pseudotsuga menziesii	Douglas Fir

Ravensara aromatica	Ravensara
Ricinus communis	Castor
Rheum palmatum	Indian Rhubarb
Rhododendron caucasicum	Rhododendron
Rhus diversiloba	Poison Oak
Rhus toxicodendron	Poison Ivy
Rhus venenata	Poison Sumac
Ribes nigrum	Black Current
Rosa damascena	Rose

Rosmarinus officinalis	Rosemary
Rumex acetosella	Sheep Sorrel
Ruta graveolens	Rue

Salvia officinalis	Sage
Salvia sclarea	Clary Sage
Santalum album	Aloes
Santalum album	Sandalwood
Sassafras albidum	Sassafras
Satureja montana	Mountain Savory
Sesamum indicum	Sesame
Solidago canadensis	Goldenrod
Syzygium aromaticum	Clove

Tagetes glandulifera	French Marigold
Tanacetum annuum	Blue Tansy
Tanacetum vulgare	Tansy
Tanacetum vulgare	Idaho Tansy
Tanacetum vulgare	Wild Tansy
Taraxacum officinale	Dandelion
Theobroma cacao	Cacao
Theobroma cacao	Chocolate
Thuja plicata	Canadian Red Cedar
Thuja plicata	Red Cedar
Thymus vulgaris	Thyme
Trifolium pratense	Red Clover
Tsuga canadensis	Canadian Hemlock
Tsuga canadensis	Tsuga

Ulmus fulva	Slippery Elm
Urtica dioica	Nettle

Valeriana officinalis	Valerian
Vetiveria zizanioides	Vetiver
Viola odorata	Sweet Violet
Vitex negundo	Vitex

Zea mays	Corn
Zingiber officinale	Ginger

♥ CHEMICAL ANALYSES OF ESSENTIAL OILS

This section tabulates more than 600 compounds found in 113 essential oils. These are representative analyses, not comprehensive ones. Each species of essential oil contains hundreds of constituents, mostly in concentrations ≤ 0.1%. To attempt a more thorough compilation of compounds in this book would contradict its title and theme which is to make the "chemistry of essential oils simple." To keep it simple, we have focused on the major ingredients, but include some minor and trace compounds as well. For more detail, including therapeutic applications, refer to the following texts, which are the sources from which Table Thirty-Two was compiled. The capital letters in front of each reference are the first letters of the author(s) name. These are used as codes to identify the texts used in Table Thirty–Two. For complete citations, see the bibliography.

B Burfield, Tony
   Natural Aromatic Materials - Odours & Origins

C Clarke, Sue
   Essential Chemistry for Safe Aromatherapy

Fl Fleming, Thomas, editor
   PDR® for Herbal Medicines

Fr Franchomme, Pierre, and Penoel, Daniel
   L'Aromatherapie Exactement

H Higley, Connie and Alan
   Reference Guide for Essential Oils

M Manwaring, Brian, editor
   Essential Oils Desk Reference

P Price, Shirley and Len
   Aromatherapy for Health Professionals

Y Young, D. Gary
   Essential Oils Integrative Medical Guide

W Williams, David G.
   Chemistry of Essential Oils

Major, Minor, and Trace Compounds

According to Sue Clarke (C), a main ingredient in an oil is any constituent that comprises at least 1% of more of the total. Minor ingredients are those in concentrations between 0.1% and 1.0%. Trace ingredients are those in concentrations of less than 0.1%.

Our omission of most trace compounds is not meant to de-emphasize their importance. There are many compounds in essential oils that contribute to their fragrance and/or healing qualities that are present only in minor or trace concentrations. As often as not, the major ingredients in essential oils are vehicles and coordinators for the therapeutically and aromatically active minor ingredients and are not the main source of fragrance and therapy themselves. For example, orange (*Citrus sinensis*) is mostly d-limonene (85-96%), which is typical of all citrus rind oils. But the character, fragrance, and healing properties of orange oil are determined by its minor and trace constituents consisting of more than 140 other compounds. These include at least 36 hydrocarbons, 34 alcohols, 30 esters, 20 aldehydes, 14 ketones, a dozen saccharides, and 10 carboxylic acids.

To list all of the compounds in the most commonly applied essential oils is impossible at this time and, if accomplished, would result in a large set of volumes describing tens of thousands of compounds. Such a body of data does not yet exist and may never exist. The vast majority of constituents in essential oils remains unknown. Not one essential oil has yet to be completely analyzed—all of its ingredients discovered and described. The best we can do here are in the tables that follow, including the last two (69 & 70) which alphabetically list more than 600 compounds and the oils in which they are found.

There is one class of trace constituents we do include in our lists—the furanoid compounds. These can sometimes lead to phototoxicity, even in traces, although this is not always the case. As mentioned in Chapter Ten, the phototoxicity potential of a furan or furanocoumarin is often quenched by the companion compounds in the oil. Such is the chemical complexity of essential oils that defies generalization.

Different Texts, Different Analyses

If you look up the chemical composition of a particular essential oil in several sources, you probably won't find any two the same, unless they were extracted from the same source. In the nine references applied in this section, the correspondence between Manwaring (M) and Young (Y) is almost exact since they were compiled by the same editors and authors. Higley's (H) data partially parallels that of Manwaring (M) and Young (Y), as well as that of Franchome and Penoel (Fr). The compilations of Price (P) and Franchomme (Fr) are similar, but also different. Franchomme (Fr), and especially Price (P), provide the most detailed and complete chemical information of the nine references. Burfield (B) contains chemical information not found elsewhere and emphasizes the compounds that provide fragrance. Burfield also provides the best source on distinguishing chemotypes. Fleming (Fl) is presented from a medical point of view and also contains considerable data not found elsewhere. Clarke (C) and Williams (W) are each unique, but only cover a few oils, less than a dozen each.

The differences between published oil compositions can be considerable in some cases. For example, an analysis of calamus oil (*Acorus calamus*) is given in both Franchomme (Fr) and Young (Y). Franchomme (Fr) describes two chemotypes of calamus: one is 75-80% β–asarone, a trimethyl ether, with 1-6% asaronal, an aldehyde. The other calamus oil is listed as 23-32% shyobunone, a ketone, and 8-19% isoasarol, a phenol. Only one chemotype is given in Young (Y) with a composition of 18-35% shyobunone and 6-12% calamuscenone, both ketones, with 16-22% α & β–asarone along with 5-9% calemendial, an aldehyde. So one (Fr) says the oil can be composed of an ether and an aldehyde, or a ketone and a phenol while the other (Y) says it is made up of ethers, ketones, and an aldehyde. Which is correct?

The answer is that all three are correct. Not only are essential oils chemically complex, they vary according to geography (i.e., climate, latitude, altitude, soil conditions, etc.) but also according to the variations from year to year (i.e. rainfall, sunshine, date of planting, date of harvest, time of day of harvest, application of fertilizers, etc.) The details of distillation also make a difference. This is discussed in Chapter Seven on chemotypes.

The point is that from the same species different authors use analyses from different batches, growers, distillers, and locations which can result in considerable differences in composition. Aromatic oils are not like precision pharmaceuticals duplicated precisely year after year, batch after batch, independent of time and geography. You could find a hundred books with analyses on, let's say, thyme or eucalyptus oil, with quite a range of compositions reported.

What we have done in this book is to combine averages and ranges of compositions from the various sources. This won't give you the exact composition of any particular sample, but will give you an idea of the common composition and general chemistry of a particular species in its main constituents.

Therapeutic and Aromatic Applications

Most books with tabulations of the chemical makeup of specific essential oils also list therapeutic and/or food/perfumery applications. We will not do that here. For therapeutic usage we recommend that you consult Franchomme (Fr), Higley (H), Manwaring (M), Price (P), and/or Young (Y). For food or fragrance applications, consult Burfield (B) and Williams (W). Fleming (Fl) offers medical and scientific information on essential oils, but is more academic than practical in its approach.

Confusion of Common and Botanical Names

Different authors list their tabulations of oil chemistry differently. Burfield (B), Franchomme (Fr), and Price (P) list their catalogs in alphabetical order by Latin names. Clarke (C), Higley (H), Manwaring (M), Young (Y), and Williams (W) list their catalogues by common names. Fleming (Fl) lists them both ways, primarily by common names, but inserting the botanical names in the list as well. We will follow the example of Fleming here, listing by both common and scientific names so no matter by what name you may personally know an oil, you can find it in a single alphabetical listing.

It is important that scientific names always be cited to reduce the confusion of common names. For example, *Achillea millefolium* goes by many common names including yarrow, yarroway, blue yarrow, bloodwort, nosebleed, devil's nettle, milfoil, staunchweed, thousand seal, carpenter's weed, and sneezewort. *Chamaemelum nobile* is known as both Roman and English chamomile. *Matricaria recutita* is known as both German and Hungarian chamomile, but is also called blue chamomile and matricaria, This last example poses yet another confusion of names.

Botanical names are supposed to uniquely identify a specific genus and species with only one name per plant. Unfortunately, this is not always true in practice. German chamomile has been assigned the botanical epithet of *Matricaria recutita*, as given above, but in some texts it is referenced by the Latin name of *Chamomilla recutita*. There is only one German chamomile plant species, yet it has two official names. This kind of error has its source in the history of plant taxonomy where botanists from different countries find, describe, and name plants unaware that what they think is a newly discovered species has actually already been cataloged and given a name. By the time the redundancy has been discovered, a number of scientific papers have already been published using one name or the other, thus entrenching both into the literature. Hence, the original scientific plan of only one botanical name per plant has been somewhat compromised.

Examples of multiple botanical names for plants are not uncommon. German chamomile is not the only one. Among essential oils we have the following examples:

White camphor oil can be labeled either *Laurus camphora* or *Cinnamomum camphora*. Either way it is the same oil from the same tree.

Juniper oil can be *Juniperus communis* or *Juniperus scopulorum*, different names, same species.

Lavandin oil is called *Lavandula x hybrida* in Manwaring (M), Young (Y) and Higley (H), while it is called *Lavandula x intermedia* in Price (P) and Burfield (B) and yet another botanical name, *Lavandula x burnatii*, in Franchomme (Fr). Their only agreement on nomenclature is in the genus (*Lavandula*) and the designation as a hybrid (x).

Cajuput oil is identified as *Melaleuca leucadendra* by Higley (H), Manwaring (M), Price (P) and Young (Y), but is labeled as *Melaleuca cajuputi* by Burfield (B) and Franchomme (Fr).

Niaouli oil bears two botanical names, *Melaleuca quinquenervia* and *Melaleuca viridiflora*. It also goes by other common names such as "MQV" and "broad-leafed paperbark."

Patchouly oil (also spelled patchouli) can be found as *Pogostemon cablin* or *Pogostemon patchouli*, depending on which book you read.

Morrocan chamomile oil (also called ormenis oil) has three technical names, *Ormenis mixta*, *Anthemis mixta*, and *Ormenis multicaulis*. Synthetic chamazulene is sometimes added to the less expensive ormenis oil and sold as the more precious oil of German chamomile.

Spruce (or black spruce) can be either *Picea mariana* or *Picea nigra*, yet are the same tree, same species.

The hemlock tree has been classified in three different genera as *Tsuga canadensis*, *Abies canadensis*, and *Picea canadensis*.

The common pine (also known as scotch pine and Norwegian

pine) has been classified as *Pinus sylvestris*, *Pinus altissima*, *Pinus borealis*, and *Pinus caucasica*.

You get the picture. These examples could go for many pages. For all the good intentions of the early scientific pioneers, botany is not as well organized, unambiguous, and unequivocal as scientists had once dreamed of. I mention these this so that if you encounter contradictory or confusing terminology, you will know that is not all your fault and will be able to know that two oils can be the same even though named differently.

As for the tabulation of compounds that follows, we have arranged it so that no matter what name you look up, common or scientific, you will be able to find your oil in a single alphabetical listing.

Summary of Compound Name Endings

Chapter Four discussed the International Union of Pure and Applied Chemists (IUPAC) who assigns scientific nomenclature to compounds as they are synthesized or discovered. Mentioned in that chapter is the fact that compounds, like plants, have both common names as well as technical ones. The technical name assigned by IUPAC actually discribes the elements and their configuration that comprises a molecule of the compound. However, some of these IUPAC names are quite long and cumbersome. The common names are much shorter and simpler. Even scientists prefer to use them in ordinary communications. As an example to refresh your memory, in Chapter Eight we defined and discussed the isoprene unit (C_5H_8). "Isoprene" is its common name. Its scientific name is 2-methylbutyl–1,3 diene. As you can appreciate immediately, "isoprene" said in three syllables is a lot easier than the sesquipedalic name of nine syllables. IUPAC also has some rules for common names, which we have used throughout this book. Let's review them briefly:

Names of **Alkanes** should end in -ane.

Names of **Terpenes** (i.e., Monoterpenes, Sesquiterpenes, Diterpenes, Triterpenes, etc.) should end in -ene.

Names of **Phenols** (including phenylpropanoids) should end in -ol, but often they don't.

Names of **Alcohols** should end in - ol, and almost always do.

Names of **Ethers** should end in -ole, -cin, or -ether.

Names of **Aldehydes** should end in -al or -aldehyde.

Names of **Ketones** should end in -one or -ketone.

Names of **Carboxylic Acids** include the word "acid."

Names of **Esters** should be double with the first name
ending in -yl identifying the parent alcohol and the last
name ending in -ate to identify the parent acid.

Names of **Oxides** usually include the word "oxide."

Names of **Lactones** should end in -olide or -lactone, but they
often end in -one, -ine, -in, -en, or -ene.

Names of **Coumarins** may incorporate the word "coumarin"
and share the same endings as lactones.

Names of **Furanoids** should incorporate prefixes such as
fur- furfur- furo-, furan-, or furano- in their names or
suffixes such as furan. The most common furanoids in
essential oils are furanocoumarins.

Common chemical names for organic compounds do not
reveal their complete formulas and structures as the technical
IUPAC names can do. However, knowing the simple rules given
above will enable you to identify the chemical class to which
most essential oil compounds belong.

Common names for compounds are not unique and can vary,
just as common names for plants can vary. For example, humulene and α-caryophyllene are the same compound. Terpinen-4-
ol, terpinen-1-ol-4, and β-terpinol are all the same compound. In
Table Thirty–One, we will use humulene and terpinen-4-ol, but
you will encounter the other names in various texts.

Important Note: The chemistry of essential oils is highly
variable. When comparing texts, you can often find a considerable range of compositions published for the same species. The
analyses in Table Thirty-Two can be considered representative
for typical samples of each species. The content of the Table has
been gleaned, averaged, and combined from the nine different
texts listed earlier. These source references are identified for
each oil by the letter codes given at the beginning of this section,
gleaned and combined from nine different texts.

The Meaning of Major: The term, "Major" as used in table
Thirty-Two refers to compounds that can occur in an essential
oil in concentrations of 1% or more. "Minor" compounds are
those in the range of 0.1% to 0.9%. "Trace compounds are those
present in concentrations of less than 0.1%.

An Average Essential Oil: Table Thirty-Two-A (page 558)
shows the composition of an "average essential oil." It is the average of the components of all 113 oils listed in Table Thirty-Two.
You might be surprised to see what an "average essential oil"
would contain. Young Living, Inc., has such an oil, a blend of
approximately 100 oils. It is called Legacy®.

Format for Table Thirty-Two	Greek Letters and Other Compound Prefixes

Botanical Name
Botanical Family
• Common Names (most popular
  common name **in bold**)
• Part of Plant Producing the Oil
• References (B, Fl, Fr, H, etc.)
Chemistry
  Alkanes, Monoterpenes
  Sesquiterpenes,
  Sesquiterpenols, Diterpenes
  Triterpenes, Tetraterpenes
  Phenols, Alcohols, Ethers
  Aldehydes, Ketones
  Sequiterpenals,
  Sesquiterpenones
  Acids, Esters, Oxides,
  Lactones, Coumarins,
  Furanoids, etc.

α = alpha
β = beta
γ = gamma
δ = delta
ζ = zeta
χ = chi
d = (+) dextrorotary
     (right-handed)
l = (−) levorotary
     (left-handed)
p = para

(See Chapter Nine for More
information.)

Table Thirty-Two
Chemical Compounds in 113 Essential Oils

1. Abies alba
Pinaceae (Pine Family)
• **Silver Fir**, White Fir
• Distilled from needles & twigs
• B, Fr, H
Monoterpenes 90-95%
  l-limonene 33-35%
  α-pinene 22-26%
  camphene 20-22%
Esters 5-10%
  bornyl acetate 5-10%

NOTE
Table Thirty-Two is 49 pages long.

2. Abies balsamea
Pinaceae (Pine Family)
• **Balsam Fir**, Idaho Balsam Fir,
  Canadian Balsam
• Distilled from needles & twigs
• B, Fr, H, M, Y
Monoterpenes 75-90%
  α-pinene 28-49%
  δ-3 carene 7-35%
  β-pinene 14-24%
  camphene 13-20%
  l-limonene 13-20%
  β-phellandrene 1-2%
Esters 9-23%
  bornyl acetate 9-23%

Abies concolor
(See *Abies grandis*)

3. Abies grandis
Pinaceae (Pine Family)
* **White Fir**, Giant Fir, Oregon Fir, Silver Fir
* Distilled from needles & twigs
* B, H, M, Y

Monoterpenes 55-75%
β-pinene 20-30%
α-pinene 8-12%
β-phellandrene 11-16%
camphene 7-15%

Sesquiterpenes 2-7%
δ-cadinene 2-7%

Alcohols 1-2%
borneol 1-2%

Esters 12-14%
bornyl acetate 11-16%

4. Achillea millefolium
Asteraceae (Aster–Daisy Family)
* **Yarrow**, Yarroway, Blue Yarrow, Bloodwort, Nosebleed, Devil's Nettle, Milfoil, Staunchweed, Thousand Seal, Carpenter's Weed, Sneezewort.
* Distilled from flowering tops
* B, Fl, Fr, H, M, P. Y

Monoterpenes 20-65%
sabinene 10-40%
β-pinene 6-12%
α-pinene 2-4%
camphene 4-6%
γ-terpinene 1-4%

Sesquiterpenes 25-55%
chamazulene 12-30%
germacrene-D 5-13%
β-caryophyllene 4-8%
humulene 3-7%

Ketones 13-30%
camphor 4-18%
isoartemisia ketone 8-10%
thujone 1-2%

Alcohols 3-13%
borneol 1-9%
terpinen-4-ol 2-5%

Oxides 3-12%
1,8 cineole 2-10%
caryophyllene oxide 1-2%

Esters 1-2%
bornyl acetate 1-2%

Lactones 1-2%
Achillin 1-2%

Sesquiterpenols 1-2%
α-cadinol 1-2%

5. Acorus calamus
Araceae (Cane Family)
* **Calamus**, Cane, Sweet Cane, Flag, Sweet Flag
* Distilled from roots
* B, Fr, Y

Ketones 29-50%
shyobunone 23-32%
calamuscenone 6-12%

Phenols 22-35%
α-asarone 2-4%
β-asarone 12-20%
isoasarol 8-19%

Aldehydes 5-9%
isocalamendial 5-9%

Aloes
(See *Santalum album*)

6. Anethum graveolens
Apiaceae (Celery-Carrot Family)
* **Dill**
* Distilled from the whole plant
* B, Fr, M, Y

Monoterpenes 35-65%
d-limonene 15-25%
α-pinene 10-20%
β-pinene 10-20%
α-phellandrene 2-4%
p–cymene 1-2%

Ketones 30-45%
d-carvone 30-45%

Ethers 9-11%
dill ether 9-11%
Coumarins 1-2%
umbelliferone 1-2%
Furanocoumarins 0-1%
ζ-ligustolide 0-1%

Angelica
(See *Angelilca archangelica*)

7. Angelica archangelica
Apiaceae (Celery-Carrot-Parsley)
• **Angelica**
• Distilled from roots
• B, Fr, H, M, Y
Monoterpenes 65-95%
d-limonene 20-40%
α-pinene 20-25%
l-limonene 10-20%
β-phellandrene 2-12%
α-phellandrene 1-4%
β-pinene 1-2%
Esters 2-4%
bornyl acetate 1-2%
verbenyl acetate 1-2%
Coumarins 1-2%
umbelliferone 1-2%
Furanoids 0-2%
angelicine 0-1%
angelica lactone 0-1%
bergaptene 0-1%
Carboxylic Acids 0-1%
angelic acid 0-1%
citric acid 0-1%

8. Aniba roseodora
Lauraceae (Laurel Family)
• **Rosewood**
• Distilled from wood
• B, Fr, H, M, Y, P
Alcohols 70-95%
linalol 70-95%
α-terpineol 2-7%
geraniol 1-3%

Oxides 2-6%
1,8 cineole 1-3%
linalol oxide 1-3%
Sesquiterpenes 1-3%
α-copaene 1-3%
Ketones 0-2%
heptanone 0-2%%

Anise
(See *Pimpinella anisum*)

Annual Tansy
(See *Tanacetum annum*)

Anthemis mixta
(See *Ormenis mixta)*

Anthemis nobilis
(See *Chamaemelum nobile*)

9. Apium graveolens
Apiaceae (Celery-Carrot-Parsley)
• **Celery Seed**
• Distilled from seeds
• B, Fl, Fr, M, Y
Monoterpenes 70-85%
d-limonene 60-65%
ocimene 9-11%
α-terpinene 3-6%
γ-terpinene 3-6%
Esters 3-23%
carvyl acetate 2-20%
geranyl acetate 1-3%
Lactones 6-16%
butylphthalide 5-10%
sedanolides 1-5%
neocilide 0-1%
Sesquiterpenes 6-12%
β-selinene 5-10%
α-selinene 1-2%
Ketones 8-10%
d-carvone 8-10%
Carboxylic Acids 3-6%
sedanolic acid 3-5%
chlorogenic acid 0-1%
Alcohols 1-2%
α-terpineol 1-2%

Furanocoumarins 0-1%
bergaptene 0-1%

Arbor Vitae
(See *Thuja occidentalis*)

Artemisia
(See *Artemisia vulgaris*)

10. Artemisia dracunculus
Asteraceae (Aster-Daisy Family)
• **Tarragon**, French Tarragon, Estragon, Russian Tarragon
• Distilled from leaves
• B, Fl, Fr, H, M, Y
Phenolic Ethers 65-85%
estragole 60-80%
anethole 5-10%
Monoterpenes 14-30%
β-ocimene 12-24%
l-limonene 2-6%
α-pinene 0-1%
β-pinene 0-1%
camphene 0-1%
Coumarins 1-4%
herniarin 1-2%
scopoletin 0-1%
scoparone 0-1%
artemidin 0-1%

11. Artemisia pallens
Asteraceae (Aster-Daisy Family)
• **Davana**
• Distilled from flowers
• B, Fr, H
Ketones 30-65%
davanone 25-55%
nordavanone 3-8%
artenone 2-5%
Ethers 1-6%
davana ether 1-6%
Furanoids 2-4%
davana furan 2-4%

12. Artemisia vulgaris
Asteraceae (Aster-Daisy Family)
• **Mugwort**, Artemisia
• Distilled from leaves & roots
• B, Fl, M
Monoterpenes 30-45%
myrcene 20-25%
sabinene 9-14%
l-limonene 1-3%
β-phellandrene 1-3%
Ketones 9-18%
α-thujone 4-8%
β-thujone 4-8%
camphor 1-2%
Oxides 1-2%
1,8 cineole 1-2%
Lactones 0-2%
vulgarin 0-1%
pilostachyin 0-1%

Autumn Rose
(See *Rosa damascena)*

Balsam Fir
(See *Abies balsamea)*

Basil
(See *Ocimum basilicum)*

Bastard Lavender
(See *Lavandula x hybrida)*

Bay (See *Laurus nobilis)*

Bay Laurel
(See *Laurus nobilis)*

Bee Balm
(See *Melissa officinalis)*

Benjamin Tree
(See *Styrax benzoin)*

Benzoin
(See *Styrax benzoin*)

Bergamot
(See *Citrus bergamia*)

Bethlehem Sage
(See *Mentha spicata*)

13. Betula alleghaniensis
Betulaceae (Birch Family)
• **Birch**, Yellow Birch
• Distilled from wood, twigs, and branches
• B, Fl, Fr, H, M, Y
Phenolic Esters 85-95%
methyl salycilate 85-95%
Carboxylic Acids 1-3%
ascorbic acid 0-1%
chlorogenic acid 0-1%
salicylic acid 0-1%
Triterpenes 1-2%
betula saponins 1-2%
Oxides 0-1%
Sesquiterpene oxide 0-1%

Bhang (See *Cannabis sativa*)

Bigarade
(See *Citrus aurantium - 28*)

Birch
(See *Betula alleghaniensus*)

Bitter Orange
(See *Citrus aurantium - 28*)

Borneol Thyme
(See *Thymus satureioides*)

Boswellia
(See *Boswellia carteri*)

14. Boswellia carteri
Burseraceae (Frankincense & Myrrh Family)
• **Frankincense**, Incense, Labonah, Olibanum, Boswellia
• Distilled from gum/resin of tree
• Fr, H, M, P, Y
Monoterpenes 64-90%
α-pinene 28-49%
α-thujene 10-22%
l-limonene 10-16%
myrcene 8-12%
sabinene 3-7%
p-cymene 2-5%
α-terpinene 1-2%
β-pinene 1-2%
camphene 1-2%
α-phellandrene 0-1%
Sesquiterpenes 5-10%
β-caryophyllene 4-8%
α-gurjunene 0-1%
α-guaiene 0-1%
α-copaene 0-1%
Alcohols 2-5%
incensol 1-2%
borneol 0-1%
olibanol 0-1%
pinocarveol 0-1%
terpinen-4-ol 0-1%
Sesquiterpenols 0-1%
farnesol 0-1%

Black Pepper
(See *Piper nigrum*)

Black Peppermint
(See *Eucalyptus radiata*)

Black Spruce
(See *Piceae mariana*)

Bloodwort
(See *Achillea millefolium*)

Blue Chamomile
(See *Matricaria recutita*)

Blue Cypress
(See *Callitris intratropica*)

Blue Gum
(See *Eucalyptus globulus*)

Blue Mallee
(See *Eucalyptus polybractea*)

Blue Tansy
(See *Tanacetum annum*)

Blue Yarrow
(See *Achillea millefolium*)

Borneol Thyme
(See *Thymus satureioides*)

Brandy Mint
(See *Mentha piperita*)

Broad-Leafed Peppermint
(See *Eucalyptus dives*)

Bulgarian Rose
(See *Rosa damascena*)

Cajuput
(See *Melaleuca cajuputi*)

Calamus
(See *Acorus calamus*)

15. *Callitris intratropica*
Cupressaceae (Cypress Family)
• **Blue Cypress**
• Distilled leaves, wood, & bark
• B, M
Sesquiterpenols 45-70%
  guaiol 10-26%
  α-eudesmol 12-23%
  β-eudesmol 6-7%
  bulnesol 5-15%

Sesquiterpenes 10-22%
  β-elemene 5-10%
  β-selinene 5-10%
  δ-guaiazulene 1-2%

Cambava
(See *Citrus hystrix*)

Camphor
(See *Cinnamomum camphora*)

Canadian Balsam
(See *Abies balsamea*)

Canadian Fleabane
(See *Conyza canadensis*)

Canadian Hemlock
(See *Tsuga canadensis*)

Canadian Red Cedar
(See *Thuja plicata - 1 & 2*)

16. *Cananga odorata*
Annonaceae (Ylang Ylang Family)
• **Ylang Ylang**
Distilled from flowers
B, C, Fr, H, M, P, W, Y
Sesquiterpenes 39-55%
  β-caryophyllene 15-22%
  germacrene-D 15-20%
  α-farnescene 8-12%
  humulene 1-5%
Esters 20-50%
  benzyl acetate 9-15%
  benzyl benzoate 6-10%
  methyl salicylate 1-10%
  methyl benzoate 3-7%
  farnesyl acetate 1-7%
  geranyl acetate 3-4%
Alcohols 15-45%
  linalol 10-40%
  geraniol 0-1%

Ethers 10-15%
paracresyl methyl ether 10-15%
Phenols 6-10%
methyl paracresol 5-9%
estragole 0-1%
eugenol 0-1%
isoeugenol 0-1%
phenol 0-1%
Oxides 4-7%
caryophyllene oxide 4-7%
Sesquiterpenols 1-2%
farnesol 1-2%

17. Canarium luzonicum
Burseraceae (Frankincense &
Myrrh Family)
• **Elemi**, Manila Elemi
• Distilled from gum/resin of tree
• B, Fr, H, M, Y
Monoterpenes 55-90%
l-limonene 40-70%
α-phellandrene 10-24%
sabinene 3-10%
β-phellandrene 2-5%
dipentene 1-2%
terpinolene 0-1%
Sesquiterpenols 5-25%
elemol 5-25%
Ethers 1-7%
elemicin 1-7%
Sesquiterpenes 1-4%
δ-elemene 1-4%
Alcohols 1-2%
α-terpineol 1-2%
Ketones 0-1%
d-carvone 0-1%

Cane (See Acorus calamus)

Cannabis
   (See Cannabis sativa)

18. Cannabis sativa
Cannabaceae (Hemp Family)
• **Marijuana**, Hemp, Bhang,
Ganja, Cannabis
• Distilled from leaves & stalk
• B, Fl, Fr
Sesquiterpenes 41-52%
β-caryophyllene 28-35%
humulene 10-12%
aromadendrene 3-5%
Monoterpenes 10-22%
myrcene 7-8%
α-pinene 2-8%
β-pinene 1-6%
l-limonene 0-1%
Oxides 4-10%
caryophellene oxide 4-10%
Triterpenols 1-2%
cannabinol 1-2%

Caraway (See Carum carvi)

Cardamom
   (See Elettaria cardamomum)

Carpenter's Weed
   (See Achillea millefolium)

Carrot Seed
   (See Daucus carota)

19. Carum carvi
Apiaceae (Celery-Carrot-Parsley)
• **Caraway**
• Distilled from seed
• B, Fr, P
Ketones 35-70%
d-carvone 35-70%
Monoterpenes 30-65%
d-limonene 10-35%
carvene 20-30%
myrcene 0-1%
p-cymene 0-1%
terpinolene 0-1%

Aldehydes 5-34%
octanal 3-20%
decanal 1-13%
cuminal 1-2%
Sesquiterpenes 1-10%
germacrene-D 1-10%
β-carophyllene 0-1%
Alcohols 5-7%
carveol 5-6%
cuminyl alcohol 0-1%
perillyl alcohol 0-1%

Cassia
(See *Cinnamomum cassia*)

Catmint
(See *Nepeta cataria*)

Catnip
(See *Nepeta cataria*)

Catswort
(See *Nepeta cataria*)

Cedar
(See *Thuja plicata -102 or 103*)

Cedar Bark
(See *Thuja plicata - 102*)

Cedar Leaf
(See *Thuja occidentalis - 101 or Thuja plicata - 103*)

Cedarwood
(See *Cedrus atlanticus*)

20. Cedrus atlanticus
Pinaceae (Pine Family)
• **Cedarwood**
•Distilled needles & branches
• B, Fr, H, M, Y, P

Sesquiterpenes 55-90%
β-himachalene 35-55%
α-himachalene 10-12%
γ-himachalene 8-15%
δ-cadinene 2-6%
Sesquiterpenols 20-40%
alantol 10-20%
α-caryophyllenol 5-10%
β-cubenol 5-10%
Sesquiterpenones 14-25%
α-alantone 8-15%
γ-alantone 6-12%
deodarone 1-2%
α-ionone 0-1%

Celery Seed
(See *Apium graveolens*)

21. Chamaemelum nobile
Asteraceae (Aster-Daisy Family)
• **Roman Chamomile,** English Chamomile
• Distilled from flowers
• B, C, Fl, Fr, H, M, P, Y
Esters 55-75%
isobutyl angelate 15-25%
isoamyl methacylate 15-25%
amyl butyrate 12-15%
allyl angelate 6-10%
methylbutyl angelate 3-7%
isobutyl butyrate 2-9%
hexyl acetate 2-5%
butyl tiglate 1-3%
propyl angelate 1-2%
isobutyl acetate 1-2%
Monoterpenes 18-35%
α-pinene 9-11%
β-pinene 2-10%
α-terpinene 1-9%
sabinene 1-8%
γ-terpinene 1-5%
camphene 1-5%
d-limonene 2-3%
p-cymene 1-4%
myrcene 1-3%

Ketones 10-15%
pinocarvone 10-15%
Sesquiterpenes 2-12%
β-caryophyllene 1-10%
chamazulene 1-2%
β-copaene 1-2%
δ-cadinene 1-2%
Sesquiterpenols 4-7%
farnesol 2-4%
nerolidol 2-3%
Alcohols 4-6%
pinocarveol 4-6%
Carboxylic Acids 0-1%
angelica acid 0-1%

Chamomile
(See *Chamaemelum nobile,
Matricaria recutita,* or
Ormenis multicaulis)

Chamomilla Recutita
(See *Matricaria recutita)*

Chaste Tree
(See *Vitex negundo)*

Chinese Parsely
(See *Coriandrum sativum)*

Chinese Sassafras
(See *Cinnamomum camphora*)

Cilantro
(See *Coriandrum sativum)*

22. Cinnamomum camphora
Lauraceae (Laurel Family)
• **White Camphor**, Japanese
  Camphor, Chinese Sassafras
• Distilled from leaves & wood
• B, Fr

Ketones 40-55%
camphor 40-50%
piperitone 1-5%
Oxides 26-38%
1,8 cineole 25-35%
linalol oxide 1-3%
Phenolic Ethers 1-18%
safrole 1-18%
Diterpenes 1-4%
α-camphorene 1-2%
β-camphorene 0-1%
hishorene 0-1%
Sesquiterpenes 0-2%
chamazulene 0-2%

23. Cinnamomum cassia
Lauraceae (Laurel Family)
• **Cassia**
• Distilled from bark
• Fr, H, M, Y
Aldehydes 75-85%
transcinnamaldehyde 70-85%
methoxycinnamaldehyde 3-15%
benzaldehyde 3-4%
cuminal 0-1%
Coumarins 6-8%
coumarin 6-8%
Phenols 4-10%
eugenol 2-5%
ethylgaiacol 1-2%
benzyl alcohol 0-1%
chavicol 0-1%
phenol 0-1%
vinylphenol 0-1%
Esters 2-6%
cinnamyl acetate 1-6%
benzyl acetate 0-1%
Alcohol 2-3%
cinnamic alcohol 2-3%
Carboxylic Acids 1-3%
cinnamic acid 1-2%
benzoic acid 0-1%

24. Cinnamomum verum

Lauraceae (Laurel Family)
- Cinnamon Bark
- Distilled from bark

Fl, Fr, H, M, Y

Aldehydes 41-52%
transcinnamaldehyde 40-50%
hydroxycinnamaldehyde 1-2%
benzylaldehyde 0-1%
cuminal 0-1%

Phenols 20-30%
eugenol 20-30%
phenol 0-1%
vinylphenol 0-1%

Alcohols 4-9%
linalol 3-7%
cinnamic alcohol 1-2%

Sesquiterpenes 3-8%
β-caryophyllene 3-8%

Carboxylic Acids 1-2%
cinnamic acid 1-2%

Coumarins 0-1%
coumarin 0-1%

Cinnamon Bark

(See Cinnamomum verum)

Cistus (See Cistus ladanifer)

25. Cistus ladanifer

Cistaceae (Cistus Family)
- Cistus, Labdanum, Rock Rose, Rose of Sharon
- Distilled from branches
- B, Fr, H, M, Y

Monoterpenes 42-65%
α-pinene 40-60%
camphene 2-5%

Alcohols 9-15%
α-terpineol 5-7%
pinocarveol 3-6%
borneol 1-3%

Esters 5-12%
bornyl acetate 3-6%
methyl benzoate 1-3%
linalyl acetate 1-2%
phenyl propanoate 0-1%
ethyl campholenate 0-1%

Ketones 5-10%
cyclohexanone 2-3%
acetophenone 1-3%
fenchone 1-2%
isomenthone 1-2%

Aldehydes 3-6%
benzylaldehyde 2-3%
campholenaldehyde 1-2%
neral 0-1%

Diterpenols 1-2%
labdanenol 0-1%
labdanendiol 0-1%

Carboxylic Acids 0-1%
campholenic acid 0-1%

Citronella

(See Cymbopogon nardus)

26. Citrus aurantifolia

Rutaceae (Citrus Family)
- Lime, Key Lime
- Cold-pressed from rind
- B, Fl, Fr, H, M

Monoterpenes 45-80%
d-limonene 34-64%
β-pinene 8-12%
α-pinene 2-5%
camphene 1-2%
sabinene 0-1%
p-cymene 0-1%

Oxides 11-22%
1,8 cineole 10-20%
1,4 cineole 1-2%

Aldehydes 10-20%
geranial 6-8%
neral 3-5%
citral 1-2%
citronellal 1-2%
lauric aldehyde 0-1%

octanal 0-1%
nonanal 0-1%
decanal 0-1%
Alcohols 2-4%
α-terpineol 1-2%
borneol 0-1%
α-fenchol 0-1%
linalol 0-1%
Coumarins 1-2%
limettine 1-2%
Furanoids 1-2%
furfural 0-1%
garanoxycoumarin 0-1%

27. *Citrus aurantium*
Rutaceae (Citrus Family)
• **Neroli**, Neroli Absolute, Orange Blossom
• Solvent extraction from flowers
• B, Fl, Fr, H, M, P, Y
Alcohols 35-60%
linalol 28-44%
α-terpineol 2-6%
nerolidol 1-5%
geraniol 2-3%
nerol 1-3%
farnesol 1-2%
Monoterpenes 21-40%
d-limonene 9-18%
β-pinene 7-17%
ocimene 3-8%
myrcene 1-4%
α-pinene 1-2%
neptadecene 0-1%
sabinene 0-1%
Esters 7-30%
linalyl acetate 3-15%
methyl anthranilate 2-10%
neryl acetate 1-3%
geranyl acetate 1-2%
Aldehydes 1-3%
benzylaldehyde 0-1%
decanal 0-1%
vinylhexanal 0-1%

Phenols 1-2%
phenylethanol 0-1%
benzyl alcohol 0-1%
Pyrroles 0-1%
indole 0-1%
scatole 0-1%

28. *Citrus aurantium*
Rutaceae (Citrus Family)
• **Bitter Orange**, Bigarade, Orange Bigarade
• Cold-pressed from rind
• B, Fl, Fr, P
Monoterpenes 85-95%
d-limonene 83-90%
α-pinene 1-2%
myrcene 1-2%
camphene 0-1%
terpinolene 0-1%
Aldehydes 3-10%
citronellal 1-2%
geranial 1-2%
neral 1-2%
nonanal 0-1%
decanal 0-1%
undecanal 0-1%
dodecanal 0-1%
Tetraterpenes 4-8%
β-carotene 3-6%
lycopene 1-2%
Esters 3-7%
linalyl acetate 1-2%
methyl anthranilate 1-2%
citronellyl acetate 0-1%
geranyl acetate 0-1%
neryl acetate 0-1%
octyl acetate 0-1%
Furanocoumarins 2-6%
bergaptene 1-2%
auraptene 0-1%
auraptenol 0-1%
bergaptole 0-1%
citrotene 0-1%

Alcohols 1-4%
α-terpineol 0-1%
citronellol 0-1%
linalol 0-1%
nerol 0-1%
Coumarins 1-3%
coumarin 0-1%
osthol 0-1%
scoparone 0-1%
Sesquiterpenes 1-2%
β-caryophyllene 0-1%
α-copaene 0-1%
β-farnesene 0-1%

---

29. *Citrus aurantium*
Rutaceae (Citrus Family)
• **Petitgrain**, Orange Leaf
• Distilled from leaves & twigs
• B, Fl, Fr, H, M, P. Y
Esters 48-65%
linalyl acetate 44-55%
geranyl acetate 2-5%
α-terpinyl acetate 1-3%
neryl acetate 1-3%
methyl anthranilate 0-1%
Alcohols 23-45%
linalol 15-28%
α-terpineol 5-8%
geraniol 2-5%
nerol 1-2%
citronellol 0-1%
terpinen-4-ol 0-1%
Monoterpenes 10-28%
myrcene 1-6%
β-cymene 3-5%
ocimene 2-5%
p-cymene 1-3%
β-pinene 1-2%
γ-terpinene 1-2%
d-limonene 1-2%
phellandrene 0-1%
sabinene 0-1%
terpinolene 0-1%
Aldehydes 1-2%
decanal 0-1%
geranial 0-1%
neral 0-1%

Phenols 0-1%
thymol 0-1%
Furanocoumarins 0-1%
bergaptene 0-1%
citroptene 0-1%

---

30. *Citrus bergamia*
Rutaceae (Citrus Family)
• **Bergamot**
• Cold-pressed from rind
• B, C, Fr, H, M, P, W, Y
Monoterpenes 40-70%
d-limonene 25-40%
γ-terpinene 6-10%
β-pinene 5-10%
p-cymene 1-4%
myrcene 1-2%
α-pinene 1-2%
δ-3-carene 0-2%
camphene 0-1%
sabinene 0-1%
Esters 25-50%
linalyl acetate 24-50
geranyl acetate 1-2%
neryl acetate 0-1%
Alcohols 5-32%
linalol 3-25%
geraniol 1-3%
nerol 1-3%
α-terpineol 0-1%
Tetraterpenes 3-7%
β-carotene 2-5%
lycopene 1-2%
Sesquiterpenes 2-5%
β-caryophyllene 1-3%
β-bisabolene 1-2%
Furanocoumarins 1-4%
bergaptene 1-2%
bergaptole 0-1%
α-bergamotene 0-1%
methoxycoumarin 0-1%
Aldehydes 1-2%
geranial 0-1%
neral 0-1%
Coumarins 0-1%
limettine 0-1%

Phenols 0-1%
p-cuminol 0-1%

31. Citrus hystrix
Rutaceae (Citrus Family)
- **Cambava**, Limette, Makrut Lime
- Distilled from Leaves
- B, Fr, M

Aldehydes 65-85%
citronellal 65-85%
Alcohols 7-15%
linalol 3-6%
citronellol 2-5%
isopulegol 2-4%

32. Citrus limon
Rutaceae (Citrus Family)
- **Lemon**
- Cold-pressed from rind
- B, Fl, Fr, H, M, P, W, Y

Monoterpenes 70-90%
d-limonene 55-75%
β-pinene 7-16%
γ-terpinene 6-14%
α-pinene 6-14%
sabinene 1-3%
p-cymene 1-2%
α-terpinene 0-1%
terpinolene 0-1%
phellandrene 0-1%
Aldehydes 4-12%
citral 1-3%
citronellal 1-2%
neral 1-2%
geranial 1-2%
heptanal 0-1%
hexanal 0-1%
nonanal 0-1%
octanal 0-1%
undecanal 0-1%
Alcohols 2-5%
decanol 0-1%
hexanol 0-1%
linalol 0-1%
nonanol 0-1%
octanol 0-1%
α-terpineol 0-1%
terpenen-4-ol 0-1%

Esters 2-5%
geranyl acetate 1-2%
neryl acetate 1-2%
methyl anthranilate 0-1%
Sesquiterpenes 2-5%
β-bisabolene 2-4%
β-caryophyllene 0-1%
Tetraterpenes 1-4%
β-carotene 1-3%
lycopene 0-1%
Coumarins 1-3%
limettine 0-1%
psoralen 0-1%
scopoletin 0-1%
umbelliferone 0-1%
Furanocoumarins 1-3%
α-bergamotene 0-1%
bergaptene 0-1%
bergamottin 0-1%
bergaptole 0-1%
citroptene 0-1%

33. Citrus nobilis
Rutaceae (Citrus Family)
- **Tangerine**
- Cold-pressed from rind
- B, H, M, Y

Monoterpenes 85-95%
d-limonene 65-80%
γ-terpinene 13-20%
myrcene 1-4%
p-cymene 2-4%
β-phellandrene 1-3%
β-ocimene 1-3%
α-pinene 1-2%
β-pinene 1-2%
α-phellandrene 0-1%
terpinolene 0-1%
Tetraterpenes 5-10%
β-carotene 3-6%
lycopene 2-4%
Alcohols 1-4%
linalol 1-4%
Aldehydes 1-2%
citral 0-1%
neral 0-1%

34. *Citrus x paradisi*

Rutaceae (Citrus Family)
- **Grapefruit**
- Cold-pressed from rind
- B, Fr, H, M, Y

Monoterpenes 90-95%
d-limonene 86-92%
myrcene 1-4%
α-pinene 0-1%
sabinene 0-1%
β-phellandrene 0-1%

Tetraterpenes 3-8%
β-carotene 1-5%
lycopene 2-3%

Aldehydes 1-3%
citral 0-1%
citronellal 0-1%
decanal 0-1%
nonanal 0-1%

Furanocoumarins 0-3%
aesculetine 0-1%
auraptene 0-1%
bergaptole 0-1%

Sesquiterpenones 0-2%
nootkatone 0-2%

Alcohols 0-1%
octanol 0-1%

Thiols 0-1%
1-p-menthen-8-thiol 0-1%

35. *Citrus reticulata*

Rutaceae (Citrus Family)
- **Mandarin**, Dancy
- Cold-pressed from rind
- B, Fr, H, M, P, Y

Monoterpenes 85-95%
d-limonene 65-75%
γ-terpinene 16-22%
α-pinene 2-3%
p-cymene 1-4%
β-pinene 1-2%
myrcene 1-2%
α-phellandrene 0-1%
terpinolene 0-1%

Alcohols 2-10%
linalol 1-6%
octanol 1-2%
α-terpineol 0-1%
citronellol 0-1%
nonanol 0-1%

Tetraterpenes 4-8%
β-carotene 3-6%
lycopene 1-2%

Aldehydes 1-4%
α-sinensal 0-1%
decanal 0-1%
perillaldehyde 0-1%
octanal 0-1%

Esters 1-3%
methyl anthranilate 1-2%
benzyl acetate 0-1%

36. *Citrus sinensis*

Rutaceae (Citrus Family)
- **Orange**, Sweet Orange
- Cold-pressed from rind
- B, Fl, Fr, H, M, Y

Monoterpenes 85-95%
d-limonene 85-90%
myrcene 1-3%
terpinolene 1-2%

Tetraterpenes 4-8%
β-carotene 3-6%
lycopene 1-2%

Aldehydes 3-8%
citral 1-2%
decanal 1-2%
citronellal 0-1%
decanal 0-1%
dodecanal 0-1%
nonanal 0-1%
octanal 0-1%
α-sinensal 0-1%

Alcohols 2-6%
carveol 1-2%
linalol 1-2%
α-terpineol 0-1%
geraniol 0-1%

Ketones 1-4%
l-carvone 1-2%
d-carvone 0-1%
Esters 2-3%
citronellyl acetate 0-1%
geranyl acetate 0-1%
linalyl acetate 0-1%
methyl anthranilate 0-1%
Furanoids 1-2%
auraptene 0-1%
bergaptole 0-1%
imperatarine 0-1%
Sesquiterpenones 0-1%
nootkatone 0-1%

Clary Sage
(See *Salvia sclarea*)

Clary Wort
(See *Salvia sclarea*)

Clove
(See *Syzygium aromatica*)

Commiphora molmol
(See *Commiphora myrrha*)

---

37. *Commiphora myrrha*
Burseraceae (Frankincense-
Myrrh Family)
• **Myrrh**, Stacte, Guggal Gum,
Didthin
•Distilled from gum/resin
• B, Fl, Fr, H, M, P, Y
Sesquiterpenes 55-75%
lindestrene 20-30%
δ-elemene 18-29%
α-copaene 10-12%
β-elemene 6-8%
β-bourbonene 4-5%
γ-elemene 2-5%
muurolene 1-2%
γ-cadinene 0-1%
humulene 0-1%
curzerene 0-1%

Furanoids 20-27%
methoxyfurogermacrene 5-9%
furoendesmadiene 4-8%
α-bergamotene 4-5%
methylisopropenylfurone 4-5%
furfural 2-3%
furanodione 1-2%
furanoguaiene 0-1%
rosefuran 0-1%
Ketones 15-20%
curzenone 8-11%
methylisobutyl ketone 5-6%
germacrone 2-4%
Monoterpenes 4-6%
ocimene 2-3%
p-cymene 1-2%
α-thujene 0-1%
l-limonene 0-1%
myrcene 0-1%
Triterpenes 4-7%
α-amyrin 2-4%
α-amyrenone 2-3%
Aldehydes 2-5%
methylbutynal 2-3%
cinnamaldehyde 0-1%
cuminal 0-1%
Arenes 2-3%
xylene 2-3%
Carboxylic Acids 1-2%
acetic acid 0-1%
formic acid 0-1%
palmitic acid 0-1%
Phenols 0-2%
eugenol 0-1%
cresol 0-1%

Conyza
(See *Conyza canadensis*)

38. *Conyza canadensis*
Asteraceae (Aster-Daisy Family)
- **Fleabane**, Canadian Fleabane, Conyza
- Distilled from leaves, stems, & flowers
- Fl, Fr, H, M, Y

Monoterpenes 63-83%
l-limonene 60-75%
β-ocimene 3-7%
β-pinene 0-1%
myrcene 0-1%

Furanocoumarins 5-11%
α-bergamotene 5-11%

Esters 3-6%
matricariamethyl ester 2-3%
methyl-lachnophyllum ester 1-2%
methyl acetate 0-1%

Alcohols 2-6%
α-terpineol 2-6%

Sesquiterpenols 2-4%
nerolidol 2-4%

Lactones 1-2%
lachnophyllum lactone 1-2%

Sesquiterpenes 1-2%
β-farnesene 1-2%

Coriander
(See *Coriandrum sativum*)

39. *Coriandrum sativum*
Apiaceae (Celery-Carrot Family_
- **Coriander**, Cilantro, Chinese Parsley
- Distilled from seeds
- B, Fl, Fr, H, M, P, Y

Alcohols 67-84%
linalol 25-45%
coriandrol 10-30%
geraniol 1-3%
terpinen-4-ol 1-3%
borneol 0-1%

Monoterpenes 10-24%
α-pinene 3-7%
γ-terpinene 2-6%
l-limonene 2-5%
p-cymene 1-3%
myrcene 1-2%
camphene 0-1%

Esters 2-7%
geranyl acetate 1-5%
linalyl acetate 0-3%

Ketones 3-6%
camphor 3-6%

Coumarins 1-2%
umbelliferone 0-1%
scopoletin 0-1%

Aldehydes 0-2%
decanal 0-2%

Furanocoumarins 0-1%
bergaptene 0-1%

Diazines 0-1%
pyrazine 0-1%

Cumin (See *Cuminum cyminum*)

40. *Cuminum cyminum*
Apiaceae (Celery-Carrot-Parsley)
- **Cumin**
- Distilled from seeds
- B, Fl, Fr, H, M, Y

Monoterpenes 43-75%
γ-terpinene 16-28%
α-terpinene 12-22%
β-pinene 12-18%
p-cymene 3-9%

Aldehydes 41-57%
p-menthadienal 25-35%
cuminal 16-22%

Phenols 1-4%
p-cuminol 1-4%

Sesquiterpenes 1-2%
β-caryophyllene 1-2%

Coumarins 0-1%
scopoletin 0-1%

41. *Cupressus sempervirens*
Cupressaceae (Cypress Family)
- **Cypress**
- Distilled from branches
- B, Fr, H, M, P, Y

Monoterpenes 58-95%
α-pinene 40-62%
δ-3-carene 12-22%
l-limonene 2-7%
terpinolene 2-6%
myrcene 1-4%
β-pinene 1-3%
sabinene 0-3%
p-cymene 0-2%

Sesquiterpenols 5-15%
cedrol 5-15%

Alcohols 4-13%
borneol 2-9%
α-terpineol 1-2%
terpinen-4-ol 1-2%
linalol 0-1%
sabinol 0-1%

Esters 6-8%
α-terpinyl acetate 4-5%
isovalerate 1-2%
terpinen-4-yl acetate 1-2%

Sesquiterpenes 1-4%
δ-cadinene 1-3%
α-cedrene 0-1%

Diterpenols 1-2%
abienol 0-1%
labdanenol 0-1%
labdanendiol 0-1%
manool 0-1%
pimarinol 0-1%
totarol 0-1%

Diterpene Acids 0-1%
cupressic acid 0-1%

Oxides 0-1%
Manool Oxide 0-1%

42. *Cymbopogon flexuosus*
Gramineae (Grass Family)
- **Lemongrass**
- Distilled from leaves
- C, Fl, Fr, H, M, W, Y

Aldehydes 55-80%
geranial 32-42%
neral 22-38%
farnesal 1-3%
decanal 0-1%

Alcohols 10-15%
geraniol 5-10%
α-terpineol 2-3%
borneol 1-2%

Sesquiterpenols 10-13%
farnesol 10-13%

Esters 9-11%
geranyl acetate 5-6%
linalyl acetate 4-5%

Monoterpenes 7-9%
myrcene 4-5%
d-limonene 2-3%
β-ocimene 1-2%

Sesquiterpenes 2-6%
β-caryophyllene 2-6%

Oxides 2-4%
caryophyllene oxide 2-4%

Ketones 2-3%
methyl heptanone 2-3%

43. *Cymbopogon martinii*
Gramineae (Grass Family)
- **Palmarosa**
- Distilled stems, leaves, flowers
- B, Fr, H, M, Y

Alcohols 74-90%
geraniol 70-85%
linalol 3-7%
nerol 1-2%

Esters 12-30%
geranyl formate 5-15%
geranyl acetate 6-10%
geranyl isovalerate 1-2%

neryl formate 0-1%
prenyl hexonate 0-1%
prenyl octonate 0-1%
Monoterpenes 1-2%
d-limonene 1-2%
Oxides 1-2%
geranyl epoxide 1-2%
Sesquiterpenols 1-2%
elemol 1-2%

---

44. *Cymbopogon nardus*
Gramineae (Grass Family)
• **Citronella**
• Distilled from leaves
• B, Fr, H, M, Y
Alcohols 33-57%
geraniol 18-30%
citronellol 8-9%
borneol 3-8%
Phenols 19-27%
methyl ether 9-10%
methyl isoeugenol 4-10%
isoeugenol 6-7%
Monoterpenes 5-10%
d-limonene 5-10%
Aldehydes 5-6%
citronellal 5-6%

Cypress
(See *Cupressus sempervirens*)

Cypress, Blue
(See *Callitris intratropica*)

Dalmatian Sage
(See *Salvia officinalis*)

Damask Rose
(See *Rosa damascena*)

Dancy (See *Citrus reticulata*)

---

45. *Daucus carota*
Apiaceae (Celery-Carrot-Parsley)
• **Carrot Seed**
• Distilled from seeds
• B, Fl, Fr, H, M, Y
Alcohols 29-47%
carotol 30-55%
daucol 3-4%
linalol 2-3%
geraniol 0-1%
Monoterpenes 20-24%
α-pinene 11-13%
sabinene 9-11%
Sesquiterpenes 14-18%
β-bisabolene 8-10%
β-caryophyllene 4-5%
daucene 2-3%
Oxides 3-5%
caryophyllene oxide 3-5%
Esters 2-4%
geranyl acetate 2-4%
Tetraterpenes 1-3%
α-carotene 0-1%
β-carotene 0-1%
γ-carotene 0-1%
ζ-carotene 0-1%
lycopene 0-1%
Phenols 1-2%
β-asarone 1-2%

Davana
(See *Artemisia pallens*)

Devil's Nettle
(See *Achillea millefolium*)

Didthin
(See *Commiphora myrrha*)

Dill (See *Anethum graveolens*)

Douglas Fir
(See *Pseudotsuga menziesii*)

Douglas Spruce
(See *Pseudotsuga menziesii*)

E. Dives
(See *Eucalyptus dives*)

E. Radiata
(See *Eucalyptus radiata*)

Elemi (See *Canarium luzonicum*)

46. *Elettaria cardamomum*
Zingiberaceae (Ginger Family)
• **Cardamom**
• Distilled from fruit and seeds
• B, Fr, H, M, Y
Esters 43-56%
α-terpinyl acetate 40-52%
linalyl acetate 3-4%
Oxides 28-35%
1,8 cineole 28-35%
Alcohols 5-10%
linalol 4-7%
α-terpineol 1-2%
terpinen-4-ol 0-1%
Monoterpenes 2-7%
l-limonene 1-3%
sabinene 1-3%
myrcene 0-1%

English Chamomile
(See *Chamaemelum nobile*)

English Lavender
(See *Lavandula angustifolia*)

Estragon
(See *Artemisia dracunculus*)

Eucalyptus
(See *Eucalyptus globulus*)

47. *Eucalyptus citriodora*
Myrtaceae (Myrtle Family)
• **Lemon Eucalyptus**
• Distilled from leaves
• B, C, Fr, H, M, P, Y
Aldehydes 40-80%
citronellal 40-80%
Alcohols 20-35%
citronellol 15-20%
geraniol 2-5%
pinocarveol 1-2%
α-terpineol 0-1%
Phenols 2-21%
isopulegol 2-20%
eugenol 0-1%
p-cuminol 0-1%
Oxides 3-18%
1,8 cineole 2-18%
linalol oxide 0-1%
rose oxide 0-1%
Esters 4-12%
citronellyl acetate 3-8%
γ-terpinyl acetate 1-2%
citronellyl butyrate 0-1%
citronellyl citronellate 0-1%
Sesquiterpenes 2-6%
β-caryophyllene 1-4%
humulene 0-1%
aromadendrene 0-1%
α-elemene 0-1%
β-cubebene 0-1%
Carboxylic Acids 3-5%
citronellic acid 3-5%
Monoterpenes 2-5%
α-pinene 1-2%
β-pinene 1-2%
p-cymene 0-1%
terpinolene 0-1%
Sesquiterpenols 0-1%
spathulenol 0-1%

48. *Eucalyptus dives*
Myrtaceae (Myrtle Family)
- **E. Dives,** Peppermint Eucalyptus, Broad-Leafed Peppermint
- Distilled from leaves
- B, C, Fr, H, M, P, Y

Ketones 35-50%
piperitone 35-50%

Monoterpenes 30-47%
α-phellandrene 20-28%
p-cymene 6-10%
α-thujene 2-6%
β-phellandrene 2-3%

Phenolic Alcohols 3-6%
terpinen-4-ol 3-6%

Alcohols 1-3%
α-terpineol 0-1%
linalol 0-1%
pipertol 0-1%

Sesquiterpenes 1-4%
α-cubebene 0-1%
β-caryophyllene 0-1%
δ-cadinene 0-1%
γ-elemene 0-1%
longifolene 0-1%

Oxides 0-1%
α-pinene oxide 0-1%
1,8 cineole 0-1%

49. *Eucalyptus globulus*
Myrtaceae (Myrtle Family)
- **Eucalyptus**, Blue Gum, Tasmanian Blue Gum
- Distilled from leaves
- B, C, Fl, Fr, H, M, P, Y

Oxides 60-75%
1,8 cineole 60-75%
α-pinene epoxide 0-2%

Monoterpenes 12-35%
α-pinene 10-22%
l-limonene 1-8%
p-cymene 1-5%
α-phellandrene 0-1%
camphene 0-1%

Sesquiterpenols 7-12%
globulol 5-6%
pinocarveol 1-5%
ledol 1-2%
viridiflorol 0-1%

Sesquiterpenes 6-9%
aromadendrene 6-8%
δ-guaiazulene 0-1%

Ketones 1-5%
pinocarvone 1-3%
d-carvone 0-1%
fenchone 0-1%

Aldehydes 1-4%
butyricaldehyde 0-1%
caproicaldehyde 0-1%
geranial 0-1%
myrtenal 0-1%
valericaldehyde 0-1%

Phenols 2-3%
myrtenol 1-2%
p-cuminol 1-2%

Alcohols 1-3%
α-fenchol 1-2%
α-terpineol 0-1%

Esters 1-2%
α-terpinyl acetate 1-2%

50. *Eucalyptus polybractea*
Myrtaceae (Myrtle Family)
- **Blue Mallee**, E. Polybractea
- Distilled from leaves & branches
- B, Fr, H, M, Y

Oxides 85-95%
1,8 cineole 85-95%

Monoterpenes 3-6%
l-limonene 1-2%
α-pinene 1-2%
p-cymene 1-2%

Ketones 1-2%
cryptone 1-2%

Aldehydes 0-1%
cuminal 0-1%

Phenols 0-1%
p-cuminol 0-1%

51. *Eucalyptus radiata*
Myrtaceae (Myrtle Family)
- **E. Radiata,** Black Peppermint, Narrow-Leafed Peppermint
- Distilled from leaves
- B, C, Fr, H, M, P, Y

Oxides 61-77%
1,8 cineole 60-75%
caryophyllene oxide 1-2%
Monoterpenes 13-24%
α-pinene 8-12%
l-limonene 4-8%
myrcene 1-2%
β-pinene 0-1%
p-cymene 0-1%
Alcohols 7-19%
α-terpineol 6-15%
geraniol 2-3%
borneol 0-1%
linalol 0-1%
Aldehydes 4-8%
citronellal 1-2%
geranial 1-2%
myrtenal 1-2%
neral 1-2%

Everlasting
(See *Helichrysum italicum*)

Fennel
(See *Foeniculum vulgare*)

Fennel, Roman
(See *Pimpinella anisum*)

52. *Ferula gummosa*
Apiaceae (Celery-Carrot-Parsley)
- **Galbanum**
- Distilled gum, stems & branches
- B, Fl, Fr, H, M, Y

Monoterpenes 50-95%
β-pinene 40-70%
α-pinene 5-21%
δ-3-carene 2-16%
myrcene 2-4%
sabinene 1-3%
camphene 0-1%
Sesquiterpenols 3-5%
galbanol 2-3%
bulnesol 0-1%
guaiol 0-1%
junenol 0-1%
Esters 1-3%
fenchyl acetate 0-1%
linalyl acetate 0-1%
α-terpinyl acetate 0-1%
Coumarins 0-3%
gummosine 0-1%
gummosenine 0-1%
umbelliferone 0-1%
Carboxylic Acids 0-1%
galbanic acid 0-1%
Diazines 0-1%
pyrazine 0-1%
Furanoids 0-1%
agarofurane 0-1%

Field Balm
(See *Nepeta cataria*)

Fir (See *Abies alba*, *Abies balsamea*, or *Abies grandis*)

Fish Mint
(See *Mentha spicata*)

Flag (See *Acorus calamus*)

Fleabane
(See *Conyza canadensis*)

---

53. *Foeniculum vulgare*
Apiaceae (Celery-Carrot-Parsley)
• **Fennel**
• Distilled from seeds
• B, Fl, Fr, H, M, P, Y
Phenolic Ethers 52-80%
anethole 50-70%
estragole 2-10%
Monoterpenes 27-50
ocimene 9-12%
l-limonene 3-12%
γ-terpinene 6-11%
α-pinene 2-10%
p-cymene 1-5%
α-phellandrene 1-4%
terpinolene 2-3%
β-phellandrene 1-3%
myrcene 1-3%
sabinene 1-2%
α-terpinene 0-1%
β-pinene 0-1%
Alcohols 12-16%
linalol 9-12%
α-fenchol 3-4%
Ketones 5-15%
fenchone 5-15%
camphor 0-1%
Oxides 1-6%
1, 8, cineole 1-6%
Phenols 1-3%
p-anol 1-3%
Furanocoumarins 1-2%
bergaptene 0-1%
seseline 0-1%
Coumarins 0-1%
psoralen 0-1%

Frankincense
(See *Boswellia carteri*)

French Marigold
(See *Tagetes glandulifera*))

French Tarragon
(See *Artemisia dracunculus*)

Friar's Balm
(See *Styrax benzoin)*

Galbanum
(See *Ferula gummosa*)

Ganja (See *Cannabis sativa*)

Garden Heliotrope
(See *Valeriana officinalis*)

Garden Mint
(See *Mentha spicata*)

Garden Parsley
(See *Petroselinum crispum*)

Garden Thyme
(See *Thymus vulgaris CT linalol*)

---

54. *Gaultheria procumbens*
Ericaceae (Heather Family)
• **Wintergreen**
• Distilled from leaves
• B, Fr, H, M, Y
Phenolic Esters 95-99%
methyl salicylate 95-99%
Carboxylic Acids 1-2%
salicylic acid 1-2%

German Chamomile
(See *Matricaria recutita*)

Geranium
(See *Pelargonium graveolens*)

Giant Fir (See *Abies grandis*)

Ginger
(See *Zingiber officinale*)

Goldenrod
(See *Solidago canadensis*)

Grapefruit
(See *Citrus x paradisi*)

Greek Oregano
(See *Origanum compactum*)

Green Mint
(See *Mentha spicata*)

Guggal Gum
(See *Commiphora myrrha*)

Heliotrope
(See *Valeriana officinalis*)

Hemlock
(See *Tsuga canadensis*)

Helichrysum
(See *Helichrysum italicum*)

55. Helichrysum italicum
Asteraceae (Aster-Daisy Family)
• **Helichrysum**, Everlasting, Immortelle
• Distilled from flowers
• B, Fr, H, M, P, Y
Esters 28-60%
neryl acetate 25-50%
neryl propionate 3-8%
neryl butyrate 1-2%
Ketones 16-22%
italidione 15-20%
β-diketone 1-2%
Sesquiterpenes 10-20%
γ-curcumene 9-15%
β-caryophyllene 1-5%
Monoterpenes 8-13%
l-limonene 8-13%
Alcohols 3-9%
nerol 2-5%
linalol 1-4%
Oxides 1-2%
1,8 cineole 1-2%
Phenols 1-2%
eugenol 1-2%

Hemp (See *Cannabis sativa*)

Hungarian Chamomile
(See *Matricaria recutita*)

Hyssop
(See *Hyssopus officinalis*)

56. Hyssopus officinalis
Lamiaceae (Mint Family)
• **Hyssop**
• Distilled from stems and leaves
• B, Fl, Fr, H, M, P, Y
Ketones 39-65%
isopinocamphone 34-50%
pinocamphone 5-17%
β-thujone 0-1%
Monoterpene 20-40%
β-pinene 13-23%
l-limonene 1-4%
ocimene 1-4%
sabinene 2-3%
α-pinene 1-2%
camphene 1-2□
myrcene 1-2%
p-cymene 0-1%
Sesquiterpenes 3-7%
germacrene-D 2-3%
β-caryophyllene 1-3%
aromadendrene 0-1%
Sesquiterpenols 1-5%
nerolidol 1-2%
elemol 0-2%
spathulenol 0-1%
Phenols 2-5%
myrtenal methylether 2-3%
myrtenol 0-2%
eugenol 0-1%
Alcohols 1-2%
borneol 1-2%
linalol 0-1%
Esters 1-3%
methyl myrtenate 1-2%
bornyl acetate 0-1%
Oxides 0-1%
linalol oxide 0-1%

Idaho Balsam Fir
(See *Abies balsamea*)

Idaho Tansy
(See *Tanacetum vulgare*)

Immortelle
(See *Helichrysum italicum*)

Incense (See *Boswellia carteri*)

Indian Valerian
(See *Nardostachys jatamansi*)

Japanese Camphor
(See *Cinnamomum camphora*)

Jasmine
(See *Jasminum officinale)*

57. *Jasminum officinale*
Oleaceae (Olive Family)
• **Jasmine**, Jasmine Absolute
• Solvent extraction from flowers
• B, H, M, Y
Esters 33-53%
 benzyl acetate 18-30%
 benzyl benzoate 14-21%
 methyl anthranilate 1-2%
Diterpenes 9-18%
 phytol 6-12%
 isophytol 3-7%
Alcohols 4-8%
 linalol 4-8%
Triterpenes 3-7%
 squalene 3-7%
Pyrroles 1-3%
 Indole 1-3%
 scatole 0-1%
Ketones 0-1%
 jasmone 0-1%

Jatamansi
(See *Nardostachys jatamansi*)

Java Frankincense
(See *Styrax benzoin)*

Juniper
(See *Juniperus communis*)

58. *Juniperus communis*
Cupressaceae (Cypress Family)
• **Juniper**, Juniper Berry
• Distilled berries, twigs, branches
• B, Fl, Fr, H, M. Y
Monoterpenes 38-70%
 α-pinene 20-40%
 sabinene 9-20%
 myrcene 6-8%
 l-limonene 3-6%
Esters 12-20%
 bornyl acetate 12-20%
Ketones 11-19%
 camphor 10-18%
 junionone 1-2 %
 pinocamphone 0-1%
Sesquiterpenes 2-3%
 muurolene 2-3%

Juniperus osteosperma
(See *Juniperus communis*)

Juniperus scopulorum
(See *Juniperus communis*)

Kaju-Puti
(See *Melaleuca cajuputi*)

Key Lime
(See *Citrus aurantifolia*)

Labdanum
(See *Cistus ladanifer)*

Labrador Tea
(See *Ledum groenlandicum*)

Lamb Mint
(See *Mentha piperita*)

Laurel (See *Laurus nobilis*)

Laurus camphora
(See *Cinnamomum camphora*)

59. Laurus nobilis
Lauraceae (Laurel Family)
• **Bay Laurel**, Bay, Laurel, Sweet Bay
• Distilled from leaves
• B, Fl, Fr, H, M, Y
Oxides 35-50%
1,8 cineole 35-50%
Alcohols 15-30%
linalol 4-16%
α-terpineol 8-10%
terpinen-4-ol 2-3%
borneol 0-1%
geraniol 0-1%
Monoterpenes 11-28%
sabinene 4-12%
α-pinene 4-10%
β-pinene 3-8%
Esters 7-18%
α-terpinyl acetate 3-10%
linalyl acetate 2-4
bornyl acetate 1-3%
geranyl acetate 1-3%
Phenols 3-9%
eugenol 3-9%
Lactones 2-4%
costunolide 1-2%
artemorine 0-1%
laurensolide 0-1%
Sesquiterpenes 2-3%
β-caryophyllene 1-2%
humulene 0-1%
β-elemene 0-1%

Lavandin
(See *Lavandula x-hybrida*)

60. Lavandula angustifolia
Lamiaceae (Mint Family)
• **Lavender**, English Lavender
• Distilled from flowering tops
• B, C, Fl, Fr, H, M, P, W, Y
Alcohols 30-58%
linalol 25-45%
terpinen-4-ol 2-6%
α-terpineol 1-2%
borneol 1-2%
lavandulol 1-2%
geraniol 0-1%
Esters 26-52%
linalyl acetate 25-45%
lavandulyl acetate 1-6%
geranyl acetate 0-1%
α-terpinyl acetate 0-1%
Monoterpenes 7-24%
β-ocimene 5-16%
d-limonene 2-5%
α-pinene 1-2%
β-pinene 0-1%
camphene 0-1%
δ-3-carene 0-1%
Sesquiterpenes 3-9%
β-caryophyllene 2-7%
χ-farnesene 1-2%
Aldehydes 2-5%
benzaldehyde 0-1%
cuminal 0-1%
geranial 0-1%
hexanal 0-1%
myrtenal 0-1%
neral 0-1%
Oxides 2-4%
1,8 cineole 1-3%
caryophyllene oxide 0-1%
linalol oxide 0-1%
Coumarins 1-4%
butanolide 0-1%
coumarin 0-1%
herniarin 0-1%
santonin 0-1%
umbelliferone 0-1%
Ketones 1-3%
octanone 1-3%

Lavandula x burnatii
(See *Lavandula x-hybrida*)

61. Lavandula x hybrida
Lamiaceae (Mint Family)
• **Lavandin**, Bastard Lavender
• Distilled from flowering tops
• B, Fr, H, M, P, Y
Alcohols 31-60%
  linalol 25-45%
  terpinen-4-ol 2-6%
  α-terpineol 1-5%
  borneol 1-3%
  geraniol 1-2%
  lavandulol 0-1%
  nerol 0-1%
Esters 32-55%
  linalyl acetate 30-50%
  geranyl acetate 1-2%
  lavandulyl acetate 1-2%
  bornyl acetate 0-1%
  neryl acetate 0-1%
Monoterpenes 7-24%
  β-ocimene 5-16%
  d-limonene 1-7%
  myrcene 1-3%
  camphene 0-1%
Ketones 5-11%
  camphor 5-11%
Sesquiterpenes 4-10%
  β-caryophyllene 3-8%
  β-farnesene 1-2%
Oxides 2-10%
  1,8 cineole 2-10%
  caryophyllene oxide 0-1%
  linalol oxide 0-1%
Coumarins 0-2%
  coumarin 0-1%
  herniarin 0-1%

Lavandula x intermedia
(See *Lavandula x-hybrida*)

Lavender
(See *Lavandula angustifolia*)

Lavender Tea Tree
(See *Melaleuca ericifolia*)

Lebonah
(See *Boswellia carteri*)

Ledum
(See *Ledum groenlandicum*)

62. Ledum groenlandicum
Ericaceae (Heather Family)
• **Ledum**, Labrador Tea,
  Marsh Tea
• Distilled from leaves
• B, Fr, H, M, Y
Monoterpenes 30-50%
  l-limonene 20-35%
  p-menthatriene 8-15%
  α-pinene 1-2%
  β-pinene 0-1%
Sesquiterpenols 13-20%
  p-menthadiene-8-ol 12-17%
  ledol 1-3%
Alcohols 1-3%
  α-terpineol 1-2%
  terpinen-4-ol 0-1%
Aldehydes 1-2%
  myrtenal 1-2%
Esters 1-2%
  bornyl acetate 0-1%
  bornyl butyrate 0-1%
Sesquiterpenones 1-2%
  germacrone 1-2%
Sesquiterpenes 1-2%
  α-selinene 1-2%

Lemon (See *Citrus limon*)

Lemon Balm
(See *Melissa officinalis*)

Lemon Eucalyptus
(See *Eucalyptus citriodora*)

Lemongrass
(See *Cymbopogon flexuosus*)

Lime (See *Citrus aurantifolia*)

Limette
(See *Citrus hystrix*)

Makrut Lime
(See *Citrus hystrix*)

Mandarin
(See *Citrus reticulata*)

Manila Elemi
(See *Canarium luzonicum*)

Marigold
(See *Tagetes glandulifera)*)

Marijuana
(See *Cannabis sativa*)

Marjoram
(See *Origanum marjorana*)

Marjoram, Spanish
(See *Thymus mastichina*)

Marsh Tea
(See *Ledum groenlandicum*)

Matricaria
(See *Matricaria recutita*)

63. *Matricaria recutita*
Asteraceae (Aster-Daisy Family)
• **German Chamomile**, Matricaria, Blue Chamomile, Hungarian Chamomile
• Distilled from flowers
• B, Fr, H, M, P, Y
Oxides 33-57%
 bisabolol oxide-A 23-32%
 bisabolol oxide-B 6-10%
 bisabolone oxide 3-20%
 1, 8 cineole 1-5%

Sesquiterpenes 34-60%
 β-farnescene 18-24%
 chamazulene 5-20%
 α-farnescene 2-13%
 δ-cadinene 4-6%
 muurolene 3-5%
 α-bisabolene 2-5%
Sesquiterpenols 3-10%
 α-bisabolol 2-7%
 farnesol 1-3%
 spathulenol 0-1%
Ethers 4-9%
 spiro ether 4-8%
 dicyclo ether 1-2%
 indole 0-1%
Monoterpenes 2-4%
 ocimene 1-2%
 α-terpinene 0-1%
 d-limonene 0-1%
 p-cymene 0-1%
Esters 0-1% .
 matricariamethyl ester 0-1%

Melaleuca
(See *Melaleuca alternifolia*)

64. *Melaleuca alternifolia*
Myrtaceae (Myrtle Family)
• **Tea Tree**, Ti Tree, Melaleuca, Snake Oil
• Distilled from leaves
• B, C, Fr, H, M, P, W, Y
Monoterpenes 35-70%
 γ-terpinene 10-28%
 α-terpinene 5-13%
 p-cymene 3-12%
 α-pinene 3-6%
 terpinolene 2-5%
 l-limonene 2-4%
 sabinene 1-3%
 β-pinene 1-2%
 myrcene 1-2%
 α-thujene 0-2%
Phenolic Alcohols 25-40%
 terpinen-4-ol 25-40%

Alcohols 2-8%
α-terpineol 2-8%
Sesquiterpenes 8-20%
δ-cadinene 2-8%
aromadrene 3-7%
viridiflorene 1-5%
β-caryophyllene 1-2%
α-phellandrene 1-2%
Oxides 5-18%
1,8 cineole 4-14%
1,4 cineole 2-3%
caryophyllene oxide 0-1%
Sesquiterpenols 1-5%
globulol 1-3%
viridiflorol 0-2%

---

65. Melaleuca cajuputi
Myrtaceae (Myrtle Family)
• **Cajuput,** Kaju-puti
• Distilled from leaves
• B, Fr, H, P, Y
Oxides 50-70%
1, 8, cineole 50-70%
1,4 cineole 1-2%
Monoterpenes 14-25%
α-terpineol 7-13%
l-limonene 3-8%
β-pinene 3-4%
α-pinene 1-3%
Alcohols 6-7%
α-terpineol 6-7%
Sesquiterpenes 5-6%
β-caryophyllene 5-6%
Sesquiterpenols 2-4%
platyphyllol 1-2%
viridiflorol 1-2%
nerolidol 0-1%
Aldehydes 1-3%
benzoicaldehyde 0-1%
butyricaldehyde 0-1%
valericaldehyde 0-1%
Esters 0-2%
α-terpinyl acetate 0-1%

66. Melaleuca ericifolia
Myrtaceae (Myrtle Family)
• **Rosalina,** Lavender Tea Tree
• Distilled from leaves
B, H, M, Y
Alcohols 37-52%
linalol 34-45%
α-terpineol 2-5%
terpinen-4-ol 1-2%
Monoterpenes 15-30%
β-phellandrene 8-10%
α–pinene 5-10%
p-cymene 2-6%
l-limonene 1-2%
γ-terpinene 0-2%
Oxides 10-20%
1,8 cineole 10-20%
1,4 cineole 0-1%
Sesquiterpenes 3-8%
aromadrene 2-6%
viridiflorene 1-2%

Melaleuca leucadendra
(See *Melaleuca cajuputi*)

---

67. Melaleuca quinquenervia
Myrtaceae (Myrtle Family)
• **Niaouli,** Nerolina, MQV,
Paperbark
• Distilled from leaves
• B, Fr, H, M, P, Y
Oxides 35-65%
1,8 cineole 35-65%
1,4 cineole 0-1%
Monoterpenes 14-29%
α-pinene 7-15%
l-limonene 5-8%
β-pinene 2-6%
Sesquiterpenols 8-22%
viridiflorol 6-15%
nerolidol 2-7%
globulol 0-1%
Alcohols 11-15%
α-terpineol 9-12%
terpinen-4-ol 2-3%

Sesquiterpenes 2-4%
β-caryophyllene 1-2%
aromadrene 0-1%
δ-cadinene 0-1%
viridiflorene 0-1%
Aldehydes 0-2%
benzaldehyde 0-1%
valeraldehyde 0-1%

Melaleuca viridiflora
(See *Melaleuca quinquenervia*)

Melissa
(See *Melissa officinalis*)

68. Melissa officinalis
Lamiaceae (Mint Family)
• **Melissa**, Lemon Balm, Sweet Balm, Bee Balm
• Distilled from leaves & flowers
• B, Fl, Fr, H, M, P, Y
Aldehydes 45-65%
geranial 25-35%
neral 18-28%
citronellal 1-3%
α-cyclocitral 0-1%
Sesquiterpenes 20-35%
β-carophyllene 12-19%
α-copaene 4-5%
germacrene-D 3-4%
β-bourbonene 1-2%
δ-cadinene 1-2%
humulene 0-1%
γ-cadinene 0-1%
β-elemene 0-1%
Oxides 5-11%
caryophyllene oxide 3-7%
1,8 cineole 2-4%
Esters 5-7%
methyl citronellate 4-5%
citronellyl acetate 0-1%
geranyl acetate 0-1%
neryl acetate 0-1%

Ketones 5-7%
methylheptanone 4-5%
farnesylacetone 0-1%
octanone 0-1%
Alcohols 4-7%
linalol 1-2%
octen-3-ol 1-2%
citronellol 0-1%
geraniol 0-1%
nerol 0-1%
isopulegol 0-1%
Monoterpenes 1-3%
ocimene 1-2%
l-limonene 0-1%
Sesquiterpenols 0-2%
elemol 0-1%
α-cadinol 0-1%
Furanocoumarin 0-1%
aesculetine 0-1%

69. Mentha piperita
Lamiaceae (Mint Family)
• **Peppermint**, Brandy Mint, Lamb Mint
• Distilled from leaves, stems and flower buds
• B, C, Fl, Fr, H, M, P, Y
Phenolic Alcohols 34-44%
Menthol 34-44%
Ketones 15-25%
menthone 12-20%
pulegone 2-5%
piperitone 1-2%
Monoterpenes 6-15%
l-limonene 2-6%
β-pinene 1-4%
ocimene 1-2%
α-pinene 0-2%
myrcene 0-1%
p-cymene 0-1%
β-phellandrene 0-1%
sabinene 0-1%
α-terpinene 0-1%
terpinolene 0-1%

Sesquiterpenes 5-10%
germacrene D 2-5%
β-bourbonene 0-1%
ζ-bulgarene 0-1%
γ-cadinene 0-1%
β-caryophyllene 0-1%
β-elemene 0-1%
β-farnesene 0-1%
muurolene 0-1%
Esters 4-9%
methyl acetate 4-9%
menthyl butyrate 0-1%
menthyl isovalerate 0-1%
Oxides 3-9%
1,8 cineole 2-5%
piperitone oxide 1-3%
caryophyllene oxide 0-1%
Furanoids 3-8%
menthofuran 3-8%
Alcohols 2-6%
terpinen-4-ol 1-3%
α-terpineol 1-2%
linalol 0-1%
Sesquiterpenols 1-2%
viridiflorol 1-2%
Furanocoumarins 0-1%
aesculetine 0-1%
Sulphides 0-1%
mint sulphide 0-1%

---

70. Mentha spicata
Lamiaceae (Mint Family)
• **Spearmint**, Garden Mint, Green Mint, Bethlehem Sage, Fish Mint Our Lady's Mint
• Distilled from leaves and stems
• B, Fl, Fr, H, M, Y
Ketones 51-70%
l-carvone 45-58%
dihydrocarvone 5-10%
menthone 1-2%
pulegone 0-1%
Monoterpenes 17-30%
l-limonene 15-25%
myrcene 1-3%

camphene 1-2%
α-pinene 0-1%
β-pinene 0-1%
Alcohols 5-10%
carveol 2-3%
linalol 1-2%
thujanol 1-2%
octanol 1-2%
borneol 0-1%
Sesquiterpenes 2-5%
β-caryophellene 1-2%
β-bourbonene 0-1%
α-elemene 0-1%
β-farnesene 0-1%
Esters 3-4%
carvyl acetate 3-4%
Oxides 2-3%
1, 8 cineole 2-3%
Sesquiterpenols 1-2%
α-cadinol 0-1%
elemol 0-1%
farnesol 0-1%
Phenolic Alcohols 0-1%
menthol 0-1%

Milfoil
(See *Achillea millefolium*)

Monk's Pepper
(See *Vitex negundo*)

Moroccan Chamomile
(See *Ormenis mixta*)

Moroccan Thyme
(See *Thymus satureioides*)

Mountain Mint
(See *Origanum compactum*)

Mountain Savory
(See *Satureja montana*)

MQV
(See *Melaleuca quinquenervia*)

Mugwort
(See *Artemisia vulgaris*)

Muscatel Sage
(See *Salvia sclarea*)

71. *Myristica fragrans*
Myristicaceae (Nutmeg Family)
• **Nutmeg**
• Distilled from fruits and seeds
• B, Fl, Fr, H, M, P, Y
Monoterpenes 55-80%
sabinene14-29%
α-pinene 15-28%
β-pinene 13-18%
myrcene 5-12%
d-limonene 2-7%
γ-terpinene 2-7%
α-terpinene 1-4%
p-cymene 1-3%
δ-3-carene 1-2%
terpinolene 1-2%
camphene 0-1%
α-phellandrene 0-1%
β-phellandrene 0-1%
Phenolic Ethers 7-16%
myristicin 5-12%
elemicin 1-3%
safrole 1-2%
eugenol 0-1%
Phenolic Alcohols 4-8%
terpinen-4-ol 4-8%
Oxides 2-4%
1,8 cineole 2-4%
Alcohols 1-2%
α-terpineol 1-2%
Sesquiterpenes 0-1%
β-caryophellene 0-1%

Myrrh
(See *Commiphora myrrha*)

Myrtle
(See *Myrtus communis*)

72. *Myrtus communis*
Myrtaceae (Myrtle Family)
• **Myrtle**
• Distilled from leaves
• B, Fl, Fr, H, M, Y
Oxides 31-48%
1,8 cineole 30-45%
caryophyllene oxide 1-3%
Monoterpenes 30-45%
α-pinene 23-30%
l-limonene 5-11
β-pinene 2-5%
Esters 8-22%
myrtenyl acetate 4-10%
geranyl acetate 1-5%
gerpenyl acetate 2-3%
methyl myrtenate 1-3%
bornyl acetate 0-1%
carvyl acetate 0-1%
linalyl acetate 0-1%
neryl acetate 0-1%
Alcohols 5-18%
α-terpineol 2-8%
linalol 2-5%
myrtenol 1-4%
myrtol 1-2%
geraniol 0-2%
nerol 0-1%
terpinen-4-ol 0-1%
Aldehydes 2-5%
myrtenal 1-2%
decanal 0-1%
hexanal 0-1%
methylbutynal 0-1%
Phenols 1-4%
myrtenol 1-4%
Furanoids 1-3%
methylfuran 1-2%
furfural 0-1%
Lactones 1-2%
myrtecommulone 1-2%

Nard
(See *Nardostachys jatamansi*)

73. *Nardostachys jatamansi*

Valerianaceae (Valerian Family)
- **Spikenard**, Nard, Jatamansi, Indian Valerian
- Distilled from roots
- B, Fr, H, M, P, Y

Sesquiterpenes 36-50%
β-gurjunene 24-30%
β-maalene 4-9%
aristoladiene 3-7%
aristolene 4-5%
seychellene 1-2%
dihydroazulene 0-1%
β-patchoulene 0-1%

Monoterpenes 27-45%
calarene 22-35%
β-ionene 4-8%
α-pinene 1-2%
β-pinene 0-1%
limonene 0-1%

Sesquiterpenols 6-11%
pachoulol 5-7%
nardol 1-2%
calarenol 0-1%
maaliol 0-1%
valerianol 0-1%

Ketones 7-10%
aristolenone 6-7%
β-ionone 1-2%
nardostachone 0-2%
valerianone 0-1%

Phenolic Aldehydes 1-2%
valerianal 1-2%

Coumarins 1-2%
coumarin 1-2%

Oxides 1-2%
1, 8 cineole 1-2%

Carboxylic Acids 0-1%
jatamanshinic acid 0-1%

Narrow-Leafed Peppermint
(See *Eucalyptus radiata*)

74. *Nepeta cataria*

Lamiaceae (Mint Family)
- **Catnip**, Catmint, Catswort, Field Balm
- Distilled leaves & flowering tops
- B, Fl, Fr, P

Alcohols 58-70%
citronellol 28-35%
geraniol 18-24%
nerol 12-20%

Lactones 8-18%
nepetalactone 8-18%

Aldehydes 7-11%
geranial 4-6%
neral 3-5%

Sesquiterpenes 2-10%
β-caryophyllene 2-7%
humulene 0-4%

Monoterpenes 1-4%
myrcene 1-2%
l-limonene 0-1%
ocimene 0-1%

Phenolic Alcohols 1-3%
carvacrol 0-2%
thymol 0-2%

Neroli
(See *Citrus aurantium - 27*)

Nerolina
(See *Melaleuca quinquenervia*)

New England Hemlock
(See *Tsuga canadensis*)

Niaouli
(See *Melaleuca quinquenervia*)

Norwegian Pine
(See *Pinus sylvestris*)

Nosebleed
(See *Achillea millefolium*)

Nutmeg
(See *Myristica fragrans*)

75. *Ocimum basilicum*
Lamiaceae (Mint Family)
- **Basil**, Sweet Basil, St. Josephwort
- Distilled leaves, stems, flowers
- B, Fl, Fr, H, M, Y

Phenols 52-90%
estragole 50-80%
eugenol 2-10%
Alcohols 7-15%
linalol 5-10%
citronellol 2-3%
α-fenchol 0-1%
α-terpineol 0-1%
terpinen-4-ol 0-1%
Oxides 3-9%
1,8 cineole 2-8%
ocimene oxide 1-2%
Esters 2-5%
methyl cinnamate 1-4%
fenchyl acetate 0-1%
linalyl acetate 0-1%
Monoterpenes 1-4%
ocimene 1-2%
α-pinene 0-1%
β-pinene 0-1%
camphene 0-1%
l-limonene 0-1%
Ketones 1-2%
camphor 0-1%
octanone 0-1%

Olibanum
(See *Boswellia carteri*)

Onycha
(See *Styrax benzoin)*

Orange (See *Citrus sinensis*)

Orange Bigarade
(See *Citrus aurantium - 28*)

Orange Blossom
(See *Citrus aurantium - 27*)

Orange Leaf
(See *Citrus aurantium - 29*)

Oregano
(See *Origanum compactum*)

Oregon Balsam
(See *Pseudotsuga menziesii*)

Oregon Fir
(See *Abies grandis*)

76. *Origanum compactum*
Lamiaceae (Mint Family)
- **Oregano**, Greek Oregano, Mountain Mint, Wild Marjoram, Wintersweet
- Distilled leaves & flowers
- B, Fl, Fr, H, M, P, Y

Phenols 60-80%
carvacrol 60-75%
thymol 0-5%
Monoterpenes 10-25%
p-cymene 5-10%
γ-terpinene 3-9%
myrcene 1-3%
α-pinene 0-1%
β-pinene 0-1%
camphene 0-1%
l-limonene 0-1%
α-terpinene 0-1%
Sesquiterpenes 2-6%
β-caryophyllene 2-5%
β-bisabolene 1-2%
Carboxylic Acids 2-5%
rosmaric acid 2-5%
Esters 3-4%
linalyl acetate 3-4%
Ketones 1-3%
camphor 1-2%
d-carvone 0-1%
Alcohols 0-2%
borneol 0-1%
linalol 0-1%
α-terpineol 0-1%
terpinen-4-ol 0-1%

77. *Origanum marjorana*
Lamiaceae (Mint Family)
- **Marjoram**, Sweet Marjoram
- Distilled leaves
- B, Fl, Fr, H, M, P, Y

Monoterpenes 28-60%
γ-terpinene 12-20%
α-terpinene 6-10%
sabinene 2-8%
myrcene 1-7%
terpinolene 1-7%
ocimene 2-6%
δ-3-carene 1-6%
p-cymene 1-6%
α-pinene 1-5%
δ-cadinene 1-4%
β-pinene 0-3%
β-phellandrene 0-2%
l-limonene 0-1%

Alcohols 9-30%
α-terpineol 5-15%
thujanol 4-12%
linalol 2-8%

Phenolic Alcohols 14-20%
terpinen-4-ol 14-22%

Esters 2-10%
geranyl acetate 1-7%
linalyl acetate 0-3%
α-terpinyl acetate 0-3%

Aldehydes 4-6%
citral 4-6%

Sesquiterpenes 2-5%
β-caryophyllene 2-5%
humulene 0-1%

Phenolic Ethers 0-1%
anethole 0-1%

Origanum vulgare
(See *Origanum compactum*)

Ormenis
(See *Ormenis mixta*)

---

78. *Ormenis mixta*
Asteraceae (Aster–Daisy Family)
- **Ormenis**, Moroccan Chamomile, Wild Chamomile
- Distilled from flowering tops
- B, Fr, P,

Alcohols 38-50%
santalina alcohol 30-33%
α-terpineol 2-4%
artemisia alcohol 2-3%
yomogi alcohol 2-3%
pinocarveol 1-3%
ormenol 1-2%
borneol 0-1%
linalol 0-1%

Monoterpenes14-26%
α-pinene 10-15%
l-limonene 4-8%
camphene 0-1%
γ-terpinene 0-1%
terpinolene 0-1%

Sesquiterpenes 7-10%
germacrene D 4-5%
α-bisabolene 2-3%
β-caryophellene 1-2%
δ-elemene 0-1%

Esters 3-5%
bornyl acetate 2-3%
bornyl butanoate 1-2%

Ketones 0-2%
camphor 0-1%
pinocarvone 0-1%

Ormenis multicaulis
(See *Ormenis mixta*)

Our Lady's Mint
(See *Mentha spicata*)

Palmarosa
(See *Cymbopogon martinii*)

Paperbark
(See *Melaleuca quinquenervia*)

Parsley
(See *Petroselinum crispum*)

Patchouly
(See *Pogostemon cablin*)

79. *Pelargonium graveolens*
Geraniaceae (Geranium Family)
• **Geranium**
• Distilled from leaves
• B, C, H, M, P, W, Y
Alcohols 50-70%
  citronellol 22-42%
  geraniol 17-25%
  linalol 10-14%
  nerol 1-3%
  γ-eudesmol 0-1%
  α-terpineol 0-1%
Esters 15-30%
  citronellyl formate 9-15%
  geranyl formate 1-6%
  geranyl acetate 1-5%
  citronellyl propionate 1-3%
  citronellyl butyrate 1-2%
  citronellyl tiglate 1-2%
  geranyl butyrate 1-2%
  geranyl tiglate 1-2%
  geranyl propionate 0-1%'
Ketones 5-10%
  isomenthone 4-8%
  menthone 1-3%
  piperitone 0-1%
Sesquiterpenes 4-8%
  guaiadene 4-8%
  α-copaene 0-1%
  δ-cadinene 0-1%
  δ-guaiazulene 0-1%
  β-farnesene 0-1%
Aldehydes 1-8%
  geranial 1-6%
  citronellal 0-1%
  neral 0-1%

Monoterpenes 2-5%
  α-pinene 1-2%
  β-pinene 0-1%
  l-limonene 0-1%
  myrcene 0-1%
  ocimene 0-1%
Sesquiterpenols 1-3%
  farnesol 1-3%
Furanoids 1-2%
  furopelargone 1-2%

Pepper, Black
(See *Piper nigrum*)

Peppermint
(See *Mentha piperita*)

Peppermint Eucalyptus
(See *Eucalyptus dives*)

Petitgrain
(See *Citrus aurantium - 29*)

80. *Petroselinum crispum*
Apiaceae (Celery–Carrot Family)
• **Parsley**, Garden Parsley
• Distilled from leaves and stems
• B, Fr
Monoterpenes 70-80%
  p-menthatriene 28-50%
  β-phellandrene 13-15%
  α-pinene 3-5%
  myrcene 3-5%
  terpinolene 3-5%
  β-pinene 2-3%
Phenolic Ethers 5-17%
  myristicin 4-17%
  apiole 1-2%
Alcohols 6-8%
  Linalol 5-6%
  carotol 1-2%
Sesquiterpenes 0-2%
  β-caryophyllene 0-2%

81. *Picea mariana*

Pinaceae (Pine Family)
• **Spruce**, Black Spruce
• Distilled leaves, needles, twigs
• B, Fr, H, M, Y

Monoterpenes 45-55%
   camphene 17-25%
   α-pinene 12-19%
   δ-3-carene 5-10%
   β-pinene 4-8%
   l-limonene 2-7%
   santene 1-5%
   tricyclene 1-5%
Esters 30-37%
   bornyl acetate 30-37%
Alcohols 1-3%
   borneol 1-2%
   longiborneol 0-1%
Sesquiterpenes 0-2%
   longifolene 0-1%
   longicyclene 0-1%

82. *Pimpinella anisum*

Apiaceae (Celery–Carrot Family)
• **Anise**, Roman Fennel
• Distilled from fruit and seeds
• B, Fl, Fr, M, P, Y

Phenolic Ethers 82-95%
   anethole 80-95%
   estragole 2-4%
   myristicin 0-1%
Alcohols 3-8%
   anisol 1-4%
   linalol 1-2%
   α-terpineol 1-2%
Aldehydes 1-2%
   anisicaldehyde 1-2%
Sesquiterpenes 0-2%
   β-caryophyllene 0-1%
   γ-himachalene 0-1%
Coumarins 0-2%
   umbelliferone 0-1%
   scopoletine 0-1%
Ketones 0-1%
   anise ketone 0-1%

Phenols 2-4%
   p-anol 2-4%
   isochavibetol 0-1%
Furanoids 0-1%
   ζ-ligustolide 0-1%

Pine

(See *Pinus sylvestris*)

83. *Pinus sylvestris*

Pinaceae (Pine Family)
• **Pine**, Scotch Pine, Norwegian Pine
• Distilled from needles
• B, Fl, Fr, H, M, P, Y

Monoterpenes 43-80%
   α-pinene 22-43%
   δ-3-carene 6-17%
   l-limonene 8-16%
   β-pinene 5-15%
   camphene 1-4%
   β-phellandrene 1-3%
   terpinolene 0-3%
   ocimene 0-2%
   p-cymene 0-1%
   γ-terpinene 0-1%
   sabinene 0-1%
Sesquiterpenes 3-12%
   β-caryophyllene 1-6%
   γ-cadinene 1-5%
   α-copaene 0-1%
   β-guaiene 0-1%
   longifolene 0-1%
   muurolene 0-1%
Alcohols 1-3%
   borneol 1-2%
   terpinen-4-ol 0-1%
Esters 1-3%
   bornyl acetate 1-3%
Sesquiterpenols 0-2%
   α-cadinol 0-1%
   muurolol 0-1%
Diterpenes 0-2%
   cembrene 0-2%
Aldehydes 0-1%
   citronellal 0-1%

84. *Piper nigrum*

Piperaceae (Pepper Family)
- **Black Pepper**, Poivre Noir
- Distilled from berries
- B, Fr, H, M, P, Y

Monoterpenes 30-70%
l-limonene 10-15%
δ-3-carene 1-15%
β-pinene 5-14%
sabinene 5-10%
α-phellandrene 5-9%
α-pinene 2-9%
α-thujene 1-4%
γ-terpinene 0-4%
p-cymene 1-3%
myrcene 1-3%
α-terpinene 0-3%
terpinolene 0-2%
Sesquiterpenes 33-60%
β-caryophyllene 25-35%
β-selinene 1-8%
β-bisabolene 2-5%
δ-elemene 2-3%
β-farnesene 1-3%
humulene 1-2%
α-copaene 0-2%
β-cubebene 0-2%
α-elemene 0-2%
β-elemene 0-2%
α-guaiene 0-1%
Oxides 3-8%
caryophyllene oxide 3-8%
Ketones 1-2%
acetephenone 0-1%
hydrocarvone 0-1%
piperitone 0-1%
Aldehydes 0-1%
piperonal 0-1%
Carboxylic Acids 0-1%
piperonylic acid 0-1%
Furanocoumarins 0-1%
α-bergamotene 0-1%

85. *Pogostemon cablin*

Lamiaceae (Mint Family)
- **Patchouly**, Patchouli, Putcha-Pat
- Distilled from leaves & flowers
- B, Fl, Fr, H, M, P, Y

Sesquiterpenes 44-63%
α-bulnesene 10-20%
β-bulnesene 8-16%
aromadrene 7-15%
α-guaiene 6-14%
seychellene 5-12%
β-patchoulene 2-7%
α-patchoulene 3-5%
β-caryophyllene 2-4%
δ-cadinene 1-3%
Sesquiterpenols 26-38%
patchoulol 25-35%
pogostol 1-3%
bulnesol 0-1%
patchoulenol 0-1%
guaiol 0-1%
Oxides 3-5%
bulnesene oxide 3-4%
caryophyllene oxide 0-1%
guaiene oxide 0-1%
Ketones 2-3%
patchoulenone 2-3%
Monoterpenes 1-2%
α-pinene 0-1%
β-pinene 0-1%
l-limonene 0-1%

Poivre Noir

(See *Piper nigrum*)

86. *Pseudotsuga menziesii*

Pinaceae (Pine Family)
- **Douglas Fir**, Oregon Balsam, Douglas Spruce
- Distilled from needles & branches
- B, Fl, Fr, H, M, P, Y

Monoterpenes 60-80%
α-pinene 25-40%
β-pinene 15-25%
l-limonene 6-18%

δ-3-carene 2-3%
camphene 1-2%
Esters 12-15%
bornyl acetate 8-15%
geranyl acetate 2-4%
bornyl coproate 1-3%
geranyl coproate 1-3%
Alcohols 6-10%
borneol 3-6%
geraniol 3-6%
Aldehydes 1-3%
benzoicaldehyde 1-2%
citral 0-1%

Putcha-Pat
(See *Pogostemon cablin*)

Ravensara
(See *Ravensara aromatica*)

87. Ravensara aromatica
Lamiaceae (Mint Family)
• **Ravensara**
• Distilled from leaves & branches
• B, Fr, H, M, P, Y
Oxides 48-61%
1,8 cineole 48-61%
Monoterpenes 16-32%
sabinene 10-15%
α-pinene 4-9%
β-pinene 1-5%
l-limonene 1-4%
Alcohols 8-10%
α-terpineol 6-7%
terpinen-4-ol 2-3%
Esters 1-3%
α-terpinyl acetate 1-3%
Sesquiterpenes 0-2%
β-caryophyllene 0-2%

Red Cedar
(See *Thuja plicata - 1 & 2*)

Red Thyme
(See *Thymus vulgaris CT thymol*)

Rock Rose
(See *Cistus ladanifer*)

Roman Chamomile
(See *Chamaemelum nobile*)

Roman Fennel
(See *Pimpinella anisum*)

88. Rosa damascena
Rosaceae (Rose Family)
• **Rose**, Rose Otto, Damask
Rose, Bulgarian Rose,
Turkish Rose, Autumn Rose
• Distilled from petals
• B, C, Fr, H, M, P, Y
Alcohols 50-70%
citronellol 30-44%
geraniol 12-28%
nerol 6-9%
linalol 1-3%
borneol 0-1%
α-terpineol 0-1%
Sesquiterpenols 0-2%
farnesol 0-2%
Monoterpenes 19-25%
stearoptene 16-22%
α-pinene 0-1%
β-pinene 0-1%
camphene 0-1%
α-terpinene 0-1%
l-limonene 0-1%
myrcene 0-1%
p-cymene 0-1%
ocimene 0-1%
Alkanes 4-19%
nonadecane 2-15%
octadecane 0-1%
eicosane 0-1%
heneicosane 0-1%
docosane 0-1%
tricosane 0-1%

tetracosane 0-1%
pentacosane 0-1%
Esters 2-5%
geranyl acetate 1-3%
neryl acetate 1-3%
citronellyl acetate 0-1%
Phenols 2-4%
eugenol 1-2%
phenylethanol 1-3%
Oxides 0-1%
rose oxide 0-1%

Rosalina
(See *Melaleuca ericifolia*)

89. *Rosmarinus officinalis CT cineole*
Lamiaceae (Mint Family)
• **Rosemary**
• Distilled from leaves
• B, C, Fr, H, M, P, W, Y
Oxides 39-55%
1,8 cineole 38-55%
caryophyllene oxide 1-2%
humulene oxide 0-1%
Monoterpenes 18-35%
α-pinene 9-14%
β-pinene 4-9%
camphene 2-8%
l-limonene 1-4%
myrcene 1-2%
p-cymene 1-2%
Ketones 8-32%
camphor 6-30%
β-thujone 1-2%
verbenone 1-2%
d-carvone 0-1%
hexanone 0-1%
heptanone 0-1%
Alcohols 4-20%
borneol 3-12%
α-terpineol 1-5%
linalol 0-2%
terpinen-4-ol 0-2%
verbenol 0-1%

Sesquiterpenes 1-3%
β-caryophyllene 1-2%
humulene 1-2%
Esters 0-2%
bornyl acetate 0-1%
fenchyl acetate 0-1%
Carboxylic Acids 0-1%
rosemaric acid 0-1%

90. *Rosmarinus officinalis CT verbenone*
Lamiaceae (Mint Family)
• **Rosemary Verbenon**
• Distilled from leaves
• B, Fr, H, P, Y
Ketones 16-50%
verbenone 15-37%
camphor 1-15%
Monoterpenes 22-45%
α-pinene 15-34%
camphene 6-10%
l-limonene 1-4%
β-pinene 0-1%
Oxides 1-15%
1, 8 cineole 1-15%
Esters 6-11%
bornyl acetate 6-11%
Alcohols 1-7%
borneol 1-7%
Carboxylic Acids 1-2%
rosemaric acid 1-2%
Sesquiterpenes 0-2%
β-caryophyllene 0-1%
humulene 0-1%

Rose
(See *Rosa damascena*)

Rosemary
(See *Rosmarinus officinalis CT cineole and/or CT verbenone*)

Rose of Sharon
(See *Cistus ladanifer*)

Rose Otto
(See *Rosa damascena*)

Rosewood
(See *Aniba roseodora*)

Russian Tarragon
(See *Artemisia dracunculus*)

Sage
(See *Salvia officinalis*)

91. Salvia officinalis
Lamiaceae (Mint Family)
* **Sage**, Dalmatian Sage
* Distilled from leaves & flowers
* B, Fl, Fr, H, M, P, Y

Ketones 18-64%
α-thujone 12-33%
camphor 4-24%
β-thujone 2-14%

Monoterpenes 10-30%
camphene 2-7%
α-pinene 1-6%
camphene 1-5%
l-limonene 1-4%
β-pinene 1-2%
p-cymene 1-2%
myrcene 1-2%
salvene 0-1%
α-phellandrene 0-1%
β-phellandrene 0-1%
sabinene 0-1%
α-terpinene 0-1%
γ-terpinene 0-1%

Alcohols 5-28%
borneol 2-14%
linalol 1-12%
α-terpineol 1-9%
terpinen-4-ol 1-4%
sabinol 0-1%
salvol 0-1%

Sesquiterpenols 2-10%
viridiflorol 2-10%

Oxides 5-13%
1,8 cineole 5-13%

Sesquiterpenes 7-12%
humulene 4-5%
β-caryophyllene 1-7%
aromadrene 0-1%
α-cadinene 0-1%
β-cadinene 0-1%
β-copaene 0-1%
ledene 0-1%
α-maalene 0-1%

Esters 1-5%
bornyl acetate 0-3%
linalyl acetate 1-2%
sabinyl acetate 0-1%

Phenols 1-2%
estragole 0-1%
thymol 0-1%

Diterpenols 0-1%
sclareol 0-1%

92. Salvia sclarea
Lamiaceae (Mint Family)
* **Clary Sage**, Clary Wort, Muscatel Sage
* Distilled from leaves, stems, & flowers
* B, Fr, H, M, P, Y

Esters 50-78%
linalyl acetate 49-75%
geranyl acetate 0-3%
neryl acetate 0-2%
bornyl acetate 0-1%

Alcohols 7-27%
linalol 7-24%
geraniol 0-3%
α-terpineol 0-1%
nerol 0-1%

Sesquiterpenes 3-14%
germacrene-D 2-12%
β-caryophyllene 1-3%
β-curcumene 0-1%
α-copaene 0-1%
β-bourbonene 0-1%

Diterpenols 3-7%
sclareol 3-7%
Monoterpenes 2-4%
myrcene 1-2%
α-pinene 0-1%
β-pinene 0-1%
l-limonene 0-1%
ocimene 0-1%
terpinolene 0-1%
Oxides 1-2%
1,8 cineole 0-1%
caryophyllene oxide 0-1%
linalol oxide 0-1%
sclareol oxide 0-1%
Ketones 0-2%
α-thujone 0-1%
β-thujone 0-1%
Sesquiterpenols 0-1%
spathulenol 0-1%
Aldehydes 0-1%
hexanal 0-1%
Coumarins 0-1%
coumarin 0-1%

Sandalwood
(See *Santalum album*)

---

93. *Santalum album*
Santalaceae (Sandalwood Family)
• **Sandalwood**, Aloes, White Santal
• Distilled from heartwood & roots
• B, Fr, H, M, Y
Sesquiterpenols 66-80%
α-santalol 47-55%
β-santalol 19-25%
Sesquiterpenes 5-11%
α-santalene 4-8%
β-santalene 1-5%
Sesquiterpenals 1-3%
teresantalal 1-3%
Carboxylic Acids 1-2%
santalic acid 1-2%

---

94. *Satureja montana*
Lamiaceae (Mint Family)
• **Mountain Savory**, Winter Savory
• Distilled from flowering plant
• B, Fr, H, M, Y
Phenols 40-58%
carvacrol 22-35%
thymol 14-24%
carvacrol methyl ether 4-9%
eugenol 0-1%
Monoterpenes 15-32%
p-cymene 7-20%
γ-terpinene 8-15%
α-terpinene 0-5%
Alcohols 14-25%
linalol 7-11%
α-terpineol 6-9%
thujenol 0-4%
borneol 0-1%
geraniol 0-1
Sesquiterpenes 3-7%
β-caryophyllene 3-7%
Oxides 1-3%
1,8 cineole 1-2%
caryophyllene oxide 0-1%
Ketones 0-2%
camphor 0-1%
damascenone 0-1%

Scotch Pine
(See *Pinus sylvestris*)

Silver Fir
(See *Abies alba or Abies grandis*)

Snake Oil
(See *Melaleuca alternifolia*)

Sneezewort
(See *Achillea millefolium*)

95. *Solidago canadensis*

Asteraceae (Aster–Daisy Family)
- **Goldenrod**
- Distilled stems, leaves, flowers
- B, Fr, H, M, Y

Monoterpenes 30-55%
α-pinene 10-18%
myrcene 8-15%
l-limonene 6-12%
sabinene 5-11%
α-phellandrene 1-2%
Sesquiterpenes 24-35%
germacrene-D 22-35%
longifolene 2-3%
Alcohols 2-5%
borneol 2-5%
Esters 2-4%
bornyl acetate 2-3%
bornyl benzoate 0-1%

Spanish Marjoram

(See *Thymus mastichina)*

Spearmint

(See *Mentha spicata)*

Spikenard

(See *Nardostachys jatamansi)*

Spruce

(See *Piceae mariana)*

Spruce, Black

(See *picea mariana)*

Spruce, Douglas

(See *Psuedotsuga menziesii)*

Spruce Pine

(See *Tsuga canadensis)*

Stacte

(See *Commiphora myrrha)*

Staunchweed

(See *Achillea millefolium)*

96. *Styrax benzoin*

Styracaceae (Storax Family)
- **Onycha**, Benzoin, Friar's Balm, Java Frankincense, Benjamin Tree, Onycha Absolute
- Solvent Extractions from gum-resin of the tree
- B, Fl, Fr, H

Esters 64-75%
coniferyl benzoate 60-70%
cinnamyl benzoate 3-5%
cinnamyl cinnamoate 1-2%
propyl cinnamoate 0-2%
Carboxylic Acids 14-25%
benzoic acid 10-20%
cinnamic acid 3-10%
hydroxyoleanic acid 1-2%
Aldehydes 1-2%
vanillin aldehyde 1-2%
Alcohols 0-2%
benzoresinol 0-1%
siaresinotannol 0-1%

Swamp Cedar

(See *Thuja occidentalis)*

Sweet Balm

(See *Melissa officinalis)*

Sweet Basil

(See *Ocimum basilicum)*

Sweet Bay

(See *Laurus nobilis)*

Sweet Cane

(See *Acorus calamus)*

Sweet Flag

(See *Acorus calamus)*

Sweet Laurel
(See *Laurus nobilis*)

Sweet Marjoram
(See *Origanum marjorana*)

Sweet Orange
(See *Citrus sinensis*)

Sweet Thyme
(See *Thymus vulgaris CT thujanol*)

St. Josephwort
(See *Ocimum basilicum*)

97. *Syzygium aromatica*
Myrtaceae (Myrtle Family)
• Clove
• Distilled from stems and buds
• B, Fl, Fr, H, M, P, W, Y
Phenols 70-85%
  eugenol 70-85%
Esters 8-16%
  eugenyl acetate 8-15%
  α-terpinyl acetate 0-1%
  methyl benzoate 0-1%
Sesquiterpenes 6-14%
  β-caryophyllene 5-12%
  humulene 0-2%
  α–cubebene 0-1%
  α-copaene 0-1%
  calamenene 0-1%
Oxides 1-3%
  caryophyllene oxide 1-2%
  humulene oxide 0-1%
Carboxylic Acids 0-3%
  oleanolic acid 0-2%
  crataegolic acid 0-1%
Ketones 0-1%
  methyl-n-amyl ketone 0-1%

98. *Tagates glandulifera*
Asteraceae (Aster-Daisy Family)
• **Marigold**, French Marigold, Taget
• Distilled leaves, stems, flowers
• B, Fl, Fr, P
Ketones 60-70%
  tagetone 40-50%
  ocimenone 20-26%
Monoterpenes 30-43%
  β-ocimene 27-39%
  d-limonene 3-7%
Coumarins 2-4%
  coumarin 0-2%
  esculetin 0-1%
  scopoletin 0-1%
  umbelliferone 0-1%

Taget
(See *Tagetes glandulifera)*)

99. *Tanacetum annum*
Asteraceae (Aster-Daisy Family)
• **Blue Tansy**, Annual Tansy
• Distilled from leaves and flowers
B, Fr, H, M, Y
Monoterpenes 35-65%
  sabinene 10-17%
  myrcene 7-13%
  d-limonene 5-11%
  β-pinene 5-10%
  α-phellandrene 5-10%
  p-cymene 3-8%
Ketones 10-17%
  camphor 10-17%
Sesquiterpenes 6-12%
  chamazulene 6-12%

100. Tanacetum vulgare

Asteraceae (Aster-Daisy Family)
• **Idaho Tansy**, Wild Tansy,
Tansy
• Distilled from leaves and flowers
• B, Fl, H, M, Y
Ketones 66-80%
β-thujone 60-75%
camphor 3-8%
α-thujone 2-5%
piperitone 1-2%
artemisia ketone 0-1%
davanone 0-1%
Monoterpenes 4-10%
sabinene 1-4%
α-pinene 2-3%
camphene 1-3%
α-terpinene 0-1%
Sesquiterpenes 3-7%
germacrene D 3-7%
Alcohols 3-6%
borneol 1-2%
α-terpineol 1-2%'
lyratol 0-1%
chrysanthenol 0-1%
vulgerol 0-1%
Sesquiterpene Lactones 1-3%
artemarin 0-1%
chrysanthemine 0-1%
crispolid 0-1%
parthenolide 0-1%
santamarin 0-1%
tatridin 0-1%
Esters 1-2%
bornyl acetate 0-1%
crysanthenyl acetate 0-1%
α-terpinyl acetate 0-1%
lyratyl acetate 0-1%
Coumarins 0-1%
scopoletin 0-1

Tangerine (See *Citrus nobilis*)

Tansy
(See *Tanacetum vulgare*)

Tansy, Annual
(See *Tanacetum annum*)

Tansy, Blue
(See *Tanacetum annum*)

Tansy, Idaho
(See *Tanacetum vulgare*)

Tansy, Wild
(See *Tanacetum vulgare*)

Tarragon
(See *Artemisia dracunculus*)

Tasmanian Blue Gum
(See *Eucalyptus globulus*)

Tea Tree
(See *Melaleuca alternifolia*)

Thousand Seal
(See *Achillea millefolium*)

Thuja
(See *Thuja occidentalis*)

101. Thuja occidentalis

Cupressaceae (Cypress Family)
• **Thuja**, Arbor Vitae, Cedar Leaf,
Swamp Cedar
• Distilled from needles
• B, Fl, Fr, H
Ketones 48-70%
α-thujone 30-60%
β-thujone 8-15%
fenchone 7-14%
camphor 2-3%
piperitone 1-2%
Monoterpenes 6-36%
sabinene 6-35%
l-limonene 0-1%
Esters 4-12%
bornyl acetate 4-12%

Sesquiterpenols 6-10%
occidentalol 2-5%
occidol 1-3%
α–eudesmol 1-2%
Phenolic Alcohols 3-6%
terpinen-4-ol 3-6%

---

102. *Thuja plicata*
Cupressaceae (Cypress Family)
• **Cedar Bark**, Western Red Cedar, Canadian Red Cedar, Red Cedar, Cedar,
• Distilled from bark and wood
• B, M
Ketones 78-95%
α-thujone 70-85%
β-thujone 5-9%
fenchone 2-3%
camphor 1-3%
Monoterpenes 2-5%
sabinene 2-5%
Ethers 3-4%
γ-thujaplicin 3-4%

---

103. *Thuja plicata*
Cupressaceae (Cypress Family)
• **Cedar Leaf**, Western Red Cedar, Canadian Red Cedar, Red Cedar, Cedar
• Distilled from leaves & branches
• B, H, M, Y
Ketones 76-95%
α-thujone 65-80%
β-thujone 5-9%
fenchone 3-7%
camphor 2-3%
tropolone 1-2%
Monoterpenes 3-7%
sabinene 2-4%
α-pinene 1-3%
β-pinene 0-1%
Esters 1-2%
methyl thujate 1-2%
Sesquiterpenols 0-2%
muurolol 0-2%

Thyme
(See *Thymus vulgaris CT linalol* or *Thymus vulgaris CT thymol*)

Thyme, Borneol
(See *Thymus satureioides*)

Thyme, Garden
(See *Thymus vulgaris CT linalol*)

Thyme, Moroccan
(See *Thymus satureioides*))

Thyme, Red
(See *Thymus vulgaris CT thymol*)

---

104. *Thymus mastichina*
Lamiaceae (Mint Family)
• **Spanish Marjoram**
• Distilled leaves & flowering tops
• B, Fr, P
Oxides 41-75%
1,8 cineole 40-75%
caryophyllene oxide 1-2%
Alcohols 18-32%
linalol 10-20%
α-terpineol 7-8%
borneol 1-4%
geraniol 0-1%
pinocarveol 0-1%
terpinen-4-ol 01-%
thujanol 0-1%
Monoterpenes 10-21%
terpinolene 3-4%
p-cymene 2-4%
α-pinene 2-3%
β-pinene 2-3%
l-limonene 2-3%
camphene 0-2%
sabinene 0-2%
α-thujene 0-1%
γ-terpinene 0-1%
myrcene 0-1%

Esters 3-7%
α-terpinyl acetate 2-3%
linalyl acetate 1-2%
bornyl acetate 0-1%
geranyl acetate 0-1%
pinocarvyl acetate 0-1%
Sesquiterpenes 2-6%
humulene 1-2%
aromadrene 0-1%
β-bourbonene 0-1%
β-caryophyllene 0-1%
β-gurjunene 0-1%
δ-cadinene 0-1%
α-copaene 0-1%
longifolene 0-1%
Phenols 1-5%
thymol 1-5%
Ketones 1-4%
camphor 1-4%

---

105. *Thymus satureioides*

Lamiaceae (Mint Family)
• **Moroccan Thyme,**
  Borneol Thyme
• Distilled leaves & flowering tops
• B, Fr, P
Alcohols 35-70%
borneol 28-50%
α-terpineol 5-21%
linalol 1-12%
terpinen-4-ol 1-5%
pinocarveol 0-1%
octanol 0-1%
Phenols 12-40%
thymol 7-23%
carvacrol 5-22%
Sesquiterpenes 3-10%
β-caryophyllene 2-7%
β-guaiene 1-2%
δ-cadinene 0-2%
aromadrene 0-1%
α-copaene 0-1%
humulene 0-1%
muurolene 0-1%

Oxides 2-7%
caryophyllene oxide 2-6%
1,8 cineole 0-1%
linalol oxide 0-1%
Ketones 2-5%
dihydrocarvone 1-2%
camphor 0-3%
verbenone 0-1%
Esters 1-5%
bornyl acetate 1-5%
linalyl acetate 0-1%
Aldehydes 0-1%
campholenic aldehyde 0-1%
Monoterpenes 0-1%
p-cymene 0-1%

---

106. *Thymus vulgaris* CT linalol

Lamiaceae (Mint Family)
• **Garden Thyme,** Thyme
Distilled leaves & flowering tops
• B, Fr, P
Alcohols 59-90%
linalol 50-75%
terpinen-4-ol 6-12%
thujanol 2-4%
geraniol 1-3%
Monoterpenes 12-21%
myrcene 4-8%
p-cymene 4-8%
γ-terpinene 4-8%
Esters 4-6%
linalyl acetate 3-5%
geranyl acetate 1-2%

107. Thymus vulgaris CT thujanol

Lamiaceae (Mint Family)
- **Sweet Thyme**
- Distilled leaves & flowering tops
- B, Fr, P

Alcohols 45-75%
thujanol 40-60%
myrcenol 1-3%
linalol 4-12%

Monoterpenes 13-24%
myrcene 6-11%
γ-terpinene 6-11%
p-cymene 1-3%

Phenolic Alcohols 3-6%
terpinen-4-ol 3-6%

108. Thymus vulgaris CT thymol

Lamiaceae (Mint Family)
- **Thyme**, Red Thyme
- Distilled leaves, stems, flowers
- B, C, Fl, Fr, H, M, P, Y

Phenols 38-60%
thymol 37-55%
carvacrol 1-10%

Monoterpenes 21-54%
p-cymene 14-28%
γ-terpinene 4-11%
terpinolene 2-6%
α-pinene 0-6%
myrcene 1-3%

Oxides 4-15%
1,8 cineole 4-15%

Alcohols 3-14%
linalol 2-8%
borneol 1-7%

Sesquiterpenes 1-8%
β-caryophyllene 1-8%

Carboxylic Acids 1-2%
rosmaric acid 1-2%

Ti Tree
(See *Melaleuca alternifolia*)

Tsuga
(See *Tsuga canadensis*)

109. Tsuga canadensis

Pinaceae (Pine Family)
- **Tsuga**, Hemlock, Spruce Pine, Canadian Hemlock, New England Hemlock, White Hemlock
- Distilled from needles and twigs
- B,Fl, H, M, Y

Monoterpenes 34-50%
camphene 12-18%
α-pinene 10-15%
β-pinene 8-10%
l-limonene 2-4%
myrcene 1-3%
β-phellandrene 0-2%
α-phellandrene 0-1%

Esters 28-38%
bornyl acetate 28-38%

Sesquiterpenes 7-14%
tricyclene 4-8%
dipentene 2-4%
δ-cadinene 1-3%

Ketones 0-3%
α-thujone 0-3%

Turkish Rose
(See *Rosa damascena*)

Valerian
(See *Valeriana officinalis*)

Valerian, Indian
(See *Nardostachys jatamansi*)

110. Valeriana officinalis

Valerianaceae (Valerian Family)
• **Valerian**, Garden Heliotrope, Heliotrope
• Distilled from roots
• B, Fl, Fr, H, M, Y
Esters 34-50%
bornyl acetate 32-44%
myrtenyl acetate 1-5%
bornyl formate 0-1%
bornyl butyrate 0-1%
bornyl isovalerate 0-1%
Monoterpenes 30-41%
camphene 14-21%
α-fenchene 9-13%
α-pinene 4-8%
β-pinene 2-6%
Alcohols 4-6%
borneol 2-3%
geraniol 1-2%
α-terpineol 1-2%
Sesquiterpenols 3-6%
germacrenol 3-6%
viterol 0-1%
Sesquiterpenes 2-5%
δ-cadinene 1-3%
vitivene 1-2%
α-farnescene 0-1%
valerazulene 0-1%
Carboxylic Acids 1-3%
valerinic acid 1-2%
isovaleric acid 0-1%
chlorogenic acid 0-1%
malic acid 0-1%
Sesquiterpenals 1-2%
valerianal 1-2%
Sesquiterpenones 0-1%
valerianone 0-1%
Sesquiterpene Lactones 0-2%
actinidine 0-1%
valerianine 0-1%

Vetiver

(See *Vetiveria zizanioides*)

111. Vetiveria zizanioides

Gramineae (Grass Family)
• **Vetiver**
• Distilled from roots
• B, Fr, H, M, P, Y
Sesquiterpenols 30-42%
isovalencenol 11-15%
bicyclovetinerol 10-13%
khusenol 6-11%
tricyclovetinerol 3-4%
vetiverol 0-1%
Sesquiterpenones 14-22%
α-vetivone 3-6%
β-vetivone 3-6%
khusimone 3-6%
nootkatone 2-5%
Sesquiterpenes 2-4%
β-cadinene 0-1%
δ-cadinene 0-1%
tricyclovetinene 0-1%
vetivene 0-1%
vetivazulene 0-1%
Sesquiterpene Esters 1-2%
vetiveryl acetate 1-2%
Carboxylic Acids 0-2%
benzoic acid 0-1%
palmitic acid 0-1%
vetivenic acid 0-1%

Vitex

(See *Vitex negundo*)

112. Vitex negundo

Lamiaceae (Mint Family)
• **Vitex**, Chaste Tree, Monk's Pepper
• Distilled bark, branches, leaves
• B, H, Y
Sesquiterpenes 52-65%
β-caryophyllene 38-40%
germacrene-B 6-10%
β-farnesene 3-7%
longifolene 3-6%
α-gurjunene 2-5%

Monoterpenes 14-20%
sabinene 10-15%
α-pinene 4-6%
l-limonene 1-3%
Oxides 7-18%
caryophyllene oxide 5-10%
1,8 cineole 4-9%
Esters 1-2%
α-terpinyl acetate 1-2%

Western Red Cedar
(See *Thuja plicata - 1 & 2*)

White Camphor
(See *Cinnamomum camphora*)

White Fir
(See *Abies alba or Abies grandis*)

White Hemlock
(See *Tsuga canadensis*)

White Santal
(See *Santalum album*)

Wild Chamomile
(See *Ormenis mixta*)

Wild Marjoram
(See *Origanum compactum*)

Wild Tansy
(See *Tanacetum vulgare*)

Wintergreen
(See *Gaultheria procumbens*)

Winter Savory
(See *Satureja montana*)

Wintersweet
(See *Origanum compactum*)

Yarrow
(See *Achillea millefolium*)

Yarroway
(See *Achillea millefolium*)

Yellow Birch
(See *Betula alleghaniensis*)

Ylang Ylang
(See *Cananga odorata*)

113. *Zingiber officinale*
Zingiberaceae (Ginger Family)
• **Ginger**
• Distilled from roots
• B, Fl, Fr, H, M, P, Y
Sesquiterpenes 50-90%
zingiberene 12-50%
α-curcumene 10-33%
β-farnesene 17-20%
β-sesquiphellandrene 2-9%
γ-bisabolene 5-7%
β-ylangene 2-3%
β-elemene 1-2%
α-selinene 1-2%
β-bisabolene 0-1%
germacrene-D 0-1%
β-curcumene 0-1%
Monoterpenes 4-22%
camphene 1-8%
β-phellandrene 1-4%
l-limonene 1-3%
p-cymene 1-4%
α-pinene 0-4%
β-pinene 0-3%
myrcene 0-1%
Alcohols 9-20%
nonanol 2-8%
citronellol 5-6%
linalol 1-5%
borneol 1-2%
butanol 0-1%
heptanol 0-1%

Sesquiterpenols 3-14%
nerolidol 1-9%
zingeberol 1-2%
elemol 1-2%
β-bisabolol 0-1%
β-eudesmol 0-1%
sesquiphellandrol 0-1%

Ketones 2-6%
heptanone 0-2%
acetone 0-1%
carvatoacetone 0-1%
hexanone 0-1%
nonanone 0-1%
cryptone 0-1%

Aldehydes 2-4%
citronellal 0-1%
myrtenal 0-1%
neral 0-1%
phellandral 0-1%

Sesquiterpenones 0-2%
gingerone 0-2%

Alkanes 0-1%
undecane 0-1%
dodecane 0-1%
hexadecane 0-1%

Table Thirty-Two-A	
Composition of an "Average Essential Oil"	
(The Averages Below are Derived from All 113 Oils in Table Thirty-Two)	
Monoterpenes	30%
Alcohols	14%
Sesquiterpenes	12%
Esters	10%
Ketones	9%
Phenols	8%
Oxides	6%
Aldehydes	5%
Ethers	3%
Di, Tri, & Tetraterpenes	0.8%
Furanoids	0.7%
Coumarins	0.6%
Carboxylic Acids	0.4%
Lactones	0.3%
Alkanes	0.2%

NOTE: There is a blend of approximately 100 essential oils sold by Young Living Oils, Inc. It is called Legacy®. Its composition would be very close to what is given above. In Table Sixty-Eight, on p. 586, you can see that the "Average Essential Oil" is also an ideal "PMS Oil."

Table Thirty-Three
Essential Oils Tabulated by Botanical Families

1. LAMIACEAE
(Mint Family)

75. Basil
74. Catnip
92. Clary Sage
106. Garden Thyme
56. Hyssop
60. Lavender
61. Lavandin
77. Marjoram
68. Melissa
105. Morrocan Thyme
94. Mountain Savory
76. Oregano
85. Patchouly
69. Peppermint
87. Ravensara
89. Rosemary
90. Rosemary verbenon
91. Sage
104. Spanish Marjoram
70. Spearmint
107. Sweet Thyme
108. Thyme
112. Vitex

2. ASTERACEAE
(Aster/Daisy Family)

99. Blue Tansy
11. Davana
38. Fleabane
63. German Chamomile
95. Goldenrod
55. Helichrysum
100. Idaho Tansy
98. Marigold
12. Mugwort
78. Ormenis
21. Roman Chamomile
10. Tarragon
4. Yarrow

3. APIACEAE
(Celery-Carrot Family)

7. Angelica
82. Anise
19. Caraway
45. Carrot Seed
9. Celery Seed
39. Coriander
40. Cumin
6. Dill
53. Fennel
52. Galbanum
30. Parsley

4. MYRTACEAE
(Myrtle Family)

50. Blue Mallee
65. Cajuput
97. Clove
48. E. Dives
51. E. Radiata
49. Eucalyptus
47. Lemon Eucalyptus
72. Myrtle
67. Niaouli
66. Rosalina
64. Tea Tree

5. RUTACEAE
(Citrus Family)

30. Bergamot
28. Bitter Orange
31. Cambava
34. Grapefruit
32. Lemon
26. Lime
35. Mandarin
27. Neroli
36. Orange
29. Petitgrain
33. Tangerine

5. PINACEAE
(Pine Family)

2. Balsam Fir
20. Cedarwood
86. Douglas Fir
83. Pine
1. Silver Fir
81. Spruce
109. Tsuga
3. White Fir

6. CUPRESSACEAE
(Cypress Family)

15. Blue Cypress
102. Cedar Bark
103. Cedar Leaf
41. Cypress
58. Juniper
101. Thuja

7. LAURACEAE
(Laurel Family)

59. Bay Laurel
23. Cassia
24. Cinnamon Bark
8. Rosewood
22. White Camphor

8. GRAMINEAE
(Grass Family)

44. Citronella
42. Lemongrass
43. Palmarosa
111. Vetiver

9. BURSERACEAE
(Frankincense/Myrrh Family)

17. Elemi
14. Frankincense
37. Myrrh

10. ERICACEAE
(Heather Family)

62. Ledum
54. Wintergreen

11. VALERIANACEAE
(Valerian Family)

73. Spikenard
110. Valerian

12. ZINGIBERACEAE
(Ginger Family)

46. Cardamom
113. Ginger

13. ANNONACEAE
(Ylang Ylang Family)

16. Ylang Ylang

14. ARACEAE
(Cane Family)

5. Calamus

15. BETULACEAE
(Birch Family)

13. Birch

16. CANNABACEAE
(Marijuana Family)

18. Marijuana

17. CISTACEAE
(Cistus Family)

25. Cistus

18. GERANIACEAE
(Geranium Family)

79. Geranium

19. MYRISTICACEAE (Nutmeg Family)

11. Nutmeg

20. OLEACEAE (Olive Family)

57. Jasmine

21. PIPERACEAE (Pepper Family)

84 Black Pepper

22. ROSACEAE (Rose Family)

88. Rose

23. SANTALACEAE (Sandalwood Family)

93. Sandalwood

24. STYRACACEAE (Storax Family)

96. Onycha

Numbers preceeding the names of oils refer to listings in Table Thirty-Two

Table Thirty-Four
Essential Oils Tabulated by Plant Parts Yielding Oil

1. LEAVES

59. Bay Laurel
65. Cajuput
31. Cambava
44. Citronella
48. E. Dives
51. E. Radiata
49. Eucalyptus
79. Geranium
62. Ledum
47. Lemon Eucalyptus
42. Lemongrass
77. Marjoram
72. Myrtle
68. Niaouli
66. Rosalina
89. Rosemary
90. Rosemary Verbenon
10. Tarragon
64. Tea Tree
54. Wintergreen

2. LEAVES & FLOWERS

99. Blue Tansy
74. Catnip
106. Garden Thyme
60. Idaho Tansy
68. Melissa
105. Moroccan Thyme
76. Oregano
85. Patchouly
91. Sage
104. Spanish Marjoram
107. Sweet Thyme

3. FLOWERS

11. Davana
63. German Chamomile
55. Helichrysum
57. Jasmine
27. Neroli
21. Roman Chamomile
88. Rose
16. Ylang Ylang

4. RIND OF THE FRUIT

30. Bergamot
28. Bitter Orange
34. Grapefruit
32. Lemon
26. Lime
35. Mandarin
36. Orange
33. Tangerine

5. LEAVES, FLOWERS & STEMS

92. Clary Sage
38. Fleabane
95. Goldenrod
94. Mountain Savory
43. Palmarosa
69. Peppermint
108. Thyme

6. SEEDS

9. Celery Seed
19. Caraway
39. Coriander
40. Cumin
45. Carrot Seed
53. Fennel

7. NEEDLES & TWIGS

2. Balsam Fir
86. Douglas Fir
1. Silver Fir
81. Spruce
109. Tsuga
3. White Fir

8. ROOTS

7. Angelica
113. Ginger
73. Spikenard
110. Valerian
111. Vetiver

9. FLOWERING TOPS

61. Lavandin
60. Lavender
78. Ormenis
4. Yarrow

10. GUM–RESIN

17. Elemi
14. Frankincense
37. Myrrh
96. Onycha

11. LEAVES & STEMS

56. Hyssop
18. Marijuana
80. Parsley
70. Spearmint

12. LEAVES, TWIGS, BRANCHES

50. Blue Mallee
103. Cedar Leaf
29. Petitgrain
87. Ravensara

13. BARK

23. Cassia
20. Cedarwood
24. Cinnamon Bark

14. FRUIT & SEEDS

82. Anise
46. Cardamom
71. Nutmeg

15. BRANCHES

25. Cistus
41. Cypress

16. NEEDLES

83. Pine
61. Thuja

17. WOOD
8. Rosewood
93. Sandalwood

18. LEAVES, WOOD & BARK
15. Blue Cypress
22. White Camphor

19. WOOD & BARK
102. Cedar Bark

20. BARK, BRANCHES, LEAVES
112. Vitex

21. WOOD, TWIGS, BRANCHES
13. Birch

22. STEMS & BUDS
97. Clove

23. BERRIES
84. Black Pepper

24. BERRIES & BRANCHES
58. Juniper

25. GUM, STEMS, BRANCHES
52. Galbanum

26. WHOLE PLANT
6. Dill

Table Thirty-Five
% Alcohol Content in Essential Oils

8. Rosewood	83%		94. Mountain Savory	19%
43. Palmarosa	82%		30. Bergamot	18%
39. Coriander	76%		92. Clary Sage	17%
106. Garden Thyme	74%		91. Sage	16%
74. Catnip	64%		113. Ginger	15%
79. Geranium	60%		53. Fennel	14%
88. Rose	60%		51. E. Radiata	13%
107. Sweet Thyme	60%		42. Lemongrass	13%
105. Moroccan Thyme	52%		67. Niaouli	13%
45. Carrot Seed	49%		25. Cistus	12%
27. Neroli	48%		72. Myrtle	12%
61. Lavandin	45%		89. Rosemary	12%
60. Lavender	44%		75. Basil	11%
78. Ormenis	44%		31. Cambava	11%
66. Rosalina	44%		87. Ravensara	9%
44. Citronella	38%		41. Cypress	8%
29. Petitgrain	34%		86. Douglas Fir	8%
47. Lemon Eucalyptus	28%		108. Thyme	8%
104. Spanish Marjoram	25%		4. Yarrow	8%
16. Ylang Ylang	25%		65. Cajuput	7%
59. Bay Laurel	22%		80. Parsley	7%
77. Marjoram	20%		70. Spearmint	7%

Continued on the next page . . .

19. Caraway	6%		23. Cassia	3%
24. Cinnamon Bark	6%		32. Lemon	3%
55. Helichrysum	6%		26. Lime	3%
57. Jasmine	6%		9. Celery Seed	2%
35. Mandarin	6%		48. E. Dives	2%
82. Anise	5%		17. Elemi	2%
100. Idaho Tansy	5%		49. Eucalyptus	2%
68. Melissa	5%		56. Hyssop	2%
21. Roman Chamomile	5%		62. Ledum	2%
64. Tea Tree	5%		71. Nutmeg	2%
110. Valerian	5%		83. Pine	2%
38. Fleabane	4%		81. Spruce	2%
14. Frankincense	4%		33. Tangerine	2%
95. Goldenrod	4%		3. White Fir	2%
36. Orange	4%		34. Grapefruit	1%
69. Peppermint	4%		76. Oregano	1%
90. Rosemary Verbenon	4%		96. Onycha	1%
28. Bitter Orange	3%			

Table Thirty-Six
% Aldehyde Content in Essential Oils

23. Cassia	80%		49. Eucalyptus	3%
31. Cambava	75%		113. Ginger	3%
42. Lemongrass	67%		60. Lavender	3%
47. Lemon Eucalyptus	60%		35. Mandarin	3%
68. Melissa	55%		82. Anise	2%
40. Cumin	49%		30. Bergamot	2%
24. Cinnamon Bark	46%		65. Cajuput	2%
19. Caraway	19%		86. Douglas Fir	2%
26. Lime	15%		34. Grapefruit	2%
74. Catnip	9%		62. Ledum	2%
32. Lemon	8%		27. Neroli	2%
5. Calamus	7%		96. Onycha	2%
28. Bitter Orange	7%		29. Petitgrain	2%
44. Citronella	6%		73. Spikenard	2%
51. E. Radiata	6%		33. Tangerine	2%
36. Orange	6%		50. Blue Mallee	1%
77. Marjoram	5%		105. Moroccan Thyme	1%
25. Cistus	4%		84. Black Pepper	1%
79. Geranium	4%		67. Niaouli	1%
37. Myrrh	4%		83. Pine	1%
72. Myrtle	4%			

Table Thirty-Seven
% Alkane Content in Essential Oils

88. Rose	11%	113. Ginger	1%

Numbers preceeding the names of oils
refer to listings in Table Thirty-Two

Table Thirty-Eight
% Coumarin Content in Essential Oils
(Including Furanocoumarins)

38. Fleabane	8%	26. Lime	2%
28. Bitter Orange	6%	84. Black Pepper	1%
32. Lemon	4%	9. Celery Seed	1%
30. Bergamot	3%	24. Cinnamon Bark	1%
60. Lavender	3%	25. Cistus	1%
98. Marigold	3%	92. Clary Sage	1%
10. Tarragon	3%	40. Cumin	1%
7. Angelica	2%	100. Idaho Tansy	1%
39. Coriander	2%	68. Melissa	1%
9. Dill	2%	36. Orange	1%
53. Fennel	2%	69. Peppermint	1%
34. Grapefruit	2%	29. Petitgrain	1%
61. Lavandin	2%		

Table Thirty-Nine
% Carboxylic Acid Content in Essential Oils

96. Onycha	19%	108. Thyme	2%
76. Oregano	4%	54. Wintergreen	2%
47. Lemon Eucalyptus	4%	7. Angelica	1%
23. Cassia	3%	84. Black Pepper	1%
110. Valerian	3%	25. Cistus	1%
24. Cinnamon Bark	2%	41. Cypress	1%
97. Clove	2%	52. Galbanum	1%
89. Rosemary	2%	73. Spikenard	1%
90. Rosemary Verbenon	2%	111. Vetiver	1%

Table Forty
% Di, Tri, & Tetraterpene Content in Essential Oils

Diterpenes

57. Jasmine	14%
92. Clary Sage	5%
22. White Camphor	3%
41. Cypress	2%
83. Pine	2%
25. Cistus	1%
91. Sage	1%

Triterpenes

37. Myrrh	6%
57. Jasmine	5%

18. Marijuana	2%
13. Birch	1%

Tetraterpenes

33. Tangerine	8%
28. Bitter Orange	6%
35. Mandarin	6%
36. Orange	6%
30. Bergamot	5%
34. Grapefruit	5%
32. Lemon	3%
45. Carrot Seed	2%

Table Forty-One
% Ester Content in Essential Oils

54. Wintergreen	97%		90. Rosemary Vervenon	9%
13. Birch	90%		25. Cistus	8%
96. Onycha	70%		47. Lemon Eucalyptus	8%
21. Roman Chamomile	65%		101. Thuja	8%
92. Clary Sage	64%		69. Peppermint	7%
29. Petitgrain	57%		1. Silver Fir	7%
46. Cardamom	50%		41. Cypress	6%
61. Lavandin	44%		77. Marjoram	6%
55. Helichrysum	43%		68. Melissa	6%
57. Jasmine	43%		28. Bitter Orange	5%
110. Valerian	42%		39. Coriander	5%
60. Lavender	39%		106. Garden Thyme	5%
30. Bergamot	37%		104. Spanish Marjoram	5%
81. Spruce	34%		75. Basil	4%
109. Tsuga	33%		23. Cassia	4%
79. Geranium	23%		38. Fleabane	4%
43. Palmarosa	21%		78. Ormenis	4%
27. Neroli	19%		88. Rose	4%
2. Balsam Fir	16%		7. Angelica	3%
58. Juniper	16%		45. Carrot Seed	3%
72. Myrtle	15%		95. Goldenrod	3%
86. Douglas Fir	14%		32. Lemon	3%
59. Bay Laurel	13%		105. Moroccan Thyme	3%
9. Celery Seed	13%		76. Mountain Savory	3%
3. White Fir	13%		91. Sage	3%
97. Clove	12%		70. Spearmint	3%
42. Lemongrass	10%		52. Galbanum	2%

56. Hyssop	2%	103 Cedar Leaf	1%
35. Mandarin	2%	49. Eucalyptus	1%
36. Orange	2%	100. Idaho Tansy	1%
83. Pine	2%	62. Ledum	1%
87. Ravensara	2%	89. Rosemary	1%
4. Yarrow	2%	63. German Chamomile	1%
65. Cajuput	1%	112. Vitex	1%

Table Forty-Two
% Ether Content in Essential Oils
(Including Phenolic Ethers)

82. Anise	88%	80. Parsley	11%
10. Tarragon	75%	6. Dill	10%
53. Fennel	66%	22. White camphor	9%
75. Basil	65%	63. German Chamomile	6%
16. Ylang Ylang	12%	11. Davana	3%
71. Nutmeg	11%	77. Marjoram	1%

Table Forty-Three
% Furanoid Content in Essential Oils
(Phototoxic Oils are Designated by an Asterisk*)

37. Myrrh	23%	26. Lime *	2%
38. Fleabane	8%	72. Myrtle	2%
69. Peppermint	5%	36. Orange	2%
28. Bitter Orange *	4%	82. Anise	1%
30. Bergamot *	3%	84. Black Pepper	1%
11. Davana	3%	9. Celery Seed	1%
7. Angelica *	2%	39. Coriander	1%
53. Fennel	2%	6. Dill	1%
79. Geranium	2%	52. Galbanum	1%
34. Grapefruit *	2%	68. Melissa	1%
32. Lemon *	2%	29. Petitgrain *	1%

• **UV RESONATORS:** The dimensions of furanoid molecules can resonate with the wave lengths of ultraviolet light, amplifying them to cause sunburn when applied to skin within 12 hours of exposure to sunshine, tanning lights, or other UV sources. The 7 oils noted by asterisks* above are known to be phototoxic in this manner. Anise and fennel oils are also considered phototoxic by some authorities. However, furanoid molecules can be configured in some oils (such as myrrh) such that they actually resonate in a way that is destructive to the energy of UV light, thus absorbing the rays and providing sunscreen protection—the opposite of phototoxicity.   (See Chapter 10 for

Table Forty-Four
% Ketone Content in Essential Oils

102.	Cedar Bark	87%	61.	Lavandin	8%
103.	Cedar Leaf	86%	73.	Spikenard	8%
100.	Idaho Tansy	73%	79.	Geranium	7%
98.	Marigold	65%	68.	Melissa	6%
70.	Spearmint	60%	39.	Coriander	4%
101.	Thuja	59%	113.	Ginger	4%
19.	Caraway	53%	105.	Moroccan Thyme	4%
56.	Hyssop	52%	49.	Eucalyptus	3%
11.	Davana	48%	36.	Orange	3%
22.	White Camphor	47%	85.	Patchouly	3%
48.	E. Dives	42%	104.	Spanish Marjoram	3%
91.	Sage.	41%	84.	Black Pepper	2%
5.	Calamus	40%	50.	Blue Mallee	2%
6.	Dill	38%	60.	Lavender	2%
4.	Yarrow	21%	42.	Lemongrass	2%
69.	Peppermint	20%	76.	Oregano	2%
89.	Rosemary	20%	109.	Tsuga	2%
55.	Helichrysum	19%	82.	Anise	1%
37.	Myrrh	17%	75.	Basil	1%
58.	Juniper	15%	92.	Clary Sage	1%
99.	Blue Tansy	14%	17.	Elemi	1%
12.	Mugwort	14%	34.	Grapefruit	1%
21.	Roman Chamomile	12%	62.	Ledum	1%
53.	Fennel	10%	94.	Mountain Savory	1%
9.	Celery Seed	9%	78.	Ormenis	1%
25.	Cistus	8%			

Numbers preceeding the names of oils
refer to listings in Table Thirty-Two

Table Forty-Five
% Lactone Content in Essential Oils
(Coumarin Lactones <u>Not</u> Included. See Table Thirty-Eight)

74.	Catnip	13%	72.	Myrtle	2%
9.	Celery Seed	11%	4.	Yarrow	2%
59.	Bay Laurel	3%	12.	Mugwort	1%
38.	Fleabane	2%	110.	Valerian	1%

Table Forty-Six
% Monoterpene Content in Essential Oils

34.	Grapefruit	93%	73.	Spikenard	36%
1.	Silver Fir	92%	110.	Valerian	35%
28.	Bitter Orange	90%	90.	Rosemary Verbenon	33%
35.	Mandarin	90%	56.	Hyssop	30%
36.	Orange	90%	27.	Neroli	30%
33.	Tangerine	90%	40.	Cumin	29%
2.	Balsam Fir	83%	80.	Rosemary	27%
7.	Angelica	80%	21.	Roman Chamomile	26%
32.	Lemon	80%	49.	Eucalyptus	24%
14.	Frankincense	78%	94.	Mountain Savory.	24%
9.	Celery Seed	77%	87.	Ravensara	24%
41.	Cypress	76%	70.	Spearmint	24%
80.	Parsley	75%	66.	Rosalina	23%
38.	Fleabane	73%	45.	Carrot Seed	22%
17.	Elemi	72%	88.	Rose	22%
52.	Galbanum	72%	10.	Tarragon	22%
86.	Douglas Fir	70%	67.	Niaouli	21%
21.	Nutmeg	68%	101.	Thuja	21%
3.	White Fir	65%	59.	Bay Laurel	20%
26.	Lime	62%	78.	Ormenis	20%
30.	Bergamot	55%	91.	Sage	20%
58.	Juniper	54%	65.	Cajuput	19%
25.	Cistus	53%	29.	Petitgrain	19%
64.	Tea Tree	52%	51.	E. Radiata	18%
83.	Pine	51%	107.	Sweet Thyme	18%
84.	Black Pepper	50%	39.	Coriander	17%
99.	Blue Tansy	50%	106.	Garden Thyme	17%
6.	Dill	50%	76.	Oregano	17%
81.	Spruce	50%	112.	Vitex	17%
19.	Caraway	48%	61.	Lavandin	16%
77.	Marjoram	44%	60.	Lavender	16%
4.	Yarrow	43%	18.	Marijuana	16%
95.	Goldenrod	42%	104.	Spanish Marjoram	16%
109.	Tsuga	42%	113.	Ginger	13%
62.	Ledum	40%	55.	Helichrysum	11%
48.	E. Dives	39%	69.	Peppermint	10%
53.	Fennel	38%	42.	Lemongrass	8%
72.	Myrtle	38%	44.	Citronella	7%
12.	Mugwort	37%	100.	Idaho Tansy	7%
108	Thyme	37%	46.	Cardamom	5%
98.	Marigold	36%	103.	Cedar Leaf	5%

Continued on the next page . . .

37. Myrrh	5%	63. German Chamomile	3%
50. Blue Mallee	4%	47. Lemon Eucalyptus	3%
79. Geranium	4%	68. Melissa	2%
75. Basil	3%	105. Morrocan Thyme	1%
74. Catnip	3%	43. Palmarosa	1%
102. Cedar Bark	3%	85. Patchouly	1%
92. Clary Sage	3%		

Table Forty-Seven
% Oxide Content in Essential Oils

50. Blue Mallee	90%	61. Lavandin	6%
51. E. Radiata	69%	69. Peppermint	6%
49. Eucalyptus	68%	16. Ylang Ylang	6%
65. Cajuput	60%	45. Carrot Seed	4%
87. Ravensara	55%	105. Moroccan Thyme	4%
67. Niaouli	50%	85. Patchouly	4%
89. Rosemary	47%	8. Rosewood	4%
63. German Chamomile	40%	53. Fennel	3%
72. Myrtle	39%	60. Lavender	3%
22. White Camphor	32%	42. Lemongrass	3%
26. Lime	17%	71. Nutmeg	3%
55. Helichrysum	15%	70. Spearmint	3%
66. Rosalina	15%	92. Clary Sage	2%
112. Vitex	12%	97. Clove	2%
64. Tea Tree	11%	94. Mountain Savory	2%
108. Thyme	10%	12. Mugwort	2%
91. Sage	9%	43. Palmarosa	2%
47. Lemon Eucalyptus	8%	73. Spikenard	2%
68. Melissa	8%	13. Birch	1%
90. Rosemary Verbenon	8%	41. Cypress	1%
18. Marijuana	7%	48. E. Dives	1%
4. Yarrow	7%	56. Hyssop	1%
75. Basil	6%	88. Rose	1%
84. Black Pepper	6%		

• **THE MOST POPULAR OXIDE:** The major oxide in all of these oils is 1, 8 cineole which is decongesting and a popular ingredient to use in over-the-counter medications for colds, flu, sinusitis, bronchitis, and other respiratory conditions. Research has shown that inhaling 1,8 cineole increases blood flow in the brain, which can relieve head pain and improve concentration. Essential oils containing 1, 8 cineole are often used as natural medicines for these therapeutic purposes. (See Tables 59 & 60.)

Numbers preceeding the names of oils
refer to listings in Table Thirty-Two

Table Forty-Eight					
% Phenol Content in Essential Oils					

54. Wintergreen	97%		59. Bay Laurel	6%
82. Anise	90%		48. E. Dives	5%
13. Birch	90%		107. Sweet Thyme	5%
97. Clove	77%		101 Thuja	5%
75. Basil	76%		56. Hyssop	4%
10. Tarragon	75%		40. Cumin	3%
53. Fennel	72%		49. Eucalyptus	3%
76. Oregano	70%		72. Myrtle	3%
108. Thyme	50%		88. Rose	3%
94. Mountain Savory	49%		104. Spanish Marjoram	3%
69. Peppermint	39%		45. Carrot Seed	2%
64. Tea Tree	33%		74. Catnip	2%
5. Calamus	29%		53. Fennel	2%
24. Cinnamon Bark	26%		55. Helichrysum	2%
105. Moroccan Thyme	26%		27. Neroli	2%
44. Citronella	23%		91. Sage	2%
77. Marjoram	19%		30. Bergamot	1%
71. Nutmeg	18%		50. Blue Mallee	1%
47. Lemon Eucalyptus	11%		49. Eucalyptus	1%
80. Parsley	11%		37. Myrrh	1%
16. Ylang Ylang	8%		29. Petitgrain	1%
23. Cassia	7%		70. Spearmint	1%
96. Onycha	7%			

• **IN MORE THAN ONE FAMILY.** Phenols are often members of other chemical families simultaneously. For example, there are phenolic alcohols, phenolic esters, phenolic aldehydes, phenolic ketones, phenolic acids, and phenolic ethers as well as phenylpropanoids. There are also diphenols and triphenols. All phenolic compounds in essential oils cleanse cellular receptor sites and detoxify the body emotionally and chemically. They also serve other functions depending on what other classes of compounds they may represent. In rare cases, some phenolic compounnds can be allergenic. (See p. 470)

• **CUSTOM BLENDED OILS.** One purpose of the many tables and cross-references in Part Two of this book is to help those who are interested to create healing blends of essential oils. Through these tables and indexes you can easily see, at a glance, what compounds are contained in which oils and in what percents. These tables also enable one to easily recognize the chemical similarities and differences between various oils to know when one may be substituted for another and not. For example, an understanding of chemistry, as revealed through these tables, shows how certain pairs of oils—like wintergreen and birch, basil and tarragon, fennel and anise—can be used interchangeably. All of the oils containing eugenol or methyl salicylate, which have analgesic and/or anesthetic properties, are also easily identified in this part of the book to assist one in creating blends that may offer relief of pain.

Table Forty-Nine
% Sesquiterpene Content in Essential Oils
(Including Oxygenated Sesquiterpenes)

20. Cedarwood	95%	100. Idaho Tansy	7%
85. Patchouly	85%	61. Lavandin	7%
93. Sandalwood	83%	105. Moroccan Thyme	7%
113. Ginger	77%	74. Catnip	6%
15. Blue Cypress	73%	92. Clary sage	6%
37. Myrrh	65%	60. Lavender	6%
111. Vetiver	59%	83. Pine	6%
112. Vitex.	58%	19. Caraway	5%
63. German Chamomile	54%	94. Mountain Savory	5%
84. Black Pepper	53%	66. Rosalina	5%
73. Spikenard	52%	70. Spearmint	5%
16. Ylang Ylang	48%	30. Bergamot	4%
18. Marijuana	46%	52. Galbanum	4%
4. Yarrow	40%	31. Lemon	4%
95. Goldenrod	28%	47. Lemon Eucalyptus	4%
68. Melissa	27%	76. Oregano	4%
62. Ledum	20%	104. Spanish Marjoram	4%
67. Niaouli	18%	48. E. Dives	3%
17. Elemi	17%	55. Helichrysum	3%
49. Eucalyptus	17%	77. Marjoram	3%
64. Tea Tree	17%	108. Thyme	3%
45. Carrot Seed	16%	3. White Fir	3%
42. Lemongrass	16%	59. Bay Laurel	2%
91. Sage	15%	34. Grapefruit	2%
41. Cypress	14%	58. Juniper	2%
21. Roman Chamomile	13%	89. Rosemary	2%
109. Tsuga	11%	8. Rosewood	2%
110. Valerian	11%	82. Anise	1%
97. Clove	10%	103. Cedar Leaf	1%
99. Blue Tansy	9%	40. Cumin	1%
9. Celery Seed	9%	71. Nutmeg	1%
69. Peppermint	9%	36. Orange	1%
65. Cajuput	8%	43. Palmarosa	1%
14. Frankincense	8%	80. Parsley	1%
79. Geranium	8%	81. Spruce	1%
56. Hyssop	8%	87. Ravensara	1%
78. Ormenis	8%	88. Rose	1%
101. Thuja	8%		

Table Fifty
Top 40 Most Popular Compounds in Essential Oils
(Based on the 113 Oils in Table Thirty-Two)

Compound Name	No. of Oils With ≥ 5%	% of Oils With ≥ 5%	Compound Classification	Rank in Top
α–Pinene	35	31.0%	Monoterpene	1st
Linalol	23	20.3%	Alcohol	2nd
1, 8 Cineole	23	20.3%	Oxide	2nd
β–Pinene	22	19.5%	Monoterpene	4th
l–Limonene	22	19.5%	Monoterpene	4th
β–Caryophyllene	20	17.6%	Sesquiterpene	6th
d–Limonene	16	14.2%	Monoterpene	7th
α–Terpineol	16	14.2%	Alcohol	7th
Sabinene	15	13.3%	Monoterpene	9th
γ–Terpinene	14	12.4%	Monoterpene	10th
Camphene	11	9.7%	Monoterpene	11th
Bornyl Acetate	10	8.8%	Ester	12th
Camphor	10	8.8%	Ketone	12th
Myrcene	10	8.8%	Monoterpene	12th
Borneol	8	7.1%	Alcohol	15th
δ–3–Carene	7	6.2%	Monoterpene	16th
Geraniol	7	6.2%	Alcohol	16th
p–Cymene	7	6.2%	Monoterpene	16th
Ocimene	7	6.2%	Monoterpene	16th
Caryophyllene Oxide	6	5.3%	Oxide	20th
Linalyl Acetate	6	5.3%	Ester	20th
α–Thujone	6	5.3%	Ketone	20th
β–Thujone	6	5.3%	Ketone	20th
α–Terpinene	6	5.3%	Monoterpene	20th
Terpinen–4–ol	6	5.3%	Phenol	20th
Citronellol	5	4.4%	Alcohol	26th
Eugenol	5	4.4%	Phenol	26th
Germacrene-D	5	4.4%	Sesquiterpene	26th
Carvacrol	4	3.5%	Phenol	29th
α–Phellandrene	4	3.5%	Monoterpene	29th
Anethole	3	2.7%	Phenol	31st
Chamazulene	3	2.7%	Sesquiterpene	31st
Estragole	3	2.7%	Phenol	31st
β–Farnesene	3	2.7%	Sesquiterpene	31st
Fenchone	3	2.7%	Ketone	31st
Geranyl Acetate	3	2.7%	Ester	31st
Humulene	3	2.7%	Sesquiterpene	31st
β-Phellandrene	3	2.7%	Monoterpene	31st
Selinene	3	2.7%	Sesquiterpene	31st
α-Terpinyl Acetate	3	2.7%	Ester	31st
Thymol	3	2.7%	Phenol	31st

Table Fifty-One
Most Popular Alcohols in Essential Oils

20.3%	of essential oils contain 5% or more of:	Linalol
14.2%	of essential oils contain 5% or more of:	α-Terpineol
7.1%	of essential oils contain 5% or more of:	Borneol
6.2%	of essential oils contain 5% or more of:	Geraniol
4.4%	of essential oils contain 5% or more of:	Citronellol

Table Fifty-Two
Essential Oils With The Most Popular Alcohols
(In Concentrations of at Least 5%)

Linalol (also spelled linalool)

8.	Rosewood	82%
27.	Neroli	36%
39.	Coriander	35%
61.	Lavandin	35%
60.	Lavender	35%
16.	Ylang Ylang	25%
29.	Petitgrain	23%
92.	Clary Sage	16%
104.	Spanish Marjoram	15%
30.	Bergamot	14%
79.	Geranium	12%
53.	Fennel	11%
59.	Bay Laurel	10%
94.	Mountain Savory	9%
46.	Cardamom	6%
105.	Moroccan Thyme	6%
24.	Cinnamon Bark	5%
108.	Thyme	5%
25.	Cistus	6%
87.	Ravensara	6%
38.	Fleabane	5%
72.	Myrtle	5%
8.	Rosewood	5%
91.	Sage	5%

α–Terpineol

47.	Lemon Eucalyptus	17%
105.	Moroccan Thyme	13%
51.	E. Radiata	11%
67.	Niaouli	11%
77.	Marjoram	10%
59.	Bay Laurel	9%
94.	Mountain Savory	8%
104.	Spanish Marjoram	8%
65.	Cajuput	7%
29.	Petitgrain	7%

Borneol

105.	Moroccan Thyme	39%
91.	Sage	8%
89.	Rosemary	7%
44.	Citronella	6%
41.	Cypress	6%
86.	Douglas Fir	5%
90.	Rosemary verbenon	5%
4.	Yarrow	5%

Geraniol

43.	Palmarosa	77%
44.	Citronella	24%
74.	Catnip	21%
79.	Geranium	21%
88.	Rose	20%
42.	Lemongrass	8%
86.	Douglas Fir	5%

Citronellol

88.	Rose	37%
79.	Geranium	32%
74.	Catnip	31%
44.	Citronella	9%
113.	Ginger	6%

Table Fifty-Three
Most Popular Aldehydes in Essential Oils

3.5%   of essential oils contain 5% or more of: Geranial
2.7%   of essential oils contain 5% or more of: Citronellal

Table Fifty-Four
Essential Oils With The Most Popular Aldehydes
(In Concentrations of at Least 5%)

Geranial

42. Lemongrass	37%
68. Melissa	30%
26. Lime	7%
74. Catnip	5%

Cinnamaldehyde

23. Cassia	85%
24. Cinnamon	46%
37. Myrrh	1%

Citronellal

31. Cambava	75%
47. Lemon Eucalyptus	60%
44. Citronella	6%

NOTE

There are many unique and different aldehydes found in essential oils. Most aromatic oils have at least traces of aldehydes. A few aldehydes are found in high concentrations in only in one or two oils, but are absent in all the rest. Citronellal and Geranial are the only aldehydes contained in concentrations of 5% or more in at least three different essential oils—which is the criterion on which Tables 50–65 are based.   .

Table Fifty-Five
Most Popular Esters in Essential Oils

8.8%	of essential oils contain 5% or more of:	Bornyl Acetate
5.3%	of essential oils contain 5% or more of:	Linalyl Acetate
2.7%	of essential oils contain 5% or more of:	Geranyl Acetate
2.7%	of essential oils contain 5% or more of:	α-Terpinyl Acetate
Only 2	essential oils contain 5% or more of:	Methyl Salicylate

---

Table Fifty-Six
Essential Oils With The Most Popular Esters
(In Concentrations of at Least 5%)

Bornyl Acetate

81.	Spruce	33%
109.	Tsuga	33%
2.	Balsam Fir	16%
58.	Juniper	16%
3.	White Fir	14%
86.	Douglas Fir	12%
90.	Rosemary Verbenon	9%
101.	Thuja	8%
1.	Silver Fir	7%
25.	Cistus	5%

Linalyl Acetate

29.	Petitgrain	50%
61.	Lavandin	40%
30.	Bergamot	37%
60.	Lavender	35%
27.	Neroli	9%
42.	Lemongrass	5%

Geranyl Acetate

43.	Palmarosa	8%
42.	Lemongrass	6%
77.	Marjoram	5%

α-Terpinyl Acetate

46.	Cardamom	46%
54.	Bay Laurel	7%
41.	Cypress	5%

Methyl Salicylate

54.	Wintergreen	97%
13.	Birch	90%

- **ESTERS COME FROM ALCOHOLS.** Note that the most popular esters— linalyl, bornyl, and geranyl acetate correspond to the most popular alcohols— linalol, borneol, and geraniol.

- **TALKING ABOUT ESTER.** Bornyl acetate prevails among the evergreen trees and shrubs. It is the fragrance we associate with a coniferous forest of pines, spruce, fir, and other needle-bearing trees. It is energizing, empowering, and mentally clearing. Linalyl acetate has a floral fragrance which you can identify in all six of the oils above that contain it. It is calming, soothing, and emotionally releasing. Geranyl acetate is also a floral fragrance, but with a sharper, greener note. It helps release tensions and leads to relaxation. α-Terpinyl acetate has a grounding effect and can help with mental, emotional, and physical detoxification.. Methyl salicylate is actually a phenolic ester with a cortisone-like effect. It is analgesic, like aspirin, and is supportive of the bones and joints. It is also a detoxifying compound and a cleanser of cellular receptor sites.

Table Fifty-Seven
Most Popular Ketones in Essential Oils

8.8% of essential oils contain 5% or more of: Camphor
5.3% of essential oils contain 5% or more of: α–Thujone
5.3% of essential oils contain 5% or more of: β–Thujone
2.7% of essential oils contain 5% or more of: Fenchone

Table Fifty-Eight
Essential Oils With The Most Popular Ketones
(In Concentrations of at Least 5%)

Camphor

22. White Camphor	45%
89. Rosemary	18%
58. Juniper	14%
91. Sage	14%
99. Blue Tansy	13%
4. Yarrow	11%
61. Lavandin	8%
90. Rosemary Verbenon	8%
100. Idaho Tansy	6%
39. Coriander	5%

Fenchone

101. Thuja	11%
53. Fennel	10%
103. Cedar Leaf	5%

α–Thujone

102. Cedar Bark	77%
103. Cedar Leaf	72%
101. Thuja	45%
91. Sage	23%
12. Mugwort	6%
100. Idaho Tansy	5%

β–Thujone

100. Idaho Tansy	67%
101. Thuja	12%
91. Sage	8%
102. Cedar Bark	7%
103. Cedar Leaf	7%
12. Mugwort	6%

• **KETONES AND PHENOLS.** While phenolic oils are known for their cleansing and detoxifying properties, ketones have many of the same cleansing and detoxifying properties. In fact, in the discussion of PMS healing oils in Chapter Nine, ketones may be substituted for phenols. Ketones are also known for their strong fragrances as well as their decongesting properties. Hyssop oil, for example, is an excellent decongestant. Simply inhaling its vapors can stimulate one to cough up phlegm and other alien fluids that need to get out of the lungs. Its principle ingredient is a ketone, pinocamphon (34-50%) which does not appear in the list of popular ketones since it is found only in hyssop. Another important, but uncommon ketone is menthone, found only in peppermint oil (12-20%). Of all known compounds in oils, menthone has been shown to have the highest rate of cell penetration. This is why peppermint is often layered over other oils to help carry them deeper into the tissues and enhance their therapeutic actions. Peppermint is one of the last oils applied in raindrop.

Table Fifty-Nine
Most Popular Monoterpenes in Essential Oils

31.0%	of essential oils contain 5% or more of:	α–Pinene
19.5%	of essential oils contain 5% or more of:	β–Pinene
19.5%	of essential oils contain 5% or more of:	l–limonene
14.2%	of essential oils contain 5% or more of:	d–limonene
13.3%	of essential oils contain 5% or more of:	Sabinene
12.4%	of essential oils contain 5% or more of:	γ–Terpinene
9.7%	of essential oils contain 5% or more of:	Camphene
8.8%	of essential oils contain 5% or more of:	Myrcene
6.2%	of essential oils contain 5% or more of:	p–Cymene
6.2%	of essential oils contain 5% or more of:	Ocimene
5.3%	of essential oils contain 5% or more of:	δ–3–Carene
5.3%	of essential oils contain 5% or more of:	α–Terpinene
3.5%	of essential oils contain 5% or more of:	α–Phellandrene
2.7%	of essential oils contain 5% or more of:	β–Phellandrene

Table Sixty
Essential Oils With The Most Popular Monoterpenes
(In Concentrations of at Least 5%)

α–Pinene

41.	Cypress	51%
25.	Cistus	50%
2.	Balsam Fir	38%
14.	Frankincense	38%
83.	Pine	33%
86.	Douglas Fir	32%
58.	Juniper	30%
72.	Myrtle	26%
90.	Rosemary Verbenon	25%
1.	Silver Fir	24%
7.	Angelica	22%
71.	Nutmeg	22%
49.	Eucalyptus	16%
6.	Dill	15%
81.	Spruce	15%
95.	Goldenrod	14%
52.	Galbanum	13%
78.	Ormenis	13%
45.	Carrot Seed	12%
109.	Tsuga	12%

67.	Niaouli	11%
89.	Rosemary	11%
51.	E. Radiata	10%
32.	Lemon	10%
21.	Roman Chamomile	10%
3.	White Fir	10%
59.	Bay Laurel	7%
87.	Ravensara	7%
84.	Black Pepper	6%
53.	Fennel	6%
110.	Valerian	6%
9.	Coriander	5%
18.	Marijuana	5%
64.	Tea Tree	5%
112.	Vitex	5%

β–Pinene

52.	Galbanum	55%
3.	White Fir	25%
86.	Douglas Fir	20%

Continued on the next page . . .

2. Balsam Fir	19%
56. Hyssop	18%
71. Nutmeg	16%
40. Cumin	15%
6. Dill	15%
27. Neroli	12%
32. Lemon	11%
84. Black Pepper	10%
26. Lime	10%
83. Pine	10%
109. Tsuga	10%
4. Yarrow	10%
84. Black Pepper	9%
99. Blue Tansy	8%
30. Bergamot	7%
89. Rosemary	7%
59. Bay Laurel	6%
21. Roman Chamomile	6%
81. Spruce	6%

l–Limonene

38. Fleabane	67%
17. Elemi	55%
1. Silver Fir	34%
62. Ledum	27%
70. Spearmint	20%
2. Balsam Fir	18%
7. Angelica	15%
84. Black Pepper	13%
86. Douglas Fir	12%
83. Pine	12%
55. Helichrysum	11%
95. Goldenrod	9%
72. Myrtle	8%
53. Fennel	7%
67. Niaouli	7%
65. Cajuput	6%
51. E. Radiata	6%
41. Cypress	5%
49. Eucalyptus	5%
58. Juniper	5%
81. Spruce	5%
10. Tarragon	5%

d–Limonene

34. Grapefruit	89%
28. Bitter Orange	87%
36. Orange	87%
33. Tangerine	72%
35. Mandarin	70%
32. Lemon	65%
9. Celery Seed	62%
26. Lime	49%
30. Bergamot	32%
7. Angelica	30%
19. Caraway	22%
6. Dill	20%
27. Neroli	14%
99. Blue Tansy	8%
44. Citronella	8%
71. Nutmeg	5%

Sabinene

4. Yarrow	25%
71. Nutmeg	22%
101. Thuja	21%
58. Juniper	14%
99. Blue Tansy	13%
12. Mugwort	12%
87. Ravensara	12%
112. Vitex	12%
45. Carrot Seed	10%
59. Bay Laurel	8%
95. Goldenrod	8%
84. Black Pepper	7%
14. Frankincense	5%
77. Marjoram	5%
21. Roman Chamomile	5%

γ–Terpinene

40. Cumin	22%
19. Mandarin	19%
64. Tea Tree	19%
77. Marjoram	16%
33. Tangerine	16%
94. Mountain Savory	12%
32. Lemon	10%
53. Fennel	9%

Continued on the next page . . .

30. Bergamot	8%
108. Thyme	7%
106. Garden Thyme	6%
76. Oregano	6%
9. Celery Seed	5%
71. Nutmeg	5%

Camphene

1. Silver Fir	21%
81. Spruce	21%
110. Valerian	18%
2. Balsam Fir	17%
109. Tsuga	15%
3. White Fir	11%
90. Rosemary Verbenon	8%
113. Ginger	5%
91. Sage	5%
89. Rosemary	5%
4. Yarrow	5%

Myrcene

12. Mugwort	23%
95. Goldenrod	12%
99. Blue Tansy	10%
14. Frankincense	10%
71. Nutmeg	9%
18. Marijuana	8%
17. Elemi	7%
58. Juniper	7%
106. Garden Thyme	6%
42. Lemongrass	5%

p–Cymene

108. Thyme	21%
94. Mountain Savory	14%
48. E. Dives	8%
64. Tea Tree	7%
76. Oregano	7%
99. Blue Tansy	6%
106. Garden Thyme	6%

Ocimene

10. Tarragon	18%
61. Lavandin	11%
60. Lavender	11%
9. Celery Seed	10%
53. Fennel	10%
27. Neroli	6%
38. Fleabane	5%

δ–3–Carene

2. Balsam Fir	21%
41. Cypress	17%
83. Pine	11%
52. Galbanum	9%
84. Black Pepper	8%
81. Spruce	7%

α–Terpinene

40. Cumin	17%
65. Cajuput	10%
64. Tea Tree	10%
77. Marjoram	8%
9. Celery Seed	5%
21. Roman Chamomile	5%

α–Phellandrene

48. E. Dives	24%
17. Elemi	17%
99. Blue Tansy	8%
84. Black Pepper	7%

β–Phellandrene

80. Parsley	14%
3. White Fir	14%
7. Angelica	7%

• **LIMONENE.** d–limonene has the mild scent of orange and is mainly in citrus oils while l–limonene has the scent of pine and is mainly in evergreen oils. There is animal research that suggests that limonene may be anti-tumerol and could have applications in cancer therapy.

Table Sixty-One
Most Popular Oxides in Essential Oils

20.3% of essential oils contain 5% or more of: 1,8 Cineole
5.3%   of essential oils contain 5% or more of: Caryophyllene Oxide

Table Sixty-Two
Essential Oils With The Most Popular Oxides
(In Concentrations of at Least 5%)

1,8 Cineole (Also eucalyptol)

50. Blue Mallee	90%
51. E. Radiata	67%
49. Eucalyptus	67%
65. Cajuput	60%
104. Spanish Marjoram	58%
87. Ravensara	55%
67. Niaouli	50%
89. Rosemary	47%
59. Bay Laurel	42%
72. Myrtle	38%
46. Cardamom	32%
22. White Camphor	30%
26. Lime	15%
66. Rosalina	15%
47. Lemon Eucalyptus	10%

108. Thyme	10%
91. Sage	9%
64. Tea Tree	9%
90. Rosemary Verbenon	8%
112. Vitex	7%
61. Lavandin	6%
4. Yarrow	6%
75. Basil	5%

Caryophyllene Oxide

112. Vitex	8%
18. Marijuana	7%
84. Black Pepper	6%
16. Ylang Ylang	6%
45. Carrot Seed	4%
105. Moroccan Thyme	4%

• **RESPIRATORY COMPOUNDS.** Oils containing camphor (a ketone), menthol (a phenol), and/or 1,8 cineole (an oxide) are traditionally the ones most often used for decongesting the lungs and sinuses during colds, flu, bronchitis, pneumonia, asthma, and other congestive conditions. All of these compounds are supportive of respiratory function. Consulting both Table Fifty-Six and Table Sixty, we see that white camphor oil is 45% camphor and 30% 1, 8 cineole while rosemary oil contains 18% camphor and 47% 1,8 cineole. The only major source of natural menthol is peppermint oil, which contains 34-44%. White camphor, harvested in the Orient, used to be a major source of commercial camphor, as well as 1,8 cineole, and peppermint was the only natural source of menthol in commercial quantities. Today, however, drug companies find it less expensive to produce these three compounds artificially in a laboratory to be added to the many over-the-counter products used for decongestion. (See Chapter 7 for a discussion on the differences between natural vs. synthetic menthol.)

Table Sixty-Three
Most Popular Phenols in Essential Oils

5.3% of essential oils contain 5% or more of: Terpinen–4–ol
4.4% of essential oils contain 5% or more of: Eugenol
3.5% of essential oils contain 5% or more of: Carvacrol
2.7% of essential oils contain 5% or more of: Anethole
2.7% of essential oils contain 5% or more of: Estragole
2.7% of essential oils contain 5% or more of: Thymol

Table Sixty-Four
Essential Oils With The Most Popular Phenols
(In Concentrations of at Least 5%)*

Eugenol*

97. Clove	77%
24. Cinnamon	25%
44. Citronella	7%
75. Basil	6%
59. Bay Laurel	6%
23. Cassia	4%
55. Helichrysum	2%
88. Rose	2%
16. Ylang Ylang	2%
47. Lemon Eucalyptus	1%
94. Mountain Savory	1%
37. Myrrh	1%
71. Nutmeg	1%

Terpinen–4–ol (Also β-terpinol and/or terpinen–1–ol–4)

64. Tea Tree	33%
77. Marjoram	18%
71. Nutmeg	6%
48. E. Dives	5%
107. Sweet Thyme	5%
101. Thuja	5%

Carvacrol

76. Oregano	67%
94. Mountain Savory	29%
105. Moroccan Thyme	14%
108. Thyme	6%

Anethole

82. Anise	87%
53. Fennel	60%
10. Tarragon	8%

Estragole (also methyl chavicol)

10. Tarragon	70%
75. Basil	65%
53. Fennel	6%

Thymol

108. Thyme	46%
94. Mountain Savory	19%
105. Moroccan Thyme	15%

• **EUGENOL.** Oils with less than 5% concentration are not normally included in these tables, but eugenol has unique locally anesthetizing properties that have been used via clove oil by dentists for centuries. In mixing blends or using essential oils, in general, knowledge of oils with anesthetizing properties may be useful. Hence, we include all oils with concentrations ≥ 1%

Table Sixty-Five
Most Popular Sesquiterpenes in Essential Oils

17.6%	of essential oils contain 5% or more of:	β–Caryophyllene
4.4%	of essential oils contain 5% or more of:	Germacrene-D
3.5%	of essential oils contain 5% or more of:	δ-Cadinene
3.5%	of essential oils contain 5% or more of:	Aromadrene
2.7%	of essential oils contain 5% or more of:	Chamazulene
2.7%	of essential oils contain 5% or more of:	β–Farnesene
2.7%	of essential oils contain 5% or more of:	Humulene
2.7%	of essential oils contain 5% or more of:	β–Selinine

• **SESQUITERPENES** have properties like hemoglobin in that they can carry oxygen molecules throughout the body and into the cells themselves. Sesquiterpenes can also delete faulty information in cellular memory that can cause disease, thus facilitating healing at the roots of the condition.

Chamazulene is not found in living plants. It results when matricene, a colorless natural sesquiterpene in certain plants, passes through the distillation process and is chemically altered by the heat into a a deep blue artifact we call chamazulene. Thus, chamazulene is a modified sesquiterpene. Chamazulene has desirable therapeutic properties that have been clinically studied. It is an artifact for which some essential oil producers alter their distillation techniques in order to maximize the production of chamazulene from matricene since it increases the value of the oil both financially and therapeutically. (See Chapter 9 for more on the above topics.)

• **THE UNPOPULAR ONES.** Tables Fifty through Sixty-Six deal with the most popular compounds in essential oils. You may have noticed that there are no tables for alkanes, coumarins, ethers, furanoids, lactones, diterpenes, triterpenes, or tetraterpenes in this section. That is because these are not very popular compounds. The criteria for being included was that for any specific compound there had to be at least three different oils containing it in concentrations of at least 5%. There were no compounds within these chemical classes that qualified by that standard. Only alcohols, esters, ketones, monoterpenes, oxides, phenols, and sesquiterpenes pass the popularity test, while aldehydes passed it too, but only barely. (See Tables 53-54)

• **WHAT IS A MAJOR INGREDIENT?** Except for oils containing eugenol compiled in Table 62, the oils listed in Tables 51-64 as containing specific compounds are ones that contain at least 5% of that compound. In most cases, the compounds listed are also found in many oils not listed in these tables because they occur in concentrations less than 5%. See Table Thirty-Two for complete analyses of all major ingredients. The definition of a major ingredient is any compound that comprises 1% or more of the oil.

Table Sixty-Six
Essential Oils With The Most Popular Sesquiterpenes
(In Concentrations of at Least 5%)*

β–Caryophyllene

112.	Vitex	39%
18.	Marijuana	32%
84.	Black Pepper	30%
16.	Ylang Ylang	19%
68.	Melissa	16%
61.	Lavandin	10%
97.	Clove	8%
21.	Roman Chamomile	8%
65.	Cajuput	6%
14.	Frankincense	6%
4.	Yarrow	6%
45.	Carrot Seed	5%
74.	Catnip	5%
24.	Cinnamon Bark	5%
60.	Lavender	5%
42.	Lemongrass	5%
105.	Moroccan Thyme	5%
94.	Mountain Savory	5%
91.	Sage	5%
108.	Thyme	5%

Germacrene-D

95.	Goldenrod	28%
16.	Ylang Ylang	18%
4.	Yarrow	10%
19.	Caraway	6%
78.	Ormenis	5%

δ–Cadinene

20.	Cedarwood	5%
63.	German Chamomile	5%
64.	Tea Tree	5%
3.	White Fir	5%

Aromadrene

85.	Patchouly	11%
49.	Eucalyptus	7%
66.	Rosalina	5%
64.	Tea Tree	5%

Chamazulene

4.	Yarrow	21%
63.	German Chamomile	13%
99.	Blue Tansy	10%

β–Farnesene

63.	German Chamomile	21%
113.	Ginger	19%
112.	Vitex	5%

Humulene (α-caryophyllene)

18.	Marijuana	11%
91.	Sage	5%
4.	Yarrow	5%

β–Selinene

9.	Celery Seed	8%
15.	Blue Cypress	7%
84.	Black pepper	5%

• **MORE COMPLETE ANALYSES** for the 113 essential oils listed in Tables 33–65 are given in Table Thirty-One.

Table Sixty-Seven
Representative Oils For
Various Classes of Compounds

Alcohols	Rosewood 70-95%; Palmarosa 74-90% Coriander 67-84%
Aldehydes	Cassia 75-85%; Lemongrass 55-80% Lemon Eucalyptus 40-80%
Alkanes	Rose 4-19%
Coumarins	Bitter Orange 3-9%; Lemon 1-5%
Carboxylic Acids	Onycha 14-25%; Lemon Eucalyptus 3-5%; Oregano 2-5%; Cassia 1-3%
Diterpenes	Jasmine 9-18%; White Camphor 1-4%; Cypress 1-3%
Esters	Wintergreen 95-99%; Roman Chamomile 55-75% Clary Sage 50-78%; Helichrysum 28-60%
Ethers	Anise 82-95%; Tarragon 65-85%; Fennel 52-80%; Basil 50-80%
Furanoids	Myrrh 20-27%; Fleabane 5-11%
Ketones	Cedar Bark 78-95%; Idaho Tansy 66-80%; Spearmint 51-70%; Hyssop 39-65%
Lactones	Catnip 8-18%; Celery Seed 6-16%; Bay Laurel 2-4%
Monoterpenes	Grapefruit 90-95%; Balsam Fir 75-90%; Angelica 65-95%; Frankincense 64-90%
Oxides	Blue Mallee 85-95%; German Chamomile 33-57% Ravensara 48-61%; Rosemary CT cineole 39-55%
Phenols	Wintergreen 95-99%; Anise 82-95%; Clove 70-85%; Basil 52-90%; Oregano 60-80%
Sesquiterpenes	Cedarwood 84-100%; Sandalwood 72-94%; Patchouly 70-95%; Ginger 50-90%; Myrrh 55-75%
Tetraterpenes	Tangerine 5-10%
Triterpenes	Myrrh 4-8%

Table Sixty-Eight
PMS Oils
Single Oils With Compounds in the Ranges of
10-50% Phenols + Ketones + Alcohols
10-60% Monoterpenes
3-20% Sesquiterpenes

Name of Oil	Phenol content	Ketone content	Alcohol content	All 3 P+K+A	Mono- terpenes	Sesqui- terpenes	Total PMS
64. Tea Tree	32%	0	5%	37%	52%	17%	100%
78. Ormenis	0	1%	44%	45%	44%	4%	93%
48. E. Dives	4%	42%	2%	49%	38%	3%	92%
77. Marjoram	17%	0	20%	37%	44%	4%	85%
56. Hyssop	3%	42%	2%	47%	30%	8%	85%
99. Blue Tansy	0	14%	0	14%	59%	9%	73%
The Average Oil *	**8%**	**9%**	**14%**	**31%**	**30%**	**12%**	**73%**
66. Rosalina	0	0	44%	44%	22%	6%	72%
60. Lavender	0	2%	44%	46%	16%	6%	68%
21. Rom. Cham.	0	12%	5%	17%	26%	12%	65%
55. Helichrysum	2%	19%	6%	27%	11%	15%	53%
67. Niaouli	0	0	13%	13%	21%	18%	52%
59. Bay Laurel	6%	0	22%	28%	20%	3%	51%
104. Sp. Marjrm.	3%	2%	25%	30%	15%	4%	49%

* The composition of an "Average Essential Oil" is detailed in Table Thirty-Two-A. There is a blend of approximately 100 essential oils sold by Young Living, Inc. whose composition closely approximates the proportions of an Average Essential Oil. It is called Legacy®. As you can see above, The Average Essential Oilt is also an ideal "PMS Oil." Notice that while the Average Essential Oil contains balanced portions of the components of PMS, it also contains 27% other compounds such as esters, oxides, aldehydes, and ethers. While the single oils listed above can each serve as a PMS anointing oil by themselves, it is usually best to combine several oils to obtain a better PMS balance than that offered by any single oil. See Chapter Nine for more on PMS.

> Numbers preceeding the names of oils
> refer to listings in Table Thirty-Two

Table Sixty-Nine
Principal Essential Oil Compounds
in Alphabetical Order

Principal = occurs in concentrations of 5% or more in at least one oil
Tables are given only for compounds ≥ 5% found in at least three oils.
Compounds with no table given are unusual—found in only 1 or 2 oils.

• When using this Table, Also Check Table 70. Some Compounds are in Both •

Compound	Category	Table	Signature Oil*
α-Alantone	Sesquiterpenone		20. Cedarwood 13%
γ-Alantone	Sesquiterpenone		20. Cedarwood 9%
Allyl Angelate	Ester		21. Roman Chamomile 8%
Amyl Butyrate	Ester		21. Roman Chamomile 14%
Anethole	Phenol	64	82. Anise 87%
Aromadrene	Sesquiterpene	66	85. Patchouly 11%
Aristoladiene	Sesquiterpene		73. Spikenard 5%
Aristolenone	Ketone		73. Spikenard 7%
β-Asarone	Phenolic Ketone		5. Calamus 12-20%
Benzoic Acid	Carboxylic Acid		96. Onycha 15%
Benzyl Acetate	Ester		57. Jasmine 24%
Benzyl Acetate	Ester		16. Ylang Ylang 12%
Benzyl Benzoate	Ester		57. Jasmine 18%
Benzyl Benzoate	Ester		16. Ylang Ylang 8%
α-Bergamotene	Furanoid		38. Fleabane 8%
Bicyclovetinerol	Sesquiterpenol		111. Vetiver 12%
β-Bisabolene	Sesquiterpene		45. Carrot Seed 9%
γ-Bisabolene	Sesquiterpene		113. Ginger 6%
Bisabolol Oxide–A	Oxide		63. German Chamomile 28%
Bisabolol Oxide–B	Oxide		63. German Chamomile 8%
Bisabolone Oxide	Oxide		63. German Chamomile 12%
Borneol	Alcohol	52	105. Moroccan Thyme 39%
Bornyl Acetate	Ester	56	81. Spruce 33%
α-Bulnesene	Sesquiterpene		85. Patchouly 15%
β-Bulnesene	Sesquiterpene		85. Patchouly 12%
Bulnesol	Sesquiterpenol		15. Blue Cypress 10%
Butylphthalide	Lactone		9. Celery Seed 8%
δ-Cadinene	Sesquiterpene	66	20. Cedarwood 5%
Cajuputol	(See 1,8 Cineole)		
Calamuscenone	Ketone		5. Calamus 9%
Calarene	Monoterpene		73. Spikenard 24%
Camphene	Monoterpene	60	1. Silver Fir 21%

* The Signature Oil for a compound is the essential oil containing more of that particular compound than any other oil. See the designated Table for a complete list of oils containing 5% or more of that particular compound.

Compound	Category	Table	Signature Oil
Camphor	Ketone	58	22. White Camphor 45%
Carotol	Alcohol		45. Carrot Seed 43%
Cedrol	Sesquiterpenol		41. Cypress 10%
α-Copaene	Sesquiterpene		37. Myrrh 11%
δ-3-Carene	Monoterpene	60	21. Balsam Fir 21%
Carvacrol	Phenol	64	76. Oregano 67%
Carvacrol Methyl Ether	Phenol		94. Mountain Savory 6%
Carvene	Monoterpene		19. Caraway 25%
Carveol	Alcohol		19. Caraway 6%
d-Carvone	Ketone		6. Dill 38%
l–Carvone	Ketone		70. Spearmint 52%
Carvyl Acetate	Ester		9. Celery Seed 11%
α-Caryophyllene	(See Humulene)		
β-Caryophyllene	Sesquiterpene	66	112. Vitex 39%
Caryophyllene Oxide	Oxide	62	112. Vitex 8%
Chamazulene	Sesquiterpene	66	4. Yarrow 21%
Cinnamic Acid	Carboxylic Acid		96. Onycha 7%
Cinnamyl Acetate	Ester		23. Cassia 5%
1,8 Cineole	Oxide	62	50. Blue Mallee 90%
Citral	Aldehyde		77. Marjoram 5%
Citronellal	Aldehyde	54	31. Cambava 75%
Citronellol	Alcohol	52	88. Rose 37%
Citronellyl Acetate	Ester		47. Lemon Eucalyptus 6%
Citronellyl Formate	Ester		79. Geranium 12%
Coriandrol	Alcohol		39. Coriander 20%
Coniferyl Benzoate	Ester		96. Onycha 65%
Coumarin	Coumarin		23. Cassia 7%
Cuminal	Aldehyde		40. Cumin 19%
α-Curcumene	Sesquiterpene		113. Ginger 22%
γ-Curcumene	Sesquiterpene		55. Helichrysum 13%
Curzenone	Ketone		37. Myrrh 10%
p-Cymene	Monoterpene	60	108. Thyme 21%
Davanone	Ketone		11. Davana 30%
Decanol	Aldehyde		19. Caraway 7%
Dihydrocarvone	Ketone		70. Spearmint 8%
Dill Ether	Ether		6. Dill 10%
β-Elemene	Sesquiterpene		15. Blue Cypress 8%
β-Elemene	Sesquiterpene		37. Myrrh 7%
δ-Elemene	Sesquiterpene		37. Myrrh 24%
Elemol	Sesquiterpenol		17. Elemi 15%
Estragole	Phenol	64	10. Tarragon 70%
Eucalyptol	(See 1,8 Cineole)		
α-Eudesmol	Sesquiterpenol		15. Blue Cypress 18%
β-Eudesmol	Sesquiterpenol		15. Blue Cypress 7%
Eugenol	Phenol	64	97. Clove 77%
Eugenyl Acetate	Ester		97. Clove 12%

Compound	Category	Table	Signature Oil
α-Farnesene	Sesquiterpene		16. Ylang Ylang 10%
α-Farnesene	Sesquiterpene		63. German Chamomile 8%
β-Farnesene	Sesquiterpene	66	63. German Chamomile 21%
Farnesol	Sesquiterpenol		42. Lemongrass 12%
α-Fenchene	Monoterpene		110 Valerian 11%
Fenchone	Ketone	58	11. Thuja 11%
Fenchone	Ketone		103. Cedar Leaf 5%
Furoendesmadiene	Furanoid		37. Myrrh 6%
Geranial	Aldehyde	54	42. Lemongrass 37%
Geraniol	Alcohol	52	43. Palmarosa 77%
Geranyl Acetate	Ester	56	43. Palmarosa 8%
Geranyl Formate	Ester		43. Palmarosa 10%
Germacrene–B	Sesquiterpene		112. Vitex 8%
Germacrene–D	Sesquiterpene	66	95. Goldenrod 28%
Globulol	Sesquiterpenol		49. Eucalyptus 6%
Guaidene	Sesquiterpene		79. Geranium 6%
α-Guaiene	Sesquiterpene		85. Patchouly 10%
Guaiol	Sesquiterpenol		15. Blue Cypress 18%
β-Gurjunene	Sesquiterpene		73. Spikenard 27%
α-Himachalene	Sesquiterpene		20. Cedarwood 11%
β-Himachalene	Sesquiterpene		20. Cedarwood 45%
γ-Himachalene	Sesquiterpene		20. Cedarwood 13%
Humulene	Sesquiterpene	66	18. Marijuana 11%
β-Ionene	Monoterpene		73. Spikenard 6%
Isoartemisia ketone	Ketone		4. Yarrow 9%
Isoasarol	Phenol		5. Calamus 14%
Isoamyl Methacylate	Ester		21. Roman Chamomile 20%
Isobutyl Angelate	Ester		21. Roman Chamomile 20%
Isobutyl Butyrate	Ester		21. Roman Chamomile 6%
Isocalamendial	Aldehyde		5. Calamus 7%
Isoeugenol	Phenol		44. Citronella 7%
Isomenthone	Ketone		79. Geranium 6%
Isophytol	Diterpenol		57. Jasmine 5%
Isopinocamphone	Ketone		56. Hyssop 42%
Isopulegol	Phenol		47. Lemon Eucalyptus 11%
Isovalencenol	Sesquiterpenol		111. Vetiver 13%
Italidione	Ketone		55. Helichrysum 18%
Khusenol	Sesquiterpenol		111. Vetiver 9%
d-Limonene	Monoterpene	60	34. Grapefruit 89%
l-Limonene	Monoterpene	60	38. Fleabane 67%
Linalol	Alcohol	52	8. Rosewood 82%
Linalyl Acetate	Ester	56	29. Petitgrain 50%
Lindestrene	Sesquiterpene		37. Myrrh 25%
β-Maalene	Sesquiterpene		73. Spikenard 7%
p-Menthadienal	Aldehyde		40. Cumin 30%
p-Menthadiene-8-ol	Sesquiterpenol		62. Ledum 15%

Compound	Category	Table	Signature Oil
p-Menthatriene	Monoterpene		80. Parsley 39%
p-Menthatriene	Monoterpene		62. Ledum 12%
Menthofuran	Furanoid		69. Peppermint 6%
Menthol	Phenol		69. Peppermint 39%
Menthone	Ketone		69. Peppermint 16%
Methoxycinnamaldehyde	Aldehyde		23. Cassia 9%
Methoxyfurogermacrene	Furanoid		37. Myrrh 7%
Methyl Acetate	Ester		69. Peppermint 7%
Methyl Anthranilate	Ester		27. Neroli 6%
Methyl Benzoate	Ester		16. Ylang Ylang 5%
Methyl Chavicol	(See Estragole)		
Methyl Ether	Phenol		44. Citronella 10%
Methyl Isoeugenol	Phenol		44. Citronella 7%
Methylisobutyl Ketone	Ketone		37. Myrrh 5%
Methyl Paracresol	Phenol		16. Ylang Ylang 7%
Methyl Salicylate	Ester	56	59. Wintergreen 97%
Myrcene	Monoterpene	60	12. Mugwort 23%
Myristicin	Phenol		80. Parsley 11%
Myristicin	Phenol		71. Nutmeg 9%
Myrtenyl Acetate	Ester		72. Myrtle 7%
Nepetalactone	Lactone		74. Catnip 13%
Neral	Aldehyde		42. Lemongrass 25%
Neral	Aldehyde		68. Melissa 23%
Nerol	Alcohol		74. Catnip 16%
Nerol	Alcohol		88. Rose 8%
Nerolidol	Sesquiterpinol		113. Ginger 5%
Nonadecane	Alkane		88. Rose 9%
Nonanol	Alcohol		113. Ginger 5%
Nordavanone	Ketone		11. Davana 6%
Neryl Acetate	Ester		55. Helicrysum 38%
Neryl Propionate	Ester		55. Helicrysum 6%
Ocimene	Monoterpene	60	10. Tarragon 18%
Ocimenone	Ketone		98. Marigold 23%
Octanal	Aldehyde		19. Caraway 12%
Paracresol Ether	Phenol		16. Ylang Ylang 13%
Patchoulol	Sesquiterpenol		85. Patchouly 30%
Patchoulol	Sesquiterpenol		73. Spikenard 6%
Piperitone	Ketone		48. E. Dives 43%
α-Phellandrene	Monoterpene	60	48. E. Dives 24%
β-Phellandrene	Monoterpene	60	80. Parsley 14%
Phytol	Diterpenol		57. Jasmine 9%
α-Pinene	Monoterpene	60	41. Cypress 51%
β-Pinene	Monoterpene	60	57. Galbanum 55%
Pinocamphone	Ketone		56. Hyssop 11%
Pinocarveol	Alcohol		21. Roman Chamomile 5%
Pinocarveol	Alcohol		25. Cistus 5%

Compound	Category	Table	Signature Oil
Pinocarvone	Ketone		21. Roman Chamomile 13%
Safrole	Ether		22. White Camphor 10%
Sabinene	Monoterpene	60	4. Yarrow 25%
α-Santalene	Sesquiterpene		93. Sandalwood 6%
Santalina Alcohol	Alcohol		78. Ormenis 32%
α-Santalol	Sesquiterpenol		93. Sandalwood 51%
β-Santalol	Sesquiterpenol		93. Sandalwood 22%
Sclareol	Diterpenol		92. Clary Sage 5%
Seychellene	Sesquitepene		85. Patchouly 9%
β-Selinene	Sesquiterpene	66	9. Celery Seed 8%
β-Sesquiphellandrene	Sesquiterpene		113. Ginger 6%
Shyobunone	Ketone		5. Calamus 28%
Spiro Ether	Ether		63. German Chamomile 6%
Squalene	Triterpene		57. Jasmine 5%
Stearoptene	Monoterpene		88. Rose 19%
Tagetone	Ketone		98. Marigold 45%
α-Terpinene	Monoterpene	60	40. Cumin 17%
γ-Terpinene	Monoterpene	60	40. Cumin 22%
Terpinen-1-ol-4	(See Terpinen-4-ol)		
Terpinen-4-ol	Phenol	64	64. Tea Tree 33%
α-Terpineol	Alcohol	52	47. Lemon Eucalyptus 17%
β-Terpinol	(See Terpinen-4-ol)		
α-Terpinyl Acetate	Ester	56	46. Cardamom 46%
α-Thujone	Ketone	58	102. Cedar Bark 77%
Thujanol	Alcohol		107. Thyme Thujanol 50%
Thujanol	Alcohol		77. Marjoram 8%
β-Thujone	Ketone	58	100. Idaho Tansy 67%
Thymol	Phenol	64	108. Thyme 46%
Transcinnamaldehyde	Aldehyde		23. Cassia 78%
Transcinnamaldehyde	Aldehyde		24. Cinnamon 45%
Tricyclene	Sesquiterpene		109. Tsuga 6%
Verbenone	Ketone		90. Rosemary Verbenon 26%
Viridiflorol	Sesquiterpenol		67. Niaouli 11%
Viridiflorol	Sesquiterpenol		90. Rosemary Verbenon 6%
Zingiberene	Sesquiterpene		113. Ginger 31%

**END OF
Table Sixty-Nine
Principal Essential Oil Compounds in Alphabetical Order**

Principal means it occurs in concentrations of 5% or more in at least one oil.
Tables are given only for compounds ≥ 5% found in at least three oils.
Compounds with no table given are rare or unusual and are
found in only 1 or 2 oils in concentrations of 5% or more.
Also Check Table 70. Some Compounds are in both Tables.

Table Seventy
Minor, Trace, & Low Concentrate Compounds (≤ 5%)
of Essential Oils in Alphabetical Order
• When using this Table, Also Check Table 69. Some Compounds are in Both •

Compound	Category	Essential Oils	%
Abienol	Diterpenol	41. Cypress	0-1%
Acetic Acid	Carboxylic Acid	37. Myrrh	0-1%
Acetone	Ketone	113. Ginger	0-1%
Acetophenone	Ketone	25. Cistus	1-3%
Acetophenone	Ketone	84. Black Pepper	0-1%
Achillin	Lactone	4. Yarrow	1-2%
Actinidine	Lactone	110. Valerian	0-1%
Aesculetine	Furanocoumarin	34. Grapefruit	0-1%
Aesculetine	Furanocoumarin	68. Melissa	0-1%
Aesculetine	Furanocoumarin	69. Peppermint	0-1%
Agarofurane	Furanocoumarin	52. Galbanum	0-1%
α- Amyrin	Triterpene	37. Myrrh	2-4%
α- Amyrenone	Triterpene	37. Myrrh	2-3%
Angelic Acid	Carboxylic Acid	7. Angelica	0-1%
Angelic Acid	Carboxylic Acid	21. Roman Chamomile	0-1%
Angelica Lactone	Furanoid	7. Angelica	0-1%
Angelicine	Furanoid	7. Angelica	0-1%
Anise Ketone	Ketone	82. Anise	0-1%
Anisicaldehyde	Aldehyde	82. Anise	1-2%

Major, Minor & Trace Compounds in Essential Oils

By definition, any compound comprising 1% or more of an oil is considered major. Minor essential oil compounds are those that occur in concentrations from 0.1% to 1.0 %. Trace compounds occur in the range of 0 to 0.1%. In this table we have tabulated essential oil compounds for which data are available that occur in the range of 0–5%, which includes trace, minor, and some of the less prevalent major compounds. These constituents (i.e. those that occur in the range of 0-5%) are called "Low Concentrate" compounds in essential oils. Most of the thousands of compounds found in essential oils are trace, minor, or low concentrate components. You will note in this table that some compounds are common to many oils, but occur only in small concentrations (i.e. rarely more than 5%, if ever). For example, Terpinolene is found in many oils, but almost never in concentrations greater than 5%. Some compounds are listed in both Tables 69 and 70. Both Tables should be used together when searching for specific compounds and oils that contain them.

Compound	Category	Essential Oils	%
Anisol	Alcohol	82. Anise	0-1%
p-Anol	Phenol	82. Anise	2-4%
p-Anol	Phenol	53. Fennel	1-3%
Apiole	Phenol	80. Parsley	1-4%
Aristolene	Sesquiterpene	73. Spikenard	4-5%
Artemarin	Lactone	100. Idaho Tansy	0-1%
Artemisia Alcohol	Alcohol	78. Ormenis	2-3%
Artemisia Ketone	Ketone	100. Idaho Tansy	0-1%
Artemidin	Coumarin	10. Tarragon	0-1%
Artemorine	Lactone	59. Bay Laurel	0-1%
Artenone	Ketone	11. Davana	2-5%
α-Asarone	Phenolic Ketone	5. Calamus	2-4%
β-Asarone	Phenolic Ketone	45. Carrot Seed	1-2%
Ascorbic Acid	Carboxylic Acid	13. Birch	0-1%
Auraptene	Furanoid	28. Bitter Orange	0-1%
Auraptene	Furanoid	34. Grapefruit	0-1%
Auraptene	Furanoid	36. Orange	0-1%
Auraptenol	Furanoid	28. Bitter Orange	0-1%
Australol	Phenol	See p-cuminol	
Benzoic Acid	Carboxylic Acid	111. Vetiver	0-1%
Benzoicaldehyde	Aldehyde	86. Douglas Fir	1-2%
Benzoicaldehyde	Aldehyde	67. Niaouli	0-1%
Benzoresinol	Alcohol	96. Onycha	0-1%
Benzyl Acetate	Ester	23. Cassia	0-1%
Benzyl Acetate	Ester	35. Mandarin	0-1%
Benzyl Alcohol	Phenol	23. Cassia	0-1%
Benzyl Alcohol	Phenol	27. Neroli	0-1%
Benzylaldehyde	Aldehyde	23. Cassia	3-4%
Benzylaldehyde	Aldehyde	25. Cistus	2-3%
Benzylaldehyde	Aldehyde	24. Cinnamon	0-1%
Benzylaldehyde	Aldehyde	60. Lavender	0-1%
Benzylaldehyde	Aldehyde	27. Neroli	0-1%
α-Bergamotene	Furanoid	37. Myrrh	4-5%
α-Bergamotene	Furanoid	30. Bergamot	0-1%
α-Bergamotene	Furanoid	84. Black Pepper	0-1%
α-Bergamotene	Furanoid	32. Lemon	0-1%
Bergamottin	Furanoid	32. Lemon	0-1%
Bergaptene	Furanoid	30. Bergamot	1-2%
Bergaptene	Furanoid	28. Bitter Orange	1-2%
Bergaptene	Furanoid	7. Angelica	0-1%
Bergaptene	Furanoid	9. Celery Seed	0-1%
Bergaptene	Furanoid	39. Coriander	0-1%

Compound	Category	Essential Oils	%
Bergaptene	Furanoid	32. Lemon	0-1%
Bergaptene	Furanoid	29. Petitgrain	0-1%
Bergaptole	Furanoid	30. Bergamot	0-1%
Bergaptole	Furanoid	28. Bitter Orange	0-1%
Bergaptole	Furanoid	34. Grapefruit	0-1%
Bergaptole	Furanoid	32. Lemon	0-1%
Bergaptole	Furanoid	36. Orange	0-1%
Betula Saponin	Triterpene	13. Birch	1-2%
α-Bisabolene	Sesquiterpene	63. German Chamomile	2-5%
α-Bisabolene	Sesquiterpene	78. Ormenis	2-3%
β-Bisabolene	Sesquiterpene	84. Black Pepper	2-5%
β-Bisabolene	Sesquiterpene	32. Lemon	2-4%
β-Bisabolene	Sesquiterpene	30. Bergamot	1-2%
β-Bisabolene	Sesquiterpene	76. Oregano	1-2%
β-Bisabolene	Sesquiterpene	113. Ginger	0-1%
α-Bisabolol	Sesquiterpenol	63. German Chamomile	2-7%
β-Bisabolol	Sesquiterpenol	113. Ginger	0-1%
Bornyl Acetate	Ester	56. Hyssop	0-1%
Bornyl Benzoate	Ester	95. Goldenrod	0-1%
Bornyl Butanoate	Ester	78. Ormenis	1-2%
Bornyl Butyrate	Ester	62. Ledum	0-1%
Bornyl Butyrate	Ester	110. Valerian	0-1%
Bornyl Coproate	Ester	86. Douglas Fir	1-3%
Bornyl Formate	Ester	110. Valerian	0-1%
Bornyl Isovalerate	Ester	110. Valerian	0-1%
β-Bourbonene	Sesquiterpene	37. Myrrh	4-5%
β-Bourbonene	Sesquiterpene	68. Melissa	1-2%
β-Bourbonene	Sesquiterpene	92. Clary Sage	0-1%
β-Bourbonene	Sesquiterpene	69. Peppermint	0-1%
β-Bourbonene	Sesquiterpene	104. Spanish Marjoram	0-1%
β-Bourbonene	Sesquiterpene	70. Spearmint	0-1%
ζ-Bulgarene	Sesquiterpene	69. Peppermint	0-1%
Butanolide	Coumarin	60. Lavender	0-1%
Bulnesene Oxide	Oxide	85. Patchouly	3-4%
Bulnesol	Sesquiterpenol	52. Galbanum	0-1%
Bulnesol	Sesquiterpenol	85. Patchouly	0-1%
Butanol	Alcohol	113. Ginger	0-1%
Butyl Tiglate	Ester	21. Roman Chamomile	1-3%
Butyricaldehyde	Aldehyde	49. Eucalyptus	0-1%
α-Cadinene	Sesquiterpene	91. Sage	0-1%
β-Cadinene	Sesquiterpene	111. Vetiver	0-1%
δ-Cadinene	Sesquiterpene	68. Melissa	0-1%
δ-Cadinene	Sesquiterpene	69. Peppermint	0-1%

Compound	Category	Essential Oils	%
γ-Cadinene	Sesquiterpene	83. Pine	1-5%
α-Cadinol	Sesquiterpenol	4. Yarrow	1-2%
α-Cadinol	Sesquiterpenol	68. Melissa	0-1%
α-Cadinol	Sesquiterpenol	83. Pine	0-1%
α-Cadinol	Sesquiterpenol	70. Spearmint	0-1%
Calamene	Sesquiterpene	97. Clove	0-1%
Calarenol	Sesquiterpenol	73. Spikenard	0-1%
Campholenic Acid	Carboxylic Acid	25. Cistus	0-1%
Campholenaldehyde	Aldehyde	25. Cistus	1-2%
Camphonelicaldehyde	Aldehyde	105. Moroccan Thyme	0-1%
α-Camphorene	Diterpene	22. White Camphor	1-2%
β-Camphorene	Diterpene	22. White Camphor	0-1%
Cannabinol	Triterpenol	18. Marijuana	1-2%
Caproicaldehyde	Aldehyde	49. Eucalyptus	0-1%
α-Carotene	Tetraterpene	45. Carrot Seed	0-1%
β-Carotene	Tetraterpene	28. Bitter Orange	3-6%
β-Carotene	Tetraterpene	35. Mandarin	3-6%
β-Carotene	Tetraterpene	36. Orange	3-6%
β-Carotene	Tetraterpene	33. Tangerine	3-6%
β-Carotene	Tetraterpene	30. Bergamot	2-5%
β-Carotene	Tetraterpene	34. Grapefruit	1-5%
β-Carotene	Tetraterpene	32. Lemon	1-3%
β-Carotene	Tetraterpene	45. Carrot Seed	0-1%
γ-Carotene	Tetraterpene	45. Carrot Seed	0-1%
ζ-Carotene	Tetraterpene	45. Carrot Seed	0-1%
Carotol	Alcohol	80. Parsley	1-2%
Carvatoacetone	Ketone	113. Ginger	0-1%
Carveol	Alcohol	70. Spearmint	2-3%
Carveol	Alcohol	36. Orange	1-2%
d-Carvone	Ketone	49. Eucalyptus	0-1%
d-Carvone	Ketone	36. Orange	0-1%
d-Carvone	Ketone	76. Oregano	0-1%
d-Carvone	Ketone	89. Rosemary	0-1%
l-Carvone	Ketone	36. Orange	1-2%
Carvyl Acetate	Ester	70. Spearmint	3-4%
Carvyl Acetate	Ester	72. Myrtle	0-1%
Cembrene	Diterpene	83. Pine	0-2%
Chavicol	Phenol	23. Cassia	0-1%
Chlorogenic Acid	Carboxylic Acid	9. Celery Seed	0-1%
Chlorogenic Acid	Carboxylic Acid	13. Birch	0-1%
Chlorogenic Acid	Carboxylic Acid	110. Valerian	0-1%
Chrysanthemine	Lactone	100. Idaho Tansy	0-1%
Chrysanthenol	Alcohol	100. Idaho Tansy	0-1%
Chrysanthenyl Acetate	Ester	100. Idaho Tansy	0-1%

Compound	Category	Essential Oils	%
1,4 Cineole	Oxide	64. Tea Tree	2-3%
1,4 Cineole	Oxide	65. Cajuput	1-2%
1,4 Cineole	Oxide	26. Lime	1-2%
1,4 Cineole	Oxide	67. Niaouli	0-1%
1,4 Cineole	Oxide	66. Rosalina	0-1%
Cinnamic Alcohol	Alcohol	23. Cassia	2-3%
Cinnamic Alcohol	Alcohol	24. Cinnamon	1-2%
Cinnamic Acid	Carboxylic Acid	23. Cassia	1-2%
Cinnamic Acid	Carboxylic Acid	24. Cinnamon	1-2%
Cinnamaldehyde	Aldehyde	37. Myrrh	0-1%
Cinnamyl Benzoate	Ester	96. Onycha	3-5%
Cinnamyl Cinnamoate	Ester	96. Onycha	1-2%
Citral	Aldehyde	32. Lemon	1-3%
Citral	Aldehyde	26. Lime	1-2%
Citral	Aldehyde	36. Orange	1-2%
Citral	Aldehyde	86. Douglas Fir	0-1%
Citral	Aldehyde	34. Grapefruit	0-1%
Citral	Aldehyde	33. Tangerine	0-1%
Citric Acid	Carboxylic Acid	7. Angelica	0-1%
Citronellal	Aldehyde	68. Melissa	1-3%
Citronellal	Aldehyde	28. Bitter Orange	1-2%
Citronellal	Aldehyde	51. E. Radiata	1-2%
Citronellal	Aldehyde	32. Lemon	1-2%
Citronellal	Aldehyde	26. Lime	1-2%
Citronellal	Aldehyde	79. Geranium	0-1%
Citronellal	Aldehyde	113. Ginger	0-1%
Citronellal	Aldehyde	34. Grapefruit	0-1%
Citronellal	Aldehyde	36. Orange	0-1%
Citronellal	Aldehyde	83. Pine	0-1%
Citronellic Acid	Carboxylic Acid	47. Lemon Eucalyptus	3-5%
Citronellyl Acetate	Ester	28. Bitter Orange	0-1%
Citronellyl Acetate	Ester	68. Melissa	0-1%
Citronellyl Acetate	Ester	36. Orange	0-1%
Citronellyl Acetate	Ester	88. Rose	0-1%
Citronellyl Butyrate	Ester	79. Geranium	1-2%
Citronellyl Butyrate	Ester	47. Lemon Eucalyptus	0-1%
Citronellyl Citronellate	Ester	47. Lemon Eucalyptus	0-1%
Citronellyl Propionate	Ester	79. Geranium	1-3%
Citronellyl Tiglate	Ester	79. Geranium	1-2%
Citroptene	Furanoid	32. Lemon	0-1%
Citroptene	Furanoid	29. Petitgrain	0-1%
Citrotene	Furanoid	28. Bitter Orange	0-1%

Compound	Category	Essential Oils	%
α-Copaene	Sesquiterpene	8. Rosewood	1-3%
α-Copaene	Sesquiterpene	84. Black Pepper	0-2%
α-Copaene	Sesquiterpene	28. Bitter Orange	0-1%
α-Copaene	Sesquiterpene	92. Clary Sage	0-1%
α-Copaene	Sesquiterpene	97. Clove	0-1%
α-Copaene	Sesquiterpene	14. Frankincense	0-1%
α-Copaene	Sesquiterpene	79. Geranium	0-1%
α-Copaene	Sesquiterpene	68. Melissa	0-1%
α-Copaene	Sesquiterpene	105. Moroccan Thyme	0-1%
α-Copaene	Sesquiterpene	104. Spanish Marjoram	0-1%
β-Copaene	Sesquiterpene	21. Roman Chamomile	1-2%
β-Copaene	Sesquiterpene	91. Sage	0-1%
Costunolide	Lactone	59. Bay Laurel	1-2%
Coumarin	Coumarin	73. Spikenard	1-2%
Coumarin	Coumarin	98. Marigold	0-2%
Coumarin	Coumarin	28. Bitter Orange	0-1%
Coumarin	Coumarin	24. Cinnamon	0-1%
Coumarin	Coumarin	92. Clary Sage	0-1%
Coumarin	Coumarin	60. Lavandin	0-1%
Coumarin	Coumarin	60. Lavender	0-1%
Crataegolic Acid	Carboxylic Acid	97. Clove	0-1%
Cresol	Phenol	37. Myrrh	0-1%
Crispolid	Lactone	100. Idaho Tansy	0-1%
Cryptone	Ketone	50. Blue Mallee	1-2%
Cryptone	Ketone	113. Ginger	0-1%
α-Cubebene	Sesquiterpene	97. Clove	0-1%
α-Cubebene	Sesquiterpene	48. E. Dives	0-1%
β-Cubebene	Sesquiterpene	84. Black Pepper	0-2%
β-Cubebene	Sesquiterpene	47. Lemon Eucalyptus	0-1%
Cuminal	Aldehyde	19. Caraway	1-2%
Cuminal	Aldehyde	50. Blue Mallee	0-1%
Cuminal	Aldehyde	23. Cassia	0-1%
Cuminal	Aldehyde	24. Cinnamon	0-1%
Cuminal	Aldehyde	60. Lavender	0-1%
Cuminal	Aldehyde	37. Myrrh	0-1%
p-Cuminol	Phenol	40. Cumin	1-4%
p-Cuminol	Phenol	49. Eucalyptus	1-2%
p-Cuminol	Phenol	30. Bergamot	0-1%
p-Cuminol	Phenol	50. Blue Mallee	0-1%
p-Cuminol	Phenol	51. E. Radiata	0-1%
p-Cuminol	Phenol	47. Lemon Eucalyptus	0-1%
Cuminyl Alcohol	Alcohol	19. Caraway	0-1%
Cupressic Acid	Diterpene Acid	41. Cypress	0-1%

Compound	Category	Essential Oils	%
β-Curcumene	Sesquiterpene	92. Clary Sage	0-1%
β-Curcumene	Sesquiterpene	113. Ginger	0-1%
Curzerene	Sesquiterpene	37. Myrrh	0-1%
α-Cyclocitral	Aldehyde	68. Melissa	0-1%
Cyclohexanone	Ketone	25. Cistus	2-3%
Damascenone	Ketone	94. Mountain Savory	0-1%
Daucene	Sesquiterpene	45. Carrot Seed	2-3%
Daucol	Alcohol	45. Carrot Seed	3-4%
Davana Ether	Ether	11. Davana	1-6%
Davana Furan	Furanoid	11. Davana	2-4%
Davanone	Ketone	100. Idaho Tansy	0-1%
Decanal	Aldehyde	36. Orange	1-2%
Decanal	Aldehyde	28. Bitter Orange	0-1%
Decanal	Aldehyde	34. Grapefruit	0-1%
Decanal	Aldehyde	26. Lime	0-1%
Decanal	Aldehyde	35. Mandarin	0-1%
Decanal	Aldehyde	72. Myrtle	0-1%
Decanal	Aldehyde	27. Neroli	0-1%
Decanal	Aldehyde	29. Petitgrain	0-1%
Decanol	Alcohol	32. Lemon	0-1%
Deodarone	Sesquiterpenone	20. Cedarwood	1-2%
Dicyclo Ether	Ether	63. German Chamomile	1-2%
Dihydroazulene	Sesquiterpene	73. Spikenard	0-1%
Dihydrocarvone	Ketone	105. Moroccan Thyme	1-2%
β-Diketone	Ketone	55. Helichrysum	1-2%
Dipentene	Monoterpene	109. Tsuga	2-4%
Dipentene	Monoterpene	17. Elemi	1-2%
Docosane	Alkane	88. Rose	0-1%
Dodecanal	Aldehyde	28. Bitter Orange	0-1%
Dodecanal	Aldehyde	36. Orange	0-1%
Dodecane	Alkane	113. Ginger	0-1%
Eicosane	Alkane	88. Rose	0-1%
α-Elemene	Sesquiterpene	84. Black Pepper	0-2%
α-Elemene	Sesquiterpene	47. Lemon Eucalyptus	0-1%
α-Elemene	Sesquiterpene	70. Spearmint	0-1%
β-Elemene	Sesquiterpene	113. Ginger	1-2%
β-Elemene	Sesquiterpene	84. Black Pepper	0-2%
β-Elemene	Sesquiterpene	59. Bay Laurel	0-1%
β-Elemene	Sesquiterpene	68. Melissa	0-1%
β-Elemene	Sesquiterpene	69. Peppermint	0-1%
γ-Elemene	Sesquiterpene	37. Myrrh	2-5%
γ-Elemene	Sesquiterpene	48. E. Dives	0-1%

Compound	Category	Essential Oils	%
δ-Elemene	Sesquiterpene	17. Elemi	1-4%
δ-Elemene	Sesquiterpene	84. Black Pepper	2-3%
δ-Elemene	Sesquiterpene	78. Ormenis	0-1%
Elemicin	Ether	17. Elemi	1-7%
Elemicin	Ether	71. Nutmeg	1-3%
Elemol	Sesquiterpenol	113. Elemol	1-2%
Elemol	Sesquiterpenol	43. Palmarosa	1-2%
Elemol	Sesquiterpenol	56. Hyssop	0-2%
Elemol	Sesquiterpenol	68. Melissa	0-1%
Elemol	Sesquiterpenol	70. Spearmint	0-1%
Esculetin	Coumarin	98. Marigold	0-1%
Ethyl Campholenate	Ester	25. Cistus	0-1%
Ethylgaiacol	Phenol	23. Cassia	1-2%
α-Eudesmol	Sesquiterpenol	101. Thuja	1-2%
β-Eudesmol	Sesquiterpenol	113. Ginger	0-1%
γ-Eudesmol	Sesquiterpenol	79. Geranium	0-1%
α-Farnescene	Sesquiterpene	110. Valerian	0-1%
χ-Farnescene	Sesquiterpene	60. Lavender	1-2%
Farnesal	Aldehyde	42. Lemongrass	1-3%
Farnesol	Sesquiterpenol	21. Roman Chamomile	2-4%
Farnesol	Sesquiterpenol	79. Geranium	1-3%
Farnesol	Sesquiterpenol	63. German Chamomile	1-3%
Farnesol	Sesquiterpenol	27. Neroli	1-2%
Farnesol	Sesquiterpenol	16. Ylang Ylang	1-2%
Farnesol	Sesquiterpenol	88. Rose	0-2%
Farnesol	Sesquiterpenol	14. Frankincense	0-1%
Farnesol	Sesquiterpenol	70. Spearmint	0-1%
Farnesyl Acetate	Ester	16. Ylang Ylang	1-7%
Farnesylacetone	Ketone	68. Melissa	0-1%
α-Fenchol	Alcohol	53. Fennel	2-3%
α-Fenchol	Alcohol	49. Eucalyptus	1-2%
α-Fenchol	Alcohol	75. Basil	0-1%
α-Fenchol	Alcohol	26. Lime	0-1%
Fenchone	Ketone	102. Cedar Bark	2-3%
Fenchone	Ketone	49. Eucalyptus	0-1%
Fenchyl Acetate	Ester	75. Basil	0-1%
Fenchyl Acetate	Ester	52. Galbanum	0-1%
Fenchyl Acetate	Ester	89. Rosemary	0-1%
Formic Acid	Carboxylic Acid	37. Myrrh	0-1%
Furopelargone	Furanoid	79. Geranium	1-2%
Furanodione	Furanoid	37. Myrrh	1-2%
Furanoguaiene	Furanoid	37. Myrrh	0-1%

Compound	Category	Essential Oils	%
Furfural	Furanoid	37. Myrrh	2-3%
Furfural	Furanoid	26. Lime	0-1%
Furfural	Furanoid	72. Myrtle	0-1%
Galbanic Acid	Carboxylic Acid	52. Galbanum	0-1%
Galbanol	Sesquiterpenol	52. Galbanum	2-3%
Geranial	Aldehyde	28. Bitter Orange	1-2%
Geranial	Aldehyde	51. E. Radiata	1-2%
Geranial	Aldehyde	32. Lemon	1-2%
Geranial	Aldehyde	30. Bergamot	0-1%
Geranial	Aldehyde	49. Eucalyptus	0-1%
Geranial	Aldehyde	60. Lavender	0-1%
Geranial	Aldehyde	29. Petitgrain	0-1%
Geraniol	ALcohol	72. Myrtle	0-2%
Garanoxycoumarin	Furanoid	26. Lime	0-1%
Geranyl Acetate	Ester	79. Geranium	1-5%
Geranyl Acetate	Ester	72. Myrtle	1-5%
Geranyl Acetate	Ester	27. Neroli	1-3%
Geranyl Acetate	Ester	28. Bitter Orange	0-1%
Geranyl Acetate	Ester	68. Melissa	0-1%
Geranyl Butyrate	Ester	79. Geranium	1-2%
Geranyl Coproate	Ester	86. Douglas Fir	1-3%
Geranyl Epoxide	Oxide	43. Palmarosa	1-2%
Geranyl Formate	Ester	79. Geranium	1-6%
Geranyl Isovalerate	Ester	43. Palmarosa	1-2%
Geranyl Propionate	Ester	79. Geranium	0-1%
Geranyl Tiglate	Ester	79. Geranium	1-2%
Germacrenol	Sesquiterpenol	110. Valerian	3-6%
Germacrone	Sesquiterpenone	37. Myrrh	2-4%
Germacrone	Sesquiterpenone	62. Ledum	1-2%
Gerpenyl Acetate	Ester	72. Myrtle	2-3%
Gingerone	Sesquiterpenone	113. Ginger	0-2%
Globulol	Sesquiterpenol	64. Tea Tree	1-3%
Globulol	Sesquiterpenol	67. Niaouli	0-1%
δ-Guaiazulene	Sesquiterpene	15. Blue Cypress	1-2%
δ-Guaiazulene	Sesquiterpene	49. Eucalyptus	0-1%
δ-Guaiazulene	Sesquiterpene	79. Geranium	0-1%
α-Guaiene	Sesquiterpene	84. Black Pepper	0-1%
α-Guaiene	Sesquiterpene	14. Frankincense	0-1%
β-Guaiene	Sesquiterpene	105. Moroccan Thyme	1-2%
β-Guaiene	Sesquiterpene	83. Pine	0-1%
Guaiene Oxide	Oxide	85. Patchouly	0-1%
Guaiol	Sesquiterpenol	52. Galbanum	0-1%
Guaiol	Sesquiterpenol	85. Patchouly	0-1%

Compound	Category	Essential Oils	%
Gummosine	Coumarin	52. Galbanum	0-1%
Gummosenine	Coumarin	52. Galbanum	0-1%
α-Gurjunene	Sesquiterpene	112. Vitex	2-5%
α-Gurjunene	Sesquiterpene	14. Frankincense	0-1%
β-Gurjunene	Sesquiterpene	104. Spanish Marjoram	0-1%
Heneicosane	Alkane	88. Rose	0-1%
Heptanal	Aldehyde	32. Lemon	0-1%
Heptanol	Alcohol	113. Ginger	0-1%
Heptanone	Ketone	113. Ginger	0-2%
Heptanone	Ketone	8. Rosewood	0-2%
Heptanone	Ketone	89. Rosemary	0-1%
Herniarin	Coumarin	10. Tarragon	1-2%
Herniarin	Coumarin	61. Lavandin	0-1%
Herniarin	Coumarin	60. Lavender	0-1%
Hexadecane	Alkane	113. Ginger	0-1%
Hexanal	Aldehyde	92. Clary Sage	0-1%
Hexanal	Aldehyde	60. Lavender	0-1%
Hexanal	Aldehyde	72. Myrtle	0-1%
Hexanal	Aldehyde	32. Lemon	0-1%
Hexanol	Alcohol	32. Lemon	0-1%
Hexanone	Ketone	113. Ginger	0-1%
Hexanone	Ketone	89. Rosemary	0-1%
Hexyl Acetate	Ester	21. Roman Chamomile	2-5%
γ-Himachalene	Sesquiterpene	82. Anise	0-1%
Hishorene	Diterpene	22. White Camphor	0-1%
Humulene Oxide	Oxide	97. Clove	0-1%
Humulene Oxide	Oxide	89. Rosemary	0-1%
Hydrocarvone	Ketone	84. Black Pepper	0-1%
Hydroxycinnamaldehyde	Aldehyde	24. Cinnamon	1-2%
Hydroxyoleanic Acid	Carboxylic Acid	96. Onycha	1-2%
Imperatarine	Furanoid	36. Orange	0-1%
Incensol	Alcohol	14. Frankincense	1-2%
Indole	Pyrrole	57. Jasmine	1-3%
Indole	Pyrrole	63. German Chamomile	0-1%
Indole	Pyrrole	27. Neroli	0-1%
Isobutyl Acetate	Ester	21. Roman Chamomile	1-2%
Isochavibetol	Phenol	82. Anise	0-1%
Isomenthone	Ketone	25. Cistus	1-2%
Isopulegol	Alcohol	31. Cambava	2-4%
Isopulegol	Alcohol	68. Melissa	0-1%
Isovalerate	Ester	41. Cypress	0-2%
Isovaleric Acid	Carboxylic Acid	110. Valerian	0-1%

Compound	Category	Essential Oils	%
α-Ionone	Sesquiterpenone	20. Cedarwood	0-1%
β-Ionone	Sesquiterpenone	73. Spikenard	1-2%
Isoeugenol	Phenol	16. Ylang Ylang	0-1%
Jasmone	Ketone	57. Jasmine	0-1%
Jatamansic Acid	Carboxylic Acid	73. Spikenard	0-1%
Junenol	Sesquiterpenol	52. Galbanum	0-1%
Junionone	Ketone	58. Juniper	1-2%
Khusimione	Sesquiterpenone	111. Vetiver	3-6%
Labdanendiol	Diterpenol	25. Cistus	0-1%
Labdanendiol	Diterpenol	41. Cypress	0-1%
Labdanenol	Diterpenol	25. Cistus	0-1%
Labdanenol	Diterpenol	41. Cypress	0-1%
Lachnophyllum Lactone	Lactone	37. Myrrh	1-2%
Laurensolide	Lactone	59. Bay Laurel	0-1%
Lauric Aldehyde	Aldehyde	26. Lime	0-1%
Lavandulol	Alcohol	60. Lavender	1-2%
Lavandulol	Alcohol	61. Lavandin	0-1%
Lavandulyl Acetate	Ester	60. Lavender	1-6%
Lavandulyl Acetate	Ester	61. Lavandin	1-2%
Ledene	Sesquiterpene	91. Sage	0-1%
Ledol	Sesquiterpenol	62. Ledum	1-3%
Ledol	Sesquiterpenol	49. Eucalyptus	1-2%
ζ-Ligustolide	Furanoid	82. Anise	0-1%
ζ-Ligustolide	Furanoid	6. Dill	0-1%
Limettine	Coumarin	26. Lime	1-2%
Limettine	Coumarin	30. Bergamot	0-1%
Limettine	Coumarin	32. Lemon	0-1%
Linalol Oxide	Oxide	22. White Camphor	1-5%
Linalol Oxide	Oxide	92. Clary Sage	0-1%
Linalol Oxide	Oxide	56. Hyssop	0-1%
Linalol Oxide	Oxide	60. Lavender	0-1%
Linalol Oxide	Oxide	47. Lemon Eucalyptus	0-1%
Linalol Oxide	Oxide	105. Moroccan Thyme	0-1%
Linalyl Acetate	Ester	75. Basil	0-1%
Longiborneol	Alcohol	81. Spruce	0-1%
Longicyclene	Sesquiterpene	81. Spruce	0-1%
Longifolene	Sesquiterpene	112. Vitex	3-6%
Longifolene	Sesquiterpene	95. Goldenrod	2-3%
Longifolene	Sesquiterpene	48. E. Dives	0-1%
Longifolene	Sesquiterpene	83. Pine	0-1%
Longifolene	Sesquiterpene	104. Spanish Marjoram	0-1%
Longifolene	Sesquiterpene	81. Spruce	0-1%

Compound	Category	Essential Oils	%
Lycopene	Tetraterpene	33. Tangerine	2-4%
Lycopene	Tetraterpene	34. Grapefruit	2-3%
Lycopene	Tetraterpene	30. Bergamot	1-2%
Lycopene	Tetraterpene	28. Bitter Orange	1-2%
Lycopene	Tetraterpene	35. Mandarin	1-2%
Lycopene	Tetraterpene	36. Orange	1-2%
Lycopene	Tetraterpene	45. Carrot Seed	0-1%
Lycopene	Tetraterpene	32. Lemon	0-1%
Lyratol	Alcohol	100. Idaho Tansy	0-1%
Lyratyl Acetate	Ester	100. Idaho Tansy	0-1%
α-Maalene	Sesquiterpene	91. Sage	0-1%
Maaliol	Sesquiterpinol	73. Spikenard	0-1%
Malic Acid	Carboxylic Acid	110. Valerian	0-1%
Manool	Diterpenol	41. Cypress	0-1%
Manool Oxide	Oxide	41. Cypress	0-1%
Matricariamethyl Ester	Ester	37. Myrrh	2-3%
Matricariamethyl Ester	Ester	63. German Chamomile	0-1%
1-p-Menthen-8-thiol	Thiol	34. Grapefruit	0-1%
Menthol	Phenol	70. Spearmint	0-1%
Menthone	Ketone	79. Geranium	1-3%
Menthone	Ketone	70. Spearmint	1-2%
Menthyl Butyrate	Ester	69. Peppermint	0-1%
Menthyl Isovalerate	Ester	69. Peppermint	0-1%
Methoxycoumarin	Furanoid	30. Bergamot	0-1%
Methyl Acetate	Ester	37. Myrrh	0.1%
Methyl Anthranilate	Ester	28. Bitter Orange	1-2%
Methyl Anthranilate	Ester	57. Jasmine	1-2%
Methyl Anthranilate	Ester	35. Mandarin	1-2%
Methyl Anthranilate	Ester	32. Lemon	0-1%
Methyl Anthranilate	Ester	36. Orange	0-1%
Methyl Anthranilate	Ester	29. Petitgrain	0-1%
Methyl Benzoate	Ester	25. Cistus	1-3%
Methyl Benzoate	Ester	97. Clove	0-1%
Methylbutynal	Aldehyde	37. Myrrh	2-3%
Methylbutynal	Aldehyde	72. Myrtle	0-1%
Methyl Cinnamate	Ester	75. Basil	1-4%
Methyl Citronellate	Ester	68. Melissa	4-5%
Methylfuran	Furanoid	72. Myrtle	1-2%
Methylheptanone	Ketone	68. Melissa	4-5%
Methylheptanone	Ketone	42. Lemongrass	2-3%
Methylisopropenylfurone	Furanoid	37. Myrrh	4-5%
Methyl-Lachnophyllum Ester	Ester	37. Myrrh	1-2%

Compound	Category	Essential Oils	%
Methyl Myrtenate	Ester	72. Myrtle	1-3%
Methyl Myrtenate	Ester	56. Hyssop	1-2%
Methyl-n-amyl ketone	Ketone	97. Clove	0-1%
Methyl Thujate	Ester	103. Cedar Leaf	1-2%
Mint Sulphide	Sulphide	69. Peppermint	0-1%
Muurolene	Sesquiterpene	63. German Chamomile	3-5%
Muurolene	Sesquiterpene	58. Juniper	2-3%
Muurolene	Sesquiterpene	37. Myrrh	1-2%
Muurolene	Sesquiterpene	105. Moroccan Thyme	0-1%
Muurolene	Sesquiterpene	69. Peppermint	0-1%
Muurolene	Sesquiterpene	83. Pine	0-1%
Muurolol	Sesquiterpenol	103. Cedar Leaf	0-2%
Muurolol	Sesquiterpenol	83. Pine	0-1%
Myrcenol	Alcohol	107. Thyme Thujanol	1-3%
Myristicin	Phenol	82. Anise	0-1%
Myrtecommulone	Lactone	72. Myrtle	1-2%
Myrtenal	Aldehyde	51. E. Radiata	1-2%
Myrtenal	Aldehyde	49. Eucalyptus	1-2%
Myrtenal	Aldehyde	62. Ledum	1-2%
Myrtenal	Aldehyde	72. Myrtle	1-2%
Myrtenal	Aldehyde	113. Ginger	0-1%
Myrtenal	Aldehyde	60. Lavender	0-1%
Myrtenalmethylether	Phenol	56. Hyssop	2-3%
Myrtenol	Phenol	72. Myrtle	1-4%
Myrtenol	Phenol	49. Eucalyptus	1-2%
Myrtenol	Phenol	56. Hyssop	0-2%
Myrtenyl Acetate	Ester	110. Valerian	1-5%
Myrtol	Alcohol	72. Myrtle	1-2%
Nardol	Sesquiterpenol	73. Spikenard	1-2%
Nardostachone	Ketone	73. Spikenard	0-2%
Neocilide	Lactone	9. Celery Seed	0-1%
Neptadecene	Monoterpene	27. Neroli	0-1%
Neral	Aldehyde	74. Catnip	3-5%
Neral	Aldehyde	26. Lime	3-5%
Neral	Aldehyde	28. Bitter Orange	1-2%
Neral	Aldehyde	51. E. Radiata	1-2%
Neral	Aldehyde	25. Cistus	0-1%
Neral	Aldehyde	30. Bergamot	0-1%
Neral	Aldehyde	79. Geranium	0-1%
Neral	Aldehyde	113. Ginger	0-1%
Neral	Aldehyde	60. Lavender	0-1%
Neral	Aldehyde	29. Petitgrain	0-1%
Neral	Aldehyde	33. Tangerine	0-1%

Compound	Category	Essential Oils	%
Nerol	Alcohol	55. Helichrysum	2-5%
Nerol	Alcohol	30. Bergamoti	1-3%
Nerol	Alcohol	79. Geranium	1-3%
Nerol	Alcohol	27. Neroli	1-3%
Nerol	Alcohol	32. Lemon	1-2%
Nerol	Alcohol	43. Palmarosa	1-2%
Nerol	Alcohol	28. Bitter Orange	0-1%
Nerol	Alcohol	92. Clary Sage	0-1%
Nerol	Alcohol	61. Lavandin	0-1%
Nerol	Alcohol	68. Melissa	0-1%
Nerol	Alcohol	72. Myrtle	0-1%
Nerolidol	Sesquiterpenol	67. Niaouli	2-7%
Nerolidol	Sesquiterpenol	27. Neroli	1-5%
Nerolidol	Sesquiterpenol	37. Myrrh	2-4%
Nerolidol	Sesquiterpenol	21. Roman Chamomile	2-3%
Nerolidol	Sesquiterpenol	56. Hyssop	1-2%
Nerolidol	Sesquiterpenol	65. Cajuput	0-1%
Neryl Acetate	Ester	27. Neroli	1-3%
Neryl Acetate	Ester	88. Rose	1-3%
Neryl Acetate	Ester	29. Petitgrain	1-3%
Neryl Acetate	Ester	32. Lemon	1-2%
Neryl Acetate	Ester	92. Clary Sage	0-2%
Neryl Acetate	Ester	29. Bergamot	0-1%
Neryl Acetate	Ester	28. Bitter Orange	0-1%
Neryl Acetate	Ester	61. Lavandin	0-1%
Neryl Acetate	Ester	68. Melissa	0-1%
Neryl Acetate	Ester	72. Myrtle	0-1%
Neryl Butyrate	Ester	55. Helichrysum	1-2%
Neryl Formate	Ester	43. Palmarosa	0-1%
Nonanal	Aldehyde	28. Bitter Orange	0-1%
Nonanal	Aldehyde	34. Grapefruit	0-1%
Nonanal	Aldehyde	32. Lemon	0-1%
Nonanal	Aldehyde	36. Orange	0-1%
Nonanol	Alcohol	35. Mandarin	0-1%
Nonanol	Alcohol	32. Lemon	0-1%
Nonanone	Ketone	113. Ginger	0-1%
Nootkatone	Sesquiterpenone	111. Vetiver	2-5%
Nootkatone	Sesquiterpenone	34. Grapefruit	1-2%
Nootkatone	Sesquiterpenone	36. Orange	0-1%
Occidentalol	Sesquiterpenol	101. Thuja	2-5%
Occidol	Sesquiterpenol	101. Thuja	1-3%
Ocimene Oxide	Oxide	75. Basil	1-2%
Octadecane	Alkane	88. Rose	0-1%

Compound	Category	Essential Oils	%
Octanal	Aldehyde	26. Lime	0-1%
Octanal	Aldehyde	34. Grapefruit	0-1%
Octanal	Aldehyde	36. Orange	0-1%
Octanol	Alcohol	70. Spearmint	1-2%
Octanol	Alcohol	34. Grapefruit	0-1%
Octanol	Alcohol	32. Lemon	0-1%
Octanol	Alcohol	105. Moroccan Thyme	0-1%
Octanone	Ketone	60. Lavender	1-3%
Octanone	Ketone	75. Basil	0-1%
Octanone	Ketone	68. Melissa	0-1%
Octen-3-ol	Alcohol	68. Melissa	1-2%
Octyl Acetate	Ester	28. Bitter Orange	0-1%
Oleanolic Acid	Carboxylic Acid	97. Clove	0-2%
Olibanol	Alcohol	14. Frankincense	0-1%
Ormenol	Alcohol	78. Ormenis	1-2%
Osthol	Coumarin	28. Bitter Orange	0-1%
Palmitic Acid	Carboxylic Acid	37. Myrrh	0-1%
Palmitic Acid	Carboxylic Acid	111. Vetiver	0-1%
Patchoulenol	Sesquiterpenol	85. Patchouly	0-1%
α-Patchoulene	Sesquiterpene	85. Patchouly	3-5%
β-Patchoulene	Sesquiterpene	85. Patchouly	2-7%
β-Patchoulene	Sesquiterpene	73. Spikenard	0-1%
Patchoulenone	Sesquiterpenone	85. Patchouly	2-3%
Pentacosane	Alkane	88. Rose	0-1%
Perillaldehyde	Aldehyde	35. Mandarin	0-1%
Perillyl Alcohol	Alcohol	19. Caraway	0-1%
Phellandral	Aldehyde	113. Ginger	0-1%
Phenol	Phenol	23. Cassia	0-1%
Phenol	Phenol	24. Cinnamon	0-1%
Phenol	Phenol	16. Ylang Ylang	0-1%
Phenylethanol	Phenol	88. Rose	1-3%
Phenylethanol	Phenol	27. Neroli	0-1%
Phenyl Propanoate	Ester	25. Cistus	0-1%
Philostachyin	Lactone	12. Mugwort	0-1%
Pimarinol	Diterpenol	41. Cypress	0-1%
α-Pinene Epoxide	Oxide	49. Eucalyptus	0-2%
α-Pinene Oxide	Oxide	50. E.Dives	0-1%
Pinocamphone	Ketone	58. Juniper	0-1%

Numbers preceeding the names of oils
refer to listings in Table Thirty-Two

Compound	Category	Essential Oils	%
Pinocarveol	Alcohol	49. Eucalyptus	1-5%
Pinocarveol	Alcohol	78. Ormenis	1-3%
Pinocarveol	Alcohol	47. Lemon Eucalyptus	1-2%
Pinocarveol	Alcohol	14. Frankincense	0-1%
Pinocarveol	Alcohol	105. Moroccan Thyme	0-1%
Pinocarveol	Alcohol	104. Spanish Marjoram	0-1%
Pinocarvone	Ketone	49. Eucalyptus	1-3%
Pinocarvone	Ketone	78. Ormenis	0-1%
Pinocarvyl Acetate	Ester	104. Spanish Marjoram	0-1%
Pipertol	Alcohol	48. E. Dives	0-1%
Piperitone	Ketone	22. White Camphor	1-5%
Piperitone	Ketone	100. Idaho Tansy	1-2%
Piperitone	Ketone	69. Peppermint	1-2%
Piperitone	Ketone	101. Thuja	1-2%
Piperitone	Ketone	84. Black Pepper	0-1%
Piperitone	Ketone	79. Geranium	0-1%
Piperitone Oxide	Oxide	69. Peppermint	1-3%
Piperonal	Aldehyde	84. Black Pepper	0-1%
Piperonylic Acid	Carboxylic Acid	84. Black Pepper	0-1%
Platyphyllol	Sesquiterpenol	65. Cajuput	1-2%
Pogostol	Sesquiterpenol	85. Patchouly	1-3%
Prenyl Hexonate	Ester	43. Palmarosa	0-1%
Prenyl Octonate	Ester	43. Palmarosa	0-1%
Propyl Angelate	Ester	21. Roman Chamomile	1-2%
Propyl Cinnamoate	Ester	96. Onycha	0-2%
Psoralen	Coumarin	53. Fennel	0-1%
Psoralen	Coumarin	32. Lemon	0-1%
Pulegone	Ketone	69. Peppermint	2-5%
Pulegone	Ketone	70. Spearmint	0-1%
Pyrazine	Diazine	39. Coriander	0-1%
Pyrazine	Diazine	52. Galbanum	0-1%
Rosmaric Acid	Caboxylic Acid	76. Oregano	2-5%
Rosmaric Acid	Carboxylic Acid	90. Rosemary Verbenon	1-2%
Rosmaric Acid	Carboxylic Acid	108. Thyme Thymol	1-2%
Rosmaric Acid	Carboxylic Acid	89. Rosemary	0-1%

IMPORTANT NOTE
Table Seventy (above) only lists compounds found in minor, trace, or low-concentration quantities in oils. Some of these same compounds occur in some oils in major quantities as well. When using Table Seventy, always also check Table Sixty Nine.

Compound	Category	Essential Oils	%
Rose Oxide	Oxide	47. Lemon Eucalyptus	0-1%
Rose Oxide	Oxide	88. Rose	0-1%
Safrole	Ether	71. Nutmeg	1-2%
Sabinol	Alcohol	41. Cypress	0-1%
Sabinol	Alcohol	91. Sage	0-1%
Sabinyl Acetate	Ester	91. Sage	0-1%
Salicylic Acid	Phenolic Acid	54. Wintergreen	1-2%
Salicylic Acid	Phenolic Acid	13. Birch	0-1%
Salvene	Monoterpene	91. Sage	0-1%
Salvol	Alcohol	91. Sage	0-1%
β-Santalene	Sesquiterpene	93. Sandalwood	1-5%
Santalic Acid	Carboxylic Acid	93. Sandalwood	1-2%
Santene	Monoterpene	81. Spruce	1-5%
Santomarine	Lactone	100. Idaho Tansy	0-1%
Santonin	Coumarin	60. Lavender	0-1%
Scatole	Pyrrole	57. Jasmine	0-1%
Scatole	Pyrrole	27. Neroli	0-1%
Sclareol	Diterpenol	91. Sage	0-1%
Sclareol Oxide	Oxide	92. Clary Sage	0-1%
Scoparone	Coumarin	28. Bitter Orange	0-1%
Scoparone	Coumarin	10. Tarragon	0-1%
Scopoletin	Coumarin	82. Anise	0-1%
Scopoletin	Coumarin	39. Coriander	0-1%
Scopoletin	Coumarin	40. Cumin	0-1%
Scopoletin	Coumarin	100. Idaho Tansy	0-1%
Scopoletin	Coumarin	32. Lemon	0-1%
Scopoletin	Coumarin	98. Marigold	0-1%
Scopoletin	Coumarin	10. Tarragon	0-1%
Sedanolic Acid	Carboxylic Acid	9. Celery Seed	3-5%
Sedanolide	Lactone	9. Celery Seed	1-5%
α-Selinene	Sesquiterpene	9. Celery Seed	1-2%
α-Selinene	Sesquiterpene	113. Ginger	1-2%
α-Selinene	Sesquiterpene	62. Ledum	1-2%
Seseline	Furanoid	53. Fennel	0-1%
Sesquiphellandrol	Sesquiterpenol	113. Ginger	0-1%
Sesquiterpene Oxide	Oxide	13. Birch	0-1%
Seychellene	Sesquiterpene	73. Spikenard	1-2%
α- Sinensal	Aldehyde	35. Mandarin	0-1%
α- Sinensal	Aldehyde	36. Orange	0-1%
Slaresinotannol	Alcohol	96. Onycha	0-1%

Compound	Category	Essential Oils	%
Spathulenol	Sesquiterpenol	92. Clary Sage	0-1%
Spathulenol	Sesquiterpenol	63. German Chamomile	0-1%
Spathulenol	Sesquiterpenol	56. Hyssop	0-1%
Spathulenol	Sesquiterpenol	47. Lemon Eucalyptus	0-1%
Tatridin	Lactone	100. Idaho Tansy	0-1%
Teresantalal	Aldehyde	93. Sandalwood	1-3%
Terpinen-4-yl Acetate	Ester	41. Cypress	1-2%
Terpinolene	Monoterpene	77. Marjoram	1-7%
Terpinolene	Monoterpene	41. Cypress	2-6%
Terpinolene	Monoterpene	108. Thyme Thymol	2-6%
Terpinolene	Monoterpene	80. Parsley	3-5%
Terpinolene	Monoterpene	64. Tea Tree	2-5%
Terpinolene	Monoterpene	104. Spanish Marjoram	3-4%
Terpinolene	Monoterpene	53. Fennel	2-3%
Terpinolene	Monoterpene	83. Pine	0-3%
Terpinolene	Monoterpene	36. Orange	1-2%
Terpinolene	Monoterpene	84. Black Pepper	0-2%
Terpinolene	Monoterpene	28. Bitter Orange	0-1%
Terpinolene	Monoterpene	19. Caraway	0-1%
Terpinolene	Monoterpene	92. Clary Sage	0-1%
Terpinolene	Monoterpene	17. Elemi	0-1%
Terpinolene	Monoterpene	32. Lemon	0-1%
Terpinolene	Monoterpene	47. Lemon Eucalyptus	0-1%
Terpinolene	Monoterpene	35. Mandarin	0-1%
Terpinolene	Monoterpene	78. Ormenis	0-1%
Terpinolene	Monoterpene	69. Peppermint	0-1%
Terpinolene	Monoterpene	29. Petitgrain	0-1%
Terpinolene	Monoterpene	33. Tangerine	0-1%
α-Terpinyl Acetate	Ester	41. Cypress	4-5%
α-Terpinyl Acetate	Ester	104. Spanish Marjoram	2-3%
α-Terpinyl Acetate	Ester	87. Ravensara	1-3%
α-Terpinyl Acetate	Ester	49. Eucalyptus	1-2%
γ-Terpinyl Acetate	Ester	47. Lemon Eucalyptus	1-2%
Tetracosane	Alkane	88. Rose	0-1%
Thujanol	Alcohol	106. Thyme Linalol	2-4%
Thujanol	Alcohol	94. Mountain Savory	0-4%
Thujanol	Alcohol	70. Spearmint	1-2%
Thujanol	Alcohol	104. Spanish Marjoram	0-1%
γ-Thujaplicin	Ether	102. Cedar Bark	3-4%
α-Thujene	Monoterpene	48. E. Dives	2-6%
α-Thujene	Monoterpene	84. Black Pepper	1-4%
α-Thujene	Monoterpene	37. Myrrh	0-1%

Compound	Category	Essential Oils	%
Totarol	Diterpenol	41. Cypress	0-1%
Tricosane	Alkane	88. Rose	0-1%
Tricyclene	Monoterpene	81. Spruce	1-5%
Tricyclovetinene	Sesquiterpene	111. Vetiver	0-1%
Tricyclovetinerol	Sesquiterpenol	111. Vetiver	3-4%
Tropolone	Ketone	103. Cedar Leaf	1-2%
Umbelliferone	Coumarin	7. Angelica	1-2%
Umbelliferone	Coumarin	6. Dill	1-2%
Umbelliferone	Coumarin	82. Anise	0-1%
Umbelliferone	Coumarin	39. Coriander	0-1%
Umbelliferone	Coumarin	52. Galbanum	0-1%
Umbelliferone	Coumarin	60. Lavender	0-1%
Umbelliferone	Coumarin	32. Lemon	0-1%
Umbelliferone	Coumarin	98. Marigold	0-1%
Undecanal	Aldehyde	28. Bitter Orange	0-1%
Undecanal	Aldehyde	32. Lemon	0-1%
Undecane	Alkane	113. Ginger	0-1%
Valerazulene	Sesquiterpene	110. Valerian	0-1%
Valericaldehyde	Aldehyde	49. Eucalyptus	0-1%
Valericaldehyde	Aldehyde	67. Niaouli	0-1%
Valerianal	Phenolic Aldehyde	73. Spikenard	1-2%
Valerianal	Phenolic Aldehyde	110. Valerian	1-2%
Valerianol	Sesquiterpenol	73. Spikenard	0-1%
Valerianine	Lactone	110. Valerian	0-1%
Valerianone	Ketone	73. Spikenard	0-1%
Valerianone	Ketone	110. Valerian	0-1%
Valeric Acid	Carboxylic Acid	110. Valerian	1-2%
Vanillin Aldehyde	Aldehyde	96. Onycha	1-2%
Verbenol	Alcohol	89. Rosemary	0-1%
Verbenone	Ketone	89. Rosemary	1-2%
Verbenone	Ketone	105. Moroccan Thyme	0-1%
Verbenyl Acetate	Ester	7. Angelica	1-2%
Vetivazulene	Sesquiterpene	111. Vetiver	0-1%
Vetivene	Sesquiterpene	111. Vetiver	0-1%
Vetivenic Acid	Carboxylic Acid	111. Vetiver	0-1%
Vetiverol	Sesquiterpenol	111. Vetiver	0-1%
Vetiveryl Acetate	Ester	111. Vetiver	1-2%
α-Vetivone	Sesquiterpenone	111. Vetiver	3-6%
β-Vetivone	Sesquiterpenone	111. Vetiver	3-6%
Vinylhexanal	Aldehyde	27. Neroli	0-1%
Vinylphenol	Phenol	23. Cassia	0-1%
Vinylphenol	Phenol	24. Cinnamon	0-1%

Compound	Category	Essential Oils	%
Viridiflorene	Sesquiterpene	64. Tea Tree	1-5%
Viridiflorene	Sesquiterpene	66. Rosalina	1-2%
Viridiflorene	Sesquiterpene	67. Niaouli	0-4%
Viridiflorol	Sesquiterpenol	65. Cajuput	1-2%
Viridiflorol	Sesquiterpenol	69. Peppermint	1-2%
Viridiflorol	Sesquiterpenol	64. Tea Tree	0-2%
Viridiflorol	Sesquiterpenol	49. Eucalyptus	0-1%
Viterol	Sesquiterpenol	110. Valerian	0-1%
Vitivene	Sesquiterpene	110. Valerian	1-2%
Vulgarin	Lactone	12. Mugwort	0-1%
Vulgerol	Alcohol	100. Idaho Tansy	0-1%
β-Ylangene	Sesquiterpene	113. Ginger	2-3%
Yomogi Alcohol	Alcohol	78. Ormenis	2-3%
Zingeberol	Sesquiterpenol	113. Ginger	1-2%

END OF
Table Seventy
Minor, Trace, & Low Concentrate Compounds ($\leq$ 5%)
of Essential Oils in Alphabetical Order

When using Table 70, also Check Table 69 which lists compounds found in concentrations $\geq$ 5%. Some compounds occur as trace constituents in some oils and major constituents in others. For example, only a trace of verbenone is found in Moroccan Thyme (Table 70) while it comprises 23% of Rosemary CT verbenon (Table 69). Hence, some Compounds are in both Tables.

To form a complete list of all oils containing a specific compound in all concentrations, you will need to compile information from Table 69, Table 70, and perhaps a third table in Part Two of this book.

For example, from Table 70 we find that citronellal is found in minor or trace concentrations (0-2%) in Bitter Orange, Geranium, Ginger, Grapefruit, E. Radiata, Lemon, Lime, Melissa, Orange, and Pine. Referring to Table 69 we find that citronellal is the major ingredient in Cambava oil (75%). Table 69 then refers us to Table 54 where we find that Citronellal is also the major ingredient in Lemon Eucalyptus (60%) and comprises 6% of Citronella oil. Hence, by consulting three different tables, we were able to compile a comprehensive list of common essential oils containing citronella in concentrations from less than 1% to as much as 75%.

END OF PART TWO

PART THREE

BEYOND
CHEMISTRY

♥ Contents of Part Three ♥

Preamble

Article One

Article Two

614   Contents

Article Three

♥ The Nature of Matter   685

Article Four

♥ Consciousness in Essential Oils   707

❤ Preamble
A BOOK IN ITSELF

Part Three of this book will introduce you to some of the realms beyond chemistry where one must go in order to understand how aromatic oils accomplish their healing and spiritually uplifting properties. It could easily be another book, in and of itself, and perhaps some day it shall become one. For present purposes, we shall keep it short, detailing only a few of the important areas one must visit to acquire a fuller wisdom of the power of essential oils.

Among the texts to which we have referred in writing this part are those \given in the list below. To deepen and expand your comprehension of what we present here, we recommend that you consult directly with the body of these works. More complete information is given for each of these references in the annotated bibliography at the end of this book. The texts are as follows:

1. The Body Electric
    by Robert O. Becker

2. Transcendental Physics
    by Edward R. Close

3. Messages from Water
    by Masaru Emoto

4. Vibrational Medicine
    by Richard Gerber

5. Radiation, Magnetism, and Living Things
    by Daniel Halacy

6. The Nature of Substance
    by Rudolf Hauschka

7. The Holy Bible
    Moses, et al., God Almighty, Editor-in-Chief

Looking for a complete explanation of how and why essential oils work within the confines of today's scientific paradigm is like confining your search to the inside of your house for a set of lost car keys you actually dropped outside in the grass on the front lawn. Confining your search to the house, you would never find them.

What follows here concerns the future science of essential oils that lies beyond the science of today. May your perusal of these pages help to crack the shell that confines your consciousness. May it release you, like a newborn eagle, fresh from the egg, into an expanded world of light and flight, of new experiences, and new understandings of God's infinite and benevolent universe.

❤ ARTICLE ONE
THE LIMITS
OF SCIENCE

In his classic book, *What Your Doctor May Not Tell You About Menopause*, John R. Lee, M.D., challenges the paradigm of currently practiced medicine in the area of hormonal biochemistry—the estrogens, androgens, and other steroids that affect our behavior— male and female.

In the spirit of a true right-brained, intuitive scientist, Dr. Lee entitled Chapter Two of his book, *The Dance of the Steroids*. He likens the ebb and flow of our hormones to the parts of a symphony in four movements: 1. Andante con molto, 2. Adagio, 3. Allegro con brio, and 4. Largo maestoso. "Understanding hormones requires a vision into the unseen," he explains. "Humans have the power to create reality beyond their normal experience. We do it all the time with music, books, stories, fantasies, dreams, and, yes, especially in science. Science is really the art of seeing forces and elements invisible to the normal senses."

The science to which John Lee refers is not the usual science as practiced today by left-brained (intellectual) scientists bent upon finding a left-brained explanation for everything, and who largely control the politics and monetary support for today's research. What Dr. Lee describes is science as it should be and as practiced by those few blessed with the right-brained (intuitive) capabilities and moral courage to seek and find truth wherever it may lead them without regard to political or monetary consequences.

True Science vs. Current Science

True science is the discovery, verification, and articulation of the laws and details of God's universe as he created it, and as he continues to create it. This includes the exploration, experience, and definition of the conscious, participating, all-permeating presence of the Creator, himself.

For spiritual explorers of God's universe, customary science as practiced today is not an instrument of discovery. It is only an instrument of verification, refinement, and description.

The great intuitive scientists work outside the traditional paradigm. They jump straight to their correct conclusions by direct perception of God's reality. They then apply the language of mathematics and the methods of scientific experimentation in order to work backwards to connect their distant vision to the body of established data and levels of current understanding for those who cannot see so far. Once these connections have been made, ordinary scientists can then apply their technical skills and lesser insights to the refinement, development, and application of these fresh gems of truth brought to them from afar beyond the perception and reach of the masses.

Ancient seers and prophets of many lands have long referred to direct perceptions of spiritual truth as visions "from the east." Thus, it has been wise men from the east, who see and follow the star of God's truth, who bring us precious gifts in the form of scientific insights that can enrich our lives on the mental and material planes, according to God's plan, and which can also enrich our souls and bring us closer to God, himself. Great and humble scientists are prophets and servants of God appointed to articulate their divinely inspired visions into a vernacular that even simple folks can use and understand.

This is what science is supposed to be and what true science is. But what exactly is the "scientific method?" And what are its capabilities and its limits?

The Limits of Science

Science has lifted us from the ignorance of the Dark Ages into the understandings we hold today. It has increased our standards of living, lengthened our life spans, and enriched our lives in every way. Music, the arts, our governments, our social customs, our religious beliefs, our educational institutions, our recreations, our modes of travel, our means of communicating, our working, our eating, our sleeping—all aspects of our culture have been transformed by the touch of technology. It is little wonder, then, that we have become conditioned to look to science for the solutions of all our problems and for the answers to life's questions.

But science, powerful as it is, is a false god. Awed by the spectacular material advancements science has brought us, we have come to expect more of science than it is capable of delivering. Many individuals, not recognizing the limitations of science, stand in expectation of results that will never come. Science does not have all the solutions. It does not have all the answers. It never has and it never will.

The purpose of this chapter is to clearly present science for what it is—no more and no less. Many answers can be obtained by the scientific method, but there are many more that cannot. It is not my intent to destroy your faith in science. As a lifetime professional scientist myself, I am duly respectful of its potential. I am also aware of its limitations. When it comes to consideration of life in its fullness, these limitations are very great. Therefore, while I don't want to destroy your faith in science, I do want to disturb it and to encourage you to question its validity as an approach to living. This brings to mind the opening verses of the *Gospel of Thomas*, who was one of the twelve (Didymus)—a beloved and close disciple of Jesus Christ of Nazareth:

> Jesus said: The seeker should not stop until he finds. When he does find, he will be disturbed. After having been disturbed, he will be astonished . . .   Thomas 1:2

While the essence of science is characterized by its inherent lack of mysticism, to the non-scientist it often bears a veil of the mystical. One of the most common persuasive devices of the advertiser is to cloak its advocacy in the jargon of science: "If it sounds scientific, it must be right," so goes the unspoken implication. And people buy it. It is my hope that this writing will serve to demystify science for those unfamiliar with its inner workings. It is not in our best interest, as human beings, to hold science in a degree of esteem that exceeds its capabilities.

Science is not the only approach of inquiry into the nature of life. In fact, it is an approach that fails in most of life's situations. While it has great capabilities, it can only do so much and no more. This chapter will assist you in obtaining a realistic expectation of science, because without a realistic expectation you will not be able to rely upon it when appropriate and you will be disappointed when it fails.

Science may be a high-speed aircraft in some ways, but an airplane cannot get you everywhere. If you want to walk about your home, visit a neighbor, enjoy a stroll through the woods, climb the heights of a mountain, fish in your favorite stream, or travel to places without airports, you cannot do it with an aircraft. Modes of locomotion must be appropriate to the circumstances. Likewise, modes of inquiry must be appropriate to the subject matter. In the case of the scientific mode of inquiry, it is inappropriate to most of life's important questions.

For example, when someone smiles at you, do you need a blood test and a urinalysis to appreciate why they smiled at you? Of course not. You simply look them in the eyes with an open heart and you know.

In order to clearly understand the limitations of science, one must first have a clear picture of what science is. Interestingly enough, there is a large fraction of scientists who do not have an accurate and complete picture of the boundaries of science. This might sound hard to believe, but it is true. It is entirely possible to practice science to a high level of success in obtaining useful, valid results, while at the same time never being fully aware of its limits.

In an analogous way, it is entirely possible, if not common, for doctors to practice medicine without being aware of its limits. In fact, it is not at all uncommon for people to confuse medicine with science. And neither is it unusual for doctors to confuse science with technology. The practice of medicine, while it may be partially described as "applied technology," is not a science.

While medicine bases some of its practices on scientifically derived data, the practice of medicine is not, itself, a science. Medicine is a discipline of opinion where accepted standards of practice are determined by a consensus of the majority, not by the scientific method.

The reason the limits of science are not widely recognized and understood lies in our educational systems, which train scientists and health care providers in how to exercise the methods of science and apply their results, but do not encourage a questioning of the fundamental assumptions behind the methods themselves. The purpose of medical training is unquestioning indoctrination, not cognitive education. It is to promote, protect, and apply the prevailing paradigm—not to question it.

The Limits of Science in a Nutshell

The limits of science can be condensed into the following nineteen statements:

1. Science explains nothing; it can only describe.
2. Science proves nothing; it can only verify or disprove.
3. Science cannot deal directly with subjective experience; it can only deal with the objective.
4. "Scientific" does not necessarily mean right, valid, or best; it only means that a certain method was followed.
5. "Objective" does not necessarily mean right, valid or best; it only means that observations are independent of the observer and can be measured scientifically.
6. "Subjective" does not mean invalid or irrelevant; it only means that observations are dependent upon the observer and cannot be measured scientifically.
7. Most of the things we experience and value in life are subjective and are, therefore, beyond science.
8. Belief in science is an act of faith and is, in itself, a choice made subjectively and personally, not scientifically.
9. Science is limited by time; tomorrow's research can not help us today and yesterday's events cannot be directly observed.

10. Science is limited in space in the infinite sense; there will always remain portions of the universe beyond its reach because of distance to the furthest reaches of intergalactic space.

11. Science is limited in space in the infinitesimal sense; there will always remain portions of the universe beyond its reach within the subspace and the subparticles of atoms.

12. Science is limited in its ability to observe natural living processes because the effect of the observer changes, if not halts, the process.

13. Science is limited by its instruments and apparati of observation. It can only study that which its apparati are designed to observe or detect.

14. Science is limited by experimental error; its results can be no better than the reliability of its data.

15. Science is limited by human bias in the application of the scientific method itself.

16. Science is limited by human bias in the choices of topics upon which the method is applied.

17. Science is limited in its impact upon society in that people, and even professionals, generally do not follow scientific facts unless the facts agree with their feelings and/or preheld beliefs.

18. The scientific method is not the only valid method of inquiry into the nature of things—there are others, and when it comes to practical inquiry into the subjective, other methods must be used because, in such experiences, science fails.

19. Science (as practiced today) is limited by the *a priori* assumption that there is no willful, conscious, participating God within the processes studied by science. Hence, God is not a factor to be considered.

What is Science?

Science, as discussed in this section, is an intellectual left-brain process dependent upon the five physical senses. This is the predominant science as defined and practiced today. We call it "materialistic science." There is also another definition of science that is intuitive and right-brained that does not depend upon the five physical senses. But in this discussion, we are referring to science as the vast majority of scientists currently understand it and practice it.

Science is an approach to the study of the universe around us—both living and inanimate. It is only one of several approaches. The purpose of science is to discover and describe the details of the universe. It does not attempt to explain, in an ultimate sense, why things are the way they are. Science merely observes and describes.

For example, Newton's Second Law states that force (F) is equal to mass (m) times acceleration (a). Or in the form of an equation: $F = ma$. The law does not explain why force, mass, and acceleration are so related. It merely states that between these three quantities, that is the way it is. It is only a description of what scientific observations have seen time and time again.

Newton's observation (stated as his second law) is no different than stating that "the average length of human pregnancies is nine months." If you ask a medical scientist why pregnancies last this long, they may reply, "Because this is how long it takes the fetus to develop into a stage where it is able to live outside the womb and yet is not too large to pass through the birth canal." But this is not really "why" in an ultimate sense. To really answer the question of "why?" one would have to explain why fetal development progresses at the rate that it does. A medical scientist might be tempted to answer this by going into the chemistry and embryology of fetal processes and how these occur in a certain sequence over a certain period resulting in a mean gestation period of nine months. But here, again, one would merely have explained "how" the growth rates resulted, not "why." At this point we could ask, "Why do these chemical and biological processes proceed at the rates and in the manners in which they do?" Trying to track down an ultimate "why" in this manner is endless. This is the reason that science does not concern itself with such considerations.

In the field of aromatherapy and essential oils, one could state as a scientific fact, derived from the data of many scientific analyses, that marjoram oil (*Origanum marjorana*) generally contains 14-21% phenols, 28-60% monoterpenes, and 2-5% sesquiterpenes. If you asked a biochemist <u>why</u> marjoram contains these types of compounds in these proportions, he or she may attempt to reply that it is due to its genetics as a member of the mint family (Lamiaceae) and because of its inbred habits of taking certain minerals from the air, water, and soil to create compounds in a certain manner in response to its environmental and nutritional needs, etc., etc. Thus, one might describe <u>how</u> marjoram makes the oils it makes. But none of these explanations would answer <u>why</u> marjoram behaves like marjoram to produce the oils it produces. "Why" is not a question that left-brain science can ever address to obtain an ultimate and final answer.

Therefore, one of the principle features that distinguishes science from other approaches to life's problems is the problems to which science limits itself. In other words, science is concerned only with "what, when, and how." When we ask, "Why?", and require an ultimate answer, we have left traditional science and have entered realms that are more properly relegated to philosophy, religion, intuition, and personal subjective judgment.

Consequently, the first limitation of science is that it does not deal with absolutes. It does not deal with "truth." It deals with facts, as perceived, but not with absolute truth. Hence, the first hope we must give up for the scientific method is that it will lead us to absolute answers about life and the universe. It cannot.

In addition to being restricted only to certain questions, science is further restricted by the approach it takes to finding answers to those questions. This approach is called the "scientific method." We shall describe this a bit later. First, let us further pursue the degree to which science is capable of dealing with "truth." In particular, let us explore the real meaning of the phrase, "scientific proof."

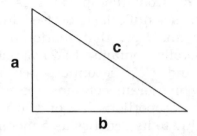

The Pythagorean Theorem: $a^2 + b^2 = c^2$

What is Proof?

Absolute proof is strictly the domain of logicians. In mathematics, for example, once a theorem is proven it is proven for all time and all circumstances. Mathematical proof is absolute. Mathematics, however, is not science. This is a point about which many are confused. Mathematics is a language used by science, but is not itself a science. Mathematical proof and scientific proof are not the same thing at all.

To see this point more clearly, consider the Pythagorean Theorem—a mathematical proof that relates the lengths of the sides (a & b) of a right triangle to the length of its hypotenuse (c). (See the figure above.)

This theorem was proven thousands of years ago once and for all time. We needn't worry that tomorrow a right triangle may be discovered that disproves the theorem. Neither should we be concerned that the theorem was proven in Greece and, therefore, may or may not apply to the United States or to astronauts on another planet. Proof of the Pythagorean Theorem is absolute—valid for all times and places. In mathematics, once proven is always proven. This is not so in science.

The reason that mathematicians can prove their theorems absolutely is because their universe of mathematics is a creation of human consciousness. The elements of this universe (numbers, functions, vectors, etc.) were all conceived and defined by mathematicians themselves. Therefore, since they created their own universe and, in principle, have knowledge of all of its parts, when they prove a theorem they are assured that the proof will stand for all time and in all places, because in making the proof they were able to consider their entire universe whose complete past, present, and future they know.

To think of it another way, mathematics, as are all systems of logic, is similar to a game with certain elements and rules devised by somebody in an arbitrary, but definite and orderly fashion. Once the game is established, the elements and the rules are not changed. If you change anything, you have a different game. When you prove a mathematical theorem you are merely playing the game as defined by the system of mathematics in which you are engaged. By agreement with other mathematicians, you must make your proof using only the elements and rules laid down for the particular mathematical system in which you are working. If you change the rules then you are not playing the game—you are inventing a new game or a new system of mathematics with different conditions.

Take baseball, for example. The elements of the game are the ball, the bat, the bases, the field, and the players. Among the established rules is that three outs constitute the end of a team's time up to bat for that inning. Now this is a completely arbitrary rule. It could have been decided that two outs would do it, or five, or seven, but for some reason, three was chosen. If we want to make it something different, then we cannot call it baseball. In any case, once the game begins, the rules remain fixed. In a mathematical sense, you could prove that if one member of your team strikes out, another pops a fly to shortstop, and a third is thrown out on first, your team is finished batting for that inning. This proof would be absolute because it is based upon a finite set of elements and rules that were invented by man. Even if afterwards someone changes the rules and elements so that three outs no longer retires the side up to bat, they will have only changed the game to something else. They will not have affected the absoluteness of your former proof since now, in effect, they are talking about a different game than the one in which you made your proof.

Just as there are many kinds of games, there are many systems of mathematics. In Euclidian Geometry the shortest distance between two points is a straight line. This follows from the manner in which the elements and rules of Euclidian Geometry are defined. In some other systems of geometry the shortest distance between two points is not a straight line. This does not disprove the Euclidian notion any more than citing the case of bowling, where the high score wins, can be used to disprove that the low score wins in golf. The two systems of geometry are entirely different games. All they have in common is that both were fashioned by the human mind.

Mathematics as Evidence of God's Image in Man

While we have compared various systems of mathematics with various games, this is not to put mathematics in the same category as games. Games are truly arbitrary—products of the whims of their creators and subject to changes by those who play the games over time. Mathematics is different. It is not arbitrary and certain fundamentals are not subject to change in time, which is the real reason mathematical proofs stand forever without fear of disproof.

The superficial aspects of mathematics are arbitrary. For example, the choices of how mathematical concepts are represented are arbitrary since these are made by humans. This includes choices such as how to represent the number one—whether in Arabic symbols, Roman numerals, Chinese characters, or the hieroglyphics of ancient Egypt. But the concept of "one" is not an arbitrary, manmade choice. It is a fixed principle of God's universe and remains unchanged regardless of the symbol by which is represented.

Mathematician and physicist, Dr. Edward Close, has pointed out that there is an uncanny correlation between mathematical systems and the observed universe, which gives physics and chemistry their quantitative basis. Close said, "I think that, as a creation of the human mind, mathematics may well be one of the best indications that man is, indeed, made in God's image, since this human creation mimics God's creation—the observable universe—so well. The truth is," Close continues, "that no logical/mathematical system can ever be complete within itself, but must be an expression of something beyond itself. This innate feature of all mathematical systems is the thrust of Godel's Incompleteness Theorem,"

In other words, if God's infinite consciousness is one of form, structure, and order, then we, as living creations made in his image (as stated in Genesis 1:26-27) would reflect a parallel form, structure, and order in our individualized consciousness. Furthermore, if the projection of God's consciousness as individualized human consciousness reflects his attributes of form, structure, and order, then all the rest of his creation (as stated in Romans 1:20) would also reflect a parallel form, structure, and order. Thus, when humans create logical systems of form, structure, and order from their own minds (such as a system of mathematics), it is not surprising that such mental constructs would find a close correlation with physical reality, as found in the quantitative sciences.

In Close's book, *Transcendental Physics*, he states this concept as follows: "If primary consciousness (God) has form and structure, it should be reflected, at least partially, in individual consciousness, and in the structure of the physical universe. If all structure is projected from primary consciousness, we can understand why logical structure, thought to originate in human minds, is repeatedly found to apply to the structure of the physical universe. The human mind and the physical universe display the same symmetry and logic because that symmetry and logic underlie all reality in the substance of primary consciousness (God)."

Thus, while mathematical systems, and logical systems of all kinds, are creations of the human mind, they are not as arbitrary as the whimsical creation of games. There is an unseen universal archetype that guides and validates the precepts of mathematics. As stated at the outset of this discussion on "What is Proof?"— Absolute proof is strictly the domain of logicians. . . Mathematical proof and scientific proof are not the same thing at all.

What is Scientific Proof?

Scientific proof is not really proof at all, in the mathematical sense, but is either verification or disproof. Since scientists deal with a universe that is not of their own creation, they cannot prove their laws absolutely as can mathematicians. Although scientists use the term "scientific proof," and I may use it in this book, what we really mean is that a particular hypothesis has been verified or disproved. We don't mean "proof" in the mathematical sense.

Scientists can never know for a certainty that the laws seemingly in effect today were always so or that they will be in effect at all future times. Neither can they know that their laws, as observed to date, within the limits of current observations, will continue to be upheld by future observations. That is to say, just because Newton's laws have been repeatedly verified during the last two centuries doesn't mean they functioned, as we observe them today, at all times in the geologic past or during the days of creation when God spoke the universe into existence.

Is the Speed of Light a Constant?

Consider the speed of light in a vacuum—186,280 miles per second or 300,000 km/sec. Twentieth-century physicists consider it to be an invariable constant of the universe. But is it? Do we really know that the speed of light was the same five-thousand or five-million years ago? Will it remain constant for all time into the future?

Some scientists, such as Barry Setterfield (*A Brief History of c* - 1987), say the speed of light used to be much faster and is gradually slowing down. Einstein's famous equation, $E = mc^2$, can be used to deduce this conclusion. Solving for c (the speed of light), we find that it equals the square-root of the energy of the universe (E) over the mass (m). ($c = \sqrt{E/m}$) If we assume that no additional energy (E) or mass (m) is being fed into the physical universe and if our observations and conclusions about the ongoing transformation of energy into mass throughout the universe is correct, then the amount of total energy in the universe (E) is continually diminishing while the total mass (m) is increasing causing the ratio E/m to get smaller and smaller in time, thus causing the speed of light to also gradually get slower and slower over the centuries. Of course, we made a few assumptions in drawing this conclusion which may turn out to be invalid. Even so, it does illustrate a point, that things we consider constant and factual today may not always have been so.

Science can only directly observe the present. We can extrapolate into the future and deduce conclusions about the past, but only the present is directly within the grasp of scientific observation. Geologists deduce that dinosaurs once thundered across the earth's surface, but no scientist has ever seen one alive. What we know of them we can only deduce from their remains.

Science is also limited in its contact with space. The universe in which we live is limitless in two opposing directions—expansively outward into the farthest reaches of unplumbed space and infinitesimally inward into the subspace of the atoms. Since absolute proof in the physical universe would require knowledge of every cubic centimeter of matter, space and energy, and since humans have no such knowledge of their universe (as mathematicians do of theirs)—absolute proofs of physical phenomena are impossible for human scientists.

If you think about it, comprehension of every speck of matter and every corner of space in the created universe is tantamount to the definitions for "omnipresence" and "omniscience"—neither of which are human attributes. In most religions, however, these are attributes of the divine. What this implies is that if you seek absolute answers about the manifested universe, they cannot be found by materialistic science. A quest for absolute truth always leads beyond science and leads into matters which are spiritual and inaccessible to our logical left brains.

The point is that scientists can never know all the elements and rules of their universe because not only did they not create it, at least a portion of it will always remain beyond them in time and/or space—where the term "space" is used here to designate the limitlessness of both the inner and the outer universes.

Unlike mathematics, the tenets of science are forever in jeopardy of ambush by a new set of facts. How many ideas formerly considered scientifically sound are now considered disproven? How many times has medical science reversed itself? How much of present-day medical practice, deemed scientific and beneficial today, will, in a few years, be demonstrated unscientific and harmful? For all we know, science may eventually invalidate them all.

Bleeding patients with leeches as a routine medical cure-all procedure sounds absurd to us now, but during the nineteenth century it was considered good medical practice. Within the framework of the scientific understanding of the time, it seemed most reasonable.

Scientific laws describe only what we see here and now within the limits of our history and of our restricted vision. Science, at best, can only provide us with a set of likely probabilities based upon and limited by current data. No matter how much data has been accumulated on growing basil or lavender over decades, or even centuries, we will never be able to predict the exact chemical composition of the next batch of essential oil harvested for a given field or from any field.

Some sciences can offer more certainty than others. Physics and chemistry are among the more certain sciences. Medical and biological science, by contrast, are among those whose probabilities are among the least certain because of the unimaginable complexity of life processes, their unknown interactions with the human mind and spirit, and the impossibility of objective and complete measurement.

Statistical Health Care vs. Personalized Care

Because of this, doctors resort to statistics. This is one of the greatest fallacies of the practicing physician—the application of statistical probabilities to individuals. We choose our personal physicians in the belief that we will receive personalized, individualized care. What doctors are actually trained to do is to give statistical care. What a left-brained doctor will do is to prescribe such that he has a certain level of statistical success among his many patients rather than striving to prescribe in a way that is optimal for each patient according to his or her unique bodily, mental, and spiritual status. In other words, an allopathic physician will be satisfied if they "lose some and win some," so long as their losses fall short of the definition of "malpractice." Winning every case and bringing relief to every patient is not his or her goal. That would be right-brained medicine, a modality in which allopaths are neither trained, encouraged to practice, nor taught to respect.

The fallacy of statistical medicine is this. Just because something is average doesn't mean it is normal, common, or necessarily desirable. Yet doctors continually fall into the logical trap of assuming that a given range of an average is normal, etc. Because of their ignorance, their fear, and their denial of the proper use of intuition, they don't know what else to do except to deal with all patients as statistics. Thus, each patient becomes a set of data to fit into the matrix of standard treatments and diagnoses taught in medical school and enforced by medical peer pressure.

For example, the average human gestation is 272 days (nine months). But that does not mean that 272 days is applicable to you and your pregnancy. Do all the apples on a tree ripen on the same day or in the same span of time from blossom to a mature fruit? Two-hundred seventy-two days may be premature for your baby, yet American doctors induce and do cesarean sections based upon this fallacy every day. As a result, six out of seven cesareans are physiologically unnecessary. Such practices are a leading cause of prematurity in the U.S. today and a leading cause of newborn and maternal mortality.

During my training in medical school, the professors repeatedly emphasized, "Don't treat the patient; treat the chart." In other words, treat the data, not the person. Health care practice will never become a true healing art until the role of right brain, non-objective science (intuition) is acknowledged, taught, nurtured, and encouraged. Only then can medical practice be customized to the client.

Proof, Disproof, and Verification

In the end, scientists can only do two things: verify or disprove. Disproof of a hypothesis is easy. All you need is one exception. To verify means that you have observed that the physical or biological law under question has been followed. You may verify again and again, but never prove, because to prove means that you have investigated every possible situation, past, present, and future throughout the entire universe—within and without. This is, of course, impossible. It is impossible now and it always will be impossible within the scope of the scientific method as defined today. Hence, when scientists say they have "proven" something, they really only mean that they have verified it enough times to be confident that if they try again, it will work, according to the stated limits; and if anyone else tries it, they, too, will make the same observations.

To state that you believe in a tenet of physical or biological science is actually an act of faith based on your experience or on the experience of other scientists in whom you hold confidence. How many people have personally verified Mendel's Laws of dominant and recessive genes in genetics? Even if you have verified it for some traits in some species, how can you be absolutely certain, without taking a leap of faith, that the laws will apply in any future specific instance?

To more clearly delineate the difference between "proof " and "verification" consider the Pythagorean Theorem again. One may verify the theorem quite easily by carefully drawing a right triangle, measuring the lengths of the sides, squaring the lengths, adding the results, and comparing the sum to the square of the measured length of the hypotenuse. Even if you drew a million different right triangles and verified the theorem for all of them, no mathematician would consider this a proof. To prove it you must, somehow, deal with all right triangles, past, present, and future, all at once. Only this would constitute absolute proof. Fortunately for mathematicians, this is possible.

Since the idea of a triangle is an abstract creation of the mind (what we draw on paper is merely a representation of that abstract idea), all right triangles can be dealt with simultaneously in the abstract so that within the realm of mathematics, absolute proof can be accomplished. Unfortunately for scientists, such accomplishments are not possible.

Therefore, it is a fallacy to assume that because something is "scientific" it is true, in an absolute sense, or that it is even better than something arrived at non-scientifically. "Scientific" only means that a certain approach has been taken (i.e. the scientific method). One can apply the method perfectly well and obtain truly "scientific" results whose application may not only rest upon an ultimately false foundation, but could, if put into practice, eventually prove to be harmful. Conversely, a "non-scientific" approach is often the best. There is a place for both science and non-science. Both must be used, but only in the right circumstances and with discretion.

Hence, only mathematicians and other types of logicians can prove things. Scientists must content themselves with verification or disproof. While mathematicians live in a comfortable realm of certainty within the universe of their own minds, scientists, courageously exploring the universe they experience, live in perpetual uncertainty. In order to make the most effective use of science, we must recognize these intrinsic limitations.

What is the Scientific Method?

A scientist's task is to invent a story to explain his or her observations and then to decide just how likely their story may be. Organizing this process into steps, we arrive at the "scientific method" consisting of three parts:

1. Observation
2. Hypothesis
3. Experimentation

These three steps may occur in any order during the scientific process, but usually a scientist first observes something that suggests a certain explanation. They then set up experiments and make further objective observations to test their hypothesis. In the beginning they may modify their hypothesis from time to time, refining it to more closely fit the data. Eventually, they may reach the point where the hypothesis fits most, if not all, observations and they feel it can be refined no more. If they have verified it repeatedly and have a great deal of confidence in the hypothesis, they may then call it a "theory." If many other scientists also verify the theory, it may become elevated to the status of a "law." A "law of nature" or a "law of chemistry or physics" is merely an accurate description of how certain parameters are related which have been verified over a period of time by many scientists. This is the scientific method.

When scientists have several theories, each of which partially describe a situation, but none completely, they may choose the theory with the fewest inconsistencies as being the "best theory." It is not unscientific to apply a theory that has not been shown to be completely accurate if it is the theory that seems to account for more observations than any other. As a scientist you never deal with absolutes. You must continually apply theories and ideas that, although not necessarily shown to be completely correct, are still workable and seem to yield acceptable results. Here, again, the idea of absolutes is one that only mathematicians can enjoy.

This lack of exactness in science is readily apparent in the life sciences where processes are so complex that precisely reproducible results are never obtained. In the limit, this lack of exactness is present even in the sciences of physics or chemistry which deal with the simpler inanimate world. The truth is that there is no such thing as an "exact" science. No science is exact. In the real world, we must always accept approximations and make choices between theories or paradigms, none of which are perfect or complete. If it were considered unscientific to use a theory that is not perfect, there would be no science. Choosing the better of two imperfects must be considered one of the most important aspects of the scientific method.

The last consideration leads us to the relative roles of objectivity and subjectivity in science because, as it turns out, the "choice" of one theory over another is primarily subjective and depends to a large extent upon the personal bias of the scientist.

Objectivity and Subjectivity in Science

The rules of the scientific method require that observations be objective. This means that, theoretically, regardless of who makes the observations, the account should be the same—within limits, of course. For example, if ten laboratories were to analyze samples from the same batch of frankincense or balsam fir, they should all get about the same results, although with some minor variations. Such data would be considered to be "scientific" and "objective."

It is from objectivity that science gains its power. It is from objectivity that science obtains its universal appeal that cuts across the barriers of language, politics, and nationality. But paradoxically, while objectivity is its greatest strength, it is also its greatest weakness, because it is also objectivity that makes science incapable of dealing with most of the important aspects of human life—the aspects that bring us warmth, affection, pleasure, and happiness. Science cannot cope with the subjective. Where subjective experience has objective consequences, the consequences can be studied scientifically, but not the experiences themselves.

Scientific objectivity assumes that the observer can be, and is, separate and independent of the observation. While this is achievable to an acceptable extent in many areas of research, in the ultimate sense, it is impossible and unachievable. This is because. at some level, the consciousness of each and every human being is connected to all things, both animate and inanimate.

Raindrop and the Scientific Method

An example of a subjective experience is that of receiving a raindrop. Raindrop technique is a procedure of applying a sequence of essential oils to the back and feet according to certain prescribed modes of massage. It is discussed in Chapter Nine of Part One in this book. The technique, itself, takes about an hour.

To objectively study the response of a client one would need to take many measurements prior to, during, and after the technique was complete. These measurements could include temperature, blood pressure, height, weight, levels of perceived pain, and various tests of the blood, lymph, saliva, and urine. One would also have to make precise determinations of the chemistry of each oil used during that particular raindrop as well as exact measurements of the quantities used, etc.

Yet no matter how many objective measurements you made, they would be inadequate to describe the experience of raindrop technique as perceived by the client. Only the receiver is in a position to observe and experience, first hand, its consequences and effects—the most significant of which would be subjective and unavailable to any objective evaluation and control. What a client takes away from their experience of a raindrop is, for the most part, not describable by parameters that lend themselves to objective documentation except, perhaps, in a very crude way.

In order to establish a body of scientific data on raindrop, the experimental data would also have to be collected from a statistically sufficient number of clients, taking into consideration the variations in the manual techniques of various raindrop facilitators. Since part of the therapy delivered in raindrop technique is also a function of the electromagnetism, energy, and attitude of the facilitator, which can vary from day to day even within the same person, this would be another subjective, immeasurable, and uncontrollable aspect of the experiment.

Even if a scientist or group of scientists were able to collect all of these kinds of data in a way that was reasonably reproducible and independent of the researchers, would it really describe the experience of a raindrop session? Nevertheless, such studies could and should be made. There is much that could be learned.

Statistics as a Means to Study the Subjective

The only scientific study of raindrop technique available, as of this publication, is *A Statistical Validation of Raindrop Technique* which is a gathering of subjective data, statistically compiled and analyzed in a way that validates, in an objective way, the general safety and efficacy of the procedure. Although the data of this study are of a subjective nature, their statistical treatment in the report are according to the methods of objective science. One can apply objective methodology to subjectively derived data. Scientific studies in the fields of psychology and sociology are almost always of this nature. Some say such studies are "soft" science and some may even say they are not science at all since their results are seldom, if ever, exactly reproducible. Reproducibility is one of the measures of objective science. This is usually an achievable goal in the fields of chemistry and physics, but not in the study of life processes or human behavior, except in a statistical sense. Nevertheless, the instrumentality of the scientific method can be applied and useful data can result.

Because something is strictly scientific does not mean it is necessarily right. And because something is strictly subjective" does not mean it is necessarily wrong. We have become conditioned in our modern society to think that if something is scientific, it must be true. But don't be intimidated by science. And don't be intimidated by professionals who hide their subjectivity behind a cloak of pseudoscience. The scientific method is merely one of several approaches to establish an understanding of the nature of things and is not the most effective approach most of the time. It is extremely limited and excludes, among other things, a universe about subjective experiences and value judgments. It does not and cannot cope with such things.

While statistical science has its place as an approach to learning certain aspects of subjective phenomena, any attempt to apply the scientific method to truly understand and describe subjective experience is invalid. It would be like attempting to take blood pressure with a thermometer, to time labor contractions with a pair of scissors, or determine the attributes of an essential oil with a yard stick. In most instances, science is simply the wrong tool. What we must realize is that just because the application of the scientific method to subjective experiences is invalid does not mean that subjective experiences, themselves, are invalid. Because an experience is subjective does not make it less real.

On the Nature of Subjectivity

"Subjective" merely means that the experience has meaning only to the person involved and is beyond scientific measurement. Take eating, for example. It is almost purely a subjective experience. The way foods taste to you is your own unique experience. No one will ever quite have your experience. No one can know what a specific food tastes like to you. I know what vanilla ice cream tastes like to me, but how can I know what it tastes like to you? As a direct experience, I can only know the sensations of my own taste buds, but not yours or anyone elses.

Tasting food can be more or less objective to the extent that given a thousand people eating lemons, they would probably universally agree that they tasted sour. However, there would be many opinions as to "how sour," what constitutes the sensation of "sour," and whether or not "sour" is a taste that is "good" or "not good."

Subjective experiences are essentially yours and, as such, cannot really be shared with others. If you smell a rose, that experience is yours. You can tell it to me in words, but until I smell it for myself, I cannot know what the smell of a rose is all about. Even after we have both smelled it, we can never know just how much each of our sensations was like the other's. If it turns out that you don't like the smell of the rose while I do, your experience does not make my experience any less pleasant or less real. Contradictory subjective experiences on the part of two people cannot invalidate the experience of either.

You can apply these concepts to your relationship with your physician regarding your own body or that of your children. If you conclude or feel one way and your doctor concludes or feels another, that does not make either of you wrong, necessarily. However, as an individual, since it is your life and body, or that of your child, you have rights that the physician does not have unless you give them up. Hence, when there is a conflict of opinion between you and your health care provider, you have the right to believe in yourself first.

There is a price to be paid for this freedom. If you do not follow the doctor's words or the hospital's policies, they may threaten you with legal action to intimidate you into compliance with their will. Ultimately, you must assume the responsibility for the consequences, legal or otherwise.

You have a right to choose, for yourself and your family, what may seem to the medical profession, a wrong choice. By following your own thoughtful inclinations, when they differ from your doctor's, you are assuming more personal responsibility than when you just go along with whatever the doctor or hospital says.

In reality, the responsibility for your health, or that of your children, is totally yours regardless of who makes the decisions in your health care. If you or your child are damaged by some medical procedure, neither the doctor nor the hospital will raise your child or care for you with your iatrogenic (doctor-caused) or nosocomial (hospital-caused) disability.

Limitations of Science in Time

One of the most severe restrictions of science is that of time. Tomorrow's research cannot benefit you today. Furthermore, we can never know what scientific principles that seem reasonable now will be disproven in the future. While some scientific conclusions are more enduring than others, in the end all scientific conclusions are tentative pending the discovery of additional data. Life, the universe, and their ramifications are infinite. Science can never get around to all of it. Published scientific studies are only progress reports. None are final. When it comes down to the problems of your own personal concerns now, scientific answers may or may not be there when you need them.

If you have cancer now, you cannot wait for science to find a cure. If you are raising your family now, you cannot wait for science to tell you how to deal with your children.

You must act now, making dozens of decisions daily, with or without the help of science. Science is a good method for research, but it's a lousy method for living.

No matter how much science studies and resolves, there will always be more that has not been studied and resolved. Science deals only with the known, which, for all we can tell, will always be relatively infinitesimal when compared with the infinite unknown.

The point is this. Science cannot help you with issues it has not yet studied and you are often in a position where you cannot wait. There will never be enough time for scientists to get around to everything in our unlimited universe. If you have a problem that needs solving now, you may have to rely on methods outside of science for assistance. Furthermore, since the choice of topics to which scientists apply their profession is a human choice, full of bias. The particular topics for which you may want scientific answers may or may not ever be chosen for study.

The choices for topics for scientific research are largely motivated by potential for long-term, unlimited profit, not by the urgency of need and the magnitude of the benefits to the public. Many topics amenable to the scientific method, whose results could be of great benefit to humankind, are deliberately avoided when it appears that such research might lead to conclusions that contradict current paradigms and threaten the security of those currently entrenched in power. The scientific community is not immune to politics.

Therefore, science is limited by time in two ways: first, because there will never be enough time to get around to studying everything; and second because humans, by their prejudices, will choose not to study many issues for fear of the truth that may be revealed thereby. The American Cancer Society is an example of this. They are afraid to invest their monies in genuine research in natural cures for cancer since a variety of such remedies already exist and have already been proven to be effective anecdotally. They prefer to believe that such cures are impossible. A scientific verification of a real cancer cure could result in the dissolution and demise of their fund-raising society, its mandate having been fulfilled.

Drug companies have the same biases and fears. They invest no research into herbs and essential oils, which cannot be patented. They fear that natural remedies could actually result in wholesale recoveries from cancer among the millions of suffering people from whom they exact their lucrative monetary tributes—a steady income which flows to them for the lifetimes of the patients so long as they are never actually cured.

Experimental Error and Human Bias

Another limitation of science involves experimental errors, which are accidental, unintentional, and due to the fallibility of human endeavor. Human bias in the scientific method is also a cause for error. Efforts are generally made to minimize human bias, such as double-blind studies, etc., but bias can still creep into the final data, slanting its implications away from truth.

There is also an incidence of deliberate fraud in the forms of manipulation, and false reporting to serve the financial objectives of corporate stockholders or the grantors of monies for research. When one realizes that medical research journals and the research that takes place in medical schools are almost all backed by grants from pharmaceutical companies, it is no wonder that a large portion of so called scientific studies published in medical journals are of flawed modalities and fallacious conclusions that favor drugs as solutions to all manner of medical maladies. The ideal of objectivity in science is difficult enough to achieve even when all motivations are pure and modalities are proper. The ideal is impossible to maintain in an environment rife with conflicts of interest.

The First Law of Medical Enthusiasm

Another perplexing problem is that when valid scientific studies do demonstrate the efficacy of natural ways to deal with disease or genuine ways to prevent them outside of the allopathic/pharmaceutical model, they are usually ignored by practicing physicians and hospitals. The entrenched incumbents of the current medical system have no enthusiasm for natural remedies because, whereas they may benefit the public, they do not benefit health professionals, nor their base of power or profit.

After decades of observing the American health care system, I have noted that new ideas do not appeal to the medical community in proportion to their scientific validity nor to the extent they may bring true relief to a suffering public. They appeal in proportion to the extent they will produce profit, maintain power, and reduce responsibility to themselves. In fact, you can predict the level of enthusiasm the medical profession will have for any new therapeutic concept, procedure, drug, or tool by the following equation,

$$E = P - R$$

where E = the Enthusiasm of hospitals and/or medical associations, P = Power and/or Profit, and R = Responsibility to be assumed on the part of the hospital and/or practitioner. Routinely prescribing drugs, surgery, radiation, chemotherapy, and other standards of allopathic medicine maximizes power and profits to the health care system and minimizes its responsibilities, liabilities, and potential for successful malpractice actions. Recommendation of vitamins, essential oils, herbal medicines, natural childbirth, breastfeeding, lifestyle changes, nutrition, and other patient-controlled means for health maintenance and dealing with disease reduces profits and transfers power to the public.

Furthermore, since natural practices are not condoned by the majority of medical practitioners, it increases the burden of personal responsibility on the rare brave health care provider who does want to empower the public and who does want to do what is morally right and in the best interest of the patient.

Hence, enthusiasm on the part of medical practitioners for natural approaches is usually negative, because such approaches cause the P part of the equation (which is positive) to be a small number while causing the R part (which is negative) to be large. The result is negative enthusiasm.

(E < 0) By comparison, when a physician sells out completely to the medical mandates of his training and his political peers, there is big P and little R on the right side of the equation, thus resulting in a big positive E for enthusiasm on the left side of the equation. (E >> 0)

Take any new medical procedure that comes along and you can take this equation and predict whether that procedure will become popular or not among allopathic health care professionals and institutions. Who would ever have thought sixty or seventy years ago that cesarean sections would be preferred by obstetricians over natural childbirth, that heart bypass surgery would prevail over nutritional and lifestyle counseling, or that chemotherapy, surgery, and radiation would become the principal modalities of cancer therapy when their actual success rates are so dismally low and when natural cancer therapies already exist that have already been proven? All of this is explained by the First Law of Medical Enthusiasm: $E = P - R$.

There are a few courageous and exceptional practitioners who serve outside of this law, but they represent fewer than 2% of American physicians today.

Peer Review and Paradigm Preservation

Refereed scientific journals such as the *Journal of the American Medical Association* (JAMA), *Nature* (published from the United Kingdom), the *New England Journal of Medicine* (NEJM), and hundreds of others spanning every field of science, are supposed to contain good and valid studies only—the best products of the scientific method. Peer reviewed journals are supposed to provide the outlets for the freshest research so that scientists can present their latest results before the world-wide scientific community in a timely fashion in an ongoing basis for critique, feedback, and independent verification. Such journals are also meant to make scientific research available for others to incorporate and develop into practical applications for people at large. Yet, refereed or peer reviewed journals comprise one of the greatest obstacles to scientific progress that exists in the world.

Peer review is a good idea in theory. It is supposed to provide a gateway through which all submissions to technical journals must pass to ensure their validity and relevance. Peer review is supposed to be a filter for sloppy science. Here is how it is supposed to work. A journal editor, upon receipt of a research paper for publication, contacts an expert in the general area of the work who is designated as the principle reviewer. In turn, the principle reviewer normally appoints at least two others known to be knowledgeable in that field. In this way, at least three scientists review the paper and make recommendations to the editor for publication, revision, conditional acceptance, or rejection with details of their reasons. The author of the paper receives copies of all of the comments and suggestions of the reviewers, but not their names. The reviewers are to remain anonymous to the researcher under review.

So long as the topic of research does not challenge any fundamental concepts of science generally agreed upon by a majority of scientists or practitioners of that field, so long as the abstract and conclusions of the article support and promote the profession and/or publisher for whom that journal is meant to serve, and so long as no leaders in that field of science or professional endeavor feel politically threatened by the thrust of the submited article—then it has an excellent chance of being published whether it is good science or bad.

On the other hand, if the article is truly breaking new frontiers of scientific understanding and expanding knowledge beyond current boundaries, it has virtually no chance of being published by any so called "respected journal of science," even if its scientific methodology is impeccable, its data flawless, and its conclusions logically irrefutable.

For the most part, peer review is paradigm preservation. It is intended to maintain the status quo. It is political protection for those who have professional turfs to guard. Since the reviewers are never revealed to the researcher, peer review can be used to stop new ideas and prevent them from seeing print. As a journal referee you are also in a position to see new ideas before they are published and, if they are close to yours, you can steal them, rejecting the article you have reviewed and later publishing your own. Scientists are human and are not, in general, any more spiritual or moral than any other segment of society.

Because of the political nature of the process of peer review and the ease with which it can be corrupted, the best of science rarely gets published and the worst of science, if it serves a political or monetary purpose, has no trouble finding a publisher. The situation is exacerbated by the fact that many medical journals are financed by drug companies, who also sponsor the bulk of the medical research whose results are published in those journals. Drug companies and other purveyors of medical paraphernalia, in cooperation with their allies, the universities to whom research grants are given, have a neat buddy system where the same commercial interests control the research, the journals that publish the research, as well as the editors and reviewers who are supposed to preserve the purity of the science that gets published. This situation is why a majority of scientific research articles published in medical journals are invalid, often bordering on fraud.

A Case in Point

For example, the U.S. Congress established an Office of Technology Assessment (OTA) in the late 1970s headed by a team of honest physicians to advise them as to what proposals by medical associations, companies, and lobbyists were actually beneficial to the public and which were actually more beneficial to the medical community and pharmaceutical industry. In 1979 a big health care issue was the employment of electronic fetal monitoring (EFM) during labor. The question was whether such devices were superior to a nurse or doctor using a simple stethoscope, as had been the practice for more than a century.

The electronic fetal monitor (EFM) is a device to record fetal heart tones during labor. To use it, the laboring woman's bag of waters has to be broken with a steel electrode inserted into the birth canal and screwed into the baby's head. Breaking the protective bag of waters exposes the baby and uterus to alien microbes that can cause infections. If the infecting microbes are a virulent strain of antibiotic-resistant staphylococcus, found only in hospitals, the result is sometimes the death of the baby and/or the mother, as well. Furthermore, when screwing the sharp metal electrode into the baby's head, the intent is to place it in the scalp on top of the head, but unavoidably sometimes doctors poke out an eye or cause a permanent scar to the baby's face. This is not to mention that a steel screw in the head (or any other place in the body) is painful. Babies are sensitive to this pain, react to it, and with EFM they have to suffer it throughout many hours of labor. The lasting emotional trauma this may cause has not been studied. These are only some of the hazards intrinsic to the technology of electronic fetal monitoring.

Let's analyze the acceptance of EFM as a standard obstetrical practice by using the First Law of Medical Enthusiasm: $E = P - R$. When first introduced back in the early 1970s, doctors, nurses, and hospitals were quick to realize that having an "objective" machine that produced a paper trace of fetal heart tones throughout labor reduced their personal responsibilities (small value for R), increased their profits (large P), and increased their power (large P) in controlling the birthing process as well as power and control (more P) over mothers during labor. Thus, we can calculate that $P - R$ would have a high positive value which would equate to a high value for E, or medical enthusiasm.

Thus, by applying the First Law of Medical Enthusiasm, one could predict in advance, before any scientific studies were done, that hospitals and obstetricians would be very enthused about the prospect of using fetal monitors. True to the predictions of the First Law, in the early 1970s, hospitals, doctors, and maternity wards everywhere adopted policies to electronically monitor every laboring mother. The medical system did not wait for scientific verification. Universal EFM had become a fact without a scientific basis to justify its use. Even though it was a technology of unproven benefit, once introduced it swept the North American continent in a matter of months.

Seeing the benefits to themselves, medical researchers, largely paid by companies that made and marketed monitors, wasted no time in publishing a plethora of papers lauding the benefits of EFM and purporting to prove that EFM was superior to nurses, midwives, and doctors actually listening to the heart of an unborn baby during labor. While it was true that a more continuous record of fetal heartbeat could be obtained by an EFM than with a human ear and stethoscope, the bottom line question from a statistical point of view is this: "Does EFM actually improve outcomes?" The answer is, "No." In fact, as pointed out above, it may actually be detrimental.

In an effort to gather some unbiased and objective insight into the EFM question, in 1979 the medical investigators of U.S. Office of Technology Assessment (OTA) reviewed every scientific paper in existence throughout the world at the time (153 of them). They found that 149 of these papers were invalid science, almost all of which promoted the use of EFM. Of the four studies that were valid, only one demonstrated any benefit of EFM as measured by outcomes of baby and/or mother. Two reports found that the use of EFM was actually detrimental to the outcome of the baby and/or the mother, while the fourth study was indeterminant in its conclusions. What almost all of these studies made clear (even the invalid ones) is that using EFM would increase the rates of cesarean section—which is a very profitable (P) surgical procedure for both hospitals and surgeons. Thus, of 153 papers published in the most respected scientific and medical journals of the world, 97% were bad science. Among the 3% that were good science, justification for routine implementation of EFM in maternity wards was not to be found.

What was the outcome of these scientific findings? Was the enthusiasm (E) of doctors and hospitals dampened by these unpromising scientific results? Did the U.S. Federal Government try to intervene?

Here is what happened. The U.S. Congress did nothing while obstetricians and hospitals quickly adopted protocols for universal application of this unproven technology.

They ignored the implications of the valid data available to them and vigorously pursued a policy that every mother should receive EFM in labor, even though no benefits had been statistically demonstrated. Why did they pursue such a course, going against the facts of science? The Law of Medical Enthusiasm explains it all. $E = P - R$

Since the late 1970s, with the universal implementation of EFM by North American hospitals, in both the U.S. and Canada, cesarean rates have more than quadrupled with no improvement in maternal-child outcomes attributable to EFM nor the increased rates of maternal surgery.

Similar narratives can be told about the introduction and proliferation of hormone replacement therapy (HRT) for menopause, bypass surgery for coronary heart disease, and chemotherapy for cancer—none of which are supported by valid science. All of these are unnecessary medical modalities because, in all of these instances, more effective, non-allopathic remedies exist, but go unprescribed (and suppressed) by allopathic doctors and their partners, the drug companies and the FDA. The list of examples goes on and on. And in every instance, $E = P - R$.

Therefore, one of the greatest limits of science is that a large percent of what is published under the name of science, particularly in medicine, is bad science and not representative of the truth. It is science full of non-scientific agendas. But even more significant is the fact that when published scientific research is good and valid, it often has little or no effect on practice. When good science is made available to health care professionals, they usually ignore it and do whatever suits them, with or without a scientific basis.

Now that you understand the First Law of Medical Enthusiasm, you can answer the big question: "Given the historic, scientific and experiential evidence, including thousands of successful case histories, that demonstrate the benefits of therapeutic applications of essential oils— what level of enthusiasm on the part of the current allopathic health care system does the First Law predict?"

Would it be positive (large P small R) or negative (large R small P)? You calculate the answer.

Thomas Preston, M.D., speaking for the U.S. Office of Technology Assessment (OTA), made the following statement at an annual meeting of the American Public Health Association (APHA): "80-90% of the medical procedures which this country trusts its lives to and spends vast amounts of money on have never been proven beneficial. Most surgeons—and a good part of the medical profession in general—rely on their beliefs, and not on scientific evidence."

Good science properly applied is a good thing. But so much of the time good science is ignored or improperly applied while bad science clutters the journals, misleading both professionals and the public. The *Bible* has a warning on being misled by pseudoscience.

> Keep that which is committed to your trust, avoiding profane and vain babblings, and oppositions of science falsely so called: which some professing have erred concerning the faith. (KJV)

> Guard what has been entrusted to you. Avoid the profane chatter and contradictions of what is falsely called knowledge; by professing it some have missed the mark as regards the faith.
> (NRSV)

Two versions of the advice given in I Timothy 6:20-21. (King James–KJV and New Revised Standard–NRSV).

So What is the Answer?

We have shown that science is limited inherently, limited in time, limited by experimental error, limited by human bias, and limited in the extent that it is actually put to use when prejudice, politics, profit, and protection of prevailing paradigms come into play. It is clear from all of this that science cannot have all the answers and never will. Science alone cannot offer us adequate guidance through the various health crises, both big and small, that we experience from day to day throughout our lives. When we are in the midst of a crisis that is beyond the current models of science to address, we cannot wait for science to find answers for us when we need them now. What do we do, then, when we must make medical decisions regarding ourselves and our loved ones and science cannot help us?

First, let us develop the habit of always seeking direct advice from God, the master physician, master scientist, and provider of all that is healthy and good. But we must not wait until a crises to seek his guidance. We must develope a relationship with him by daily prayer and attunement, practicing his presence in all that we do. A great saint once said, "If you don't make God your summertime friend, he won't come in the winter of your life." It isn't exactly that he won't come, but what you must do is to develop your lines of communication with God during times of calmness and learn to hear his still quiet voice during the peacetime of daily practice. Otherwise, you may not be able to hear him during the battle din of a real emergency.

Second, let us look to nature as our teacher. Nature is permeated with God's intelligence, humbly and patiently waiting for us to seek his advice and wisdom as he speaks to us through what he has made. (Job 12:8; Romans 1:20) Let us assume that nature knows best. Learn her ways, and harmonize with her in a conscious, intelligent way always praying to God for his perfect guidance.

Thirdly, let us also follow science appropriately when good data are available and let us apply the scientific method wherever possible to test the relative merits of alternatives in health care. But let us realize that science cannot lead us to the right answers unless we lead science to the right topics for research. When presented with a firm fact that contradicts current theory, let us be willing to accept the fact and give up the theory.

Fourthly, let us also understand and recognize where the efficacy of science ceases and rely on other means to base our judgements. Don't be intimidated when what appears to be science contradicts your own true feelings in a crisis situation. Learn to trust yourself as the best judge in personal or family situations. Let us openly restore and practice our faith in our God-guided feelings and our common sense. Let us learn how to refine and develop the gift of divine intuition by practice, experience, reinforcement, and association with others that use it.

Let us also recognize and respect the natural nurturing and healing gifts that God manifests through women and the nurturing sides of men. Let us honor mothers appointed by God as natural healers for their families.

There is an intelligence and an order in our universe that already has all of the answers and to which we can directly appeal for solutions to all of life's problems—now and whenever we are in need. There is a consciousness in creation that transcends science and the senses—a source of wisdom and knowledge to which we can apply for help at any time. Its name is God. Its language is prayer. Its condition for receiving is humility. Its channel is love.

It can never be through science, as we know it today, that the optimization of health care practice will be realized in the world. Science is a powerful ally, a gift from God that can be used for good or abused for ill. God leaves that choice to us, his children.

The limits of science today are a reflection of the limits of consciousness held by today's scientists and the practitioners of professions that are supposed to be based on science. As individuals of the scientific community develop spiritually, expand their awareness, and become able and willing to see and recognize the reality of things beyond the physical that underly the manifested universe, then the limitations of the scientific method will become less constrained. Even the definition of "objectivity" will be modified to include experiences deemed "subjective" today. We won't elaborate on that here, but the concept of "inner objectivity" is discussed in many books, including *Transcendental Physics* by Edward Close.

The point is this. Until scientists learn to pray and commune with God, in humility, they will lack the necessary awareness to perceive a more complete vision of the true nature of reality. Until scientists develop their spiritual gifts along with their intellectual gifts, the methods of science will remain limited and incapable of discovering the true nature of this world in which we dwell. The day must come when students of mathematics and the sciences will be educated in institutions that offer a balance between cerebral education and spiritual discipline. Then, and only then, will a true science come into being, the fruit of which is the truth of God.

♥ ARTICLE TWO
BIOTRANSMUTATION
OF ELEMENTS

During the Middle Ages (500–1450 A.D.) alchemists labored in their laboratories on a quest to discover three things: 1. An elixir of eternal youth, 2. A cure for all diseases, and 3. A method to transmute base metals (like tin, lead, and iron) into precious gold. It was from these medieval motivations that the science of modern chemistry was born. The word, "alchemy," stems from the ancient Egyptian word, *chemi,* which referred to "knowledge of secret, hidden, and obscure things." *Chemi* was later adopted into the Arabic language as the word *al-kimiya,* where "*al*" is the Arabic article, "the," and "*kimiya*" means "pouring together to form a juice or potion." The English word, alchemy, thus comes to us from Egypt via Arabia. The science of chemistry derives its name from alchemy by dropping the "al."

By modern definitions and standards, the practice of alchemy was not an application of the scientific method, but more of a ritualistic application of superstitious arts. The goals of alchemy were never achieved by alchemists and have been all but abandoned by today's scientists who consider them to be impractical and/or unachievable.

Nevertheless, in the back of their minds, but not necessarily admitted to their colleagues, some scientists still entertain the notions of the ancient alchemists that, perhaps, there really is an elixir of youth, a universal remedy for disease, and/or a means of transmuting the elements, one into another—including base metal into gold.

In this chapter we will discover that with respect to transmutation of the elements, the alchemists of old were closer to the truth than they ever realized.

The Chickens of Brittany

On the shores of northwestern France, in the province of Brittany, a few years before the start of World War I, a young boy by the name of Louis Kervran, made an interesting observation of his father's chickens. They lived in a geologic terrain that was devoid of calcium and the chickens were not fed any calcium supplements, yet they laid eggs daily with calcium shells. He also wondered how they acquired the calcium needed for their bones and beaks.

The underlying bedrock and their outcrops in that region of Brittany are mostly granites and the soils are composed of the decomposition products of granite. This includes certain clays, grains of feldspar, silica sand, and small flakes of mica—none of which contain calcium. Louis noticed that the chickens selectively ate the mica, vigorously pecking the mineral flecks from the ground when exposed following a rain. The presence of mica on the land surface is easy to spot in bright sunshine since its flat sided crystals sparkle in sunlight like thousands of tiny mirrors. Louis also noted that when his mother dressed the chickens for a family meal, their gizzards contained grains of sand and feldspar, but not mica. "What happened to the mica?" he thought.

Louis later became a high official in the French government, a research chemist, an author of many scientific publications, and a lecturer at several European universities. But he did not discover the answer to his chicken-calcium conundrum until after 1955, when he was 50 years old. This was after he had several other experiences that could not be explained by conventional science.

The Case of the Mystery Monoxide

Chickens were not the only thing that aroused his boyhood curiosity. In the public school which Louis attended, heat in the winter was provided by a rudimentary stove made of cast iron. When the fire began to roar and the hot stove began to glow red, everyone would begin to complain of headaches. The teacher explained that the headaches were due to carbon monoxide (CO). The vents regulating oxygen supply to the stove would then be closed, the temperature of the hot iron would cool, and the headaches would disappear.

What puzzled young Louis was how a fast-burning stove could produce carbon monoxide when production of CO was thought to be the result of a slow-burning situation where oxygen supply was limited? Furthermore, if there was CO being produced inside the stove, how could it leak into the room when the air flow was all rushing into the stove and up the flue into the atmosphere outside? None of the teacher's explanations made sense to him. What remained a fact was that a red hot stove could result in carbon monoxide poisoning and teachers and students needed to be cautious in keeping a wood stove below certain temperatures for their own safety.

Later, in 1935, as a government scientist involved with the environmental safety of French workers, Louis was assigned to investigate a mystery. A welder had been overcome with carbon monoxide (CO) poisoning, yet no carbon monoxide gas could be detected anywhere in the air in the vicinity of where he had worked and died. Yet, an autopsy left no doubt that his blood contained the deadly gas and that it was the cause of his demise. The mystery remained unsolved for more than twenty years. Meanwhile, more French welders died in the same way while other deaths were reported among welders in Russia, Germany, and other European countries—all mortalities from CO asphyxiation with no detectable source for the CO.

In 1955, Kervran ordered the blood to be tested on other welders, still alive, and found that they all had dangerously high levels of CO gas in their blood, but not enough to cause death. Yet every effort to find the source of CO in the air breathed by the welders as they applied their torches found nothing. Kervran could only conclude that the source of the CO was endogenous, formed internally inside of the welders. They had all inhaled air free of carbon monoxide. Therefore, the fatal gas had been created inside their lungs and/or their blood by some heretofore unknown biological process. This conclusion was a major departure from classical science.

Here is the problem. The air they inhaled contained plenty of oxygen, which comprises half of the CO molecule, but where did the carbon come from? Why, how, and where, did such a carbon/oxygen reaction occur? Was elemental carbon being created at the site of the alveoli in the lungs? Was there a catalyst for such a phenomenon, an enzyme previously unsuspected and previously unknown?

Challenging Lavoisier

Remembering his childhood dissatisfaction with his teacher's explanations for CO formation from a red hot stove in the school room, as well as the unsolved puzzle of the chickens who seemed to manufacture their own calcium, Kervran eventually realized that to solve the CO crisis with the welders he would have to step outside of the paradigm of normal chemistry and physics and prove a case for the creation of new elements by biological processes involving reactions within the nuclei of atoms. This would be a proposal deemed scientifically impossible by his colleagues. He also knew that to suggest such a radical idea would threaten his professional credibility and, perhaps, his career.

The fundamental unchallenged doctrine of chemistry, as a science, had long been based on Lavoisier's Law, articulated centuries ago, in the 1700s, and discussed in Chapter Three, Part One, of this book. In chemical reactions, the prevailing wisdom had always been that "Nothing is lost. Nothing is created. Everything is transformed." That is to say, in chemistry, no elements are created and no elements are destroyed. A carbon or an oxygen atom may move from one molecule to another, forming different compounds or uniting with atoms of its own kind, but it still remains a carbon or an oxygen atom.

Lavoisier's theorem that "Matter can be neither created nor destroyed," was not something one would want to challenge lightly. Within the bounds of chemistry, Lavoisier's postulate continues to be true and has been proven right, over and over again, by countless experiments for more than 200 years. To suggest otherwise would be to make a fool of oneself in the eyes of the scientific community.

However, outside of the field arbitrarily defined as classical chemistry, matter was created and destroyed by nuclear reactions such as natural radioactive decay, nuclear fusion in the stars, and the creation of new elements by high-energy bombardment with atomic particles. But these phenomena had been delegated to the realm of nuclear physics (also called nuclear chemistry)—not normal chemistry. In the experiences of physicists, nuclear reactions that resulted in transmutations of elements, or their destruction and transformation into energy, were all high energy processes, far too intense to take place within living matter.

The unanimous consensus among life scientists was that nuclear processes never took place as an integral part of any living form. Biochemists, biophysicists, biologists, and medical doctors were all in agreement on that.

Blasphemy and Heresy

If Kervran's hunches were right, he was about to commit a blasphemy and a heresy which would expose him to the possibility of ridicule, professional ostracism, and excommunication from the church of science.

In grappling with the deadly problem of monoxide poisoning among welders, Kervran wrote, "Notwithstanding the current respect for official paradigms, there were nonetheless many people who had met death by carbon monoxide intoxication. I decided to cross the Rubicon and undertook a long series of experiments. I abandoned my long-held attachment to the traditional tenets of science concerning the invariance of matter and sought to confirm or nullify my hypothesis about the real cause of death, intending to concentrate only on results, whatever they might be."

These are the courageous words of a true scientist and true servant of humanity. Risking everything, he set out dauntlessly in search of the truth, whatever and wherever that may be—regardless of the personal or professional price he may be required to pay.

Kervran's revolutionary findings brought predictably violent opposition from many entrenched leaders of the scientific community, but they also brought accolades and approval from the scientists open enough and insightful enough to recognize the truth and genius of his work. Fortunately for Kervran, and for the world, he was able to keep his high position as a scientist for the French government and was able, through that position, to obtain unique privilege, financing, and assistance for his research endeavors from many laboratories, universities, and top scientists of his day. His research has ultimately led to a new and exciting paradigm that is neither chemistry, biology, nor physics, but something new and heretofore unknown in the field of science.

Kervran was to discover that transmutations of the elements is a routine and daily process in all living forms, including human beings. The processes, energy transformations, and reactions between matter that constitute life for all plants, animals, and microorganisms cannot be fully explained by chemistry, physics, and the paradigms of material science as we know them today. Adequate descriptions of living organisms must go well beyond chemistry and physics.

This is a major paradigm shift for biologists and biochemists to swallow since their science has long been based on the belief that life is chemistry and can be completely described and explained by chemistry. Transmuting elements, a process essential to all life, is not traditional chemistry. Neither is it physics as physics is usually defined. Kervran called it *"Transmutations Biologiques,"* in French. In English we can call the new field "Biological Transmutation" or, simply, "Biotransmutation."

The Case of the Mystery Monoxide Solved

In the instances of carbon monoxide poisoning from red hot wood stoves and welding torches applied to sheets of iron, Kervran and his colleagues eventually established the following explanation which has been experimentally proven to be correct and whose understanding and application has resulted in no more deaths to welders.

The atmosphere we breathe is mostly nitrogen (about 80%) and only about 20% oxygen. Nitrogen is necessary to life inasmuch as proteins and amino acids cannot be manufactured without it. Yet atmospheric nitrogen is not directly available to most living creatures. As human beings, we breathe it in and breathe it out without any chemical reactions or absorption into our bodies. We acquire some of our essential nitrogen by eating plants that contain it, acquired with the help of nitrogen-fixing bacteria in the soil. We also receive nitrogen from meat, fish, fowl, and dairy products, but the ultimate transfer of nitrogen from the atmosphere into the biosphere is through the agency of microbial activity.

A typical atom of nitrogen (N) has 7 protons, 7 electrons, 7 neutrons, and a mean atomic weight (A.W.) of 14.01 amu. (See Table Seventy-One on the next page.) However, nitrogen never occurs in nature as a single atom. Atmospheric nitrogen is always in the form of a diatomic molecule composed of two N atoms with the formula of N_2, consisting of a pair of N atoms joined side by side, N–N.

In the excerpts from the Periodic Table on the next page (Table Seventy-One) notice that nitrogen (N) falls in between carbon (C) and oxygen (O), which differ from nitrogen by one proton and one electron. This is designated by their atomic numbers in the tops of the boxes. The atomic number of an element is merely the number of protons (or electrons) in an atom of that element. Take a proton and an electron away from an N atom (#7) and you get a C atom (#6). Add a proton and an electron to an N atom (#7) and you get an O atom (#8). One proton with one electron paired up by themselves is a hydrogen (H) atom whose atomic number is 1. (See Table One.) Hence, nitrogen, and all elements of the periodic table, are different from their neighbors on either side by one hydrogen atom.

What Kervran discovered and repeatedly verified with a

Table Seventy-One
Selected Elements from the Periodic Table*

11	12
Na	**Mg**
22.99	24.31

19	20
K	**Ca**
39.10	40.08

6. C - Carbon
7. N - Nitrogen
8. O - Oxygen
11. Na - Sodium
12. Mg - Magnesium
14. Si - Silicon
15. P - Phosphorus
16. S - Sulfur
19. K - Potassium
20. Ca - Calcium
25. Mn - Manganese
26. Fe - Iron

6	7	8
C	**N**	**O**
12.01	14.01	16.00
14	15	16
Si	**P**	**S**
28.09	30.97	32.07

25	26
Mn	**Fe**
54.94	55.85

6
C
12.01

— Atomic Number = # of Protons in Nucleus of an Atom
— Chemical Symbol
— Mean Atomic Weight (A.W.) in amu's (atomic mass units)
A.W. = # of Protons + # Neutrons in Nucleus of an Atom

* See Table One, Chapter Three, page 82, for the complete Periodic Table.

team of scientists and engineers between 1955 and 1959 was that when air, containing diatomic nitrogen (N_2) comes into contact with iron heated to at least 400° C (752° F) glowing red, the nuclei of the two nitrogen atoms move closer to one another. This is in response to a resonance that is created by the infrared and visible spectrum emmitted from the incandescent iron. A molecule of diatomic nitrogen has a specific and known frequency and normal distance between its two nuclei of 1.12 Å (where Å is an angstrom unit, a tiny distance equal to one hundred millionth of a centimeter or 0.00000001 cm). It takes 250 million Å to equal 1 inch. The resonance of the hot iron pushes the two N nuclei closer to a distance of 1.09 Å, which is a state of higher energy. At this point, we still have nitrogen in the air.

When the welder breathes this energized, activated nitrogen into his or her lungs, a biological transmutation takes place at the contact with the alveoli and the pulmonary blood. A proton and an electron (one H atom) is transferred from one N atom to the other. Now, instead of a diatomic molecule composed of two nitrogen atoms (N_2) we have a new molecule composed of one carbon (C) and one oxygen (O)—a toxic and deadly molecule of CO. One of the N atoms has lost a proton and an electron to become a C atom while the other N atom has gained a proton and an electron to become an O atom. The normal distance between the nuclei of a C atom and an O atom in a molecule of carbon monoxide is 1.09 Å, the distance to which the two N atoms had been pushed by the influence of the incandescent iron. The actual transfer of a hydrogen atom (H) from one N atom to the other was accomplished in the lungs via an enzyme. The transmutation from diatomic nitrogen to carbon monoxide can be written as an equation as follows:

$$N_2 = {}_7N + {}_7N = {}_6C + {}_8O = CO$$

where the subscripts to the left of N, C and O represent the atomic numbers (number of protons) in atoms of the corresponding elements. Notice that the protons add up equally on both sides of the equation: $7 + 7 = 6 + 8 = 14$. In this example, the conversion was first catalyzed by the heated iron and then finalized by an enzymatic biological process within the body of the welder.

Chemistry, as discussed in Chapter Three, is the science of the displacement of electrons situated in the peripheral layers of atoms. It is the science of molecules, not of the nuclei of the atoms.

Physics is the science of energy transformations including those resulting from nuclear reactions within atoms. However, the nuclear reactions studied under the banner of physics involve no biological processes and all take place at energy levels too high to be part of a living process.

Biology is the science of living things. Biochemists say, "Life is chemistry," and espouse the belief that all living processes are explainable by the laws of chemistry. The digestion of food, the contraction of a muscle, the healing of a broken bone—it all comes down to interactions among chemicals that follow Lavoisier's Law—or so they believe. Biologists see no need for nuclear reactions or elemental transmutations to explain life processes. Doctors and other health professionals, along with nutritionists and agronomists, all agree and practice accordingly.

There is nothing wrong with defining (or restricting) chemistry, physics, and biology in these ways, since definitions are human constructions and largely arbitrary anyhow. It is only wrong to conclude that the processes we call life fall within these man-made definitions. It is invalid to conclude that healing, the actions of essential oils, and the life and spirit of humankind can be circumscribed by the limited viewpoints that define these sciences.

Kervran has discovered a new field that is not chemistry, since it involves the nuclei of atoms and involves phenomena outside the scope of Lavoisier's Law. Neither is it physics inasmuch as a biological process is necessary to complete a given transmutation. Physicists and nuclear chemists are naturally skeptical of Kervran's work because he has discovered nuclear processes occuring within normal living organisms producing conditions that they have thus far failed to achieve in a lab except by high energy particle acceleration or extreme temperatures. The dream of "cold fusion"—nuclear exchanges at low temperatures—has never been accomplished in a laboratory, even though millions of dollars and many years of research have been expended toward the effort by many scientists. The difference is the presence of life.

The laws of physics and chemistry do not apply to living processes the same way they do to the dead processes of a lab or to the inorganic world around us. There are two ways to crack a safe: you can apply high energy technology and blow it up with dynamite; or you can simply know the combination, requiring minimal energy. Nuclear transformations in sterile, lifeless physics labs, or other environments devoid of life, are only possible with considerable expenditures of energy. But the intelligence innate to living organisms knows the combinations to the hearts of atoms. Thus, Kervran's work leads us to a new field of science exploring a heretofore unknown phenomenon requiring a new name. Biotransmutation is the intersection of three classical fields: chemistry, biology, and physics.

By stepping outside the prevailing paradigm, Kervran was able to solve the deadly problem of the mystery monoxide for the cast iron stove in his early school as well as for the red hot welder's plate. As a result, there have been no deaths among French welders from this cause since 1959.

Chickens Without Calcium

When young Kervran pondered the puzzle of chickens with no calcium in their soil, water, or food who yet laid calcium coated eggs and had healthy bones, he also noticed that they selectively ate mica, carefully pecking out the mineral flakes exposed on the ground following a rain. He wondered if there was a connection between the mica and the calcium, which seemed to materialize from nowhere. But the connection was not obvious since mica contains no calcium.

Muscovite mica is a mineral found in igneous rocks that occurs in thin flat sheets or flakes. It is composed of potassium (K), Aluminum (Al), Silicon (Si), Oxygen (O), and Hydrogen (H). Its formula is: $KAl_3Si_3O_{10}(OH)_2$. Muscovite, or muscovy glass (also called isinglass) is a light tan transparent mineral, used to make fireproof windows in wood stoves and applied as an insulator in electrical equipment.

What Kervran and others have verified by a number of experiments is that there is a biological process within chickens that can transmute potassium into calcium.

Take another look at Table Seventy-One and notice the cluster of four elements on the left side extracted from the Periodic Table. Notice that potassium (K) and calcium (Ca) are adjacent and that the atomic number (number of protons) in a $_{19}K$ atom is 19 and in a $_{20}Ca$ atom is 20. In other words, the difference between them is only a hydrogen atom ($_1H$). Apparently, with the help of appropriate enzymes natural to their systems, chickens can make their own calcium from potassium through biotransmutation.

In experiments performed by Kervran, and later verified by other researchers, chickens were deprived of both Ca and K whereupon they began to lay soft-shelled eggs. When given Ca supplements (and no K), their eggs had normal hard shells containing Ca. The surprise finding was when they were given K supplements (and no Ca), their eggs were still normal—composed of Ca. The $_{19}K$ had been transformed into $_{20}Ca$.

Thus, God has designed his creatures to make the minerals they need from what is available (within limits) when they are not provided by their natural environments nor in their diets. One cannot generalize, however. Not all living creatures can make their own calcium.

The biotransmutation equation for turning K into Ca is as follows:

$$_{19}K + {_1}H = {_{20}}Ca$$

Notice that the number of protons is the same on both sides of the equation, $19 + 1 = 20$, but the elements are different. As for a source of H atoms, plants and animals can get all they want from water, H_2O.

It All Comes from Hydrogen

The idea of transmutation of elements is not new. Astrophysicists have long known that the elements that make up the stars, including our sun, consists almost entirely of hydrogen (H) and helium (He), the two lightest elements—atomic numbers one ($_1H$) and two ($_2He$). All heavier elements are formed from H and He by some form of nuclear fusion. (See Periodic Table on page 82.)

Hydrogen ($_1H$) consists of one electron (e) and one proton (p). Fuse these together and you have a neutron (n). Thus, neutrons are formed by the collapse of a hydrogen atom.

$$_1H = e + p = n$$

Helium consists of two electrons and two protons plus two neutrons. Thus, one helium atom can be constructed by the fusion of four hydrogen atoms, as follows:

$$4(_1H) = {_1}H + {_1}H + {_1}H + {_1}H = 2(_1H) + 2n = {_2}He$$

One $_2$He atom plus one $_1$H atom can make one lithium ($_3$Li) atom. Two $_2$He atoms can fuse and be transmuted into berylium ($_4$Be). Three $_2$He atoms can fuse and be transmuted into carbon ($_6$C). Four He atoms can fuse and be transmuted into oxygen ($_8$O). . . and so forth. Thus all of the 92 natural elements were made from simple hydrogen and helium, the stuff stars are made of.

Although they do not yet fully understand the manner in which these fusions and transmutations take place, scientists generally agree on the idea that this is how our physical universe of 92 natural elements was formed and they agree that in some way this creation of heavier elements is still taking place in the stars. Where scientists today do not agree is that transmutations of one element into another continue to take place on a daily, ongoing basis, as a natural biological process essential to life.

The Dance of the Daisies

In order to grow an attractive lawn, you need calcium in the soil. When soils become deficient in calcium, daisies spontaneously spring up. Daisies require no calcium in their soil. Experienced gardeners know that when daisies appear, it is time to add more calcium.

In a number of experiments, scientists have analyzed the elemental composition of daisies and in every analysis they found calcium in the plant. This was found to be true even when there was no calcium whatsoever in the soil where the daisies grew. When daisies grow in calcium poor soil, each year as they die and contribute their wilted stalks and leaves to the soil, they gradually increase the calcium content, thus enriching the soil of its deficient elements.

Apparently, just like chickens, daisies can make their own calcium. But they don't necessarily need potassium to do it. There are several other elements that can be biotransmuted into calcium.

Making Your Own Calcium

Calcium is the fifth most abundant element in the crust of the earth (See Table Four), exceeded only by oxygen, silicon, aluminum, and iron. Even so, mineral calcium as it occurs in natural soils and groundwater, is virtually unassimilatable by humans. Organic compounds of calcium are more absorbable, but it turns out that the best way to assimilate calcium into the essential biological processes of your body may not be to simply take calcium, itself.

There are at least three ways that have been documented for plants and animals to make their own calcium from other elements. Look again at Table Seventy-One (or the Periodical Table on page 82). You have already noticed that $_{19}K$, just to the left of $_{20}Ca$, only lacks one $_1H$ atom to become Calcium. Also notice that magnesium $_{12}Mg$ is directly above $_{20}Ca$ and only lacks 8 protons (electrons) of being a Ca atom. An atom with 8 protons is an oxygen atom. Combine $_8O$ with $_{12}Mg$ as a biotransmutation and you get $_{20}Ca$. The equation is as follows:

$$_{12}Mg + {_8O} = {_{20}Ca}$$

Notice that the number of protons is the same on both sides of the equation, $12 + 8 = 20$, but the elements are different. As for a source of O atoms, plants and animals can get all they want from water, H_2O, as well as from air.

Return to Table Sixty-Seven once again and this time notice silicon (Si) which has 14 protons per atom. Then notice Carbon (C) which has 6 protons per atom. Here is another means to get calcium. Combine $_{14}Si$ with $_6C$ as a biotransmutation and you get $_{20}Ca$. The equation is as follows:

$$_{14}Si + {_6C} = {_{20}Ca}$$

Notice once again that the number of protons is the same on both sides of the biotransmutation equation, $14 + 6 = 20$, with calcium the resultant new element. And as a source of C atoms, every living body is full of them and, if they are lacking, C atoms can be made from N atoms by subtracting an H atom. They can also be made from Si atoms by subtracting an atom of O from the silicon.

Thus God has provided at least three ways for plants and animals to receive their necessary calcium when calcium, itself, is unavailable. In fact, the biotransmuted forms of calcium are much more readily utilized by our bodies than that which is directly available in nature.

None of these biotransmutations are possible in a scientific laboratory dedicated to pure chemistry or pure physics. It takes living intelligence at cellular levels to accomplish these feats.

Calcium is Not Always the Answer

The biotransmutations for calcium just given have implications in the fields of nutrition, medicine, and the maintenance of health. For centuries it has been known by herbalists that regular intake of horsetail helps prevent bone loss and will speed up the repair of broken bones. Yet horsetail contains little or no calcium.

What it does contain is rich amounts of silica. Apparently, the Si atoms in horsetail can be converted into Ca atoms by the body. Even some physicians have come to recognize the value of taking horsetail supplements in healing bone fractures.

However, the body cannot transmute just any old silicon into calcium. In fact, ingesting inorganic silicon will cause decalcification of the bones.

Natural sources of both Si and Mg, such as various herbs, have long been known for their benefits in other bone and joint ailments, such as rheumatism, osteoporosis, and arthritis. A diet rich in calcium does not necessarily strengthen bone or repair joints or build teeth. Children on normal diets, including calcium-rich milk and cheese, have been known to suffer delayed dental growth until placed on diets of fruits, meat, and vegetables (with no dairy products). Within weeks, their tooth development was restored to normal.

Fresh green leafy vegetables contain significant amounts of silicon. In fact, cows excrete more calcium than they ingest and can live on a diet of various grasses rich in silicon and poor in calcium. Pregnant and breast-feeding mothers would also be wise to eat plenty of fresh produce for its silicon in order to meet their babies' need for calcium without any decalcification of their own bodies.

Another secret to healthy calcium content in your body is magnesium (Mg). Magnesium is the core element around which the chlorophyll molecule is built. Eating any green vegetable is consuming magnesium. Notice that magnesium is one of the biotransmutable sources of calcium. ($_{12}Mg + _8O = _{20}Ca$). But more than that, it seems that without the presence of magnesium most organisms cannot properly utilize calcium. Looking at Table Seventy-One, we see a foursome of elements—Sodium ($_{11}Na$), Magnesium ($_{12}Mg$), Potassium ($_{19}K$), and Calcium ($_{20}Ca$). These four vital elements must all maintain a delicate balance to maintain a healthy, functioning body. They are all close to one another in the Periodic Table, differing by either an H atom or an O atom, each biotransmutable into any of the other three. The necessary balance between these in our bodies is maintained, to a great extent, by continuous and daily biotransmutations—a process beyond chemistry—and as yet unrecognized by nutritionists and health care professionals.

A Word About Silicon

Silicon is the second most abundant element on the surface of the earth, comprising 26% of the earth's crust. Also known as silica, it is an element found in all the sands of all the beaches and in all the clays of all the soils of the world. As discussed in Chapter Three, silicon (Si) is necessary for our bones, teeth, blood vessels, hair, skin, and nails. As discussed in the previous section, silicon ($_{14}Si$) also plays a role, through biotransmutation, in the calcium needs of our bodies.

The chemistry of essential oils consists entirely of carbon compounds. If you look at the Periodic Table (Table One, page 82) you see that $_{14}Si$ is directly below $_6C$. They are in the same chemical family. They have the same valence. While carbon is unique in its ability to form the chains and rings that comprise the skeletal structures of organic molecules, silicon possesses many of the same properties. Si can make chains and rings, too, as well as sheets and various three-dimensional shapes to form a variety of crystals. All of modern electronics, including the chips that make cell phones and computers, depend on silicon compounds—the operational ingredient of virtually all commercial semiconductors.

Silicon is the essential element in making glass, china dishes, and ceramics, as well the most common element found in precious stones and crystals. Crystals of silicon compounds have the capability of resonating with energies beyond the physical to bring healing to our bodies. In vitreous form, long chains of silicon compounds make fiber glass and conduits for fiber optics while flat sheets of silicon compounds make plate glass. The flat flaky transparent chips of mica, eaten by Kervran's chickens, are compounds, not only of potassium ($_{19}K$) which the chickens turned into calcium ($_{20}Ca$) by adding a hydrogen ($_1H$), but also of silicon ($_{14}Si$) which the chickens could have also biotransmuted into $_{20}Ca$ by adding a $_6C$ atom.

Elemental silicon ($_{14}Si$), itself, is formed by the transmutation of a carbon atom ($_6C$) by the addition of an oxygen atom ($_8O$). While carbon is absolutely essential to all living forms as we know them, silicon may be more important to our bodily functions than we currently appreciate, because it biotransmutes between carbon and calcium, and perhaps other elements like phosphorus (P), which are vital to life.

The Mysteries of Potassium

The balance between potassium (K) and sodium (Na) in your body fluids and tissues is vital to life and health. Too much potassium causes electrical dysfunctioning of the heart and can lead to heart attack and death. On the other hand, the heart and body cannot function when K is too low.

A major mystery, thus far unexplained by biologists and biochemists, is the fact that more sodium (Na) is absorbed into cells than is excreted. Meanwhile, more potassium (K) comes out of the cells than is taken in. What happens to the sodium and where does the excess potassium come from?

Attempting to find an answer within Lavoisier's Law has been impossible. Rather than admit that chemistry as it is presently defined has no explanation, biochemists simply say that their analyses have been too inaccurate to identify the discrepancies, so far, and that at some future time, when technology improves enough, they will find an explanation for the K-Na imbalances within current paradigms.

A series of carefully controlled experiments in the Sahara desert were performed on men working for an oil company under extreme heat. They drank lots of water and consumed quantities of sodium as table salt (NaCl). Their sweat evaporated so fast that their skin was always completely dry. It was initially thought that this evaporation was what kept them cool enough to stand the heat so well as they did. However, some anomalies came to light in the analysis of their intake and outtake of salts and fluids.

For one thing, they excreted less sodium than they were ingesting while they excreted more potassium than they consumed. Furthermore, in calculating the calories of heat dissipated by the evaporation of their water intake, it was significantly insufficient to produce the cooling they actually experienced.

It was found that their bodies were converting sodium (Na) into potassium (K) by biotransmutation, which not only explained the surplus of K excreted and the shortage of Na, but also explained their healthy regulation of body heat.

Look at Table Seventy-One and note that sodium ($_{11}$Na) is directly above potassium ($_{19}$K). There are 8 protons difference between the two. In other words, they differ by one oxygen ($_8$O) atom. By combining an Na atom with an O atom through the process of biotransmutation, you get a K atom. This process is endothermal. It absorbs heat. The equation is as follows:

$$_{11}Na + {_8}O + heat = {_{19}}K$$

Again, notice that the number of protons is the same on both sides of the biotransmutation equation, $11 + 8 = 19$, with potassium the resultant new element. In this case, heat was necessary which was absorbed from the oil worker's body, thus cooling him. Measurements of the excess potassium and calculations of the cooling afforded by this biotransmutation proved that the ability of these men to work unprotected in the hot desert sun and keep their bodies at a safe temperature was not only the evaporation of sweat, but necessitated the endothermic conversion of Na into K. The value of sodium salt in a desert culture is so great it is sometimes used as money, a medium of exchange like gold. Its mechanism of cooling is biotransmutation characterized by the disappearance of Na, the appearance of K, and the consumption of O.

This finding offers an explanation of why ingesting salty vegetable broth or chicken soup when we are sick will lower a fever.

Another observation made in the Sahara experiment was that the men excreted 320 mg more calcium every day than what they ingested. If the excess calcium would have come from their bones and other body parts, they would all have been crippled in a short time. Since they remained strong and healthy, other elements eaten with their food and drink must have been biotransmuted into Ca.

Seeds and Sprouts

Numerous experiments on seeds and their germinated sprouts have found that the amount of calcium in the sprout is greater than what was in the seed even when the seed was germinated in a medium without calcium.

If you have access to a chemistry laboratory, you could perform such an experiment on your own that will verify the biotransmutation process. Take a set of 200 seeds of wheat or oats. Divide into two equal parts of 100 seeds each. Analyze one set for calcium content. Take the other and germinate them in an environment without calcium in the water or soil. Then measure the calcium content of the germinated plant and compare.

The data from one such experiment reported by Kervran showed a 3.34 times increase in calcium for wheat and a 4.51 increase in calcium for the oats. When rye seed was used, there was no increase in Ca. Not all plants can make their own calcium.

More than a dozen studies have compared the content of phosphorus (P) in seeds compared to germinated plants of wheat, vetch, lentils, and sunflowers. It was found that P content was always less in the sprouted plant than in the original seed. Some of the missing P was accounted for by the biotransmutation into sulfur (S).

Again, looking at Table Seventy-One, we see that phosphorus ($_{15}P$) is only one hydrogen atom ($_1H$) short of sulfur ($_{16}S$). The biotransmutation equation would be:

$$_{15}P + {}_1H = {}_{16}S$$

Here, again, the protons add up to the same number on both sides of the equation with different elements on both sides.

Compost, Apricots, and Worms

An average earthworm ingests 1/10 of a gram of earth per second as they burrow through the soil. This amounts to 3 tons per year per worm. Every gardener knows that earthworms are good for the soil. Agronomists have attributed this to the worms aerating the soil with their tunnels and their bringing fresh mineral material to the surface from depth. They also point out that the glands of the worm also excrete calcium carbonate ($CaCO_3$) which raises the pH of the soil, making it more permeable and suitable for growth. But these are not the only reasons earthworms are good for your garden.

The fact is that what goes into the front of the worm is not the same as what comes out the back. The difference is not just chemical. It is elemental. The excrement of earthworms has been measured to be 5x richer in nitrogen (N), 2x richer in calcium (Ca), 2.5x richer in magnesium (Mg), 7x richer in phosphorus (P), and 11x richer in potassium (K) than the soil it takes into its mouth. Only biotransmutation could do this.

It has also been found that the microorganisms at work in a compost heap create new elements not present in the original material contributed to the pile.

Dried fruits also acquire new elements and lose old ones through biotransmutation. Dehydration from plums into prunes, grapes into raisins, cranberries into craisins®, and fresh apricots into dried fruit is more than the simple loss of water. New elements are formed, biotransmuted from the original elements of the fresh fruit.

Fallowing the Land

Allowing land to lie fallow and unfarmed is another example of biotransmutation. When tons of harvest are removed from cropland every year, how does the soil replenish its stores of essential nutrients for next year's crop? A typical experience of those that till the land is that, unless regularly replenished in some way, it will produce less and less in time unless measures are taken to restore its mineral nutrients. God had a solution for this problem expressed in the *Old Testament* where the Hebrews were instructed to leave the land fallow every seventh year.

> "The Lord spoke to Moses, saying . . . Six years you shall sow your field, and six years you shall prune your vineyard, and gather in their yield; but in the seventh year there shall be a sabbath of complete rest for the land, a sabbath for the Lord. You shall not sow your field or prune your vineyard. You shall not reap the aftergrowth of your harvest or gather the grapes of your unpruned vine. It shall be a year of complete rest for the land."
>
> Leviticus 25:1-5

Farmers for thousands of years have known that when land loses its fertility, leaving it fallow, unplanted, and unharvested for a time will restore its mineral losses. Agricultural experts have long explained the restored fertility by wind, rain, birds, and animals bringing minerals from outside to replenish the soil. But these opinions are not based on actual measurement or scientific experimentation.

What has been found is that the microorganisms in the soil perform feats of biotransmutation during the fallow years, turning the available elements into those that are absent or in short supply, thus restoring balance to the soil.

When farmers use chemical fertilizers, herbicides, and pesticides on the soil, they kill the living organisms of the earth, thus destroying its capability for natural regeneration via biotransmutation. The capability for natural regeneration can be restored by the cessation of chemicals and inorganic fertilizers and the application of live manures and composts.

Iron or Manganese? Which Should I Take?

Many stone monuments eventually become streaked with black stains consisting of manganese (Mn) compounds. Analyses of some of these monuments find virtually no manganese in the stone, but find, instead, abundant stores of iron (Fe). Iron ($_{26}$Fe) is only one hydrogen atom away from manganese ($_{25}$Mn). (See Table Seventy-One.) It has been concluded that it is the iron in the stone that has been biotransmuted into manganese via microorganisms according to the following equation:

$$_{26}\text{Fe} - {}_1\text{H} = {}_{25}\text{Mn}$$

The bacteria that turn iron into manganese have already been put to practical use by some mining companies. They use them to enrich iron ore into commercial quantities of manganese.

Manganese levels in the human body have been closely related to iron levels. It appears that the human organism contains enzymes which allow iron to change into manganese and vice versa in order to maintain a healthy balance. So what do you need in your diet? More iron? More manganese? Or both?

Boron in Apples, Germanium in Beans

There are traces of cadmium and fluorine in coffee, but are these elements always in the soil or are could they also have been manufactured by the coffee plant via biotransmutation? Have you ever wondered how it is that you are supposed to be able to metabolize boron from apples, iron from peaches, magnesium from bananas, nickel from chocolate, vanadium from radishes, germanium from beans, selenium from broccoli, etc.? Is it because these plants selectively choose and filter certain elements from the soil, water, and air, and concentrate them in their tissues? Or is there more than chemistry going on here?

For example, if you grew apple, peach, banana, and coco trees all in the same soil in the same acre, would the apples have more boron than the peaches? Would the peaches have more iron than than the bananas? Would the bananas have more magnesium than chocolate? And if you harvested beans, radishes, and broccoli from the same garden, would there be more germanium in the beans, more selenium in the broccoli, etc. And if they each did contain more or or less of one element than the other fruits and vegetables, would it all be due to selective chemistry? Or would biotransmutation be a factor?

The biologists, chemists, physicians, and nutritionists of today would virtually all say that any element that does not enter an organism (plant or animal) from the outside cannot and will not be found inside. They would say, "Life is chemistry. Nothing is created. Nothing is destroyed. Matter is conserved. The atoms of elements can move from one compound to another, but remain the same elements throughout all reactions. Lavoisier's Law still holds true," and they would agree, "Nuclear transformations of elements do not exist as a biological process."

But these are all statements of belief. Not statements of proven science. There are no studies and no body of published data to substantiate such a position. Just because it is a majority opinion, does not make it true. The Chinese have a saying: "If 1,000 people believe in a foolish thing, it is still a foolish thing." Truth cannot be determined by majority vote. But for the most part, throughout the scientific community, the majority rules—usually with the facts in their favor, but sometimes not.

The truth is that no one at this time can state, as a verified fact of science, that all of the elements found in a plant come directly from the soil, water, and air in which that plant was nurtured and grown. Until scientists have performed enough experiments of sufficient scale to find out exactly what elements in living organisms come from the outside and what elements appear by some non-chemical process from the inside, no scientist can rationally argue that biotransmutation does not happen. To discount and dismiss the idea of biotransmutation without applying the scientific method to check it out would be an unscientific reaction. Unfortunately, the history of science is replete with unscientific reactions by scientists.

A scientific response to the proposition of biotransmutation on the part of those first confronted with the concept would be to say, "Before I draw any conclusions let's see what the data ultimately say. Let's explore existing evidence thoroughly and impartially and then let's design and carry out some experiments to see if biotransmutation can be verified or disproven. While biotransmutation certainly does not fit the current model of how we think the universe works, maybe our paradigm is incomplete, perhaps even mistaken. This could be an opportunity to make corrections in our viewpoint, expand its scope, and trade it for a better one."

There is a growing number of scientists with the courage, integrity, and spirituality to express such an attitude in the face of a new concept. These will be the scientists and truth seekers who will lead us into a future of increased enlightenment that will bring a better world to us all.

There is already enough data collected by enough scientists from enough places to say that biotransmutation is a plausible theory. In fact, it is a lot more than a theory. It is the only logical explanation for a host of experimental data that the classical theories of chemistry have yet to explain and cannot explain. Chemists, physicists, and biologists can keep looking for explanations within their paradigm, but that is like looking for a lost wallet in the office when it was dropped in the parking lot. What must ultimately happen is for someone to step outside into the fresh air of a larger space where the lost wallet they seek actually exists, ready to be discovered.

Protein from Carbohydrates

All living cells, both plant and animal, need nitrogen to form proteins. Proteins are built of amino acids. There are 20 amino acids that we need to support biological functions, 10 of which we manufacture in our bodies and 10 of which we must take in through our diet. Amino acids all contain an amine functional group (NH_2) and a carboxylic acid functional group (COOH).

Carnivorous animals get plenty of amino acids in their diets since the flesh they eat is composed of proteins. Herbivorous animals must acquire their necessary amino acids in a different way. Consider elk, moose, deer, cattle, elephants, and horses. They eat no meat. Even some of the largest dinosaurs were herbivores. Did you ever wonder how large grazing animals like these, living exclusively on grass and other green vegetation, are able to grow into such masses of muscular bulk? Can protein be manufactured from grass alone? The truth is that large herbivores contain a great deal more nitrogen in their bodily tissues than they eat. Since they can't take it directly from the atmosphere, how do they acquire it?

Carbohydrates are compounds whose formulas consist of carbon atoms (C) combined with water molecules (H_2O). Carbohydrates include sugars and starches. Glucose is a simple sugar metabolized by the cells of our bodies for energy. Its formula is $C_6H_{12}O_6$ which is sometimes written as $C_6(H_2O)_6$ showing that it is composed of six carbons and six water molecules. But how can compounds containing only C, H and O be used to build proteins that require nitrogen?

The story of the monoxide poisoning of welders, reported earlier in this chapter, demonstrates that nitrogen in the air can be biotransmuted into carbon and oxygen by the following equations:

$$_7N + {}_1H = {}_8O$$
$$_7N - {}_1H = {}_6C$$

Add an H atom to an N atom and you get an O atom. Subtract an H atom from an N atom and you get a C atom. It is interesting to note that the proportions of C, H, and O in a fructose molecule $C_6H_{12}O_6$ are exactly right to produce three amine groups 3 x (NH_2) and three carboxylic acid groups 3 x (COOH). This totals to 3 C atoms, 9 H atoms, 6 O atoms, and 3 N atoms.

The fructose molecule already has six O atoms and a surplus of C and H atoms. If we take 3 of the 6 carbons and 3 of the 9 hydrogens, we can make the 3 nitrogens and everything will add up perfectly. The biotransmutation equation for turning C and H into N is as follows:

$$_1H + {}_6C = {}_7N$$

Thus, carbohydrates can be converted into amino acids via biotransmutation, which is how grass-eating animals produce some of their necessary proteins. Humans probably do it too, only to a lesser extent.

The CHOSN Ones

We concluded back in Chapter Four that the principle elements important to essential oils were five in number: Carbon (C), Hydrogen (H), Oxygen (O), Sulfur (S), and Nitrogen (N) ("The CHOSN Ones") with the vast majority of oil compounds consisting entirely of the first three elements only: C, H, and O.

You may have already noticed that the three elements most frequently involved with biotransmutations are the same three: C, H, and O, that comprise 99% of the composition of essential oils. New elements are most frequently created by adding or subtracting one of these three. In some biotransmutation processes, an atom of N, S, or lithium ($_3Li$) is involved. Sulfur (S), you may have noticed, can be formed from two O atoms as follows:

$$_8O + {}_8O = {}_{16}S$$

Go back to Table One in Chapter Three, p. 82. We have already pointed out that every element on the sequence of the Periodic Table is merely the previous element with an H atom incorporated into it, plus, perhaps, a neutron or two. Now notice that every element from left to right in Period 2 (from lithium (Li) to neon (Ne)) has exactly 8 protons less than every element from left to right in Period 3 (from sodium (Na) to argon (Ar)). This difference of 8 protons also includes the first two elements of Period 4 (K and Ca), which are both 8 protons more than the Na and Mg atoms directly and respectively above them. Every element in Period 3 can be obtained from the elements in Period 2 by simply adding an O atom to each one while every element in the periodic table can be created from its next door neighbors by adding or subtracting an H atom.

Turning Lead into Gold

The alchemists' dream of transmuting base metals into gold still remains elusive and unachieved. The research in biotransmutation to date reveals limits to the process. Not just any element can be transmuted into any other. The decisions as to what elements are to be transmuted into others are made by living organisms at cellular levels. When a plant, animal, or microorganism finds it necessary to turn base metals into gold as a matter of survival or wellbeing, then it will be done, and, perhaps, it is already being done. It could be that biochemists have just not discovered it because they have never looked for it.

Whether gold (Au) is a necessary trace element for human life (or any other form of life) is a matter of debate. Some authors, such as Gerber (*Vibrational Medicine*), and Harting & Bergstrom (*Chronobiotic Nutrition*) believe gold is a necessary nutrient as yet unrecognized. If this is so, then our bodies may very well be transmuting base metals into gold on a small scale, as yet undetected.

For example, if you look in Table One, you see that gold or aurum ($_{79}$Au) is only three elements to the left of lead or plumbum ($_{82}$Pb). That is a difference of one lithium atom ($_3$Li). Lithium is one of the elements known to participate in biotransmutations of the elements. The equation showing lead turning into gold would be as follows:

$$_{82}Pb - _3Li = _{79}Au$$

This is a biotransmutation that is both feasible and theoretically possible. If found to be operable, you can be sure that countless commercial companies would plunge into research to develop living organisms to turn masses of cheap lead into fortunes of pure gold. Such an occurrence would have profound consequences for the gold standard that most countries have as a basis of value and stability for their money. Herein lies another theme for a good science fiction movie. Let's hope it remains a fiction.

It is also interesting to note that the atomic number of silver or argentum ($_{47}Ag$) is 47 which is exactly 32 protons short of gold ($_{79}Au$) which has 79 protons. Thirty-two protons is the number possessed by two sulfur atoms ($_{16}S$). Hence, if two sulfur atoms combined with a silver atom, through some form of transmutation, it would produce a gold atom. At the same time, if the equivalent of two sulfur atoms were removed from a gold atom by transmutation, it would produce silver. It is interesting to note that it is not unusual for gold, silver, and sulfur to all be found together geologically in the same deposits.

Biotransmutation and Aromatherapy

Most biotransmutations occur by adding or subtracting an O or an H atom, and sometimes a C. Nitrogen (N) and Sulfur (S) are also involved, as well as Lithium (Li). Except for lithium, it appears that the elements chosen for most biotransmutations are also the ones chosen to compose essential oils.

The chemical activities of essential oil compounds are only part of what they do in our bodies. We know by experience that they help restore balance to our bodies—in terms of hormones, pH, frequencies, and in a host of other ways. Achieving these balances is not all chemical. It is also biotransmutational. The most common elements in essential oils, C, H, and O, are also the most common participants in the biotransmutation of elements. Biotransmutation is an ongoing, every day process in our bodies. Essential oils become a part of this process—bringing us health and well being by means both chemical and non-chemical, both by interactions between electrons as well as the nuclei of the atoms.

For more detailed information on biotransmutation, read *Biological Transmutations: A New Science* by Louis Kervran, translated from the French by Michel Abehsera and published by Swan House, Binghamton, New York. The book is actually out of print, but can be obtained on the internet from various sources. Kervran's book cites 78 scientific papers published by more than 40 research scientists that provide abundant verifying evidence for the existence and prevalence of biotransmutations in living organisms. This book contains much more than I have presented in this brief chapter.

We must also add a word of caution here. Nothing stated in this chapter should be taken as a suggestion to modify one's dietary habits or to choose healing modalities other than those already proven effective. While the existence of biotransmutation has been proven and documented, as a new science it is only an infant and remains to be refined and developed into a full-fledged paradigm for applications. But that will come in due time.

The subject matter of Kervran's book is not hard to understand. However, it is hard to believe since it contradicts a lifetime of misinformation taught in traditional chemistry books and science classes. Once you have cleared away the mental handicaps and emotional blocks of your previous education and have mustered up the courage to go wherever truth leads, you will find that Kervran's data and theories explain a lot that will remain forever unexplainable by current science.

At this time, the concept of biotransmutation is not mentioned in any conventional chemistry, biology, or physics book (in English) of which I am aware. There may be such texts in French or Russian. Neither is biotransmutation mentioned in any academic course taught in

English. But that will change soon. Commercial corporations, like the Dow Chemical Company, are already aware of Kervran's work and are secretly seeking ways to use biotransmutation to create marketable products. With the prospect and possibility of potential profit, professional prejudice disappears.

Water, Wine, and Essential Oils

When Jesus turned water into wine at the wedding in Cana of Galilee, there was obviously a transmutation of elements that took place (John 2:1-11). Water containing only hydrogen and oxygen (H_2O) was transformed into a beverage containing alcohol (C_2H_6O), lycopene ($C_{40}H_{64}$), methyl anthranilate ($C_8H_9NO_2$) and other esters, various saccharides ($C_6H_{12}O_6/C_{12}H_{22}O_{11}$), and other fragrant, flavorful compounds composed of elements, such as sulfur and nitrogen, not present in the original water. In this case, the transmutation of elements was a miracle wrought by Jesus' divine will and consciousness. Perhaps, some day, there will be a scientific explanation for how Jesus accomplished this feat, but it won't diminish the wonder of the miracle that it was.

When biotransmutation becomes widely known, accepted, understood, and well integrated into the mainstream of science and society, it will profoundly influence the fields of agriculture, nutrition, medicine, biology, chemistry, physics, ecology, geology, health care, and even our daily eating habits.

Kervran was familiar with essential oils. He suggests that one of the reasons aromatherapy works so successfully is that essential oils activate certain enzymatic activities in the body that facilitate beneficial biotransmutations, which restore health and vitality. Though long unrecognized as such, it appears that biotransmutation has always been a part of the healing power of essential oils and one of the secrets of their remarkable powers of regeneration, balance, and restoration.

But chemistry and biotransmutation are not all there is to the actions of essential oils. There is more.

♥ ARTICLE THREE
THE NATURE
OF MATTER

We stated at the beginning of Chapter Three that "Chemistry is the study of matter." We defined matter as anything that has mass and occupies space. But is this all there is to matter?

Solid matter is not what it appears to be to our five senses. Its physical properties and visual appearance are manifestations of a more subtle template, a parallel universe invisible to the human eye, composed of energies beyond physical measurement, yet more real than the tangible world around us. To understand the nature of matter, including its chemical properties, one must study the nature of the subtle substrate of light and consciousness that underlies all of God's creation.

Physicists and chemists agree that solid matter is not really solid in the sense that it is composed of substantative material. Electrons, protons, and neutrons fill less than 1% of the space occupied by an atom. Is the remaining 99% of matter a vacuum? In a material sense, we can say, "Yes it is," since there are no particles there. But is it an empty vacuum? The answer is, "No." There is energy there. And there is consciousness.

The gross energies of the material world are detected and measured with the instrumentation of material science. But the subtle energies that underlie this world and determine its form are beyond physical measurement—no matter how sophisticated the apparatus. So long as our instruments of scientific investigation are built on material technology, so long will their utility be confined to the measurement of material phenomena and nothing beyond.

Only consciousness can measure and detect consciousness. Thus, it is in the development, refinement, and fine tuning of our own consciousness that the future frontiers of science will be explored.

The Meaning of Omniscience

If God's omniscience and omnipresence are to be believed, then he is consciously present throughout the physical universe. He is conscious in every atom, in the subspace of every atom, and in the space surrounding every atom. He is also consciously present in the subtle energies and vibrations, beyond the physical, which are the frequency fields, blueprints, and templates that make physical manifestation possible and determine its forms.

In Job 12:8 it says, "Ask the plants; speak to the earth, and they will teach you." This scripture is telling us to ask God, who is conscious in the plants, and to speak to God, who is conscious throughout the material substance of the earth, and he will teach you. In practical terms, this is what God's omniscience and omnipresence mean.

When we pray to God, he can answer and respond directly by his listening presence in the energy fields and atoms of physical matter—bringing us the guidance, the cures, the healings, and the phenomena we call miracles. Thus, Jesus turned water into wine, caused the blind to see, the dead to be raised, and multiplied some small loaves and a few fishes into a feast for thousands. (John 2:1-12; Matthew 9:27-31; 14:13-21)

The material sciences of physics, chemistry, and biology which form the basis for allopathic medical practice, are defined in terms of things discernable by our five senses. This includes phenomena such as x-rays and microwaves, invisible and undetectable to our five senses, yet measurable by instruments that produce data or information discernable by our five senses and for which there is a material explanation. There is a tendency among scientists to believe that the entire universe consists only of subjects amenable to the tools of material science. In other words, if it cannot be seen, heard, touched, tasted, smelled, or measured by physical instrumentation, it does not and cannot exist. Nothing could be further from the truth.

Putting Life into Iron Filings

If you take a china plate and sprinkle unmagnetized iron filings upon it, they will scatter and pile up in a random disordered incoherent manner. If you place a large magnet under the plate the filings will suddenly take on an apparent life, lining themselves up in an orderly fashion, moving and waving in phase with the movements of the hidden magnet beneath. Remove the magnet and the filings collapse into a lifeless, discordant, incoherent heap again.

The visible behavior of the filings is in response to the invisible magnetic field from below where, from above, even the metal magnet (the source of the field) cannot be seen. Without the field of magnetic energy, the iron filings manifest no movement, no form, and no apparent life. However, without the gross filings as a vehicle, the magnetic field cannot manifest its presence, motion, and form in a visible way.*

This is exactly the way it is between our visible bodily vehicles and the invisible energy fields that support and shape them. These subtle fields are the blueprints, templates, and sources of life force, that energize and determine the forms and movements that our bodies manifest as visible vibrating, physical life. Similar unseen fields underlie all living forms as well as the compounds that compose them.

Our bodies, as well as all physical substances, have a visible manifestation discernable to one or more of our five senses. But their behaviors, attributes, and/or apparent life is due to dynamic invisible energy fields not detectable by any of our physical senses nor by any physical instrumentation. These fields are vibrational in nature, just as

---

* NOTE: If you want to do this experiment, and need some iron filings, go to a hardware store or key maker. You can get filings for free from the castaway cuttings where keys are made. You can also get filings from a welder or metal worker that grinds implements of iron.

visible light, audible sound, electromagnetism, the rhythms of nature, and the atoms themselves are all vibrational. All the objects in God's creation have a spectrum of frequencies that account for their essential qualities and makeup. This spectrum is spoken of as light in the *Old Testament*, and is mentioned as light, and also as God's Word, or *Logos*, in the *New Testament*.

> In the beginning God created the heaven and the earth . . . And God said, Let there be light: and there was light. And God saw the light, that it was good.   Genesis 1:1,3

> In the beginning was the Word, and the Word was with God, and the Word was God. The same was in the beginning with God. All things were made by him; and without him was not anything made that was made. In him was life; and the life was the light of men. And the light shineth in darkness and the darkness comprehended it not.   John 1:1-5

In these passages, the phrase, "God said" refers to the divine vibration by which "God created the heaven and earth" and by which "all things were made." The terms, "Word" and "light," are also references to vibrations that not only give form and physical existence to all things, but also imbue all living things with life, itself.

In the scripture above, "Word" is an inadequate attempt in English to express the Greek "Logos." It has many meanings and interpretations among theologians and scholars, both Christian and non-Christian. In ancient Greek philosophy, *Logos* was the underlying principle, consciousness, template, or vibration that gives the material world its character and coherence. This definition of *Logos* is in concordance with the creation story of Genesis where God spoke the universe into existence by his vibratory "Word." The Hebrew equivalent of *Logos* is *Dabar*, which in the original Greek translation of the *Old Testament* (*Septuagint*) is translated as *Logos*, and which, in English, is rendered as "Word" or "Word of God."

Thus, the ancients, both secular and nonsecular, were of the belief that the visible, tangible universe is underlain by a more subtle realm that determines its nature and form. They did not have and did not need scientific instrumentation to discern this reality. They perceived it themselves directly by their own spiritual senses. Thus, *Logos* or *Dabar* was not an intellectual construct, a fabrication of the human mind. It was a reality seen and perceived directly by the spiritually developed individuals of those times. Humankind in general has temporarily lost those abilities since ancient times, but is now regaining them. There are many people today who see and understand what the ancients saw. Many are scientists and mathematicians who are currently working to express, in scientific terms, what had formerly only been expressable by allegory, esoteric teachings, or scriptural symbolism.

Seeing the Light

The scripture just quoted (John 1:5) remarks that even in the presence of light, darkness does not comprehend it as the light that it is. This is the state of most people. Immersed in God's light, like a fish in the ocean, they yet fail to perceive his surrounding, all-encompassing presence. However, some people who have developed themselves spiritually through prayer, devotion, humility, surrender, and daily communion with God can actually see the subtle lights, sense the subtle energies, and hear the subtle sounds beyond the physical that comprise God's secret vibrations that permeate the universe. Such sights, sensations, and sounds are not perceived by our five physical senses, but only by developing our spiritual senses which are gifts of the spirit. St. Paul urges us to seek these gifts.

> Concerning spiritual gifts... there are diversities of gifts, but the same Spirit... covet earnestly the best gifts.
> I Corinthians 12:1,4,31

When people pray or direct their attention heavenward, they automatically tend to focus upwards with their eyes toward the center of their foreheads. This happens naturally whether one prays with eyes open or closed. Many prayerful individuals have testified to seeing light behind the darkness of their closed eyes when focused at the single point between the eyebrows. This is not the flickering of residual images on the retina that you may experience when you first close your eyes in darkness for sleep at night. This is described as a real supernal light in which one's body and the universe can seem to merge as one. It can be a joyful experience that speaks of the nearness of God and Christ as well as a true witness to the heavenly realms beyond the physical. It is an enriching experience one does not forget. It is a blessing and a gift from God.

There is a *Bible* quote from a sermon that Jesus delivered on a hillside overlooking the Sea of Galilee that says:

> The light of the body is the eye: If therefore thine eye be single, thy whole body shall be full of light.   Matthew 6:22

This verse from the Sermon on the Mount, about a single eye seeing the body as an expression of light, seems to describe the experience mentioned above and shared by so many who have seen and know, firsthand, of the subtle realms of light of God's universe.

Today's scientists consider spiritual perception as subjective and unverifiable by the scientific method. When enough scientists have developed their spiritual senses that they can all share a common vision of the unseen ocean of light and energy in which we live and have our being, such perceptions will be considered objective. Thus, the scientific method will be modified to apply to phenomena currently considered beyond the scientific method.

Oils as Liquid Crystals

Liquid crystals are familiar to most of us. We find them as liquid crystal displays (LCDs) in our clocks, watches, calculators, laptop computers, and a host of other devices. Crystals are normally solids, built atom by atom, or molecule by molecule, into the most perfect of natural forms. Our most prized gem stones are crystals such as ruby, amethyst, emerald, sapphire, and diamond, where the invisible atomic structures of the molecules are replicated in visible, geometric forms. The entire industry of solid state electronics is based on crystals which are mostly compounds of silicon (Si) doped with trace elements.

Liquids are normally amorphous and fluid, possessing no fixed geometric forms, their molecules rotated and oriented in all directions randomly. Crystals are solids where the atoms or molecules are all oriented in fixed, mathematically precise patterns and directions. Substances that can exist in a liquid-crystalline phase simultaneously possess some properties of liquids as well as some properties of solids. Liquid crystals are substances whose molecules have certain freedoms to slide and move (like a liquid) but are also partially restricted in that they are restrained to certain planes or orientations (like a solid crystal). Liquid crystals manifest either their fluid or crystalline properties in response to heat, magnetism, and/or electric fields. When such liquids express their crystalline qualities, they often do so in colors or shades of light and dark that are different than those of their liquid qualities. LCDs consist of thin layers of liquid crystal material under transparent glass or plastic beneath which are various sources of heat, voltage, or magnetism. When these hidden, invisible energy sources are configured as numbers, pictures, or symbols, the reaction of the liquid crystal above is to assume these shapes in visible forms.

The energy field behind the liquid crystal in our watch face is invisible. Without the field, the liquid appears lifeless, grey, featureless, and inert. The liquid crystal manifests form and motion only when it can pulsate with the vibrations of the energy field from behind or below. On the other hand, the energy field, the source of the apparent life and movement on our watch face, needs the liquid crystal as a vehicle through which to manifest as readable symbols and communicate the time of day to a human observer.

Like the iron filings on a plate, activated by a magnetic field from below, liquid crystals are another analog of the relationship between our etheric body and our physical body where an unseen field determines the form of that which is seen.

This analogy also applies to essential oils. Our directed thoughts and spiritual intentions are subtle magnetic fields that write readable symbols upon essential oils as if they were liquid crystals. These messages travel throughout our bodies, carried by the absorption of the oils, which are then communicated to our cells to facilitate healing.

Is There an Ether?

Ancient sages, prophets, wise men, healers, and philosophers of many cultures—from the Orientals of the Far East, to the alchemists of Europe, to the tribes of indigenous peoples of North America—have traditionally categorized earth materials into five classes: 1. earth, 2. water, 3. air, 4. fire, and 5. ether, where earth refers to solids, water to liquids, air to gases, fire to energy, and ether to an ocean of subtle material permeating all matter and all space. According to those with the spiritual vision to directly experience and witness the subtle energies of the universe, ether-permeated space is the boundary line between earth and heaven, between the physical and the non-physical. All the finer forces God has created are composed of light, energy, vibration, or thought-forms, which are merely hidden behind a particular set of high frequencies that manifest as ether.

Scientists of recent centuries, including Isaac Newton (1642-1727), considered ether to be a theoretical invisible medium that occupied what appeared to be empty space by which light, gravity, magnetism, and cosmic rays could propagate, reach out, and act at a distance. After the failure of repeated experiments to detect and verify the existence of ether during the late nineteenth and early twentieth centures, scientists in general abandoned the idea of an ether as being a necessary medium for the transmission of electromagnetic energy in a vacuum and simply adopted the theory that light could pass through a space without any supporting medium. Some scientists, misinterpreting the work of Einstein, concluded that Einstein's theories did away with the need for an ether to explain the passage of light and other forms of radiant energy between stars, planets, and galaxies.

Scientists are now changing their minds. In an article in *Physics Today* (January 1999), Dr. Frank Wilczek, a physics professor at the Massachusetts Institute of Technology (MIT), had this to say: "There is a myth, repeated in many popular presentations and textbooks, that Albert Einstein swept the ether into the dustbin of history . . . The truth is nearly the opposite. Einstein first purified, and then enthroned, the ether concept. As the twentieth century has progressed, its role in fundamental physics has only expanded. At present, renamed and thinly disguised, it dominates the accepted laws of physics."

Dr. Edward Close, author of *Transcendental Physics*, (1996) comments, "While Einstein's Special Theory of Relativity assumed no preferred reference frame, which many misinterpreted as doing away with ether, his General Theory of Relativity established an ether in the form of the gravitational field. Quantum physics reveals the way that pervasive field (or ether) functions. It is just that the term 'ether' fell out of favor."

Physicists today refer to the ether as "the quantum vacuum," "the quantum field," and/or "the zero-point energy field." In Lynne McTaggart's book, *The Quest for the Secret Force of the Universe* (2002), she describes it as follows: "The very underpinning of our universe is a heaving sea of energy, one vast quantum field. What we believe to be our stable, static universe is, in fact, a seething maelstrom of subatomic particles fleetingly popping in and out of existence."

As predicted by Einstein's theories relating energy to mass ($E = mc^2$), all elementary particles interact with each other by exchanging energy through subtle quantum particles. These are particles that are beyond the simple electrons, protons, and neutrons of basic chemistry. Called "virtual particles," these quantum entities appear to come out of nowhere, combining and annihilating each other in fractions of an instant. During their brief moments of existence, they radiate energy. Physicists call it "zero-point energy." While the life span of a single subatomic particle is unimaginably short, when you add up all the particles of all kinds in the universe constantly popping into and out of physical being, you find a vast, inexhaustible source of energy unobtrusively occupying all of empty space around us. This concept has become the twenty-first century equivalent of what scientists a century ago called "ether."

Dr. David Bohm is considered one of the great physicists of the last century. In a biography entitled *The Life Work of David Bohm: A River of Truth* by Dr. Will Keepin (1993), Bohm is quoted as saying, "Calculations of the quantity known as zero-point energy suggest that a single cubic centimeter of empty space contains more energy than all of the matter in the known universe. This enormous energy inherent in empty space can be viewed as theoretical evidence for the existence of a vast, yet hidden realm. The vast physical universe we experience is but a set of ripples on the surface of the implicate order. The manifest objects that we regard as comprising ordinary reality are only the unfolded projections of the much deeper, higher dimensional implicate order, which is the fundamental reality."

What Sustains Life?

All the knowledge, wisdom, experience, experimental data, theories, and laws of science to this point in history support the idea of an ether—regardless of what name you may call it. Discarded decades ago, the theory of the existence of a quantum vacuum, a zero-point energy field, or an ether has now become the cornerstone of modern physics. Without such a postulate, the rest of what we now understand about the universe makes no sense.

> The stone that the builders rejected has become the chief cornerstone.   Psalm 118:22; Matt. 21:42; Luke 20:17;I Peter 2:7

Enlightened scientists today have incorporated an ether into their conceptual paradigm of the universe. Some have done so by intellectual deduction, others by direct personal perception of the etheric realm. itself. Few people are able to consciously experience and comprehend this fundamental reality. Most humans are experientially unaware that they are walking, breathing, moving, sleeping, living, and are literally submerged and swimming in a limitless sea of subtle energy in which we exist as physical beings.

Our bodies and minds are continuously exchanging energies from this sea. In fact, we cannot remain physically alive without such exchanges. We draw upon it daily and unconsciously recharge our batteries from it at night when we sleep. We feed our bodies food and drink, but fats, fluids, proteins, minerals, and carbohydrates, alone, will not sustain us. The continuous flow of force through our bodies to sustain life is from a higher source of energy than that which we access through the food we eat. Our sustaining energy is only partially provided by our physical intake. This concept is expressed in the *Bible* as follows:

> Man shall not live by bread alone, but by every word that proceedeth from the mouth of God. Matthew 4:4

The subtle etheric universe, coexisting with and superimposed upon the grosser physical universe, is an ocean of God's Word, God's vibrations, God's conscious presence, and God's infinite energy. This limitless reservoir of Divine energy secretly sustains and maintains us as it flows into our bodies through the portal of the brain from whence it is distributed and stepped down in frequency via the chakras (see glossary) to nourish our muscles and organs. Some people have developed their spiritual sensitivities to the point that they can personally perceive and experience the heavenly realms of vibration and can consciously plug into them. Such highly developed individuals don't need physical food any more. They live on light. There are more people on earth that have achieved this than you would suspect. Unfortunately, this is not going to be the solution to feeding the starving masses of humanity that suffer in hunger throughout the world today.

With respect to today's scientific community, there are only a few exceptional persons who can grasp and accept these concepts, but their numbers are growing. Most scientists are still practicing on the premise of secular materialism.

The Second Law of Thermodynamics

One of the cornerstones of classical physics is the Second Law of Thermodynamics or the Law of Entropy. The law expresses the notion that there is an inherent direction in which natural processes occur. While there are precise mathematical expressions of this law used by scientists and engineers, suffice it to say here that, in a nutshell, the Second Law simply states that "in all spontaneous processes within a closed system there is an increase in the overall disorder of the system where useful energy available to do work is irreversibly transformed into useless energy unavailable to do work."

To put it another way, most natural processes are irreversible, occuring in one direction only. Otherwise we could unstub a toe, unshatter a broken mirror, unsalt the salty soup, unwilt a rose, unburn the chocolate pudding, unspill the beans, unfry an egg, uncurdle sour milk, uneat the meat that didn't agree, be a year younger next year, find needles in a haystack as easily as we can lose them, or build a perpetual motion machine. The fact that none of these things have ever been observed attests to the apparently universal application of this law.

Of course, order can always be restored to a chaotic situation within limits. But the Second Law says there is always a price such that, in the end, more disorder results in the universe as a whole even though, in one corner, it may have been reordered. For example, gas and oil occur in only certain places in the earth while iron, gold, and other metals are found in only certain environments, etc. This is a certain amount of order. But consider the ultimate end of these carefuly sorted natural resources. We mine them, manufacture with them, use them in our homes and cities, and ultimately throw them away, whereupon they eventually find themselves in a landfill. What could be more random than a dump? Now theoretically we could go back to a dump and separate all the metals, plastics, bottles, etc., and reuse all these resources, thus undoing some of the disorder we have created. But the Law of Entropy says that, all things considered, we will never be able to completely recapture the order that was destroyed by our consumption, no matter how advanced our technology or conscientious our efforts. 100% recycling is impossible. There will always be wasted and unrecyclable energy and matter, much in the form of increased heat and the random motion of atoms and molecules.

If a tornado were to rip through a landfill containing all the metals and materials found in an airplane could it accidentally assemble an airplane? If an explosion were to happen in an auto parts store with every item present to make a car, could it ever happen that a complete automobile would be accidentally created by the explosion? In both instances, according to the Second Law, the answer is never—not in a trillion tornados or explosions could such things happen! This line of thought has been used to argue that the Big Bag Theory of the origin of the cosmos is an impossible explanation for the creation of the order we see in the universe. If you think of the Big Bang as a typical explosion, it would be a direct contradiction of the Second Law to say that an orderly universe was, thereby, created. If you believe in the Second Law, and scientists universally do, then to be consistent you would have to conclude that the act of creation was beyond the laws of physics as we know them today. In scientific terms, to admit to an ordered universe, that was created at some point in time, is to admit to an intelligent power that created everything, endowed it with life, and is, itself, both within and above the physical universe. In this statement, we have just described God.

But you can think of the Big Bang another way. It is a fact that the observed universe appears to be expanding from a point as if some at time in the past it exploded from that point. What if the universe did start with a Big Bang, but it was not an ordinary explosion. It was the booming voice of God speaking the cosmos into creation? Such a "Bang" would produce order and life as we know it. (See p. 190 for more on this.)

The key point of the Second Law is that it applies only to closed systems. In physics, a closed system is one with boundaries through which no energy passes in or out. The experiences of many scientists seems to have verfied to the satisfaction of the scientific community that, within such systems, the randomness or disorder within the system always increases. Hence, according to the Second Law, when we, as humans, bring order to our corner of the universe through our activities and technology, it is always at the price of creating disorder elsewhere such that the aggregate total of our actions has increased disorder in the universe. In other words, no process that produces order in a system can proceed without producing an even greater disorder in its surroundings.

For example, if you have a messy desk and you straighten it up, you have increased the order of things on your desk. But in the process you expended energy obtained through the air you breathed and the food you have eaten involving respiration and metabolic processes that increased disorder. Furthermore, as you exerted yourself, your body produced heat that was lost to the air and to your surroundings which increased the disorderly motions of their atoms and molecules.

Is Life a Violation of the Second Law?

We have said earlier in this book that living processes are a violation of the Second Law since the hallmark of life is to bring order from chaos while the Second Law says that natural processes create chaos from order. It was pointed out in the opening lines of Chapter Five that the very word, "organic," comes from the Latin root, *organum*, which means to organize. Life, in all forms, is an organizing process. Even the tiniest microbe brings a high degree of order to its speck of the universe. The way scientists explain this seeming contradiction is that even though we see order in living processes, their formation and ongoing existence creates even greater disorder all around them such that when it is all added up, the universe has moved closer to total disorder. In other words, when a highly ordered organism eats, moves, breathes, metabolizes food, gives off heat, eliminates waste, recreates, assimilates, and procreates, it scatters disorder all around itself everywhere it goes such that when one subtracts the amount of disorder it makes from the amount of order it creates, you get a negative number.

The truth is that this interpretation of the Second Law, assumed by most scientists, is not a proven fact. It is an assumption—a matter of chosen belief. No one has ever been able to take a living being and prove that the order they bring to the world adds up to a value less than the disorder their existence causes in the world. The reason this has never been proven in a real life example is because one would need to have the ability to measure all energy transformations in the world simultaneously and quantitatively, including all energies radiating to and from the earth. This is an impossible experiment.

The assumption of material science is that the physical universe is the only universe there is, and is, hence, closed—no energy going in, no energy going out. But this is not true. The physical universe is not a closed system. Energy comes and goes into and out of it all the time, particularly when it comes to the energies that sustain life. There is a non-material universe beyond the material, and energy passes between the two continuously. In fact, were it not for these subtle energies passing into the physical from the non-physical, life, as we know it, including our own, could not exist.

Therefore, living entities in the physical world are not living in a closed material system, as scientists assume. As human beings, we are both subject to the Second Law, and at the same time, beyond it. This statement also applies to essential oils which act as intercessories and channels between us and our bodies in the physical world and the universe of subtle energies beyond.

Newton, Einstein, and Quantum Physics

The frequencies of gross matter obey Newtonian physics. In other words, they follow physical laws, including the Second Law of Thermodynamics, the conservation of matter and energy (Lavoisier's Law), and the inverse square laws of gravity, electricity, and magnetism where fields fall off in intensity with distance. According to Einsteinian physics, physical matter operates within the frequency limits of the speed of light as its boundary and ceiling. The frequencies (f) possible for physical matter and energy are defined and limited by the equation, $f = c/\lambda$, where c = the speed of light and (lambda) λ = wavelength.

In the physical universe, nothing travels faster than light. Thus, the light from distant stars and galaxies we see on earth today was beamed from their sources countless eons ago and we have no visible way of knowing, by physical means, what is happening on these distant bodies in present earth time. Every star we see in the night sky is a statement of history, not a report of current events. If a bright visible star in outer space exploded in a supernova today, it would be many generations before humans on earth would receive visible evidence of its spectacular demise traveling at the speed of light. If the sun, our closest star at 97 million miles distance, were to instantly go out, it would be 8 minutes and 40 seconds before we knew it on earth. Light travels at the rate of 300,000,000 meters per second (or 186,280 miles per sec), which is pretty fast, but it still takes time to traverse a distance.

By contrast, the frequencies and velocities of the subtle etheric worlds which comprise the fields that underlie the physical world, and give life to our bodies, they obey laws outside of classical physics. In other words, they do not follow physical laws, including the law of entropy and the conservation of matter and energy. Neither do the intensities of etheric fields diminish with distance, inverse to the square. With inverse square laws, as they apply to electric, magnetic, and gravitational fields, as well as to light propagation, doubling the distance from the source reduces the field intensity to $(1/2)^2$ or one-fourth of what it was.

Etheric matter and energy operate at frequencies and velocities much higher than those possible for material substances and visible light. Etheric fields are not limited by the speed of light. The underlying worlds of subtle energies are best described by totally new concepts suggested by quantum physics—such as non-locality and participatory, self-referential reality. (See glossary.)

The Speed of Thought

The world of thought is within these subtle spheres of higher vibrations. It has been shown by scientific experiments that thoughts not only travel through space from person to person, and from persons to animals or things, but they do so at velocities exceeding the speed of light. In some experiments, thoughts have even appeared to travel instantaneously—i.e., at infinite speed. Hence, if a person on a distant planet, say 100,000 light years away, were to send a thought to an earthling, it would be received instantaneously. Whereas, a beam of physical light from that same planet would take 100,000 years to get here. Furthermore, the thought would arrive undiminished in force and clarity while the intensity of the light beam reaching earth would be diminished to virtual undetectability by the inverse square of that great distance. Furthermore, by the second law of thermodynamics, various stellar gases and other fields in the path of that ray of light would cause it to disperse and become less and less coherent. Whereas, a thought traveling that distance would arrive focused and completely intact as if sent from a person just across the room.

Thus, the higher and higher levels of vibrational frequencies that underlie our physical existence get closer and closer to transcending all of time and space. The highest level is God, himself, who can communicate simultaneously with every being and particle of his creation throughout the whole universe. There is no time lag between the instant of your prayer and its receipt by God, as is the case in a long distance broadcast, an email, or a telephone call.

The basic concepts discussed above are given in much greater detail in the book, *Vibrational Medicine*, by Richard Gerber, M.D. Another book I also highly recommend is *Transcendental Physics* by Edward R. Close, Ph.D., available via www.amazon.com or www.iuniverse.com on the internet.

Why Synthetic is Different than Natural

In several chapters of this book we discussed differences between natural and synthetic substances. As mentioned earlier, one reason essential oils cannot be artifically synthesized in a laboratory is because their composition is so complex no one has been able to completly analyze even a single oil. It is impossible to synthesize something whose list of ingredients is incomplete. Even so, many companies create artificial essential oils by taking a selected number of the known main ingredients (those that provide flavor and/or fragrance), synthesize them in a lab, and mix them to make an imitation. In this case, the difference between a synthetic and a natural oil is that the man-made version is lacking many ingredients—including those that must be present for healing to result.

There is also a difference between synthetic compounds and natural ones which has to do with isomers. Laboratories can produce compounds with exactly the same chemical formula as, say, natural menthol. But there are a number of isomers for the formula of menthol, only one of which is produced in the peppermint plant. Laboratories have not figured out how to make only that isomer. What they get is a mixture containing the one found in the plant plus some unlike those in the plant. (See Chapter Seven.) Hence, another difference between a synthetic and a natural essential oil is in the isomers they contain. They may contain compounds of the same formula, but not necessarily of the same isomeric mix.

But these are not the most important differences between natural and unnatural aromatic oils. The chemical formula and isomeric structure of a compound do not completely describe that compound in all of its aspects. This is particularly true of the aspects that have to do with human interaction and healing.

The Law of Constant Composition

There is a fundamental law (assumption) of chemistry called "The Law of Constant Composition," also called "The Law of Definite Proportions." The law is stated as follows: "The elemental composition and the properties of a pure substance or compound is always the same, regardless of its source." In other words, a specific isomer of a specific compound whether produced by nature or in a laboratory or by any other means would have exactly the same properties in every way. In other words, they would be identical and indistinguishable. This is the fundamental basis in science of why allopathic physicians and pharmaceutical companies believe that they can reproduce compounds in a lab that will have all of the properties of the one produced in nature. This is why when a drug company finds an effective herb or natural medicine that actually works, they analyze it to find "the active ingredients" so they can then synthesize them in a lab, mass produce them in a patented form, and make a fortune.

The law of constant composition is also the basis of how and why the U.S. FDA has ruled that a compound manufactured in a chemical factory can be labeled as "natural" when sold as long as that compound is also produced by nature. Hence, when your drinks or foods say that they contain "natural flavorings," that usually means they are flavored by artificial substances synthesized in a commercial laboratory. But since they are also found in nature, they can be called "natural," even though man-made.

When chemists state the law of constant composition, saying that a given compound of given formula and structure is a given compound of given formula and structure— identical in all respects, independent of its origin, they may be right when they limit themselves to inorganic chemistry. They may even be right to some extent when they limit themselves to organic chemistry outside of living processes. They err when it comes to biochemistry and the interaction of living systems and the creation of chemical compounds by life processes, including the alterations in the behavior of chemical compounds in therapeutic applications.

When it comes to how compounds and mixtures of compounds (such as essential oils) respond and behave—their origin and source counts, as well as their history. They may be chemically identical, but they are not therapeutically identical because they are not spiritually identical. Natural organic substances, created by God, are endorsed by him and contain his signature. Synthetic compounds do not contain his endorsement and signature. Natural is different than synthetic in ways that go beyond chemistry.

Essential Oils as Cosmic-Biological Creations

There is an interesting book entitled *The Nature of Substance* by a German scientist, Rudolf Hauschka, D.Sc. The premise of his book is that matter is a physical precipitate of spirit. In this context he discusses a wide variety of topics—from the structure of the cosmos to the structure of the atom. He calls the oils of a plant "perfect plant substances . . . products of cosmic-biological synthesis." According to Hauschka, essential oils are the outgoing oils by which plants interact with other plants and with animals by their extended aromas, while the fatty acids are the life-force preserving oils that focus inward in order to preserve the species.

In his book he also analyzes the elements of the Periodic Table for their individual and unique places in the created universe—from the perspectives of both chemistry and spirit. In Hauschka's view, every element and every compound carries spiritual counterparts. Hauschka also discusses the biotransmutation of elements as a part of natural life processes. The main point of Hauschka's treatise is the same point we have been making in this chapter, that all physical matter has a non-physical counterpart that determines the form and nature of the physical precipitate, as well as its behavioral properties when applied therapeutically.

With respect to compounds of the same formula, same isomer, same physical characteristics in every way this concept has important implications. The history of the compound is hidden beneath its form, including its spiritual history. The law of constant composition which scientists have verified to their satisfaction with the chemistry in a lifeless lab does not apply to the chemistry in a living organism, including people. Synthetic compounds have different ethereal counterparts than natural compounds of the same formula and structure. Secularly produced compounds do not have the same healing properties as those that have been prayed over, or created by God, himself, as a natural substance. These are factors never tested nor considered by materialistic science, which is why they are unaware of them.

Hence, the compounds of a natural oil, birthed by the cosmic-biological processes of a living plant possess a different spiritual blueprint than the same compound made in a lab. Different thoughts, different intents, different etheric imprints underlie natural compounds than those that underlie synthetic ones. This is one of the main reasons natural medicines are better—more able to offer benefits without unwanted side effects.

Natural Benzoic Acid vs. Synthetic

Homeopathy is a system of medicine where therapeutic substances are successively diluted as 1–10% solutions with prescribed numbers of rhythmic concussions delivered to the diluted fluids between each dilution. The process of repeated dilutions and periods of rhythmic excitations of the solution continues until the concentration of the substance originally dissolved in the water has been reduced to virtual zero, while the spiritual essence of the substance has been transferred to the water. This is the way homeopathic remedies are made. The process of making homeopathic remedies is not describable by classical laws of chemistry or physics. It is beyond chemistry.

Hauschka carried out a series of experiments with benzoic acid of two types. One was synthesized from coal tar while the other was from a natural plant source. Hauschka wanted to see if synthetic and natural benzoic acid were both processed into a homeopathic remedy in the same way whether they would result in remedies with the same potentcies. At the start of the process, the two benzoic acids were chemically indistinguishable. At the end of the process, two quite different homeopathic preparations resulted. The one made from the natural benzoic acid had all the desirable healing properties a homeopath would expect, while the one made from the synthetic benzoic acid had no healing properties.

Hauschka concluded that synthetic derivatives cannot be etherealized by rhythmic potentization. "They have forfeited all relationship to cosmic and terrestrial rhythms." he says. "A basic biological difference exists between natural and synthetic products despite their chemical identity," he concludes,

Hauschka goes on to say, "The two benzoic acids are off-spring of two realms. . . These realms are governed by different laws. The living plant belongs with its whole spectrum of substances to the realm governed by the laws of life. . . In the second realm the laws of physical, atomic, and molecular chemistry prevail. In one case we are dealing with organisms, in the other with mechanisms. Hence, the laws of matter are entirely valid in the mechanical realm, but not in the organic."

Onycha oil (*Styrax benzoin*), discussed in Chapter Ten, contains up to 20% benzoic acid. In that chapter, we mentioned that natural oil of onycha dissolved in ethyl alcohol was more effective as an antiseptic than synthetic benzoic acid in a tincture of similar concentration. Now you know another reason why the natural tincture of onycha possesses superior therapeutic properties by comparison to the synthetic version. The reason is more than chemistry.

The Nature of Matter

Every piece of material matter—organic, inorganic, living or dead—is underlain by a spiritual/ethereal counterpart, an archetype, a blueprint, a template, a substrate, a hidden thought-pattern. The visible, tangible, and measurable forms of the physical universe are all determined by the invisible, intangible, and immeasurable forms in the ether. Spirit is primary. Material manifestation is secondary. The nature of matter is determined by ethereal factors manifested as material.

❤ ARTICLE FOUR
CONSCIOUSNESS
IN ESSENTIAL OILS

The foundations of secular science, as practiced today, rest upon two assumptions:

(1) The universe came into existence by chance, requiring neither a creator nor a pre-existing intelligence; and

(2) The objective world exists independent of the perceiving subject.

Thus, materialistic scientists make an atheistic assumption about the origin of the universe as well as an assumption about our place, as humans, in that universe. In other words, scientific practice today allows no consideration for an intelligent creator with a loving plan for the enfoldment of his creation. Neither does the current practice of science allow for the participation and interaction of the experimenter with the experiment. In other words, the current scientific paradigm states that we, as individual humans, are not connected with the universe around us. By presupposing this, scientists act in the belief that we are detached and can carry out "objective" experiments that are independent of the experimenting researcher.

These are the assumptions of present-day science and both of them are false. When scientists presume them, they are not doing so by any method of science. It is a simple matter of blind belief, no different than a person's blind belief in or unquestioning acceptance of a particular dogma of a particular religion. Thus, scientists start from a premise they have not verified by the scientific method.

The truth is that there is a consciousness that pre-existed creation, that is responsible for creation, that has a plan and a motive in bringing creation into existence, and continues to operate consciously throughout the created universe. Call this consciousness God, if you will. Call it an assumption, if you will. All of current science is based on assumptions. So what is wrong with you choosing different ones, ones that provide a better fit to the universe as we see it and know it?

The truth is also that we are all part of that universal consciousness. We truly are created in God's image. God is omnipresent and we are connected with that omnipresence, whether we realize it or not. No matter what we do by way of scientific experimentation, we are always part of the experiment, part of God's omnipresence and, hence, our presence within the objects of the experiment. Our consciousness plays a role in the outcome, try as we may to make it otherwise. In other words, complete objectivity, as defined by materialistic scientists, is impossible. Unless scientists take into account their role in their experiments, their interpretations of their data will always be somewhat flawed and incomplete. Scientists use the mathematics of statistics to obscure and overcome this fact.

Spiritual Implications of Physical Science

Edward Close, PhD, has written an insightful book entitled *Transcendental Physics*. He took all of the most significant experimental and theoretical work of the 20th century and integrated it into two conclusions (see p. 710). A brief summary of the scientific foundations, data, and principles he integrated, analyzed, and took into account is given below:

1. Max Planck's discovery of the discrete quantum nature of physical energy as measured by Planck's constant and the development of quantum physics. (1900)

2. Albert Einstein's special and general theories of relativity, along with his explanation of the photoelectric effect and Plank's quantum observations. (1905-1915)

3. Neils Bohr's model of the atom and development of quantum theory. (1914-1930)

4. Werner Heisenberg's uncertainty principle and development of quantum probability matrices. (1925-1930)

5. Erwin Schroedinger's wave equation is derived and verified enabling more precise and complete descriptions of atoms and their quantum energy levels. (1926-1935)

6. Albert Einstein, Boris Podolsky, Nathan Rosen, and Neils Bohr debate a paradox (so called "EPR paradox") resolution of which showed that matter does not exist without the participation of an observer. (1935)

7. John Bell formulates a theorem that provides an experimental means to resolve the debate between Rosen, Podolsky, Einstein, and Bohr so that the issue of "what is matter" can be definitively resolved. (1964)

8. George Spencer Brown published a new calculus in a book, *Laws of Form*, which provided a means to express the concepts of modern physics in mathematical language necessary to describe the nature of matter as both particulate (quantum) and wavelike (continuous). (1969)

9. John A. Wheeler proposes the delayed-choice, double-slit experiment where the nature of a light beam enroute to a target can be made to manifest as a beam of particles (quanta) or as a wave form (frequency) depending on the choices of the observer after a light beam is already on its way to a target. (1978)

10. Alain Aspect and his colleagues demonstrate, experimentally, that quantum phenomena must be observed before they may be said to exist as physical objects. All matter composed of particles (electrons, protons, and neutrons) manifests as both quantum and wave phenomena. Physical energy by Planck's constant is a quantum phenomenon, but is also a wave with frequencies. (1982)

11. Edward R. Close combines all of these scientific theories, experiments, mathematical models, and achievements into a logical sequence that proves that a pervasive form of consciousness not only must exist throughout the universe in order for the universe to exist, but necessarily preceded physical creation. (1996)

Ed Close and his co-researcher, Vernon Neppe, MD, PhD, are currently (2013) completing an even more profound treatise entitled, *Reality Begins with Consciousness*, that for the first time provides a scientifically complete mathematical theory, in nine dimensions, relating space, time and conscious. No longer can physics, psychology, and spirituality be considered as separate unrelated fields.

Non-Local Reality and Infinite Velocity

You would have to read Close's well written 365 page book, *Transcendental Physics*, to see how he ties all of this together in a rigorous and irrefutable way. Besides a scientific proof of an all-knowing consciousness (which theologians would call "omniscience"), Close has also demonstrated the "non-locality" of that consciousness. The concept of non-locality in physics means that something appears to exist everywhere at once. Quantum physicists have already encountered this. The consciousness required to explain the creation and continued existence of the universe is a non-local reality. When we earlier discussed the experiments that implied that thought travels at infinite speeds, that was another way to say that thought is a non-local reality, existing simultaneously everywhere. That which is described as "non-locality" in the jargon of science is described as "omnipresence" in the language of theology. Thus, the precepts of science have unintentionally proven the existence of God. The bottom line of Close's work can be summarized by the two conclusions given immediately below:

(1) There is a consciousness that pre-existed creation that has a plan and continues to be conscious throughout all creation.

(2) We who manifest human consciousness are inextricably connected to the universe such that the so called "objective world" does not exist independent of we who observe it. That is, we and the universe are actually integral parts of one whole.

As you can see, these two conclusions are diametrically opposite to the two basic premises of secular science stated earlier. Yet, these conclusions follow logically and inescapably from the principles of science already known to describe the physical universe. In other words, if you are a scientist who comprehends and accepts the natural laws of physics and chemistry as they have been developed and come to be understood during the last century, you would have to come to the same two conclusions stated above or be logically and scientifically inconsistent. In other words, atheistic science is a self-contradiction.

God's existence, omnipresence, and omniscience form the foundation for the universe as implied by the tenets of science. The laws of physics tell us that without a continuously conscious God everywhere there can be no physical universe. Our very existence and the ultimate validity of science depends on the presence of an infinite, eternal being. Thus, science and scripture are in agreement.

> The eyes of the Lord are in every place, keeping watch on the evil and the good.   Proverbs 15:3

> Indeed he is not far from each one of us. For in him we live and move and have our being.   Acts 17:27-28

> Where can I go from your spirit? Or where can I flee from your presence? If I ascend to heaven, you are there; if I make my bed in Sheol, you are there.   Psalm 139:7-8

For more scripture along these lines, read Psalm 139 in its entirety.

The Next Step

The accomplishments of secular science over the past three centuries have been spectacular, even though they rest upon an incomplete and faulty foundation that is only partially true. But, as mentioned in the Article One of Part Three on *The Limits of Science*, the scientific method is not capable of arriving at absolute answers. No scientific study is final. All scientific publications are but progress reports that will ultimately be refined or discarded as new knowledge and insight becomes available and known.

While current scientific understanding is flawed and incomplete, this is nothing new. Science will forever be flawed and incomplete. It is the nature of scientifically derived data to be so. The only pathway to a complete and flawless understanding of the universe is by a spiritual path, not a scientific one. But science is a great tool and can be integrated into a spiritual path. Humbly recognizing the limits of secular science, true scientists who live by prayer and devotion to God remain unattached to present and past accomplishments and are ever seeking to take the next step—to break through to the next, more inclusive paradigm for the benefit of life on this planet.

The next step for secular science is to renounce its atheistic assumptions and adopt a position closer to the reality of the universe that includes a proper understanding of God and our proper place and function in his creation. When that happens, the seemingly spectacular accomplishments of science over the past three centuries will seem trivial in light of what will be discovered when scientists remove the self-imposed blinders that most of them wear today. We are currently on the brink of that new era when science and spirituality will be reunited.

Waves or Particles?

The items of the physical universe we observe with our eyes and ears are sometimes perceived in forms that seem continuous and other forms that seem to be constructed of discrete units. In other words, we can see a concrete wall that consists of one continuous slab of poured stone while a wall of brick is composed of discrete units, all the same size, yet together forming a wall.

Physical matter seems to be continuous to us. Tables and chairs seem solid. Water and beverages seems to be fluids that flow and mix together as continuous streams or liquids in a cup. The atmosphere seems to be a continuous medium of gases we can breathe and feel as a waft of wind on our faces. But the truth is that none of these items are continous. They are composed of particles—atoms and molecules. In turn, atoms and molecules are composed of smaller particles—electrons, protons, and neutrons which are composed of even smaller, more fundamental particles called quarks. However, there is an end to this descent into divisions of smaller and smaller units of substance. Ultimately, all matter seems to be composed of discrete particles which, at some point, are no longer divisible into smaller units. These are called "quanta."

Light and other forms of electromagnetic radiation generally behave as wave phenomena, which is based on a continuum concept. Waves vibrate in a continuous spectrum of frequencies, phases, and levels of intensity and energy. But light can also be observed as being composed of photons, an indivisible smallest unit measured by multiples of Planck's constant. The things of this universe all seem to manifest either the properties of particles or the properties of waves, but not both simultaneously. Thus, even light beams, normally perceived as waves, can behave as streams of quantum particles.

Classical Physics vs. Quantum Physics

Both classical and quantum physics are true descriptions of the world around us. It basically depends on whether you are looking through a telescope or a microscope which viewpoint prevails and holds true.

Classical physics views the universe as a continuum that can be conceptually divided and subdivided into smaller and smaller units ad infinitum where even the smallest unit can still be divided into still smaller ones. In Classical physics, there is no "smallest unit." In classical mechanics, the experimenter is separate, detached, and independent of the experiment. The test of validity in classical physics is whether or not other researchers can conduct the same experiment and obtain the same results. Replication of results, independent of the observer, is the criterion for proof in classical science.

Quantum physics is the study of the universe viewed as being composed of discrete indivisible units. In quantum physics, there is always a "smallest unit" of energy or matter beyond which there can be no further divisions. In quantum mechanics the experimenter is always part of the experiment. The test of validity in quantum physics is more difficult since the separateness, detachment and independence of the experimenter cannot be achieved. In quantum physics, lack of replication may not be an indication of disproof, but only an indication of different attitudes and choices on the part of different experimenters.

Since 1900, it has come to be understood that particulate matter can also manifest as waves and that waves of electromagnetic energy can also manifest as particles. Thus is the innate duality of this universe. The universe is accurately described by Newtonian physics on a scale of normal experience, low frequencies, and reasonable velocities. It is described by Einsteinian concepts at velocities approaching the speed of light. It is described by quantum physics on a scale of atoms, photons, quarks, and Planck energy units. The same phenomena can manifest as either waves or particles, but not both at the same time. Thus light can propagate as discrete photons in a quantum manner or as rays in the manner of waves. Matter can also exist as particles (electrons, protons, and neutrons) in a quantum manner or as a beam of electrons or protons that has all the properties of waves including frequency, amplitude, spectra, and phase.

Whether we experience the universe as vibrational wave forms or bundles of particles depends on our choices as human beings. Our manner of observation actually determines what we see. Our observation is part of the picture. Matter and energy exist as sets of probabilities in the etheric world before they manifest as form and energy in the physical world. Of the various probabilities present in the ether, the determination of what manifests is set by human choice. In other words, our thoughts and intentions are part of the creative process by which nature manifests itself. Whether we know it or not, we live in a participatory universe. Our choices, words, thoughts, doubts, and intentions have an effect on everything—including essential oils.

Oils and the Uncertainty Principle

With respect to essential oils, back in Chapter Six we introduced the benzene ring—a set of six carbons linked in a hexagon with six hydrogen atoms attached. As carbon and hydrogen atoms composed of electrons, protons, and neutrons, the benzene ring is a form of particulate matter—an ordered configuration of quanta (atomic particles). However, as mentioned in that chapter, scientists have discovered, that when six carbons join with six hydrogens in the manner of a benzene ring, the resultant no longer behaves like matter. It takes on the properties of a standing wave with frequency, amplitude, spectra, and phase. In other words, matter has become energy. This is Einsteinian physics. (There is a rainbow representation of a benzene ring as a wave form on the back cover.)

Within classical physics, which now includes the concepts of both Newton and Einstein, all particles and objects have definite and specific locations, velocities, moments, spins, etc. Within this paradigm, there can be certainty. All things can be known and measured, provided the instrumentation is sensitive and sophisticated enough. In classical physics the observer is regarded as separate from the phenomena of investigation. Einstein's new ideas did not refute those of Newton. They added to Newton. According to the Theory of Relativity, the line between energy and matter is not fixed while time and space are not absolutes. Even so, through Einstein's equations, all transformations and distortions of energy, matter, time and space are still predictable, knowable, and exactly measurable.

Within quantum physics, things are different. There are no longer any definite locations, velocities, moments, spins, etc., only probabilities. In quantum mechanics there is uncertainty. All things cannot be known. Knowing some things precludes knowing others. This is true no matter how sensitive or sophisticated our instrumentation. This is true because in quantum physics the observer is part of the observation, which unavoidably alters the process under observation. The better the observer measures one part of a phenomena, the less able they are to measure another. Thus, in studying the motion of an atomic particle, one can know its precise location, but not its spin. Or one can know its precise spin, but not its location. This uncertainty is an intrinsic property of matter and not the fault of inadequate technology or inaccurate scientific measurement. Knowing one quantity renders uncertain the other parameters. This discovery was first articulated by Werner Heisenberg in 1925 as a twenty-four-year-old graduate student. It is called the "Heisenberg Uncertainty Principle." In a quantum experiment, among the set of possible outcomes or observations, only one will manifest to an observer in any given session. The specific probability that manifests depends on the choice of the observer.

Therefore, essential oils should not be thought of as having fixed and specific chemical or physical qualities and characteristics. That is classical thinking. They should be thought of as consisting of sets of probabilities. The specific probability that ultimately manifests is determined by the intentions of and choices made by the person applying and/or receiving the oil. Until these choices are made, the oil does not possess any particular property—only a set of possibilities. (See *Quantum Physics, Essential Oils, & the Mind-Body Connection* by Stewart in the Bibliography.)

Quantum Answers to Aromatherapy Questions

From now on, when a friend asks you what a particular oil <u>will</u> do, what issues it <u>will</u> address, what diseases it <u>will</u> alleviate, etc., give them a quantum physics answer. Just say, "I don't know. This bottle of oil is only a container of possibilities. You decide which one you want to manifest."

You can then elaborate to your friend that within a bottle of essential oil there are only a finite set of probabilities. They don't do everything. Based on past experiences that others have had, you can say what a particular oil <u>may</u> do, what issues it <u>may</u> address, what diseases it <u>may</u> alleviate, etc. But as to what it <u>will</u> do, that is a choice to be made by the receiver as well as by the one applying the oil. That choice can be made before, during, or after the oil is applied. Depending on the choices made, the oil will manifest one or more of its possibilities—but not all of its possibilities in any given application.

This means that when researchers study oils, they won't all get the same results from the same oils because they all have different expectations. In other words, the outcomes of the experiments will vary according to the prejudices, desires, beliefs, intents, and choices of the experimenter. Unless such factors are taken into account, no scientific study of an essential oil is completely valid.

Different people receive different results from the same essential oils. This is partly explained by differences in personal chemistry—which is classical thinking. A more complete explanation must consider the subatomic and quantum aspects of the oils where their properties are mere probabilities until choices are made by the participants who use them. It is on this level that oils respond to our prayers and intentions, not on the level of gross chemistry.

The properties manifested by essential oils are a combination of chemistry, quantum physics, and the faith of the user. It is a blend of both the wave mechanics and partical mechanics of the physical world along with the non-physical attributes of the ethereal world.

The Substance of Faith

In this and the last chapter we have been laying the groundwork to show that both science and scripture support the same conclusions, namely, that God's consciousness is present in all of creation, and that he can hear and respond anywhere, any time, at the level of the atoms. The fundamental requirement for us to exercise these spiritual/scriptural/scientific laws of God's creation is faith.

In the book of Hebrews of the *New Testament* we find the the following statement:

> Faith is the substance of things hoped for, the evidence of things not seen.   Hebrews 11:1

Faith is a substance. This means that even though its initial form is ethereal (not physical), it is as real as tangible matter, as real as something solid you can feel and touch and grasp in your hand. This verse means that with faith the object of one's hope is already formed. It begins instantly in invisible, unmanifested form, before it appears physically, but it is already a reality in God's consciousness. It is only a matter of time before it manifests materially. The very fact of your faith is, itself, the evidence and the proof that the unseen ethereal form of your hope has already come into being, waiting to become physical reality in God's time and in your time, when you are receptive and spiritually ready to receive it.

There is a chronological order to the creative process, including the creation of a hope or a healing. The order of creation is that the unseen comes first. Your hope is first conceived in the ethereal and vibrational realms and then, and only then, can it manifest in the physical earthly realms. It is the vibrations of the unseen realms that bring all things into physical reality. God first conceived of his creation, then spoke it as vibration which then became manifested as light, air, water, earth, plant, animal, and human.

Faith is the opposite of fear. They cannot coexist. You have one or the other, but not both. Faith is total trust in the benevolent creator as your father, provider, and protector. In the book of Romans we read the following:

> Whatsoever does not proceed from faith is sin.
> Romans 14:23

One can just as well say, "Whatsoever does not proceed from faith is fear." Fear is doubting God. Fear is blindness to God. Fear is denial of God. Fear is disbelief of God. That is why Paul called it "sin." Sin is any act, thought, emotion, or deed that places a separation between you and God. (cf. Isaiah 59:2; II Chronicles 24:20) Nothing creates separation more than fear. Fear is at the root of virtually every disease—physical, mental, spiritual, and social. While fear drives out faith, its opposite is love. The opposite of love is not hate. It is fear.

> There is no fear in love; but perfect love casteth out fear.
> I John 4:18

The foundation of faith is love. But faith is more than mere belief. One can believe and fear at the same time. Belief can be mental while faith must be spiritual. Belief can be a head-only thing. Faith is a thing of the heart. Faith originates from a higher vibrational level of consciousness than belief.

So how does one gain real faith? A faith that goes beyond belief? A faith that is real and substantive? A faith that is, in fact, a real substance? A substance of things hoped for? The evidence and the proof of things unseen?

Mark 9:17-29 tells of a father with a son suffering severe seizures who came to Jesus pleading, "If you are able to do anything, have pity on us and help us."

Jesus replied, "If you are able!—All things can be done

for the one who believes."

Tearfully, the father of the child responded to Jesus, saying, "Lord, I believe; help thou mine unbelief."

In this example, when Jesus referred to "the one who believes," he was actually referring to faith in the sense spoken in Hebrews 11:1. The man's response is a good description of where most of us are. We believe with our minds, but in our hearts we harbor some unbelief. We have feelings of doubt. We have fears. The question is, how do we go from belief to faith? How do we clear the heart so that it will be capable of expressing true faith?

A proper intellectual belief is good. It is the first step toward faith. Intellectual belief may be the best we can do in the situation at hand, but if we cling to that belief it can be turned into the faith that moves mountains. The key is love. Devotion and love for God. Devotion and love for ourselves and our fellow human beings. Devotion to God is surrender to God. Surrender to God requires humility. Humility is recognizing God as the sole doer in the universe and giving God the credit for everything.

In the story of the man with the epileptic son told in Mark, he had his doubts and fears which he confessed honestly in complete surrender to the will and mercy of Jesus. His devotion to the Lord, as well as to his afflicted child, were true and pure. His request to Christ was cleansed with the tears of his sincerety. The genuineness of his simple supplication touched the heart of the Lord. Through the father's belief and unbelief, transformed into faith, the demon that had possessed the boy was cast out.

The father's frank confession to Jesus of his doubt is a key element in this story. In James 5:16, the congregation is admonished to "Confess your faults one to another . . . that ye may be healed." Sincere introspection and recognition of one's shortcomings is a condition for healing. In the exercise of one's faith, denial of one's doubt does not clear it from one's consciousness. One must be honest with one's self, and with others, in order to manifest a faith by which all things are possible.

Receiving Gifts of Spirit

In I Corinthians 12 St. Paul describes the gifts of the spirit and urges us to earnestly seek them, saying that they are "given to every man." Paul lists nine of them: (1) Wisdom; (2) Knowledge; (3) Faith; (4) Healing; (5) Miracles; (6) Prophecy; (7) Discernment; (8) Diverse Tongues; and (9) Interpretation of Tongues. God intends for everyone to have these gifts, but you have to ask for them and prepare yourself to receive them.

The third gift of the spirit is faith. The way to acquire the gift of faith is to ask for it. Pray for it. Pray without ceasing for it. And then surrender yourself to God in order to receive it. The Gospel of Thomas quoted near the beginning of the chapter on the *Limits of Science* quotes Jesus as saying: "The seeker should not stop until he finds." The Gospel of Matthew quotes Jesus as saying:

> Ask, and it shall be given you; seek and ye shall find; knock and it shall be opened unto you: For every one that asketh receiveth; and he that seeketh findeth; and to him that knocketh it shall be opened.   Matthew 7:7-8

These are promises from God. They are guarantees. They are laws of the universe as God has created it. But they are only guarantees of God's side of the bargain. To keep our side we must first ask. Then we must persist. Persistence achieves all it strives for. We fail only when we give up. This is the way to the faith that can do all things. (Matthew 17:20) True faith is more than an article of intellectual belief. It is more than a mental construct. Faith is the experience of being in contact with God's presence within ourselves, around ourselves, and in everything.

Consciousness in Matter

Hundreds of scientists in thousands of experiments over the past century have demonstrated that material matter responds to our thoughts, our motives, and/or our prayers. Yet, to read the textbooks of science used in our classrooms, you would never know that this was true. The reason such a vast body of data has not been incorporated into traditional scientific texts is because of the fundamental assumptions of scientific materialism stated at the beginning of this chapter that accept, *a priori*, that there is no God and that humans and their thoughts do not interact with physical substance. Until this prejudicial stance of the majority of scientists has been repealed, you won't find much in standard texts on mind over matter nor will you find much about the consciousness within matter that makes communication between humans and the elements possible.

Nevertheless, such consciousness does exist. The nonbelief of scientists does not make it nonexistent. The earth is round and revolves around the sun whether humans believe it or not, and there was a time when most people did not believe these things. Disbelief in the truth does not negate it.

In all ages of history, there have always been exceptional individuals who see beyond what the general population can see. They are the heralds of progress that lead the way to greater and greater understandings for us all, both spiritual and temporal.

Let us now review some of the data and experiments (currently omitted from textbooks) that testify to consciousness in matter and how matter can, and does, respond to human thought and direction.

The Power of Prayer on Plants

A summation of the concepts of modern physics, as articulated by Edward Close in his book, *Transcendental Physics*, as well as works by many other authors, including those of Rudolf Hauschka, *The Nature of Substance*, and Richard Gerber, *Vibrational Medicine*, leads to one and only one conclusion: All creations, both animate and inanimate, possess consciousness at some level. Without innate consciousness nothing exists. Consciousness is the fundamental substance that underlies every proton, electron, neutron, thoughtron, and lifetron in the universe and is what makes the manifested universe possible. That consciousness existed before the universe was formed and continues without interruption as an omnipresent all knowing part of creation today. In fact, if there was even the briefest break in the concentration of that consciousness, the universe would dissolve in an instant. These are conclusions drawn entirely from science—not from religion and not from scripture.

However, scripture concurs with science with regard to the unbroken continuity of God's consciousness. In Psalm 121 we read these words:

> The Lord is your keeper . . . He who keeps you will not slumber. He who keeps Israel will neither slumber nor sleep.
>
> Psalm 121:3-5

The presence of a universal consciousness in all things has been established both from science and from scripture. Therefore, it should be no surprise that when we consciously communicate with plants, they can and do consciously respond.

The life work of Rev. Franklin Loehr is summarized in his brief book entitled *The Power of Prayer on Plants*. Loehr was originally trained as a research chemist, but then became a Presbyterian pastor. His dual background eventually led him to establish the Religious Research Foundation in California while employed as a staff minister of the First Congregational Church of Los Angeles, the largest Congregational church in the world. By means of thousands of carefully controlled experiments on plants, many of which were validated and replicated by others, Loehr established a firm scientific verification that plants do, indeed, respond to people and their prayers and thoughts.

One example of the type of experiments Loehr carried out was to study the effect of prayer on seed germination. He would plant identical sets of seeds (usually corn or wheat) to be attended and watered in identical ways but with one difference: One set would receive positive prayers for their early germination and vigorous growth, the other set would be ignored. In all experiments, the prayed-for seeds and plants did better. They germinated earlier and grew faster in both height and depth of root than the ignored seeds. These results occurred when single people prayed but were more pronounced when groups prayed. Distance was also not found to be a factor, whether those praying were in the same room or miles away. The odds of

Loehr's results were calculated to be approximately 1 in 2,000,000 by chance. Science generally accepts an experimental result as valid proof of a hypothesis when the odds are consistently at least 1 in 100.

In many of Loehr's experiments a third set of plants was engaged toward which negative thoughts were aimed. In most of these instances the seeds did not sprout at all or were delayed and stunted in their growth compared to the neutral control set of seeds.

After numerous experiments over a period of years Loehr was able to make three statements, not as faith, but as established fact:

(1) Prayer can make a difference in the speed of seed germination and in the rate and vigor of plant growth.

(2) Prayer is an objective energy as real as sunlight or electricity. Prayer is not merely a state of mind.

(3) Scientific laboratory research can be done in religious fields with demonstrable, replicable results.

Plants as Lie Detectors

Cleve Backster was America's foremost lie-detector expert back in the 1960s. The polygraph is a sensitive galvanometer that can detect minute changes in electric current. When attached to a person, a lie-detector passes a tiny current through the skin which varies according to the variable resistance of the skin. Variations in skin resistance occur according to one's level of calmness or agitation. The theory is that if one is telling the truth, one maintains a degree of even-mindedness and galvanic skin resistance remains steady. If one is telling an untruth, they will be internally agitated causing changes in organic skin activity that alters the chemistry, by subtle secretions of the sweat glands, which changes skin resistance. These fluctuations are transduced as variations in readings traced on the polygraph recording paper. An experienced examiner can interpret these wiggly lines as evidence of truth or falsehood.

Backster was a plant lover and kept a large house plant called *Dracaena massangeana* in his office. Dracaena is a tropical plant similar to a palm tree. It is known as the "dragon tree." One day, after he had been up all night in his school for polygraph examiners where he teaches policemen and security officers from around the world, he attached the electrodes of one of his lie detectors to the leaf of the dragon tree. He was curious to see if the leaf would register the effect of pouring water on the soil about its roots. He expected that the absorption of water by the plant would reduce its electrical resistance by increasing the conductivity of the fluids in the plant. Much to his surprise, the plant registered an increase of resistance, up and down in an occilatory motion, similar to the response of a human being experiencing an emotion. "Was the plant expressing an emotion, perhaps one of pleasure upon receiving a refreshing drink of water?"

His curiosity aroused, Backster then initiated a series of hundreds of experiments over the next several years on plant responses to a variety of circumstances. Among his discoveries, he found that when he threatened the plant with something unpleasant, it would trace an excited message on the polygraph, a statement of fear. For example, if he poured hot coffee on one of the leaves or cut off a piece of a limb, the tree would express a dramatic tracing of excitement. More amazingly, Backster found that if he even thought of doing violence to the plant, it would respond to his mind before he carried out the actual act. When Backster would only pretend in his mind that he was going to harm the plant, it would not react as if it knew when he was serious and when he was only kidding. The plant could discriminate between real and pretended intent. Over a period of years, Backster tested more than 2,000 different varieties of plants and fruits. All of them tested as if they had consciousness in response to human actions, thoughts, and intentions.

Backster found that plants communicate, not just with people, but with other plants as well. In one of Backster's most creative experiments, he put two large plants in a room and had a student enter the room and destroy one of them by smashing its pot and ripping up its leaves and limbs. The only witness to the violence was the remaining plant. Backster then attached a polygraph to the surviving plant and let a series of students walk through the room one at a time. When the student guilty of murdering the other plant entered the room the galvanometer readings went wild. Thus, a living plant was able to identify the killer from a line up. Backster was convinced that plants at a crime scene could correctly identify key parties to the crime. When Backster tried to sell the idea of using plants to identify criminals to police departments, it did not fly.

Like Rev. Franklin Loehr, Backster also found that once a plant had formed a relationship with a particular individual, the thoughts and actions of that individual could be recorded in real time at a distance, even when measured in miles. The forces and transmissions involved did not seem to fall off inverse to the square like the signals of ordinary radio.

Another amazing finding of Backster was that even when a leaf was cut from the living plant, it still manifested a conscious response to various forms of experimentation, just as if it were still attached to the living stem. Even when the leaf was shredded, it would emit the same appropriate responses. Thus, the consciousness of a plant seems to extend down to its very cells and molecules—including the compounds of its oils.

Backster was to conclude that the consciousness of plants is more than the simple concept we hold about humans with brains as central processors of consciousness. Plant awareness seemed to extend well beyond the physical dimensions and space occupied by the plant form itself. It appeared to be part of a much larger whole that enabled it to respond to stimuli, not only in its vicinity, but also at a distance.

The Spirituality of Scientists

Many of the experiments performed by Cleve Backster on the East Coast of America were replicated by a research chemist working for the International Business Machine corporation (IBM) in California on the West coast. Marcel Vogel had originally trained to become a Franciscan priest, but spent most of his adult career as a research scientist. In one of his first attempts to repeat one of Backster's experiments, he assigned a group of students in one of his classes to each attempt to replicate Backster's results. Vogel had replicated Backster's results several times, himself, but found that his students could not. "What was the difference," he wondered.

According to the principles of the scientific method, a fact is not considered to have been verified until it can be repeatedly demonstrated by many experiments by many experimenters. How could it be that different experimenters performing the same experiment in every detail would obtain conflicting results.

Vogel concluded that the consciousness of the experimenter was part of the experiment. In particular, in experiments with living plants, the spiritual development of the researcher must be at such a level as to enable the experiment to work. Because Vogel had spent a lifetime of discipline in prayer, fasting, and meditation, his spiritual sensitivities were more finely tuned than those of his students. Plants would perform for him, but not for his students.

Backster had actually discovered the same thing. When negative people or skeptical scientists came to witness Backster's plant experiments, they would often shut down and refuse to perform. To the unbelieving visitors, it was proof that Backster's experiments had no basis, but to Backster it was further proof that plants could sense whether those present were friendly or not. When the unwelcome visitors left, the plants would then respond again.

Scientists are trained to prove before one believes, but in experiments involving consciousness, it appears that one must believe before one can prove. It apparently takes an atmosphere and environment of faith for experiments of this nature to succeed. We are disciplined as left-brained scientists to say "I'll believe it when I see it," but as the physicist Henry Swift, editor of *Science Within Consciousness*, has said, when it comes to perceiving the subtle realities that underly the material universe, scientists must learn to accept the idea that, "I'll see it when I believe it."

In a simple experiment involving gross matter and energy at macroscopic levels, the separation of experimenter from the results of the experiment can usually be achieved within a repeatable consistency acceptable to science. This is the definition of "objective" science.

However, in experiments involving subtle energy and consciousness, the scientific method must be modified to include the influence of the experimenter since, in these circumstances, it cannot be avoided. This includes all phenomena on microscopic levels such as cellular activity and the responses of cells to molecules of essential oils.

Vogel concluded that there must be a "life force or cosmic energy surrounding all living things that is sharable among plants, animals, and humans. Man can and does communicate with plant life. Plants are living objects, sensitive, rooted in space. They may be blind, deaf, and dumb in the human sense, but there is no doubt that they are extremely sensitive instruments for measuring man's emotions. They radiate energy forces that are beneficial to man. One can feel these forces. They feed into one's own force field, which in turn feeds back energy to the plant."

Native Americans and all people who live close to nature know this. Gardeners with a green thumb know this. It is nice, however, to have scientific verification for what one experiences and feels. But not everyone experiences and feels in the same way. Just as people have different levels of intellectual capability, people have different levels of spiritual sensitivity and perception. Many scientific experiments on plants, including extracts of plants such as essential oils, cannot be carried out by ordinary scientists who lack the spiritual development to provide, by their consciousness, a subtle environment for such experiments to be carried out with clear results. To truly study plant behavior, the scientists must be able to mingle their consciousness with that of the plants and experience the consciousness of the plants first hand, as if they were temporarily one. All of the great botanists and plant scientists speak of experiences like this.

In some of the experiments carried out by Vogel, he and his helpers were able to "get inside" of plants to such an extent that they could see the inner workings of the oils and fluids in the capillaries, the gyrations of the cells, and even the detailed organizations of the DNA, itself.

Scientists of the future won't need mechanical or electronic microscopes to study the infinitesimally small. They will discipline and train themselves to see such details by their own spiritually developed faculties. The published data from remote viewing experiments has already demonstrated the human capability to see things at a distance and peer into the subspace of cells and molecules. When scientists develop and apply these latent abilities, science and spirituality will be reunited as they should be. It will ultimately be found that the furthest reaches of scientific endeavor are attainable only through faith and love. Without gifts of the spirit secular science remains locked in an opaque box, blind to the vast universe outside.

Is Inorganic Matter Conscious?

We have given several examples of how living plants respond to human thoughts. There are many more you can read about in the book, *The Secret Life of Plants* by Tompkins and Bird, as well as the book on prayer by Franklin Loehr mentioned earlier. But what about inorganic matter? Can it respond to thoughts and emotions as plants do? We have presented a detailed discussion of how modern science, by way of quantum physics, provides the theoretical basis by which matter could and should be resposive to human will and direction. We have also presented a scriptural basis by which matter could and should respond to people. The miracles of Jesus and his disciples are examples of the molecules of matter adjusting and rearranging themselves according to the intent of a person.

Among the experiments of Franklin Loehr were some on water. He found that persons who had demonstrated healing powers through their hands could hold water, bless it, and that their healing powers were transferred into the water. Richard Gerber, in his book, *Vibrational Medicine*, also speaks of transferring consciousness or etheric impressions into water and other substances such as crystalline minerals. It appears from the concepts of physics and the data of many experiments that every particle of physical matter and every manifestation of physical life has an energetic blueprint in a non-physical realm we call the "etheric" realm or universe. It is a physically invisible universe, but even more real than this one since it is fundamental to physical manifestation and essential to physical existence. Thus, there are certain forms of physical matter that can take on the etheric imprint of substances and carry the qualities of that substance without carrying a single molecule of the substance. This is the basis of homeopathic medicine where substances are diluted to the point to where not even one molecule is present in the solution, but the water, itself, maintains the etheric blueprint or energy imprint of the substance.

Substances that can take on energetic imprints include water, crystals, and essential oils. Loehr and others have found that when water is blessed, the bonding angles between the two hydrogen atoms and the oxygen atom of each molecule are changed from their normal 114°. Thus, when blessed waters crystallize, they form a variety of geometric shapes representative of their new bonding angles.

Your Car, Yourself

Another book that verifies the consciousness in material matter is entitled, *My Car, Myself*. Dr. Narayan Singh (aka Michael Lincoln), the author, is a practicing psychologist in the State of Washing-ton. As his clients came in for counsel, they would often complain about troubles with their cars. He began to notice that their car problems bore a correlation with their psychological problems. After years of observation he compiled his book. It is uncanny how accurately the psychological state of the car owner matches the mechanical state of the car.

For example, when your air conditioner goes out, it means "you are losing your cool." Whereas you had been the calm collected one of the family, circumstances have pushed you to your limit and you have become over-reactive and hot under the collar about everything—or would like to. As another example, when your right front door ceases to open, that indicates "input-avoidance." You are closed to external input and won't let people past the entrance of your "cave." It is reflective of untrustworthy parenting, says Dr. Singh. His book contains hundreds of such correlations.

Singh postulates that since people spend so much time in their automobiles the machine absorbs the vibrations and consciousness of the person to the extent that it eventually manifests the condition of the driver/owner in the form of various disrepairs. This is a book you would enjoy and could learn much about yourself. Be careful what you say, think, or do in your car. Evidently, it sees and hears you and, to those who can read its symbols (thanks to Singh's book), it can reveal a lot about yourself that you thought was hidden. (See bibliography for info to obtain a copy of *My Car, Myself*.)

Messages From Water

Water is special. It is unique among earth substances. It is the universal solvent. It exists in all three states, solid, liquid, and gas, at normal earth temperatures. It is the creator of clouds and weather. It is the medium for trillions of life forms in seas and rivers. It is one of the only liquids that expands when it freezes, enabling ice to float instead of sink. It is the vehicle for baptism in many religions. It is the cleanser of physical dirtiness. It is the fluid facilitator of all living processes in both plants and animals. As a newly formed embryo attached to our mother's womb, we were 95% water. As an adult, our bodies are still 70–80% water. The formula of water is simple—H_2O. But its behavior is complex beyond imagination. And now we find that water is also capable of storing thought and responding to human intent and emotion.

Professor Masaru Emoto is a Japanese Doctor of Alternative Medicine. He has spent many years researching the effects of words and thought on water. Some of his extraordinary work is recorded in graphic color photographs in his book, *Messages from Water.*

Emoto conducts his experiments by taking vials of water and either sending thoughts or taping words to the bottles, freezing them, and then photographing the crystals. What he found is that the geometric forms of ice reflect the thoughts aimed at the water before and as it becomes ice. With words or phrases addressed to the water, like "thank you," "love," "appreciation," "soul," "angel," or "beautiful," the crystals were attractive artistic expressions of these thoughts. With words or phrases such as "you fool," "you make me sick," "I will kill you," "demon," "devil," or "dirty," the ice crystals were ugly and distorted. The water responded appropriately regardless of the language in which the thought was expressed.

Emoto also sampled different waters from different locations. Water from clear springs and calm lakes made beautifully balanced crystals, while water from industrial sources or polluted lakes formed mis-shapen crystals. Emoto also found that water responds to sound. Beautiful classical music of the masters, such as Mozart and Chopin, formed lovely crystals in some ways representative of the themes of the music.

Emoto also developed ways to impart the imprint of other substances into water before freezing. In one experiment he imprinted the essence of Roman chamomile oil and the crystals came out in little white daisy-like forms close to the appearance of the blossoms of a chamomile plant (*Chamaemelum nobile*). In another experiment he imprinted the essence of fennel oil and the crystals formed were yellow and fine in detail, like lace, similar in appearance to the flowers of the fennel plant (*Foeniculum vulgare*).

In another experiment, Emoto sampled the natural waters where a major earthquake had just occurred, where many people had been killed or injured. The ice crystals were confused, chaotic, grotesque, and fearful-looking, reflecting the fear and apprehension of the victims. Months later he sampled the same water and more ordered, coherent, graceful, and peaceful-looking ice crystals resulted.

You would have to read Emoto's book and see his pictures of ice crystals yourself to appreciate the implications of his research. One fact is firmly established by his work. Inanimate, inorganic matter, such as simple water, does have consciousness and will respond to conscious intent from humans.

Are Any Two Snowflakes Identical?

You have probably heard that among the countless trillions of snowflakes that have fallen on earth, no two have ever been exactly alike. Of course, this is an untestable hypothesis since no one could possibly collect, photograph, and inspect every snowflake, present and past to see if this is true. One thing is certain. Snowflakes from frozen water vapor yield countless variations in form. This is unusual among natural substances. Most minerals crystallize in only one form or, at the most, two or three. Water is unique.

One reason snowflakes always seem to be different is because the earth's waters are constantly absorbing the billions of thoughts from humans every day. Thus, when it snows, the crystalline forms assumed by the flakes represent the myriad varieties of human thoughts and emotions present and absorbed at the times they fall, which is changing constantly and cover the spectrum of contrasts—from clarity to confusion, kindness to cruelty, love to hate, confidence to fear, harmony to conflict, prayers to curses, peace to war, life to death. Question: What would snow flakes look like if everyone in the world felt only spiritual, unselfish, kind, and loving thoughts?

Here's another question: With respect to water as an absorber of human consciousness, capable of carrying the imprints of subtle energies, what about our human bodies? They are 70–80% water. In several research experiments with plants, aiming negative or hateful thoughts toward plants killed them or stunted their growth. Were these thoughts transferred through the water in the plants? What are your thoughts doing to the waters of your body? Or to the waters of others around you?

Vibrating Matter into Life

Hans Jenny lived in Switzerland (1904-1972). He was a Renaissance man in every sense. A medical doctor, painter, pianist, philosopher, historian, scientist, and researcher. His boundless curiosity embraced all fields of endeavor. Among his most far-reaching areas of research was in the field of sonic vibrations and their effects upon matter, both living and non-living. His work is colorfully documented with text and photographs in the book entitled, *Cymatics*, as well as in several videos: *Cymatics*, *Cymatic Soundscapes*, and *Sound, Mind and Body*. All of these are available through the website, www.cymatic-source.com. The term, "cymatics," refers to the study of waveforms fashioned by mechanical vibration. It comes from the Greek word, *kyma*, meaning "wave."

During his many years of research, Jenny would place various finely divided powders on a surface and then submit that surface to mechanical vibrations, usually in the band of audible sound. Sometimes he employed one specific frequency (like a middle C) and sometimes several or a spectrum of frequencies. He carefully controlled and recorded the frequencies applied. His data were compiled in the form of still photographs and, in some cases, motion pictures. While the photographs are stunning in both form and color, the dynamic movements that can be seen only in the videos are breath-taking.

What Jenny demonstrated over and over is that simple vibrations can turn amorphous lifeless matter into the most intricate and complex forms that, on video, appear to possess the motions of life. Jenny's work has been developed into a system of vibrational medicine where musical tones, either sung or played, can be directed to sick body parts in ways that heal them.

What you will learn from Jenny's work is that life is vibration and is described by frequency. Higher frequencies and higher energy vibrations produce higher forms of life, including life beyond the physical and beyond the measurement of physical instruments. You and I and essential oils are all created by vibrations, the spoken word of God. The healing power of essential oils is more than chemistry. It is vibrational in nature, the resonance of the healing vibrations in the oils that carry their creator's benevolence, seeking harmony with the vibrations that comprise our bodies, minds, and souls.

Consciousness in Essential Oils

If plants, water, crystals, and even our vehicles can respond to human thought and direction, what about essential oils? The answer is a definite yes. Oil molecules are both receivers and transmitters of thought. They can receive and respond to our thoughts and, in turn, broadcast messages back to us and to our bodies. In fact, the best way to learn about essential oils is to talk to them and let them teach you as you use them. Sleep with them and pray with them and they will reveal their secrets to you. They can do this because they contain consciousness and vibration to a very high level, the level of God's very word.

You don't have to wait for science to prove this to you. There is already enough scientific data to strongly support the idea. You can discover the subtle language of essential oils through your own personal use. You don't need science to tell you to believe or not to believe. You can verify everything said here for yourself. All it takes is for you to become sensitive enough to hear the still small voices of God's nature and of the natural substances he has created for our health and healing.

If you don't feel that you have developed your spiritual sensitivities sufficiently to learn the Godly art and science of applying healing oils directly from the oils themselves, pray for such gifts. In I Corinthians 12:31 St. Paul says we should "earnestly covet the best gifts," that we should "strive for the greater gifts of spirit." Jesus said "ask and you shall receive." James 4:2 says "You do not have because you do not ask." In I Corinthians 2:14 St. Paul admonishes us saying, "Those who are unspiritual do not receive the gifts of God's Spirit," to which James 4:3 adds, "You ask and do not receive, because you ask wrongly."

In summary, what this all says is that we must make spiritual effort to attune ourselves to God and his will in order to receive, use, and express God's gifts. We don't earn such gifts, but we must prepare ourselves to manifest them on God's behalf. You can't expect God to give you a gallon of his grace when all you present to him is a one-ounce cup. Through intense and daily prayer we can expand the size of our cups that we may more generously receive from his infinite bounty, which he is ever ready to bestow upon each and every one of us.

The ultimate depths of God's universe can only be plumbed by the Spirit of God, himself. When we attune ourselves to the Spirit of God through love, then and only then can we become true scientists.

The scientists of the future will start their research with prayer, asking for God's guidance and grace, requesting the gifts of spirit necessary to accomplish the bringing of God's truth into human consciousness to the benefit of all people. It is hoped that this book will encourage scientists everywhere to start now spiritualizing their research into works for God. When a sufficient number of scientists work in that manner, the scientific discoveries of the last 1,000 years will pale by comparison to what remains to be seen. Our paltry libraries contain only the meekest hint of what remains to be seen of God's creation.

> Eye has not seen, nor ear heard, neither have entered into the heart of man, the things which God has prepared for them that love him. These things God has revealed to us through the Spirit; for the Spirit searches everything, even the depths of God. For what human being knows what is truly human except the human spirit that is within? So also no one comprehends what is truly God's except the Spirit of God. Now we have received not the spirit of the world, but the Spirit that is from God, so that we may understand the gifts bestowed on us by God. And we speak of these things in words not taught by human wisdom but taught by the Spirit, interpreting spiritual things to those who are spiritual.   I Corinthians 2:9-13

Thus it will be with the scientists of tomorrow. men and women searching everything in the Spirit of God to interpret research in the light of spiritual understanding. It is only through spiritual endeavor that the secrets of essential oils, beyond chemistry, will be understood. Only by combining spirituality and science can we hope to understand how essential oils work their healing miracles.

Conclusion

The healing knowledge being revealed and brought to light at this time in history is but a resurrection of knowledge that was once known and only temporarily lost. The newly discovered truths of today regarding the spiritual and emotional roots of disease, as well as their treatment and prevention by spiritual and natural means with herbs and oils, were once common knowledge in the ancient times before Moses and Abraham. Much of what is being called "New Age" today is actually "Old Age Rediscovered."

> What has been is what will be, and what has been done is what will be done; there is nothing new under the sun. Is there anything of which it is said, "See, this is new?" It has already been in the ages before us. Ecclesiastes 1:9-10

The vast herbal knowledge of Native Americans has, for the most part, been lost. The living repositories of this healing wisdom have largely died off without suitable heirs to carry it on to future generations. However, we need not grieve that such lore is lost forever, because it isn't.

Wisdom is inherent in nature because God put it there. Even when humans forget and lose it for a while, nature stands patiently by, always ready to teach a new generation what ancient generations once knew and intervening ones forgot.

Peter Gorman is a writer and regular adventurer into the jungles of South America. He has written a book entitled *Between the Canopy and the Forest Floor.* "While everyone who lives in the Amazon has a knowledge of the plants they need for survival," he writes, "those with the most refined knowledge of plants are those whom

Westerners call shamen, curanderos, healers, medicine men, and medicine women."

During one of Peter's early stays in the jungle, he accompanied one of the tribal healers, Pablo, on an excursion to set an animal trap.

"I had a headache," recounts Peter, "and Pablo noticed it. Moments later he pulled two leaves off a vine growing up a tree trunk and rubbed them vigorously into my temples. He actually rubbed the skin raw enough to draw a little blood, then had me hold the leaves in place there. In minutes the headache vanished. His cure worked so well that I asked if he had others. He laughed and said he did, and began to point things out as we walked."

As they trod through the rain forest, Pablo would show a plant to Peter and then act out the infirmity for which that herb was effective. Realizing that he had stumbled upon a great opportunity, Peter collected leaves, flowers, and bark from the plants Pablo discussed.

After the trap was set and they were back at the village, Peter laid out all of the plants, got his tape recorder and camera, and asked Pablo if he would discuss the plants again, explaining their curative applications. Pablo was silent for a minute, then broke into a wide grin.

"I have introduced you to the plants," he said, "but now you have to make your own friends with them."

"But I don't understand what you mean," said Peter, to which Pablo replied, "You should go sleep with them. Make friends with them. Dream them. Then you won't need me to explain what they are for."

Peter later found that the customary manner by which the curanderos acquired their knowledge of plant medicines was exactly what Pablo had described. Their belief was that plants are sentient beings, capable of listening and responding to human inquiry. What they knew of the plants and their curative powers was gained directly from the plants, themselves, who were their teachers. This was often accomplished through dreams and visions experienced while sleeping with the plants.

Apparently this manner of learning herbal medicine was also known to the healers of ancient Israel. In the *Old Testament*, Job 12:8 instructs us to "talk to the plants and they will teach you." Great botanists, such as Luther Burbank and George Washington Carver knew how to talk to plants and listen to them. That is how they conducted their research. Spiritual men and women who grow and distill therapeutic oils also know that a good way to learn what a specific oil will do and how it should be applied to people is to talk to the plants from which the oils are extracted and they will tell you.

As for learning how oils extracted from plants respond to human thought and intent, a good way is to study how plants respond to human thought and intent. There is plenty of research available on that. *The Secret Life of Plants* by Tompkins and Bird is a good place to start.

What this all means is that so long as there are living plants, the knowledge of their healing powers, including their oils, can never be lost. Even if lost and forgotten from antiquity, hidden in the vaults of time, the information is always still there in the plants, themselves, who are always ready to share what they know with anyone willing to befriend them and learn to speak and comprehend their native tongue.

Their silent language is one of the spirit and can only be heard through the spirit. But plants won't teach just anyone. They have entrance requirements and pre-requisites before you can be accepted into their special university of flowers, fields, and forests. Their entrance exam is patience. Their pre-requisite is love. Their code of conduct is respect for nature. Their tuition is a commitment to serve and share with others.

The true and complete chemistry of essential oils cannot be learned from a book like this. It can only be learned from God speaking directly to you through his loving creations—the oils and the plants, themselves.

END OF PART THREE

PART FOUR

APPENDICES AND RESOURCES

♥ CONTENTS ♥

❤ Appendix A
A Short Course
On Essential Oil
Chemistry

This is the text book and resource for a course on the chemistry of essential oils offered by the Center for Aromatherapy Research and Education (CARE) and taught by Certified CARE Instructors (CCIs)—who are members of the CARE faculty. The course is taught in two parts: Part I (Chem I) - three hours; and Part II (Chem II) - two hours—usually as a morning session followed by an early afternoon session.

You may visit www.RaindropTraining.com for a schedule of such classes taught by Dr. Stewart or other CCIs. You may also learn from that site how you may become a Certified CARE Instructor and, perhaps become trained member of the CARE Faculty and teach this course yourself.

The outline given on the next nine pages is the course guide, as it is currently offered. The outline is addressed to instructors teaching the course. Wherever you see the instruction, "pass around such and such oils..." that is a cue for you (as a reader) to do the same as you read this book (provided you have the oils). The material and page numbers to which this outline corresponds are from Part One of this book. Supporting data and information for the class is given in Part Two of this book. Except for brief comments on quantum physics, Part Three of this book is not part of the material presented in this class.

We hope you have fun browsing and studying this book. The actual classes are a lot of fun. We hope the book will be just as enjoyable and that, in the process, you gain an appreciation and feeling for the chemistry of essential oils and what wonderful gifts they are, created especially for you and me by God, himself.

INTRO TO CHEMISTRY OF ESSENTIAL OILS

(Text: *The Chemistry of Essential Oils Made Simple*)

Chem One

(The First Three Hours: 9:00 am – 12:00 noon)

I. INTRODUCTION   9:00–9:45 am

A. **Introduce yourself** Pass * *Valor®* (for courage to learn chemistry), *peppermint and lemon* (to increase alertness and retention), and *cedarwood* (to be applied to the right thumb (and roof of mouth) to help remove any mental blocks to acquiring new information and learning science.

B. **Get a show of hands** asking who has never had a chemistry course, who had it in high school, college, or graduate school, who has a degree in chemistry, who has training in organic chemistry, and who actually feared chemistry and avoided it in high school and college

C. **Set the tone for the class and quick browse through the book**
  1. **Read first part of the Introduction** from text, pp. xxix–xxx (down to "My Life as a Chemist.").
  2. **Quickly Review Part Two.** pp. 494-611.
     a. **Table32.** pp. 509-558. Explain indexing with both common and scientific names. Use Yarrow (*Achillea millefolium*), p. 510, as an example of multiple names. Pass *yarrow oil* if you have it.
     b. **Table 32A,** p. 558. Legacy and the Average Oil.
     c. **Tables 33 & 34.** pp. 559-563. Plant families & plant parts.
     d. **Table 50.** p. 573. Top 40 List. Mention a-pinene
     e. **Table 67.** p. 585. Representative Oils. *Pass 1 or 2 examples.*
     f. **Table 68.** p. 586. PMS oils, to be discussed in Chapter Nine.
  3. **Briefly Touch on Part Three.** pp. 6̀121-737.
     a. **Quantum Physics and Uncertainty Principle.** pp. 714-717. Classical physics deals with particles of atomic size and larger. Quantum physics deals with subatomic particles, i.e. electrons, protons, neutrons, quarks, neutrinos, etc. In classical science there are definite laws and predictable outcomes independent of the experimenter or observer. In quantum physics there are probabilities and, unpredicatble outcomes, dependent on the thoughts of the experimenter or observer. Science has shown that human thought influences electron behavior.
     b. **The Mind-Body-Oil Connection.** All bodily processes involve electron behavior. It is at the level of electrons that the body and mind connect and psychosomatic effects begin. It is also where the human mind connects and influences the behavior of essential oils. When asked, "What will this oil do for me?" give two answers: one based on classical chemistry (mentioning phenols, sesquiterpenes,

---

* Oils to be passed around are underlined and in italics throughout the outline.

etc. and their actions) and another based on quantum physics saying, "What do you want it to do?" (See p. 716).

Mention the booklet entitled *Quantum Physics, Essential Oils, and the Mind Body Connection*, and that if not available inn class, it is available at www.RaindropTraining.com.

   b. **Review Conclusion.** pp. 735-737. Quote Ecclesiastes (p. 735). Briefly tell Peter Gorman story in jungles of S.A. (pp. 735-736). Read last three paragraphs, "What this all means . . ." down through ". . . the oils and the plants, themselves."

   4. **Read "Why Do You Need to Know Chemistry."** pp. xxxiv–xxxv (down to "What This Book Has for You"). (This is optional. Omit this if you are running short on time.)

II. REVIEW & CRITIQUE OF RESOURCES – CH 1   9:45 –10:05

A. **Define four portals** for essential oils to enter body. (p. 2)
B. **Define three schools** of aromatherapy (pp. 3–6)
C. **What is a Therapeutic Grade Oil?** (pp. 6–9)
D. **Point out pitfalls** of British school
   1. Contrast British and French schools(pp. 4–5)
   2. Forbidden Oils (pp. 18–20)
   3. Animal (vs. human) and isolated compound (vs. whole oil) studies. Examples of misusing scientific data. (pp. 21–24)
E. **Choose a few books** to mention, but not too many. Refer students to Chapter One and Bibliography for more information. Point out recommended/non-recommended books at end of Chapter One (p. 50, Key Points 10 & 11.)

TAKE A SHORT RECESS   10:05–10:20

III. CHEMISTRY MADE EASY – CH 3   10:20 –10:45

A. **The Scent of Grapefruit.** Pass around samples of *several citrus oils including grapefruit*. Present the information on p. 124–125 on the scent of grapefruit to illustrate the following points:
   1. Just because different oils all contain the same main ingredient (d-limonene in this case) does not mean they have the same therapeutic actions or fragrances.
   2. Just because a compound is present as only a trace (less than 0.1%) doesn't mean it isn't important and may, perhaps, be the key ingredient for the fragrance and therapeutic action of the oil.
   3. One must always use therapeutic grade oils that are complete with
      all trace compounds carefully preserved in the extraction and bottling process.
   4. Our noses can be quite sensitive to a trace compound in an oil even when comprising less than a billionth of the total oil.

B. Basic Chemistry Concepts:
1. Define scope of chemistry as the "Study of Matter." (p. 78)
2. Define electron, proton, and neutron as basic particles of matter.
3. Define and make drawings of hydrogen, heavy hydrogen, deuterium, tritium, helium, carbon, and oxygen. (pp. 79–81)
4. Point out that all chemical reactions are electrical, involving only electrons in the outer shells of atoms. Any process involving changes in the nucleus of an atom is physics, not chemistry. (pp. 80–81)
5. Periodic Table of Elements, atomic number, atomic weight, (God's Plan for Creation in a Table) (pp. 82–84, 100)
6. Explain what makes the Periodic Table periodic and how elements arranged in vertical columns have similar chemical properties and can replace each other in compounds. (pp. 82, 100–101)
7. Quickly indicate the 27 elements we need for human life as the light, small atoms in the upper part of the periodic table and that iodine (I) is the heaviest element we need. (p. 91)
8. Define molecule, compound, and molecular weight. (pp. 107–110)
9. Discuss how atomic weight, molecular weight, viscosity, volatility, and half-life are related. Pass *myrrh or sandalwood*, which are mostly large sesquiterpene molecules and *frankincense or cypress* (which are mostly smaller monoterpene molecules. Ask students to see which is most aromatic (most volatile) and which is thickest (most viscous) noting how that correlates with molecular weight. (pp. 107–112)

IV. THE CHOSN ONES – CH 4   10:45–11:10

A. Identify the five life sustaining elements—C,H,O,S,N (The Chosen Ones). (pp. 121–123)
B. Give the CHOSN valences and illustrate with cartoon drawings how H+O makes water, C+O makes carbon dioxide, C+H makes methane, H+N makes ammonia, and H+S makes rotten egg gas. (pp. 132–136)
C. Point out that O and S are in the same vertical column of the periodic table and, therefore, have the same valence. This illustrates why all elements in same vertical column in Periodic Table have similar chemical properties—all have same valences. (p. 82, 134–135)
D. Mention that sulfur and nitrogen are not major players in essential oils but when sulfur is present, it almost always influences fragrance (examples: garlic, onion, and grapefruit), (pp. 123–128)
E. Mention that oils contain virtually no amino acids and are devoid of protein molecules which are too large to pass through distillation. However, oil compounds often do start out in plants as amino acids before they are metamorphosed into the hydrocarbons and oxygenated hydrocarbons that comprise essential oils. (pp. 127–131)
F. Allergies and nitrogen compounds. Here is a good place to mention the topic of allergies, saying that allergies are thoroughly covered in Chapter Twelve, pp. 451-470. Simply say that allergies are mostly

caused by reactions to peptides, polypeptides, amino acids, or proteins, noe of which are found in essential oils. Carrier oils and expressed oils, which are not distilled, can be allergenic because they do contain traces of protein, etc. Some people are allergic to Valor because of the almond oil, but not because of the essential oils in that blend. Unpleasant reactions to essential oils that mimic the symptoms of allergies are either detoxes, chemical irritations, or emotional reactions with the exception of phenolic compounds (like oregano or thyme) that, on rare occassions, can result in true allergies. (See pp. 466-470)

G. **Conclude Chapter with single sentence mantra** (to be read out loud by the whole class) summarizing essential oil chemistry. (p. 138)

V. ORGANIC CHEM MADE EASY – CH 5   11:10–11:35

A. **Define organic chemistry.** Explain how the word, "organic" means one thing to a chemist and quite something else to the public at large in considering "organic" products for purchase. (pp. 142–144)

B. **Present alkane series** from methane to pentane, mentioning octane, giving general formula for an alkane. Mention that a number of alkanes are found in oils but usually only in trace amounts. Mention Rose's affair with the alkane family. (pp. 146–153)

C. **Introduce Methyl, Ethyl, Propyl, and Butyl** (pp. 153–155)

D. **Oxygenate the alkanes into alcohols.** Define hydrocarbon, oxygenated hydrocarbon, alcohol, methanol, ethanol, propyl alcohol, isopropyl alcohol, isomer, as well as the prefixes, methyl, ethyl, propyl, and butyl, Make sure they know the difference between "hydrocarbon" and "carbohydrate." (pp. 156–159)

E. **Define isomers** with propyl and isopropyl alcohol. Have 5 Yellow, 8 Red, and 3 Blue Legos® ($Y_5R_8B_3$) to illustrate, pointing out how, with only 16 legos, there are trillions of possibilities. (pp. 165–166)

F. **Restate single-sentence summary** of essential oil chemistry. (p. 138, end of Chapter Four) now with all terms defined.

VI. LORD OF THE RINGS – CH 6   11:35–12:00

A. **Kuekele's dream of dancing snakes,** define benzene (aromatic) ring showing three ways to write in shorthand. (pp. 172–175)

B. **Define non-localized electrons** and the origin of electromagnetic frequencies in oils, mentioning that aromatic rings cease to have the properties of particles (matter) only, but also take on the properties of a wave (energy) as well. Refer students to rainbow colored representation on the back cover depicting a benzene ring as a wave form with resonance energy. (See pp. 176–177 & p. 716, on Quantum Physics.)

C. **Define phenol molecule/functional group,** phenolic compounds, and what is a phenylpropanoid. Explain that phenolics and phenylpropanoids cleanse receptor sites. (pp. 191–195)

D. **Learn to read structural formulas** with C atom locations indicated by line ends, angles, intersections, etc., and with H atoms not shown but deducible by using valences (H = 1, O = 2, C = 4). (pp. 195-196)

E. **Reiterate one statement summary** of essential oil chemistry, read together out loud: "The chemistry of essential oils consists of simple hydrocarbons, oxygenated hydrocarbons, and their isomers." (p. 198)

End of Chem I
Twelve Noon or Therabouts

Chem Two
(The Second Three Hours: 9:00 am – 12 noon)

VII. REVIEW CHEM ONE CONCEPTS   9:00–9:20 am

A. **Define snake oil.** Pass _Tea Tree or "snake oil" and/or Purification®_, which contains Tea Tree (_Melaleuca alternifolia_). (p. 246)

B. **Quickly review valence,** molecular weight, phenols, and isomers.

C. **Practice reading formulas from structures:** Choose from formulas given on pp. 750-751. This is a confidence building exercise and helps them to not be bewildered when structural formulas are flashed up during Power Point presentations at YLEO functions.

VIII. BIOCHEMISTRY MADE EASY – CH 7   9:20–9:45

A. **Define biochemistry** and how is it different from organic chem. (pp. 203–204)

B. **Define chiral molecules** and show structural diagrams of d-carvone and l-carvone. (Pass around _dill and spearmint_ oils to demonstrate how sensitive our noses are.) (pp. 212–215)

C. **Discuss receptor sites** and how they work like keys and locks., Show structural diagrams of thymol, carvacrol, menthol, terpen-1-ol-4, and how they are all similar except for placement of OH radical and the bending of some of the parts (comparing them to different keys). (Pass _thyme, oregano, peppermint, and tea tree_ oils.) (pp. 216–221)

D. Practice reading formulas of six molecules just shown in B and C, explaining how to read bent symbols for menthol. (p. 218)

IX. SPECIES & CHEMOTYPES - CH 8   9:45–10:00

A. **Define genus and species.** Pass around various species of _eucalyptus or melaleuca_, emphasizing that these are different species, not chemotypes. (pp. 234–239)

B. **Define chemotype.** Pass around whatever chemotypes you may have such as those of *Thyme, Basil or Rosemary* emphasizing that chemotypes are the variations of the same species. (pp. 239–242)

C. **Summarize chemotypes by saying** "Chemotypes are to oils what vintages are to wines." (p. 252, Key points #9 & #10)

X. ISOPRENES & PMS - CH 9   10:00-10:25

A. **Define isoprene and terpene units.** Discuss terpenes, monoterpenes, sesquiterpenes, diterpenes, triterpenes, tetraterpenes, carotene, vitamin A, lycopene, rubber, and the CARE logo (subliminal chemistry). (pp. 255–266)

B. **PMS—Phenolics, Monoterpenes, Sesquiterpenes.** The Triple Whammy of Essential Oils. Phenolics cleanse receptor sites. Sesquiterpenes delete bad information in DNA memory, Monoterpenes reprogram or reinstate the correct information (God's image) for proper cellular function. PMS oils can work together to bring about permanent healing, sometimes instantaneously, because together they can remove the root source of some problems at a cellular level. (pp. 290–297)

C. **Chemistry of Raindrop Technique,** an example of PMS where you apply more P than M, and more M than S. (pp. 297–301)

D. **Conclude CH 9 by Reiterating** one sentence summary: "The chemistry of essential oils consists of simple hydrocarbons, oxygenated hydrocarbons, and their isomers." Ask students if they now understand what that statement means and if they see how true it is.

SHORT RECESS   10:25–10:40

XI. COMMON COMPOUNDS IN OILS – CH 10   10:40–11:25

A. **Explain how oil compounds behave like people.** (p. 311–312)

B. **Define alcohols, ethers, aldehydes, ketones, carboxylic acids, esters** – Table Seventeen (p. 314) Choose oils from Table Sixty Seven (p. 585) to pass around as examples of each of the six classes of compounds just listed.

C. **Define oxides.** (Pass *Blue Mallee, Eucalyptus, E. Radiata, Ravensara, Rosemary cineole, and/or German Chamomile* as oils principally composed of oxides.) (pp. 362-368)

D. **Define lactones and coumarins.** Explain difference between coumarin and coumadin®. (pp. 369–375) Point out how drug companies take generic or natural substances and alter them slightly to create patentable drugs and obtain a monopoly. (pp. 375-79)

C. **Define furan, furanoids, and furanocoumarins**—mostly found in citrus oils, but not in all citrus oils. Explain the phototoxicity of furanoids and the role they play in ripening fruit. (Pass *bergamot* which contains bergaptene, a furanocoumarin) (pp. 379–383)

XII. PRACTICAL ANSWERS – CH 12   11:25–11:45

A. **Discuss as many of the topics of CH 12 as time will allow,** pointing out that detailed, easily understood discussions are given in the book: (pp. 430–493). If there is time, let students choose which topics to discuss. Mention that Allergies, a topic in CH 12, was discussed in Chem I along with nitrogen and the CHOSN Ones.

XIII. CONCLUSION   11:45–12:00 noon

A. **Pass Around** *Oil of Joy*® **and Summarize:** "The chemisty of essential oils consists of simple hydrocarbons, oxygenated hydrocarbons, and their isomers" . . . but their behavior cannot be explained by chemistry, alone. Direct the students to Part Three of this book (Beyond Chemistry) for more discussion on this.

B. **Quickly list what has been covered during the course:**
   1. Review of Literature
   2. Basic Chemistry
   3. The Chosen Ones
   4. Basic Organic Chemistry
   5. Aromatic Rings and Phenols
   6. Basic Biochemistry
   7. Chemotypes
   8. Terpenes
   9. PMS
   10. Twenty-Two Categories of Compounds in Essential Oils, and
   11. Practical Answers to Frequently Asked Questions

C. **Review Scriptures** on p. xxviii (where Introduction begins). Ask students if they perceive a deeper meaning in these scriptures than before this course. Ask if they can see now how a proper understanding of science truly "tells the glory of God" and truly "proclaims his handiwork" and that "God's nature is revealed in what he has made." (cf. Psalm 19:1 and Romans 1:20)

D. **Concluding Statement:**
   1. According to the *Bible*, God created plants (and their oils) on the third day (Genesis 1:11–13), but didn't create man and woman until the sixth day (Genesis 1:26–31). Plants came before people
   2. Comment that if one subscribes to the Geologic Model for creation, plants and people happened in the same order. Plants were growing on earth long before people came to dwell.
   3. The molecules of essential oils fit human receptor sites so perfectly and our bodies accept and metabolize them so readily and with such benefits, that one can only conclude that God created them with his children in mind.
   4. In other words, God loved us before he ever created us. The chemistry of essential oils is God's love manifest in molecules.

End of Chem II
12 Noon or Therabouts*

COURSE HANDOUTS: Make Copies of This 12-page Outline to Hand Out to all of the Students at the Beginning of Class, Including the Molecular Diagrams. Also hand out copies of Periodic Table. (Table One). For a complete set of additional notes, students need to purchase the book: *The Chemistry of Essential Oils Made Simple*.

SUGGESTION: Delegate Someone in Class to take Charge of the Oils to Open Them, Pass them Around at the Right Times (by taking ques from you and/or the outline), and Recapping the Bottles with the Right Caps as They Complete Their Rounds of the Students.

* A NOTE ON SCHEDULING: The outline here is for presenting Chem I and Chem II as two consequetive morning sessions, thus avoiding the afternoon right after lunch when people tend to sleep. However, this course has been successfully taught in afternoon sessions. It works both ways. You may need to use extra peppermint in the afternoons.

Before-Class Things to Bring and Do

- **Before Class:** Be well prepared. Anoint yourself with Valor®, and other appropriate oils. Pray for wisdom to answer questions according to God's will.

- **Molecular diagrams to draw on board or chart during Chem I break:** d-Carvone & l-Carvone (p. 205), Carvacrol,Thymol, Menthol, and Terpinen-1-ol-4 (p. 211)). (See Next Page.)

- **Molecular diagrams to draw on board or chart before Chem II:** Isoprene unit (p. 249); d–Limonene, Myrcene, δ–3–Carene, Camphene, α–Pinene, β–Pinene, Sabinene, (p. 265;) β–Farnesene, β-Caryophyllene (p. 270); Cembrene (p. 277) Camphor (p. 320); Thymol & Menthol (p. 211); 1,8 Cineole, 1,4 Cineole, numbered template (p. 350). (See Next Page.)

- **Bring to Class:** Lecture Notes, Cutouts of isoprene units, White board or flip chart with markers. Handouts: Course Outline and Periodic Table.

- **Oils to be passed during Part I (Introduction):** Valor®, Peppermint, Lemon, Cedarwood (for courage, alertness, retention, and openness to learning)

- **Oils to be passed during Part III (Basic Chemistry Made Easy):** Grapefruit, Orange, Lemon, Tangerine (smelling trace compounds) Myrrh, Sandalwood, Frankincense, Cypress (viscosity & volatility)

Legos®: 3 Yellow, 8 Red, 5 Blue, Part V to demonstrate the trillions of possibilities for isomers with only three elements: C, H, & O.

- **Oils to be passed during Part VII (Review & to Snake Oil):** Tea Tree or Snake Oil (*Melaleuca alternifolia*) or Purification®. Draw structural diagrams on board before class begins.

- **Oils to be passed during Part VIII (Biochemistry Made Easy):** Dill, Spearmint, Oregano, Thyme, Peppermint, Tea Tree (*Melaleuca alternifolia*) (detecting isomers by nose)

- **Oils to be passed during Part IX (Species and Chemotypes):** Various Eucalyptus and Melaleuca oils (different species) Rosemary CT Verbenon, Rosemary CT Cineole, Basil CT Estragole (Methyl chavicol), Basil CT Linalol, or any other chemotype examples you can get. (detecting different chemotypes)

- **Oils to be passed during Part XI (Classes of Compounds):** Roman Chamomile, Wintergreen (mostly esters) Blue Gum (*Eucalyptus globulus*), Black Peppermint (*Eucalyptus radiata*), Blue Mallee (*Eucalyptus polybractea*), German Chamomile (mostly oxides), and Bergamot (furanocoumarins-phototoxic)

- **Oil to be passed during Conclusion:**   Oil of Joy®

Structural Diagrams to Present in Class

Note: These may be drawn on a white-board, flip-chart, or chalk-board just before each class (which is temporary), or they may be drawn on large posterboards once to be reused each time the class is taught. Oil examples listed are those with the highest concentration of that particular compound. See Part Two for more complete listings of oils containing these compounds.

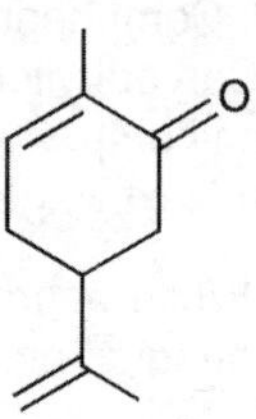

l-Carvone
Spearmint 52%

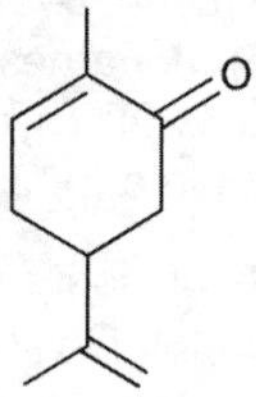

d-Carvone
Dill 38%

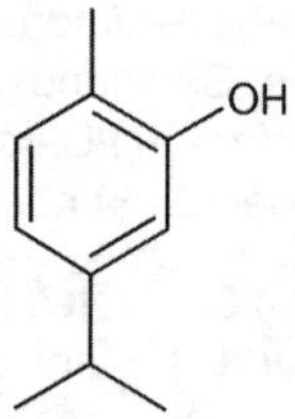

Carvacrol
Oregano 67%

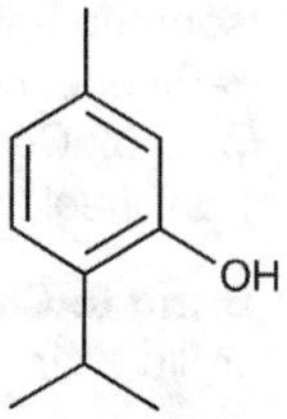

Thymol
Thyme 46%

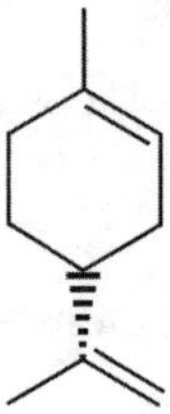

d–Limonene
Grapefruit 89%

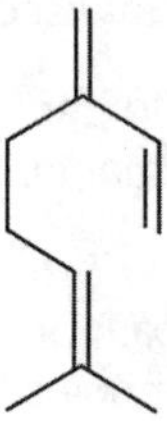

Myrcene
Mugwort 23%

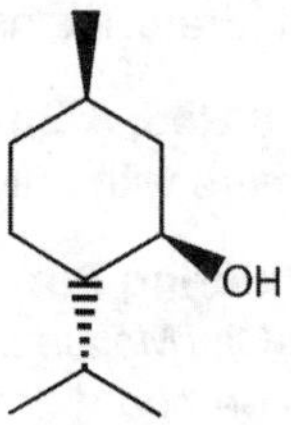

Menthol
Peppermint 39%

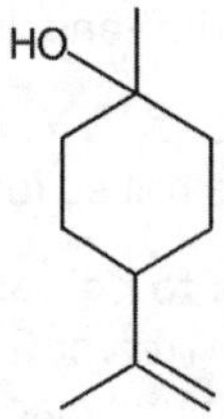

Terpinen-1-ol-4
Tea Tree 33%

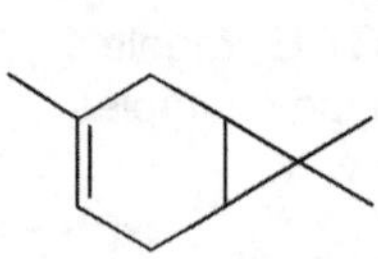

δ-3-Carene
Balsam Fir 21%

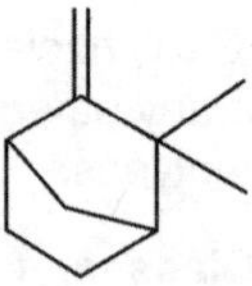

Camphene
Silver Fir 21%

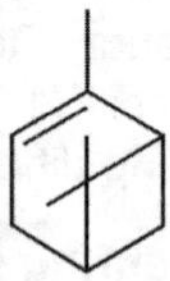

α–Pinene
Cypress 51%

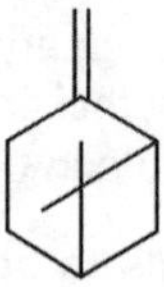

β–Pinene
Galbanum 55%

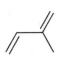

Isoprene
Unit

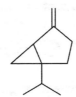

Sabinene
Yarrow 25%

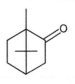

Camphor
White Camphor 45%

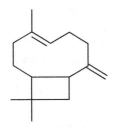

β–Caryophyllene
Vitex 39%

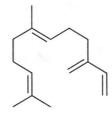

β–Farnesene
German Chamomile 21%

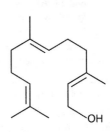

Farnesol
Geranium 2%

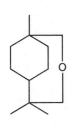

1,8 Cineole
Blue Mallee 90%

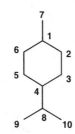

Molecular
Numbering System

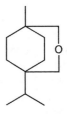

1,4 Cineole
Tea Tree 3%

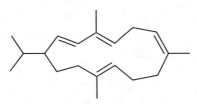

Cembrene
Pine 1%

♥ GLOSSARY

absolute. Aromatic oil extracted from plant material by solvents.

absolute zero. −273° Celsius or −434° Fahrenheit. At this temperature, not yet ever achieved in a laboratory, observed in nature, or detected anywhere in the universe, all motion ceases, including the motion of electrons in an atom.

acid. A substance that is able to donate H+ ions (protons) when dissolved in water. Opposite of base or alkali.

acyclic. A molecule with no rings.

adaptigen. An oil or oil compound whose therapeutic action is such that it can increase a body function, reduce a body function, or have no effect depending on the body's needs. eg. an adaptigen could raise blood pressure, lower blood pressure, or have no effect if one's blood pressure were normal. The ability for essential oils to be adaptigens is because they possess homeostatic intelligence.

adulteration. The adding of synthetic compounds to a natural essential oil.

AFNOR. Association French Normalization Organization Regulation. The French agency that sets standards for therapeutic grade essential oils accepted by the European Community or EC. Also known as *Norme Francaise.*

alcohol. A hydrocarbon group (R) with a hydroxyl radical (OH-) attached. Alcohol names end in -ol.

aldehyde. A carbonyl group (C=O) with a hydrocarbon group (R) attached to one side of the carbon and a hydrogen atom (H) attached to the other side. Aldehyde names usually end in -al.

alkali. A substance that produces an excess of OH- ions (hydroxyl radicals) when dissolved in water. Same as base. Opposite of acid.

alkane. A hydrocarbon fitting the general formula of C_nH_{2n+2}, where n = any integer. Alkane names end in -ane.

alkane alcohol. An alkane group with a hydroxyl radical attached (OH-) fitting the general formula of $C_nH_{2n+2}O$, where n = any integer.

allergy. A hypersensitive reaction to common, often intrinsically harmless, substances contacted in the environment or ingested as food. The triggering substance for an allergic reaction is called an allergen. Allergies are a malfunction of the immune system which usually has an emotional or spiritual root.

allopath. A health care provider focusing on drugs, surgery, radiation, and other conventional medical procedures. MDs are allopaths as are most DOs.

allopathy. Conventional medical practice emphasizing drugs, surgery, and radiation therapy.

amino acid. A carboxylic acid containing an amino functional group ($-NH_2$) and a carboxylic acid group (COOH+).

amino group. An incomplete ammonia molecule ($-NH_2$) incorporated into every amino acid molecule. Also called an amino radical.

amplitude. The height or magnitude of a wave at its peak.

amu. See atomic mass unit.

Glossary 753

androgen. A class of hormonal steroid compounds that promote the development of male secondary sex charactgeristics. There are only four natural androgens manufactured by the human body: DHEA, androstenediol, androstenedione, and testosterone.

angstrom. A unit of length, denoted Å, used to measure atomic dimensions. $1Å = 10^{-10}$ meters.

antibacterial. Able to destroy or inhibit the growth of bacteria.

antibiotic. Antimicrobial agents manufactured by drug companies that can destroy or interfere with the development of a spectrum of bacteria.

antibody. Complex designer proteins created by the immune system and attached to special lymphocytes (white corpuscles) designed to destroy or disable a specific pathogen, microorganism, or alien agent in the body.

anticarcinogenic. Able to destroy or inhibit the growth of tumors, particularly malignant or cancerous tumors.

antifungal. Able to destroy or inhibit the growth of fungi.

antimicrobial. Able to destroy or inhibit the growth of micro-organisms.

antioxidant. A substance that inhibits or absorbs free radicals. Essential oils are among the most powerful antioxidants in the world. The antioxidant capacity of a substance is measured by the ORAC scale. Many free radicals are incomplete oxygen molecules with an imbalance of electrons—thus the term, "antioxidant."

antiparasitic. Able to destroy or inhibit the growth of parasites.

antiseptic. Able to destroy or prevent the development of microbes.

antiviral. Able to destroy or inhibit the growth of viruses.

aqueous solution. A solution in which water is the solvent. (See tincture.)

aromatic oil. Fragrant oil extracted from a plant by distillation, expression, or solvents.

aromatic ring. Any ring (or polygon) of carbon atoms containing double bonds. They can be 3, 4, 5, 6 or any number of sides on the polygon.

atom. The smallest particle of an element that still retains the properties of that element.

atomic mass. The number of protons and neutrons in an atom expressed in amu.

atomic mass unit. The mass of a proton or neutron which has been assigned a value of 1.000. Same as a dalton. Abbreviated: amu.

atomic number. The number of protons in the nucleus of an atom. (which is equal to the number of electrons orbiting the nucleus)

atomic weight. Same as atomic mass. Sometimes abbreviated as A.W. Measured in amu.

atomize. To vaporize a liquid into the atmosphere as molecular-sized units by forcing it through a pinhole at high pressure. Nebulizing diffusers are based on the atomizing principle.

base. A substance that produces an excess of OH- ions (hydroxyl radicals) when dissolved in water. Same as alkali. Opposite of acid.

base oil. A fatty oil in which an essential oil has been mixed or an essential oil containing large molecules.

bicyclic. A molecule with two rings.

biochemical half-life. The time required for the concentration of a chemical substance to decrease or metabolize to half its initial quantity within a living organism.

biochemistry. The study of the chemical processes in living systems.

biodegradable. Organic material that bacteria are able to break down and decompose.

biological half-life. Same as biochemical half-life.

biology. The study of living things and life processes.

biotransmutation. Changing of elements into other elements through biological processes.

benzene. A compound with the chemical formula C_6H_6 and the structural formula of a hexagon.

blood-brain barrier. A wall of capillaries and membranes that separate the passage of blood from the nerve tissues of the brain that prevents or slows the passage of certain substances. Abbreviated BBB. The BBB protects the brain from virusis, bacteria, and other disease-causing organisms as well as radioactive ions, and various toxins, including some drugs. In general, a molecule or particle must be less than 500 amu in weight and lipid-soluble to pass through the BBB. All of the molecules of pure essential oils will pass through the BBB.

bond. A strong attractive force between atoms in a molecule due to exchanges or sharing of electrons. Same as chemical bond.

bond angle. The angle made by the lines joining the nuclei of atoms in a molecule.

BP. British Pharmacopoeia. British agency that sets standards for British drug manufacturing processes.

buffer. Same as buffered solution.

buffered solution. A solution that undergoes a limited change in pH upon addition of a small amount of acid or base.

butyl radical. A functional group consisting of an incomplete methane molecule. C_4H_8 or C_4H_7. Any compound whose name includes "butyl" has incorporated one or more butyl radicals in its molecules..

carbohydrate. A compound of carbon atoms and water molecules with the general formula—$nC + mH_2O$—where n and m are integers. Carbohydrates include sugars (saccharides), starches, polysaccharides, and cellulose.

carbonyl group. A carbon double bonded to an oxygen—C=O—found in aldehydes, ketones, carboxylic acids, and esters.

carboxylic acid. An organic acid containing the carboxyl radical, COOH+.

carboxyl radical. A functional group consisting with the formula, COOH+.

carcinogen. A substance or agent that produces or creates cancer.

carrier blend. A blend of essential oils mixed with a carrier oil. The blend can be mostly essential or mostly carrier.

carrier oil. Any vegetable oil in which essential oils are mixed.

catalyst. A substance that enables or changes the speed of a chemical reaction without itself undergoing a chemical change in the process.

Celsius scale. The metric scale of temperature measurement, abbreviated C. Fomerly called the Centigrade scale. Water freezes at 0°C. and boils at 100°C.

chakra. Everyone has an electromagnetic field associated with their physical body. The details of this field correspond to our physical body. There are neural centers (plexuses) along the physical spine. Chakras are the electromagnetic correlates of our neural plexuses.

chemical bond. A strong attractive force between atoms in a molecule due to exchanges or sharing of electrons. Same as bond.

chemical change. A process where one or more substances are converted into other substances. (Same as chemical reaction.)

chemical equation. A representation of a chemical reaction using the chemical formulas of the chemical reactants and products.

chemical formula. A list of chemical symbols with numerical subscripts to convey the relative proportions of atoms of the constituent elements in a compound.

chemical products. The resultant substances of a chemical reaction.

chemical reaction. A process where one or more substances are converted into other substances. (Same as chemical change.)

chemical symbol. Abbreviations for the elements in the form of one or two letters, the first capitalized when there are two. eg. H, He, C, N, O, Mg, Ca, etc.

chemistry: The study of the properties, compositions, and transformations of matter.

chiral. A term describing an isomeric pair of molecules where the mirror image of one is identical to the actual image of the other, like the mirror image of our left hand is identical to the actual right hand. This feature is determined by where "right-handed" molecules must be rotated to the right (*dextro-rotation*) and "left-handed" molecules mujst be rotated to the left (*lev-orotation*) to line up with the polarized light.

chirality. Possessing the chiral property.

chiral molecules. Pairs of isomers whose only structural difference is that one is the mirror image of the other.

classical physics. See continuum mechanics.

closed system. A system in which no energy enters or exits. The physical universe, as a whole, is assumed to be a closed system by material scientists. This assumption does not take into consideration the possibility of non-physical energies outside the physical universe that may come and go.

complex. Same as a metal complex or coordination compound.

compound. A substance composed of two or more elements united chemically in definite proportions. Compounds are composed of molecules.

continuum mechanics. The study of energy and matter as a contiuum or wave phenomenon. Also called wave mechanics, classical physics, or Newtonian physics. Also see quantum physics.

coordination compound. Same as a metal complex.

Coumadin®. A synthetic, patented anti-coagulating coumarin drug with the formula, $C_{19}H_{15}NaO_4$, owned by Bristol-Meyers-Squib, Inc. used as a prescription blood thinner and anti-stroke medication. Not to be confused with coumarin, which is a natural compound found in minor or trace amounts in some essential oils.

coumarin. 1. A class of compounds which are lactones with a benzene ring. 2. A specific compound (a coumarin) with the formula $C_9H_6O_2$. Not to be confused with Coumadin®, a synthetic patent medicine. The biochemical properties of coumarin are not the same as Coumadin®.

cps. Cycles per second, a measure of frequency. Same as hertz.

cutaneous. Pertaining to the skin.

cytokine. Information-carrying proteins secreted by cells involved in cell-to-cell communication, coordinating antibody activity, and amplifyuing immune reactivity.

dalton. Same as atomic mass unit or amu.

delocalized electrons. Same as non-localized electrons.

deoxyribonucleic acid. See DNA

deuterium. An isotope of hydrogen containing a neutron in the neucleus of each atom.

dextrorotary. A right-handed chiral isomer usually designated with the prefix, d, as in d-limonene or d-carvone. See levorotary and chiral.

diterpene. A compound consisting of or containing a functional group with the formula, $C_{20}H_{32}$—which is two terpene units.

DNA. Abbreviation for deoxyribonucleic acid. A large, double-stranded, helical molecule composed of nucleotides that are the carriers of genetic information and cellular intelligence.

double bonds. When two atoms are joined chemically by two bonds (involving two electrons) instead of one.

double helix. The structure for a DNA molecule such that two helical chains of polynucleotides appear to be twisted clockwise when viewed from either end.

EC. European Community. Regulating agency for cosmetics, perfumes, herbs, essential oils and other products, both natural and synthetic.

electromagnetic spectrum. Radient energy ranging in frequency from ELF waves (less than 10 hz), to visible light (10^{14} hz), to x-rays (10^{18} hz), cosmic rays (10^{24} hz), and beyond.

electromagnetism. A form of energy that has wave characteristics and propagates at the speed of light.

electron. A negatively charged atomic particle orbiting the nucleus of an atom and also the moving charge in electrical currents and in lightning. The mass of an electron is 1/1840th of that of a proton or neutron or 0.00054 amu.

electron shell. A layer of orbiting electrons around the nucleus of an atom. Also referred to as "outer shell" or "shell."

element. A substance that cannot be separated into simpler substances by chemical means. Elements are composed of atoms.

endothermic. A process that absorbs heat.

energy. The ability to do work or transfer heat

entropy. The tendency of a closed system to change from a state of order to a state of disorder, expressed in physics as useful energy available to do work being transformed into useless energy unavailable to do work. Entropy is the idea that spontaneous processes occur in irreversible directions, always in the direction of greater disorder. When entropy increases, disorder increases. Hence, entropy is always a positive quantity in all spontaneous processes.

entropy, law of. Same as the second law of thermodynamics.

enzyme. An organic substance that enables or changes the speed of a biochemical reaction without itself undergoing a chemical change in the process.

ERT. Estrogen replacement therapy. The prescription of synthetic estrogenic steroids to address an alleged deficiency of natural human hormones. See HRT and estrogen.

essential oil. Oil extracted from plant matter by distillation.

ester. An organic compound resulting from the reaction of an alcohol and a carboxylic acid. Ester molecules consist of a carbonyl group with a hydrocarbon group (R) attached to one side of the carbon and an oxygen atom (O) to the other side of the carbon to which is attached another hydrocarbon group (R'). Esters have double names the first ending in -yl, the second ending in -ate.

estrogen. A class of hormonal steroid compounds that promote the development of female secondary sex characteristics. There are only three natural estrogens manufactured by the human body: estrone, estradiol, and estriol.

ether. An organic compound in which two hydrocarbon groups are bonded to one oxygen. Names of ethers end in -ole, -cin- or ether.

ethereal oils. Same as an essential oil.

ethyl radical. A functional group consisting of an incomplete methane molecule. C_2H_5 or C_2H_4. Any compound whose name includes "ethyl" has incorporated one or more ethyl radicals in its molecules..

exothermic. A process that gives off heat.

expressed oil. An oil obtained from plant material by cold pressure. The most common expressed oils are from citrus rinds.

Fahrenheit scale. The English scale of temperature measurement, abbreviated F. Water freezes at 32°F. and boils at 212°F.

fatty acid. A long chain hydrocarbon with a carboxylic group (COOH) on one end. Vegetable oils are mixtures of fatty acids.

fatty oil. A vegetable oil or or mixture of fatty acids.

FDA. U.S. Food and Drug Administration. Regulates drugs and sets standards for food additives, etc.

fission. Splitting of an atom with a heavy nucleus into smaller atoms.

flavor grade essential oil. An aromatic oil grown and produced and manipulated for its favor. Such oils are usually missing the therapeutic compounds normally present in a particular species and may contain synthetic ingredients.

food grade essential oil. Same as flavor grade essential oil.

force. A push or a pull.

formula. Same as chemical formula.

fragrance grade essential oil. An aromatic oil grown and produced and manipulated for its fragrance. Such oils are usually missing the therapeutic compounds normally present in a particular species and may contain synthetic ingredients.

free radical. An incomplete molecule carrying an electric charge. (i.e., a substance with one or more unpaired electrons.) Same as "radical." Also see ion. Free radicals in the body can cause disease, cancer, and accelerate the aging process. Free radical scavengers are called antioxidants.

free radical scavengers. See antioxidants. Essential oils are antioxidants.

frequency. The number of times per second that one complete wavelength passes a given point. Measured in hertz. Frequency is the reciprocal of wave length.

functional group. A group of associated atoms acting as a unit in the formation of compounds.

furan. A functional group consisting of a pentagonal, heterogeneous ring with the formula C_4H_4O. As a part of a molecule in essential oils, it can amplify UV light and result in phototoxicity.

furanocoumarin. A coumarin molecule containing a furan group. Can be phototoxic, but not always.

furanoid. Any molecule containing a furan functional group. Furanoids can be phototoxic, but not always.

fusion. Joining of two light atoms to form a more massive atom.

GRAS. "Generally Regarded As Safe." A designation assigned by the U.S. FDA and appllied to most essential oils in common usage.

half-life. 1. The time for the concentration of a chemical substance to decrease to half its initial value. 2. The time for half of a sample of a particular radioisotope to decay.

Heisenberg uncertainty principle. See uncertainty principle.

helix. A spiral.

hemoglobin. An iron-containing protein responsible for oxygen transport in the blood.

hemostatic. Arrests bleeding.

hertz. A measure of frequency as cycles per second. Abbvreviated as hz.

heterogeneous. In organic ring chemistry, heterogeneous means the ring is formed of carbon atoms with at least one atom of element other than carbon. The most common heterogeneous rings contain an oxygen (O) or nitrogen (N) atom.

homeostasis. A state of physical health, harmony, balance, or wellbeing where all bodily systems work properly and normally.

homeostatic intelligence. A characteristics of essential oils wherein their action upon a person is in the direction of balance, harmony, or wellbeing. eg. Whether a person suffers from hyperthyroidism, hypothyroidism, or no thyroid problems, administration of an essential oil that addresses the thyroid system can act in whatever way the person needs or not at all if the person is healthy.

homochirality. Molecules of all the same rotary properties, either all left (levo) or all right (destro). All amino acids, polypeptides, enzymes, and proteins of all living systems on earth are of the same chirality—viz. left (or levorotary). See chiral and levorotary.

homogeneous. In organic ring chemistry, homogeneous means the ring is formed entirely of carbon atoms.

HRT. Hormone replacement therapy. The prescription of synthetic estrogenic steroids to address an alleged deficiency of natural human hormones. Formerly called ERT.

hydrocarbon. A compound containing only carbon and hydrogen atoms.

hydroxy acid. A compound with a hydroxyl radical on one end (OH-) and a carboxylic acid radical (COOH+) on the other end making it both alkaline and acid.

hydroxyl radical. An incomplete water molecule, OH- possessing a negative charge.

hz. Abbreviation for hertz.

IACET. International Association for Continuing Education Training. Certifies CARE for CEUs for professionals.

iatrogenic. Caused by a doctor. (used in reference to iatrogenic diseases or medical conditions.)

immiscible liquids. Liquids that don't mix. eg. oil and water.

inorganic acid. An acid containing no carbon atoms. Same as mineral acid.

ion. An electrically charged atom or group of atoms which can be positively or negatively charged, depending on whether electrons are lost (positive) or gained (negative) by the atoms.

IP. International Pharmacopoeia. International agency in Geneva, Switzerland, that sets standards for drug manufacturing processes.

ISO. International Standardization Organization in Geneva, Switzerland, that sets standards for many products and procedures in some 130 countries, including the definitions and Latin names for various species of essential oils.

isomer. Compounds with the same chemical formula but different structural formulas.

isoprene unit. The most common functional group in nature. Its formula is C_5H_8. Two isoprene units acting as a functional form a terpene unit, $C_{10}H_{16}$.

isotope. Atoms of the same element with differing numbers of neutrons in their nuclei and, hence, possessing different atomic masses, but the same chemical properties.

IUPAC. International Union of Pure and Applied Chemistry. The agency that sets the rules for naming organic compounds.

ketone. A carbonyl group (C=O) with two hydrocarbon groups (R & R') attached one on each side of the carbon. Ketone names end in -one.

lactone. An ester with one of its oxygen atoms incorporated into a heterogeneous ring. Lactones are formed from hydroxy acids.

law of constant composition. A law that states that for a given compound, the elemental composition and properties of are always the same, regardless of the source or history of the compound. This law assumes that there are no ethereal properties to a physical substance, that its physical parameters completely describe it and its potential behavior. Also called the law of definite proportions.

Lavoisier's law. In a chemical reaction, nothing is created, nothing is lost, everything is transformed. Also called the law of conservation of matter.

Lego®. A patented form of children's building blocks made of plastic and designed to interlock and stick together. Legos come in different colors including red, yellow, blue, and green.

levorotary. A left-handed chiral isomer usually designated with the prefix, l, as in l-limonene or l-carvone. See dextrorotary and chiral.

ligand. The word's root is Latin, *ligare*, meaning "to bind." There is a biological and a chemical definition. 1. An organic message-carrying molecule that brings information to cells or passes information between cells. This includes various hormones, steroids, peptides, enzymes, vitamins, neurotransmitters. Essential oil molecules also act as ligands. 2. An ion or molecule that coordinates to a metal atom or a metal ion to form a complex. Cholorophyll is a complex where ligands coordinate to a magnesium atom (Mg) while hemoglobin is a complex where ligands coordinate to an iron atom (Fe).

lipid-soluble. Able to dissolve in a fat or an oil. All fats and oils are lipid-soluble.

liquid crystal. A substance that exhibits one or more partially ordered liquid phases above the melting point of the solid form and which responds to voltages, magnetic fields, and/or heat in ways that alters its shade, hue, or color. Used in many devices as LCDs.

LCD. Liquid crystal display.

mass. A the amount of material in an object as measured by the force required to move it or by the force of gravity that attracts it.

matter. Anything that has mass and occupies space.

metal. A substance that is usually solid at room temperature, has a high electrical and heat conductivity, is usually malleable and ductile, and appears lustrous. Most of the elements are metals. Mercury (Hg) is the only metallic element that is liquid at room temperatures while the gas, hydrogen (H), is actually a metal, but manifests its metallic properties only at temperatures approaching absolute zero. In the normal range of temperatures on or near the earth's surface, hydrogen is a gas, behaves as a nonmetal, and is considered as such.

metal complex. A compound with a central metal atom surrounded in three dimensions by attached ligands. Chlorophyll and hemoglobin are metal complexes also known as coordination compounds. Chlorophyll molecules are built on magnesium (Mg) atoms while hemoglobin molecules are built on iron (Fe) atoms.

methyl radical. A functional group consisting of an incomplete methane molecule. CH_3 or CH_2. Any compound whose name includes "methyl" has incorporated one or more methyl radicals in its molecules..

megahertz. One million hertz (10^6 cps). Abbreviated as Mhz. Radio waves fall in the Mhz range of frequencies.

microbe. A minute living organism, expecially pathogenic bacteria, viruses, etc.

microbiological agent. A microscopic living entity such as bacteria, virus, fungi, or parasite.

mineral acid. An inorganic acid. An acid containing no carbon atoms. See organic acid.

miscible liquids. Liquids that can mix in any proportion. eg. fatty oils and essential oils are miscible. Essential oils and the lighter alkane alcohols are miscible.

mixture. A combination of two or more substances in which each retains its own chemical identity.

molecule. The smallest particle of a compound that still retains the properties of that compound. Molecules are composed of atoms.

molecular weight. The sum of the atomic weights of the atoms in a molecule. Sometimes abbreviated M.W. Measured in amu.

monocyclic. A molecule with one ring.

monoterpene. A hydrocarbon molecule or functional group with the formula $C_{10}H_{16}$, which is the formula for one terpene unit.

natural. 1. Created by nature. 2. Any substance, even though synthetized artificially in a laboratory, that exists in nature.

NCBTMB. National Certification Board for Therapeutic Massage and Bodywork. Certifies CARE for CE hours.

neat. Application of a pure essential oil directly without dilution with a carrier oil, usually to the skin.

nebulizing diffuser. A cold diffuser that vaporizes essential oils by atomization by passing the oil through a pin hole at high velocity by means of an air pump. Nebulizing diffusers are superior in that they vaporize all of compounds in the oil simultaneously, thus maintaining the oil's natural balance. They also employ no neat, which can be damaging to an essential oil.

neutron. An electrically neutral (or uncharged) particle in the nucleus of an atom with approximately the same mass as a proton, or 1 amu.

non-localized electrons. Electrons in a molecule no longer associated with a particular atom. Non-localized electrons are present in all double bonds. Also called delocalized electrons.

nonlocal reality. A reality in which apparently separate regions are connected by instantaneous interactions.

nonmetals. Substances that do not display the properties of metals—i.e. they are generally poor conductors of heat and electricity, are neither malleable or ductile, and have no metallic luster. Elements in the upper right corner of the periodic table are nonmetals.

nosocomial. Caused by a hospital. (used in reference to nosocomial diseases or medical conditions.)

nucleotide. A molecule composed of nitrogen groups, phosphate groups, and pentose sugars.

nucleus. 1. The central controlling body within a living cell. 2. The central, very dense body of an atom composed of protons and neutrons and possessing a positive electrical charge (associated with the proton).

ORAC scale. Oxygen radical absorbance capacity. A measure of antioxidant capability. All essential oils have very high ORAC values. Wolfberries (*Lycium barbarum*) have the highest known ORAC scale value of any known fruit or vegetable. Clove oil (*Syzygium aromaticum*) has the highest ORAC scale value of any known substance—approximately 400 times higher than even wolfberries.

organic. 1. Containing or consisting of carbon compounds; 2. plants, produce, or livestock raised without chemicals.

organic acid. An acid containing the carboxyl radical, COOH. Same as a carboxylic acid. See inorganic acid.

organic chemistry. The study of carbon compounds, especially those with carbon to carbon bonds.

outer shell. See electron shell.

oxide. Organic oxides are formed when an oxygen atom (O) is chemically bonded to an organic compound or hydrocarbon group such that the two bonds of oxygen are attached to two different carbon atoms.

participatory reality. A reality in which consciousness participates as a formative agent.

pathogen. A microbiological agent harmful to human beings.

peptide. A molecule composed of amino acids. Peptides are one of the principle types of hormones or ligands in the human body and come in unlimited varieties as the lexicon for intercellular communication.

perfume grade essential oil. Same as fragrance grade essential oil.

periodic. Properties that repeat themselves.

periodic table. A list of the elements in ascending order of atomic number with those of similar chemical properties lined up as vertical columns.

petrochemical. Products manufactured from petroleum or natural gas.

petroleum. A naturally occurring combustible liquid composed of hundreds of hydrocarbons and other organic compounds. A raw material from which tens of thousands of products are manufactured or extracted including many drugs, pesticides, herbicides, plastics, and fuels—including gasoline and kerosene.

pH. Potential Hydorgen. A measure of acidity or alkalinity. 7.0 is neutral.

phase. 1. A physical state, such as solid, liquid or gas. 2. A chemical state. 3. The point at where a wave begins.

phenol. 1. A compound consisting of a hydroxyl radical (OH-) attached to a benzene ring (C_6H_6). Its formula is (C_6H_6O). 2. A family of compounds containing a phenol molecule as a functional group. Members of this family are also called phenolics.

phenolpropanoid. A compound containing a phenol functional group and a propyl radical (C_3H_7 or C_3H_5).

pheromone. An aromatic substance secreted by an organism that elicits a particular response from another individual of the same species, uisually of the opposite sex. Pheromones may be sexual stimulants or attractants or alarm or trail-making substances. In social insects they have a role in the determination of castes.

photon. The smallest unit (quantum) of radient energy. The energy of a photon is its frequency times Planck's constant.

phototoxicity. A property of some substances that when applied to the skin amplify UV light and cause sunburn or other damage, sometime permanent. In essential oils, these substances all contain compounds incorporating the furan functional group.

physics. The study of energy and all of its ramifications and interactions with matter.

Planck's constant. A measure of the quantum nature of energy. Its value is 6.6×10^{-34} Joule-seconds. It is usually represented by the symbol, h.

PMS. A paradigm for applying essential oils for therapeutic purposes where oils are used such that the combination of them provides certain amounts of phenols (P), monoterpenes (M), and sesquiterpenes (S). Few single oils contain these three classes of compounds in the right proportions. Blends of oils or layering of oils one after the other are usually necessary to achieve a PMS anointing. See PMS blend.

PMS anointing. Applying essential oils for therapeutic purposes such that a certain proportion of the oils (as an aggregate) contain phenols, monoterpenes, and sesquiterpenes. See PMS blend.

PMS blend. A therapeutic combination or sequence of essential oils with a 10-50% phenols, 10-60% monoterpenes, and 3-20% sesquiterpenes, where ketones or alcohols may be substituted for phenols.

polymer. A large molecule formed by the joining together (polymerization) of a large number of smaller molecules.

polymerization. The formation of large molecules by the joining together of many small molecules. Essential oil molecules polymerize when exposed to light for extended periods of time.

polypeptide. A large molecule composed of peptide molecules which, in turn, are built from amino acids. Polypeptides combine to make proteins.

polysaccharide. A large molecule composed of several sugar molecules. Cellulose and starch are a polysaccharide.

precipitate. An insoluble substance that forms in, and separates from a solution.

propyl radical. A functional group consisting of an incomplete methane molecule. C_3H_7 or C_3H_5. Any compound whose name includes "propyl" has incorporated one or more propyl radicals in its molecules..

Glossary 763

protein. A large organic molecule composed of polypeptides which are, in turn, built from large numbers of amino acids.

protium. Another name for hydrogen as the isotope containing no neutrons.

proton. A positively charged atomic particle in the nucleus of an atom whose atomic mass is 1.000 amu.

psychosomatic. Physical symptoms caused by mental or emotional states.

quantum. The smallest increment of radient energy that may be absorbed or emitted as measured by its frequency times Planck's constant.

quantum physics. The study of energy and matter manifested as discrete particles or quanta. Also called quantum mechanics and Einsteinian physics. Also see continuum mechanics.

quenching. A term used to describe the modification of the chemical behavior of a compound in an essential oil as a result of the other compounds in the oil. It is the phenomena of quenching, among other things, that invalidates single component studies of essential oils.

racemic mixture. A mixture of equal amounts of dextrorotary and levorotary forms of a chiral molecule. When laboratories attempt to synthesize a single chiral form (either dextro or levo) in a lab, they usually get a racemic mixture and not the pure isomer created by nature.

radical. An incomplete molecule or ion carrying an electric charge. (i.e., a substance with one or more unpaired electrons.) Same as "free radical." Also see ion.

raindrop technique. A structured protocol, which takes about an hour, of applying a suite of essential oils to the back and feet. The oils applied include oregano, thyme, basil, wintergreen, mar-joram, cypress, and peppermint plus certain specific blends. Many therapeutic benefits have been claimed for raindrop technique, which has been performed on hundreds of thousands of people since first developed and introduced by D. Gary Young in the 1980s. The only published scientific study, to date, on the outcomes of raindrop technique is *A Statistical Validation of Raindrop Technique*, available from a variety of sources. (See back of this book for info on this study as well as training programs on how to do raindrop.)

receptor sites. Portals on the surface of a cell through which hormones and other ligands can pass or through which information can pass into and out of a living cell.

ring. Three or more atoms connected in a manner to form a polygon such as a quadrilateral, pentagon, hexagon, etc. In organic chemistry rings are mostly or completely composed of carbon atoms. A ring completely composed of carbon atoms is called homogeneous. A ring of carbons containing at least one atom of another element is called heterogeneous. Rings can have any number of sides.

saccharide. A sugar. (See carbohydrate.)

scientific law. A concise verbal statement or a mathematical equation that summarizes a broad variety of observations and experiences.

scientific method. The general process of advancing scientific knowledge by making experimental observations and by formulating laws, hypotheses, and theories.

second law of thermodynamics. Closed systems tend to change from a state of order to a state of disorder where useful energy available to do work is irreversibly transformed into useless energy unavailable to do work. In physics this law is mathematically expressed in terms of heat exchanges. Can also be expressed as a statement of our experience in that there is a direction to the way events occur in nature. When a process occurs spontaneously in one direction, it is nonspontaneous in the reverse direction. It is possible to state the second law in many different forms, but they all relate back to the same idea about spontaneity. A common form found in chemical texts is that in any spontaneous process the entropy of the universe increases. Also called the law of entropy.

self-referential reality. All-inclusive reality, outside of which no reference is possible.

sesquiterpene. A compound consisting of or containing a functional group with the formula, $C_{15}H_{24}$—the joining of three isoprene units or one-and-a-half terpene units.

shelf life. The amount of time an essential or fatty oil remains chemically stable and maintains its desirable properties at normal room temperatures. Pure essential oils have an unlimited shelf life while fatty oils eventually break down and lose their original character.

single component studies. A scientific study of the chemical behavior of a single compound in an essential oil as opposed to study of the behavior of the whole oil. Single component studies are not valid measures of the properties of a whole oil. See quenching.

spectrum. The range of frequencies of a wave.

speed of light. 300,000,000 meters per second or 186,280 miles per second. (In a vacuum). The speed of light is slightly slowed when passing through a transparent or translucent medium such as glass or water.

spontaneous process. A process that is capable of proceeding in a given direction, without needing to be driven by an outside source or energy. Spontaneous processes are irreversible. i.e., they do not automatically right themselves. Example: Iron nails exposed to weather spontaneously rust. Then never unrust on their own.

strong nuclear force. The force that opposes the repulsive force of like charges on protons and holds them together in the nucleus of an atom. At very close proximities the strong nuclear force is greater than the natural repulsion of like electrical charges.

structural formula. A diagram of the atoms in a molecule showing their spatial relationships.

shell. See electron shell.

synthetic. Manufactured by humans.

terpene unit. A common functional group found throughout nature formed from a pair of isoprene units and having the formula, $C_{10}H_{16}$. Countless natural organic compounds are built from multiples of terpene units.

tetraterpene. A compound consisting of or containing a functional group with the formula, $C_{40}H_{64}$—which is four terpene units.

therapeutic. Capable of facilitating a healing process.

therapeutic grade essential oil. An essential oil grown, distilled, and packaged for therapeutic purposes that fulfills the AFNOR standards for such oils. Less than 5% of the products sold as essential oils in the world are therapeutic in grade. Most aromatic oils are for the fragrance or flavor industries and are not suitable for therapeutic applications.

thrombosis. Formation of a blood clot.

thrombus. A blood clot.

tincture. A solution in which an alcohol is the solvent—usually a light alkane alcohol such as methyl, ethyl, propyl, or butyl. (see aqueous solution)

transmutation. Changing elements into other elements.

tricyclic. A molecule with three rings.

triterpene. A compound consisting of or containing a functional group with the formula, $C_{30}H_{48}$—which is three terpene units.

tritium. An isotope of hydrogen containing two neutrons in the nucleus of each atom.

Ultraviolet light. That portion of the electromagnetic spectrum just beyond visible violet that can be damaging to the skin. eg. sunburn. Abbreviated UV. The frequencies of UV radiation fall in the range of 10^{15} hz.

USP. United States Pharmacopoeia. An American agency that sets standards for British drug manufacturing processes.

uncertainty principle. There is an inherent uncertainty in the precision with which we can simultaneously specify the position and momentum of a particle. This uncertainty is significant only for exremely small particles, such as electrons. This uncertainty is a property of matter and not due to any limitations in scientific measuring apparati. Also called the "Heisenberg uncertainty principle."

UV. Ultraviolet light.

warfarin. A synthetic, generic anticoagulating coumarin drug with the formula, $C_{19}H_{16}O_4$, developed by the Wisconsin Alumni Research Foundation (WARF) as a hemorrhagic rodenticide (rat poison).

wave. A periodic function described by amplitude, frequency (or spectrum), and phase.

waveform. Anything that manifests some or all of the properties of a wave.

wavelength. The distance between identical points on successive waves. Abbreviated as lambda λ. Wavelength is the reciprocal of frequency.

wave mechanics. See continuum mechanics. Also called wave physics.

weak nuclear force. The force of repulsion that keeps electrons from falling into the proton or nucleas of an atom. At very close distances, the weak force over-powers the electromagnetic attraction due to electron being negatively charged and the proton being positively charged.

work. A force acting through a distance or the movement of an object against resistance.

valence. The tendency of an element to give, receive, or share electrons which can be expressed as a number. Knowing the valence (or valences) of an elements enables chemists to predict which other elements it will chemically bond with, which it will not, and if so, in what proportions.

vegetable oil. Any fatty oil pressed from the seed of a plant.

viscosity. A measure of the resistance of fluids to flow. Fatty oils are more viscous than essential oils.

volatile oil. Same as essential oil.

volatility. A measure of the tendency of a liquid to readily evaporate. Essential oils are volatile. Fatty oils are not.

x-rays. Electromagnetic radiation with frequencies in the neighborhood of 10^{18} hz. X-rays can pass through most materials and can break compounds into free radicals which can, in turn, be damaging to the tissues of the body.

❤ ANNOTATED BIBLIOGRAPHY
WITH RECOMMENDATIONS

List of References
Alphabetical By Title
(For Complete Bibliographic Information on each Title,
See the Alphabetical List by Author that Immediately Follows.)

1. **Advanced Aromatherapy: The Science of Essential Oil Therapy**
   by Kurt Schnaubelt

2. **Aromatherapy for Health Professionals**
   by Shirley and Len Price

3. **The Aromatherapy Practitioner Reference Manual**
   by Sylla Sheppard-Hanger

4. **Aromatherapy Scent and Psyche**
   by Peter and Kate Damian

5. **Bible (King James and Revised Standard Versions)**
   by Moses, David, Isaiah, Matthew, John, Paul, et al. (Editor-in-Chief, God)

6. **Biological Transmutations**
   by C.L. Kervran (Translated by Crosby Lockwood)

7. **Biological Transmutations: A New Science**
   by C.L. Kervran (Translated by Michel Abehsera)

8. **Body Electric**
   by Robert O. Becker

9. **Chemistry of Isoprenoid Compounds**
   by A.J. Haagen-Smit and C.C. Nimmo

10. **Chemistry: The Central Science**
    by Theodore L. Brown, H. Eugene LeMay, Jr., and Bruce E. Bursten

11. **Chemistry of Essential Oils: Introduction for Aromatherapists, Beauticians, Retailers, & Students.**
    by David G. Williams

13. **Clinical Aromatherapy: Essential Oils in Practice**
    by Jane Buckle

14. **Clinical Aromatherapy for Pregnancy and Childbirth**
    by Denise Tiran

15. **Complete Book of Essential Oils & Aromatherapy**
    by Valerie Ann Worwood

16. **Cymatics**
    by Hans Jenny

17. **Dr. Whitaker's Guide to Natural Healing**
    by Julian Whitaker

18. **Encounter with the Earth**
    by Leo F. Laporte

19. **Essential Chemistry for Safe Aromatherapy**
    by Sue Clarke

20. **Essential Oil Safety**
    by Robert Tisserand and Tony Balacs

21. **Essential Oils Desk Reference**
    edited by Brian Manwaring

22. **Essential Oils Integrative Medical Guide**
    by D. Gary Young

23. **Five Standards for Safe Childbearing**
    by David Stewart

24. **Freedom Through Health**
    by Terry Shepherd Friedmann

25. **God's Existence: Can Science Prove It?**
    by David Stewart

26. **The Gospel of Thomas**
    by Thomas the Disciple (Translated by Stevan Davies)

27. **Handbook of Chemistry and Physics**
    edited by David R. Lide

28. **Healing Oils of the Bible**
    by David Stewart

29. **The Holy Science**
    by S.S. Yukteswar

30. **Hormone Replace Therapy: A Theory Run Amok**
    Anonymous

31. **Illustrated Encyclopedia of Essential Oils**
    by Julie Lawless

32. **Integrated Aromatic Medicine 1998**
    English version edited by Brian Manwaring

33. **Integrated Aromatic Medicine 2000**
    English version edited by Brian Manwaring

34. **Integrated Aromatic Medicine 2001**
    English version edited by Brian Manwaring

35. **L'Aromatherapie Exactement**
   by Pierre Franchomme and Daniel Penoel

36. **Medical Aromatherapy: Healing with Essential Oils**
   by Kurt Schnaubelt

37. **The Merck Index: An Encyclopedia of Chemicals, Drugs, and Biologicals**
   edited by Susan Budavari

38. **The Merck Manual of Diagnosis and Therapy**
   edited by Mark H. Beers and Robert Berkow

39. **Merck's Manual of the Materia Medica, 1899 edition** anonymous (Merck & Company)

40. **Messages from Water**
   by Masaru Emoto

41. **Metabolism of Isoprenoid Compounds**
   by H.J. Nicholas

42. **Metabolism of Steroid Hormones and Bile Acids**
   by D.B. Gower

43. **Molecules of Emotion: The Science Behind Mind-Body Medicine**
   by Candace B. Pert

44. **Mosby's Medical, Nursing & Allied Health Dictionary**
   by Douglas Anderson,

45. **My Car, Myself**
   by Narayan Singh

46. **Natural Aromatic Materials - Odours & Origins**
   by Tony Burfield

47. **Natural Home Health Care Using Essential Oils**
   by Daniel and Rose-Marie Penoel

48. **The Nature of Substance: Spirit and Matter**
   by Rudolf Hauschka

49. **Organic Chemistry**
   by Francis A. Carey

50. **Organic Chemistry: A Crash Course**
   by Herbert Meislich, Howard Nechamkin, Jacob Sharefkin, and George Hademenos

51. **Pharmacognosy and Pharmacobiotechnology**
   by James Robbers, Marilyn Speedie, & Varro Tyler

52. **PDR® for Herbal Medicines**
   Chief Editor, Thomas Fleming

Annotated Bibliography 769

53. PDR® for Nutritional Supplements
Chief Editors, Shelden Hendler and David Rorvik

54. PDR® for Pharmaceuticals (Physician's Desk Reference)
Chief Editor, David W. Sifton

55. Plant Aromatics: Oral and Dermal Toxicity of Essential Oils and Absolutes
by Martin Watt

56. Powerful New Research on the Highest Antioxidant Foods
anonymous (Young Life Research Clinic)

57. The Power of Prayer on Plants
by Franklin Loehr

58. The Practice of Aromatherapy
by Jean Valnet

59. Prescription for Nutritional Healing
by James F. Balch and Phyllis A. Balch

60. Principles of Physical Geology
by Arthur Holmes

61. Quantum Physics, Essential Oils, and the Mind-Body Connection
by David Stewart

62. Radiation, Magnetism, and Living Things
by Daniel Halacy, Jr.

63. Reference Guide for Essential Oils
by Connie and Alan Higley

64. Reference Guide to Precautions in the Use of Aromatic Extracts from Plants
by Martin Watt

65. Science and Application of Essential Oils, Level I
by D. Gary Young.

66. Science and Application of Essential Oils, Level II
by D. Gary Young

67. Secret Life of Plants
by Peter Tompkins and Christopher Bird

68. A Statistical Validation of Raindrop Technique
by David Stewart

69. Structure and Function of the Body
by Gary A. Thibodeau and Kevin T. Patton

70. Theory and Problems of Organic Chemistry
by Herbert Meislich, Howard Nechamkin, Jacob Sharefkin, and George Hademenos

71. **Thieves, Deceivers, Killers: Tales of Chemistry in Nature**
by William Agosta

72. **375 Essential Oils and Hydrosols**
by Jeanne Rose

73. **Transcendental Physics**
by Edward R. Close

74. **Unlocking the Mysteries of Creation**
by Dennis R. Peterson

75. **USP27-NF22, 2004**
anonymous (U.S. Pharmacopoeia Convention)

76. **Vibrational Medicine**
by Richard Gerber

77. **What Your Doctor May Not Tell You about Menopause**
by John R. Lee

78. **Yes, No, Maybe: Chronobiotic Nutrition**
by Marcella Vonn Harting and G.I. Bergstrom

Bibliography of References
Alphabetical By Author
(With Commentary and Recommendations)

Agosta, William. (2002) *Thieves, Deceivers, and Killers: Tales of Chemistry in Nature.* 3rd printing. Princeton University Press, Princeton, NJ. 241 pp. (This fascinating book describes how plants and animals communicate through chemical compounds called pheromones, which relates to the way certain molecules of essential oils communicate information to us and to the systems of our bodies at a cellular level.)   ISBN 0-691-09273-7

Anderson, Douglas, et al. (2002) *Mosby's Medical, Nursing & Allied Health Dictionary*, Mosby, St. Louis, MO, 2134 pages. (A definitive and up-to-date resource for currently used medical terminology—probably the best resource of its kind. Includes excellent drawings and color photos. Defines medical jargon in easy-to-understand terms. Works well with Beers & Berkow, *The Merck Manual*—see listing below.)   ISBN 0-323-01430-5

Anonymous. (1899) *Merck's Manual of the Materia Medica,* Merck & Co., New York, 192 pp. (This facsimile edition was reprinted in 1999 by Merck as a centennial celebration. Compared to the current modern 1999 edition of the same manual (see Beers & Berkow below) one can see much that has changed in medicine and much that has not changed. Compare the length of the two: 192 small pocket-sized pages in 1899 versus 2833 full sized pages today. This 19th century medical guide actually suggests prescriptions for the following eleven essential oils: bitter almond, cajuput, eucalyptus, wintergreen, juniper, mustard, mountain pine, scotch fir, rosemary, sandalwood, and thyme. Today, bitter almond is not used by aromatherapists because of its potentially lethal cyanide content. Mustard oil is also not used today because its vapors can damaging to the lungs and nasal tissues. In all instances, the essential oils recommended by Merck are U.S.P. grade (U.S. Pharmacopoeia) which are not true therapeutic grade oils with healing qualities. USP means the oils have been manipulated by refining, denaturing, rectification, or adulteration with synthetics to fit a USP standard. USP grade oils are usually produced by drug companies.)   No ISBN.

Anonymous. (2003) *Hormone Replacement Therapy: A Theory Run Amok.* Essential Edge, Young Living, Lehi, Utah, November 2003, pp. 2-22

Anonymous. (2001) *Powerful New Research on the Highest Antioxidant Foods,* Natural Medicine Alert, Feb-Mar 2001, pp. 2-14, Young Life Research Clinic, Springville, Utah.

Anonymous. (2004) **USP27-NF22, 2004.** U.S. Pharmacopoeia Convention, www.USP.org. 3500 pp. (Provides the latest FDA-enforceable standards of identity, strength, quality, and purity for prescription and nonprescription drug ingredients and dosage forms, dietary supplements, medical devices, and other healthcare products. It includes tests, analytical procedures, and acceptance criteria. The main edition of USP–NF is published every November and becomes official January 1 of the next year. Supplements are published in February (official on April 1) and June (official on August 1). USP–NF is available in print, online, intranet, and CD formats. Price for hard-bound copy $633. Available via www.USP.org.

Balch, James & Balch, Phyllis. (1990) *Prescription for Nutritional Healing.* Avery Publishing Group, Garden City Park, NY. 368 pp. (James Balch is an MD and Phyllis is his wife. This is an encyclopedia from A to Z on dealing with diseases and maintaining health by natural means. This text, found in most health food stores, has become a classic reference for those who seek natural approaches to health and healing. While it contains considerable information on diet and herbal medicine, it only mentions essential oils once but places them in a very positive light. We used this book primarily for its information on the trace minerals in the body. Highly recommended for its guidance in health matters, not for its oil content, which is negligible.)   ISBN 0-85929-429-X

Becker, Robert O., and Selden, Gary. (1985) *The Body Electric.*
William Morrow, New York. 364 pages. (The best book there is on
the electromagnetic properties of the human body. Highly recommended.)   ISBN 0-688-06971-1

Beers, Mark H., & Berkow, Robert. editors. (1999) *The Merck Manual
of Diagnosis and Therapy.* Seventeenth edition. Merck Research
Laboratories, Whitehouse Station, New Jersey. 2833 pages.
(Describes every known disease and their prevailing allopathic
treatments. This is a reference used by physicians everywhere
and useful for anyone who wishes to take charge of their own
health care and be able to properly interpret a doctor's diagnosis.
This book does not support or recommend the use of essential
oils and contains misinformation on oil of wintergreen. Besides
being a publisher of medical references, Merck is also a major
drug company with a vested interest in promoting everything that
is allopathic and pharmaceutically oriented. Nevertheless, it is a
good book to have when you want to check up on your doctor.)
                                                  ISBN 0-911910-10-7

Brown, Theodore, LeMay, Eugene, & Bursten, Bruce (2000)
Chemistry: The Central Science 8th edition. Prentice Hall,
Upper Saddle River, New Jersey. 1040 pages. (An excellent up-
to-date, easy to follow basic text on General Chemistry. Well illustrated and student-friendly.)   ISBN 0-13-010310-1

Buckle, Jane. (2003) *Clinical Aromatherapy: Essential Oils in
Practice.* second edition. Churchill Livingston, London. 416 pp.
(Jane Buckle, RN, PhD., is British born, but has become an
American leader in the field of aromatherapy. Her perspective and
her publisher are both British. However, this book contains excellent chemistry and is a thoroughly informative book listing more
than 30 professionals as reviewers and/or editors.This book is
the outgrowth of her first book, *Clinical Aromatherapy in Nursing,*
(1995) also published in England, but this one is not from a
nursing perspective. Its appeal is to health care providers, both
individual and institutional. Its intent is to provide credible documentation for incorporating aromatherapy into today's medical
practice. The book contains a brief, well written section on essential oil chemistry. Her British perspective is evident in her overly
conservative contraindications for certain oils such as wintergreen, calamus, cassia, fennel, and tansy (which we know to be
harmless when top grade oils are used with common sense). She
is also against neat applications of oils such as oregano, which is
one of the principal oils applied undiluted in raindrop technique,
a safe, effective and beneficial procedure that applies oils neat
has helped hundreds of thousands of Americans, but is not widely practiced in England. This is a great book with a wealth of
well-organized, clearly written information not found in any other
text. If you are planning to study for the (ARC) Aromatherapy

Registration Council exam, familiarity with this book, alone, would probably get you through the test. Dr. Buckle is one of the people who helped write this exam. To pass that exam, some of the answers have to be politically correct (and factually wrong) in order to pass. For information on this exam, by which one can become a "Registered Aromatherapist" or "R.A.," visit the web site, www.aromatherapycouncil.com or call (212) 356-0668. We recommend this book. Just don't believe all of her precautions against using certain oils or against using essential oils orally or neat. Her safety comments do not apply to genuine therapeutic grade oils.) ISBN 0-443-07236-1

Budavari, Susan. editor. (1996) *The Merck Index: An Encyclopedia of Chemicals, Drugs, and Biologicals.* Twelfth edition. Merck Research Laboratories, Whitehouse Station, New Jersey. 2425 pp. (First published in 1899, this is the most comprehensive reference on the organic compounds comprising natural substances and developed as medicines. More than 10,000 compounds are described, including virtually every constituent found in essential oils, and including their structural diagrams, indications, and toxicities. Also lists many herbs.) ISBN 0-911910-13-1

Burfield, Tony. (2000) *Natural Aromatic Materials - Odours & Origins.* 2 vols. Edited by Sylla Sheppard-Hanger. Atlantic Institute of Aromatherapy (AIA), Tampa, Florida. 525 pp. (Dr. Burfield is a thoroughly trained British plant biochemist and this book is one of the most thorough compilation of chemical information on essential oils available. Although more qualitative than quantitative, Burfield's book contains chemical profiles of more than 500 essential oils and includes an index of both common and latin names. His long career with essential oils has been with the perfume industry and his expertise is in fragrance. I recommend this book to serious students as an unparalleled resource on the olfactory chemistry of essential oils.) No ISBN

Carey, Francis A. (2000) *Organic Chemistry*, 4th edition. McGraw-Hill, Boston, MA. 1108 pages. (Good basic text. Good section on terpenes. Cites numerous natural substances as examples of various types of molecules. Recommended only for serious organic chemistry students or those seeking in-depth understanding of essential oils. See books by Meislich, et al., listed elswhere in this bibliography are for simpler more student-friendly organic texts.) ISBN 0-07-290501-8

Clarke, Sue. (2002) *Essential Chemistry for Safe Aromatherapy.* Churchill Livingston, London. 231 pages. (An excellent resource for essential oil chemistry. Includes many photos of molecular models along with structural diagrams. Well written and very comprehensive. Includes a good glossary. However, it is written from the British point of view on aromatherapy which means that the safety advice in this book is inappropriately restrictive and does not apply to pure therapeutic grade oils. British aromatherapists generally frown on undiluted oils applied to the skin and discourage oral usages. We recommend this as an excellent source for essential oil chemistry, but don't believe all of the safety advice given here.)   ISBN 0-443-06485-7

Close, Edward R. (1997) *Transcendental Physics.* Paradigm Press, Jackson, Missouri. 371 pp. (This book takes the laws of physics as proven and accepted by scientists and shows by impeccable logic, as surely as 2+2 = 4, that to accept the precepts of science leads to the inevitable conclusion that there is a God and we are his children. This book is probably 100 years ahead of its time and presents a long and involved set of arguments from the classical laws of physics through relativity and quantum mechanics that lead to God as the conclusion. Dr. Close is a gifted writer/teacher and has broken forever the barrier between science and religion. Highly recommended for serious students who seek the reconciliation of science and religion. To purchase a copy, go to www.amazon.com or www.iuniverse.com.)   ISBN 0-934426-78-3

Damian, Peter, and Damian, Kate. (1995) **Aromatherapy Scent and Psyche.** Healing Arts Press, Rochester, Vermont. 244 pp. (There are no formulas, lists of chemical constituents, or diagrams of molecules in this book, but it contains information on chemistry woven throughout the text with numerous insights that I have not encountered in any other source.)   ISBN 0-89281-530-2

Emoto, Masuru (2003) *Messages from Water.* HADO Publishing, Amstel, The Netherlands. 147 pp. (Printed in Czechoslovakia, published in Holland, this book was originally released in Japanese and is now translated into English. Dr. Emoto froze water and photographed the crystals at 200-500 magnifications under a microscope in a photo lab that was kept at $-5°$ C. He and his staff made tens of thousands of photos before and after various phenomena to see how water responded. For example, water exposed to classical music had no crystalline patterns before but developed them afterwards. Water that was prayed over responded with beautiful designs when there had been none before. By a magnetic resonance device, Emoto would resonate things like an essential oil and imprint those frequencies onto a water sample to see how these imprints changed the crystalline patterns. Oil of Roman Chamomile, for example, stimulated the water to produce white crystals that imitated the white flowers of the chamomile plant. Oil of fennel stimulated the water to form yellow crystals in patterns that were like those of clusters of fennel blossoms. Polluted water in a reservoir that made ugly crystals were prayed over for an hour by a priest which then caused the water to form pretty crystals that were pure. Even saying or writing different words and placing them on the glass water container caused the waters to reflect the words to which they had been exposed, regardless of the language. This book proves that inanimate matter responds to human thought and human intent, which is what oils do when applied with thought and intent. An excellent indirect scientific confirmation of the manner of interaction between human consciousness and essential oils. Contains dozens of excellent color photos of ice as it communicates with us through its infinitely variable crystalline patterns. Highly recommended.

ISBN 9-080742-13-9

Fleming, Thomas, editor. (2000) **PDR® for Herbal Medicines.** Second edition. Thomson Medical Economics, Montvale, New Jersey. 854 pp. (Contains over 800 large pages of fine print and is a gold mine for the herbalist as well as a good reference on many essential oils. This is true even though the book is presented from an allopathic point of view, since it is specifically compiled for allopathic physicians (MDs) and pharmacists. Thousands of herbs are listed along with color photos of the flowering plants along with excellent descriptions of their therapeutic applications. In many cases, the herb is featured, not only as a plant, but also as the source of an essential oil. The descriptions of the oils are thorough in their treatment of the chemical components contained therein. This is a valuable resource in gathering information on the chemistry of essential oils. Thousands of research publications are cited in support of the therapeutic benefits, indications, administrations, and the effects of herbs and their oils. Even though this is an allopathic resource, most of the commentary is positive toward the use of essential oils.)

ISBN 1-56363-361-2

Franchomme, Pierre, & Penoel, Daniel. (2001) *L'Aromatherapie Exactement*, Roger Jollois, Editor/Publisher, Gassendi-Dietetique, Paris, France. 522 pp. ("Exact Aromatherapy" is the title in English. The subtitle (in English) is "Encyclopedia of Therapeutic Utilization of Aromatic Extracts." An additional subtitle is "Foundations, demonstrations, Illustrations, and Applications of the Science of Natural Medicine." This is the best book on essential oil chemistry in the world written by two of the world's leading authorities—Franchomme (a chemist) and Penoel (a physician). However, it is in French. If you don't read French, you won't get much from the text, but you can still understand most of the information on chemical compounds found in oils. A must reference for serious researchers into essential oil chemistry. Available via the following web site, www.biogessendi.com.)

ISBN 2-87819-001-7

Friedmann, Terry S. (1998) **Freedom Through Health.** revised edition. Harvest Publishing, Northglenn, Colorado. 280 pp. This book does not contain much about essential oil chemistry, but contains a great deal about healing applications of essential oils. Dr. Friedmann is a practicing allopathic physician who is also a founder and officer of the American Holistic Medical Association (AHMA). His one-of-a-kind book integrates allopathic medicine with homeopathy, acupuncture, reflexology, herbology, nutrition, vibrational medicine, chiropractic manipulation, emotional release, and, to a great extent, aromatherapy. It is the best book available in English on applying essential oils with a medical/ holistic perspective. Dr. Friedmann has not only successfully used essential oils for years in his practice, but has conducted considerable research into their benefits. This is a practical, how-to-do-it book, not only for health care practitioners, but for the public at large. Easy to read and contains a glossary for unfamiliar terms. Highly recommended). ISBN 0-9638366-8-4

Gerber, Richard. (2001) **Vibrational Medicine.** third edition. Bear & Company, Rochester, Vermont. 607 pp. (This is the best and most comprehensive book on vibrational medicine available. Well written and easy to understand, Dr. Gerber has done a monumental work in assembling this material for everyone to use. Essential oils are mentioned only once on page 512. However, in that one paragraph Dr. Gerber, who is an MD, sees much promise in essential oils as part of vibrational medicine. This is an excellent book to familiarize one's self with the changing paradigm of medicine, which has traditionally been based on manipulating matter through chemistry. While allopathy is based on a chemical model for life processes, Gerber presents a host of data to show that life processes are also electrical, magnetic, and involve even more subtle energies not yet named nor discovered by science. Gerber believes medical doctors will eventually move toward consideration of life as energy. The author refers to this as "Einsteinian Medicine," in reference to Einstein's famous equation that equates energy and matter through the speed of light. This book is for those who want to understand the physics and current scientific understanding of energy or vibrational medicine. Those who understand how essential oils work will recognize that essential oil therapy is truly another aspect of vibrational medicine. When Dr. Gerber realizes this, he will, no doubt, add a new chapter to his already encyclopedic book. Highly recommended.) ISBN 1-879181-58-4

God, Almighty. Editor-in-chief. **The Holy Bible.** The King James Version (KJV) was first published in 1611, the New International Version (NIV) in 1978, and the New Revised Standard Version (NRSV) in 1989. (The Bible is an anthology of spiritual works by more than 50 inspired authors spanning more than a thousand years in the making. A great source of insight and inspiration to the workings of God in man and nature as expressed through the writings of his prophets, disciples, and humble servants—none of whom were PhDs, MDs, or college graduates. Unrecognized and uncertified by any academic institution of humankind, they were, instead, authorized and recognized by God. Highly recommended.) Available under many ISBNs depending on translation, publisher, and edition.

Gower, D.B. (1968) **Metabolism of Steroid Hormones and Bile Acids.** Chapter II, Vol. 20, *Comprehensive Biochemistry* (in 29 vols.), Elsevier Publishing Company, London. pp. 63-124. (A highly technical, but thorough, discussion of steroid compounds, including some diterpene plant molecules that copy certain estrogens. Recommended only for thoroughly dedicated organic chemists.)　　　LCCN 62-10359

Haagen-Smit, A.J., and Nimmo, C.C. (1968) *The Chemistry of Isoprenoid Compounds.* Chapter V, Vol. 9, *Comprehensive Biochemistry* (in 29 vols.), Elsevier Publishing Company, London. pp. 114-164. (A highly technical, but thorough, discussion of terpene compounds found in essential oils from monoterpenes through tetraterpenes with some additional information on polyterpenes (really big molecules). Recommended only for thoroughly dedicated organic chemists.)　　LCCN 62-10359

Halacy, Daniel, Jr. (1966) *Radiation, Magnetism and Living Things.* Holiday House, New York. 196 pp. (A good introduction to the electricities and magnetisms of plants, animals, and humans and the responses of living organisms to external fields.) No ISBN.

Harting, Marcella Vonn, & Bergstrom, G.I. (2004) **Yes, No, Maybe: Chronobiotic Nutrition.** Warm Snow Publishers, Torreon, New Mexico. 275 pp. (This book says that for optimal health it not only matters what you eat, but when you eat it. The body, they say, is best adapted to digest fruits, nuts, and things that grow high on trees in the morning, four-legged meats and things that grow on bushes at mid-day, with fish, eggs, ground crops and vegetables that grow on or beneath the soil in the evening. Foods that can cause weight gain can also cause weight loss, depending on the time of day eaten. Even specific essential oils have their best and worst times of the day. A fascinating concept, the validity of which one can test themselves. As for minerals and elements, this is the first source I ever read that says that all natural elements, including heavy metals, are essential to the body. Caution: This book may stretch your mind and benefit your health.)　　　ISBN 0-9710684-2-9

Hauschka, Rudolf. (2002) *The Nature of Substance: Spirit and Matter.* Sophia Books, an imprint of Rudolph Steiner Press, East Sussex, United Kingdom, 233 pp. (This book was first published in the German language, in Frankfurt in 1950. It was first translated into English in 1966 and again in 1983 by Rudolph Steiner Press. There is one short chapter on "Scents, Etheric Oils, and Resins." The entire book has to do with the chemistry of plants and their relationship to the earth, the elements, the sun, the moon, and to spiritual forces.Hauschka was also one of the first scientists to recognize that transmutation of the elements does take place routinely in biological processes. This book brings to light the little-known, almost forgotten, work of Austrian scientist, Baron Von Herzeele, published in 1875, that for the first time offered quantitative evidence of elements transforming into other elements by common, natural processes. This book will expand your thinking about relationships between what we term as the animate and inanimate aspects of our universe and demonstrates that inanimate matter responds to consciousness and behaves in ways beyond the currently accepted laws and paradigms of physical science. This is relevant information when attempting to explain how essential oils interact with people to effect healing.) ISBN 1-85584-122-3

Hendler, Shelden, and Rorvik, David, editors. (2001) *PDR® for Nutritional Supplements.* Thomson PDR Company, Montvale, New Jersey. 575 pp. (Only the products of participating companies are included in this tome, which may not include your favorite brands. Many of the most commonly used brands of nutritional supplements are not included because those companies choose not to participate. While the book is for and by allopathic physicians and pharmacists, there is a lot of valuable information on specific supplements and minerals contained here you won't find elsewhere. Contains hundreds of citations of scientific research. Most large libraries will have this book. Includes latest findings on nutrition and cancer, aging, immunity, fitness and other aspects of nutritional supplementation. Lists all Poison Control Centers in the U.S.) ISBN 1-56363-364-7

Higley, Connie, and Higley, Alan. (2001) *Reference Guide for Essential Oils,* 8th edition. Abundant Health, Orem, Utah, (888) 718-3068. 578 pages. (Excellent reference on therapeutic essential oils and their usage. Contains considerable information on the chemical constituents of essential oils as well as the science behind their effectiveness. All the oils and blends of oils mentioned in this book are sold by Young Living Essential Oils, Inc., an American grower, distiller, and vendor of high quality therapeutic essential oils. Highly recommended.) ISBN 0-9706583-0-3

Holmes, Arthur. (1965) ***Principles of Physical Geology.*** Second edition, revised. Ronald Press, New York, NY. 1287 pp. (A thorough and exhaustive basic geology text.) LCCN 65-21811

Jenny, Hans (2001) ***Cymatics.*** MACROmedia, Newmarket, New Hampshire. 295 pp. (Translated from German, the book title, "Cymatics," is taken from a Greek word meaning " vibration" or "wave form." It has been said by many, from ancient philosophers to modern physicists, that "everything is vibration." Even the Book of Genesis says that God "spoke" the universe into existence. To speak is to create vibrations. While it is easy to visualize simple vibrations producing simple manifestations, it is difficult to see how a complex entity like our human body could be the result of complex vibrational patterns. This book shows how life forms, including complex life forms, can be produced by vibration. The way one object or entity relates to another is by the degree of resonance they share. This is crucial to understanding how oils work. They have their own vibrational patterns which, when they resonate with our bodies, minds and spirits, can bring about healing. Dr. Jenny was a medical doctor who was also an accomplished artist and musician. This book contains numerous stunning photographs that make vibrations visible. This book is highly recommended to those who want to gain a better understanding of the vibrational nature of essential oils, of ourselves, and of the universe. ISBN 1-888-13807-6

Kervran, Louis. (1972) ***Biological Transmutations: A New Science.*** Translated from the French by Michael Abehsera in 1972. Swan House Publications, Binghamton, New York. 163 pp. (This is some of the works of Louis Kervran who spent his life in the study of cold temperature nuclear processes in plants and animals, proving that life processes do not consist merely of chemistry, but of atomic processes as well. This discovery sheds light on a lot of unexplained biochemical processes as well as some of the unexplained behaviors of essential oils.. This book has the same title as the next one listed below, but they are not the same book. Both are translations of Kervran's research and writings, but not the same research and writings. They are both worth study. With respect to essential oils, the most common elemental transformations almost always involve the transfer of hydrogen or oxygen atoms. Add or subtract a hydrogen (1 proton and 1 electron) to any element and you get the next element before or after in the periodic table. Thus you can combine a hydrogen with a potassium and get calcium. Or you can subtract an oxygen (8 electrons and 8 protons) from silicon and get carbon. etc. Since essential oil molecules are composed mostly of hydrogen atoms with carbons and oxygens, they could be participants in the creation and transmutations of elements, which adds another dimension to the role of essential oils in therapy. Highly recommended for those who are unafraid to expand their thinking outside of the self-created shell that confines classical science.

ISBN 0-913010-03-0

Kervran, Louis. (1980) *Biological Transmutations*. Translated from the French by Crosby Lockwood in 1971. Beekman Publishers, Woodstock, New York. 134 pp. (This important book is the result of a lifetime of research on the part of C.L. Kervran who has demonstrated conclusively that elements can be changed one into another through biological processes. In other words, cold fusion and other low intensity nuclear processes never achieved in a laboratory, are daily occurrences in the lives of plants and animals. This book proves that life, as we know it, is far more than a chemical process (as is currently taught in schools of medicine and biology) or even an electromagnetic process. It is also a matter of nuclear biophysics which explains a lot concerning the behavior of essential oils. This book is similar to the one above, but it's not the same book. Both are translations of Kervran's work, but are not the same works. Both need to be read to grasp the significance of his discoveries. Chemists, physicists, and biologists could all expand their field of vision for their respective sciences by studying Kervran's books. His well documented studies profoundly contradict the limited paradigms by which chemistry, physics, and biology are understood today. Highly recommended.)

ISBN 0-8464-0195-9

Laporte, Leo F. (1975) *Encounter With the Earth.* Harper & Row, New York, NY. 538 pp. (A good basic text on environmental geology—the effects of natural forces on society and human life and the effects of human society on the planet.) ISBN 0-06-384780-9

Lawless, Julia. (1995) *Illustrated Encyclopedia of Essential Oils*. Element Books Ltd., An Imprint of Harper-Collins Publishers, London. 256 pp. (Beautifully illustrated throughout in full color, this is a book to put on your coffee table. But it is also a valuable reference on essential oil remedies from A to Z. Contains detailed information on more than 160 specific oils and a short, but clearly written, summary of basic chemistry. It has been adopted as the primary recommended text for aromatherapy training in the United Kingdom. While British in its point of view toward the safe use of oils, safety is not a primary focus of this book. Contains many insights not found elsewhere. Recommended.)

ISBN 1-85230-721-8

Lee, John. R. (1996) *What Your Doctor May Not Tell You About Menopause*. Warner Books, New York. 372 pp. (This book tells the truth about the dangers of hormone replacement therapy

(HRT) and what measures women can take to achieve a balance in their hormones without synthetic drugs. Highly recommended.) ISBN 0-446-67144-4

Lide, David R., Editor-in-Chief. (2003) *Handbook of Chemistry and Physics*, 84th Edition. CRC Press, New York, 2700 pages. (This is the world's most comprehensive and up-to-date reference book on elements, compounds, and their physical/chemical properties. Contains thousands of structural formulas of organic compounds. It has been republished and updated 84 times since 1918. It is expensive—$135 wholesale for the 2003 edition. A great reference, but unless you are going into chemistry as a profession, you don't need it.) ISBN 0-8493-0484-9

Loehr, Franklin. (1969) *The Power of Prayer on Plants*. Second edition. Signet Books, New York. 127 pp. (Franklin Loehr was a professional research chemist who became a Presbyterian minister with a passion for both God and science. He ultimately left the ministry and founded the Religious Research Foundation through which he conducted well controlled experiments on 27,000 seeds and seedlings, taking more than 100,000 measurements, that prove conclusively that prayer exerts a measurable force and dramatically affects the growth of plants. Loehr sees science as a great tool to confirm and support spiritual faith. This book provides indirect evidence of how prayer also affects the behavior of oils and how they heal. Highly recommended.) LCCN 58-11320

Manwaring, Brian, English version editor (2000) *Integrated Aromatic Medicine 1998* Introduction by Daniel Penoel, MD. Proceedings from the First International Symposium on Aromatic Medicine, Grasse, France, March 21-23, 1998. Translated into English and published by Essential Science Publishing, Orem, Utah. 150 pp. (A collection of 22 scientific papers on such diverse topics as oil chemistry, oil production, oils applied in gynecology, fatigue, allergies, prostate cancer, neurology, HIV cases, Fibromyalgia, acupuncture, removing dental amalgams, emergency care, tinnitus, ADHD, melanoma, and other topics. Most topics are authored by MDs. Recommended for serious students seeking information on the leading edge of scientific research in aromatherapy.) No ISBN

Manwaring, Brian, English version editor (2001) *Integrated Aromatic Medicine 2000*. Editorial management, Daniel Penoel, MD. Proceedings from the Int'l Symposium on Aromatic Medicine, Grasse, France, March 19-21, 2000. Translated into English and published by Essential Science Publishing, Orem, Utah. 124 pp. (A collection of 23 scientific papers on on such diverse topics as oil chemistry, natural medicines, intestinal parasites, hospital disinfection, oils as insect repellents, treatment of acne, gengivitus, energetic aromatherapy, candida, UV filtering, athletes foot, aromaceuticals, and other topics. 8 papers authored by MDs, 1 by an ND, 1 by a DDS. Recommended for serious students seeking info on the leading edge of research in aromatherapy.) No ISBN

Manwaring, Brian, English version editor. (2002) *Integrated Aromatic Medicine 2001.* Editorial management, Daniel Penoel, MD. Proceedings from the International Symposium on Aromatic Medicine, Grasse, France, March 2-4, 2001. Translated into English and published by Essential Science Publishing, Orem, Utah. 165 pp. (A collection of 20 scientific papers on such diverse topics as oil chemistry, respiratory infections, stress relief, DNA, inflammation, psoriasis, rheumatoid arthritis, natural cosmetics, ayurvedic medicine, cancer, ear infections, and other topics. Half the papers are authored by MDs or PhDs. Recommended for serious students for information on the leading edge of scientific research in aromatherapy.)   No ISBN

Manwaring, Brian, editor. (2002) *Essential Oils Desk Reference,* 2nd edition. Essential Science Publishing, Orem, Utah. 466 pp. (Excellent reference on therapeutic essential oils and their usage. Contains considerable information on the chemical constituents of essential oils as well as the science behind their effectiveness. All the oils and blends of oils mentioned in this book are sold by Young Living Essential Oils, Inc., an American grower, distiller, and vendor of high quality therapeutic essential oils. Highly recommended.)   ISBN 0-943685-25-7

Meislich, Herbert, et al. (1999) *Theory and Problems of Organic Chemistry (Schaum's Outline Series),* 3rd edition. McGraw-Hill, New York. 468 pages. (Excellent learning resource for organic chemistry. Very student friendly. Highly recommended for introduction to the field.)   ISBN 0-07-134165-X

Meislich, Herbert, et al. (2000) *Organic Chemistry: A Crash Course.* (*Schaum's Easy Outlines*) McGraw-Hill, New York. 138 pages. (An abbreviated, simplified version of the book, *Theory and Problems of Organic Chemistry* mentioned immediately above. Highly recommended as an introduction to organic chemistry.)   ISBN 0-07-052718-0

Nicholas, H.J. (1968) **Metabolism of Isoprenoid Compounds.** Chapter I, Vol. 20, *Comprehensive Biochemistry* (in 29 vols.), Elsevier Publishing Company, London. pp. 1-62. (A highly technical, but thorough, discussion of terpenes as they occur and are metabolized in plants. Recommended only for thoroughly dedicated biochemists.)   LCCN 62-10359

Penoel, Daniel, and Penoel, Rose-Marie. (1998) *Natural Home Health Care Using Essential Oils.* Brian Manwaring, Editor. Essential Science Publishing, Orem, Utah. 235 pp. (This excellent book is revised, enlarged, and translated from the French publication "*Pratique Aromatique Familial.*" Daniel Penoel, MD, is the world's leading authority on the medical application of essential oils. This book is both practical and inspirational. He weaves information on chemistry throughout the book, as well as insights on the healing properties of essential oils that cannot be explained by chemistry. He represents the epitome of the French school of aromatherapy to which we also subscribe in this book. Highly recommended.) ISBN 2-909531-02-3

Pert, Candace B. (1997) *Molecules of Emotion: The Science Behind Mind-Body Medicine.* Simon & Schuster, NY. 368 pages. (Excellent enjoyable reading on the complex biochemistry of the body and how hormones and receptor sites work. Although oils are not mentioned, the book gives insight into how essential oils work at cellular levels thru receptor cites. Highly recommended.) ISBN 0-684-84634-9

Peterson, Dennis R. (2002) *Unlocking the Mysteries of Creation.* Creation Resource Publications, El Dorado, California. 239 pp. (This is the best creation science book I have ever read. Both scriptural and scientific, it contains a wealth of rewarding and intellectually stimulating material. Beautifully illustrated with full color photos and graphics that enhances its easy-to-read format. A true classic. Recommended.) ISBN 0-89051-371-6

Price, Shirley, and Price, Len. (1999) *Aromatherapy for Health Professionals*, 2nd edition. Churchill Livingstone, London. 391 pages. (Excellent general reference for technical aspects of essential oils and applications. These are British authors with a viewpoint more French than British. The foreword is by Daniel Penoel, MD, of France. While their safety indications are more liberal than most British authors, they may be more conservative than necessary when using top grade therapeutic oils. Contains excellent detailed chemical information on 66 different oils. Highly Recommended.) ISBN 0-443-06210-2

Robbers, James E., Speedie, Marilyn K., Tyler, Varro E. (1996) *Pharmacognosy and Pharmacobiotechnology.* Williams & Wilkins, Baltimore. 337 pages. (Highly technical, but a good source of chemistry on natural substances, including essential oils. The ancestral roots of this book go back to when pharmacies had natural herbs on their shelves along with the other medicines. Much of the content of this book has to do with manipulating plants to produce pharmaceuticals (i.e. pharmacobiotechnology). This book explains many processes for synthesizing or extracting the compounds of essential oils—like how to extract or manufacture menthol, thymol, camphor, etc. It is used by companies that adulterate natural oils to make them fit certain standards or who sell synthetic versions for flavors, fragrances, or medicines. Unless you really wish to plunge deeply into the field of biochemistry, you don't need this book.)

ISBN 0-683-08500-X

Rose, Jeanne. (1999). *375 Essential Oils and Hydrosols.* Frog Limited, Berkeley, California. 251 pp. (An excellent reference for botanical information on aromatic plants and their oils, including the main chemical components. A good general reference. Recommended.)
ISBN 1-883319-89-7

Schnaubelt, Kurt. (1995) *Advanced Aromatherapy: The Science of Essential Oil Therapy.* Healing Arts Press, Rochester, Vermont. 138 pages. (Excellent and readable text on the science and chemistry of essential oils. Translated from German. Schnaubelt studied under Daniel Penoel, MD, in France and writes from the French point of view of aromatherapy, which we think is the best point of view. Recommended.)
ISBN 0-89281-743-7

Schnaubelt, Kurt. (1999) *Medical Aromatherapy: Healing with Essential Oils.* Frog, Ltd., Berkeley, California. 296 pages. (Excellent and readable text on the science and chemistry of essential oils. A German by birth, Schnaubelt studied under Daniel Penoel, MD, in France and writes from the French point of view of aromatherapy. Recommended.)
ISBN 1-883319-69-2

Sheppard-Hanger, Sylla. (1994) *The Aromatherapy Practitioner Reference Manual.* 2 vols.12th printing 2000. Atlantic Institute of Aromatherapy (AIA), Tampa, Florida. 577 pages. (This manual contains hundreds of pages of detailed chemistry on over 350 essential oils. This publication, though American, reflects the British school of aromatherapy, which tends to be ultraconservative in its attitude toward what is safe in applying essential oils. Don't believe all of the precautions given. They do not apply to therapeutic grade oils. With these reservations in mind, I recommend this book as a valuable resource on the chemistry of essential oils and their applications. There is a great deal of quantitative chemical information here you won't find anywhere else.)
ISBN 0-9643141-0-X

Sifton, David W., editor. (2003) *Physicians' Desk Reference (PDR®)*, 57th edition. Thomson PDR Company, Montvale, New Jersey. 3550 pages. (The only complete reference on American prescription pharmaceuticals. Contains information on prescribing protocols for prescription drugs with some discussion of their chemistry, biochemical mechanisms, and structural formulas. It is not a resource for over-the-counter drugs. There is another PDR for that. Only about 20% of the book has to do with indications, effects, dosages, routes, and administration while 80% of the book has to do with warnings, hazards, contraindications. side effects, and precautions. A good book to have if you want to know the possible consequences of any specific drug. Contains a complete list in the back of the book of Poison Control Centers in the United States. The emergency number to call for any or all of these Poison Centers is (800) 222-1222. Info on the PDR can be found at www.PDR.net) ISBN 1-56363-445-7

Singh, Narayan. (2002) *My Car, Myself.* Lynn Henderson Publications, Vancouver, BC. 178 pp.(Dr. Singh is a practicing psychologist who noticed that when his clients came in and complained about some of their car problems that there was a correlation between their personal problems. He compiled these correlations over a period of years and produced this book. He postulates that since you spend so much time in your automobile, it absorbs your vibrations and conciousness such that whatever troubles you may have start manifesting as troubles with your car. It is available from Lynne Henderson Publications, Vancouver, BC, email, empath@direct.ca or phone, (604) 261-0801 No ISBN

Stewart, David. (1976) *God's Existence: Can Science Prove It?* Dwapara Herald Publications, Hillsborough, NC. 51 pp. (This treatise applies the second law of thermodynamics to prove, by applied physics, the existence of an intelligent creator that functions both within the laws of nature as we know them, as well as outside of those laws. It also demonstrates that science as we know it can never disprove the existence of a personal God because this area of inquiry is outside of and not amenable to the scientific method. In fact, the scientific method is very restrictive in its capabilities and cannot be applied to the majority of life situations. One cannot live by the scientific method. While the science is an effective way to sort out certain types of facts and verify or disprove certain kinds of information, it is a poor and ineffective technique by which to live. In fact, it is impossible to live entirely by science. Our daily decisions must be made by other means.) ISBN 0-917952-00-6

Stewart, David. (1998) *The Five Standards for Safe Childbearing.* Fourth edition. Napsac Reproductions, Marble Hill, MO, 586 pp. (Originally published in 1981 and revised and updated in 1998, this book contains exhaustive documentation (more than 1000 cited articles and publications) that proves the superiority and safety of the following five aspects of childbirth: 1. Good Nutrition in Pregnancy, 2. Midwifery, 3. Home Birth, 4. Natural Birth, and 5. Breastfeeding. It conclusively demonstrates by citing published scientific and technical data that midwives are safer than doctors and home is a safer place to give birth than a hospital. The book contains a chapter entitled "The Limits of Science in Childbirth," which has been adapted as a portion of this book.) ISBN 0-934426-72-4

Stewart, David (2002) *Healing Oils of the Bible.* Care Publications, Marble Hill, MO, 324 pp. (This book cites more than 500 Bible verses in documenting the use of essential oils and other aromatic substances by the people of Biblical times, both Old and New Testament. While not possessing a science of chemistry as we have today, the ancients seemed to understand many of the medical and healing properties of oils.)   ISBN 0-934426-98-8

Stewart, David. (2003) *A Statistical Validation of Raindrop Technique.* Care Publications, Marble Hill, MO. 60 pp. (This is the only scientific study yet published on raindrop technique. Raindrop is an hour-long procedure applying 8 single oils undiluted and 2-3 blends to the feet and back. Summarizing data from several thousand raindrop experiences, this study clearly demonstrates the safety and effectiveness of raindrop technique as a healing modality. Besides statistical information, there are 74 brief testimonials of individuals who received raindrop which provides additional insight into the benefits and results of raindrop not possible through numbers alone.)   ISBN 0-934426-38-4

Stewart, David. (2009) *Quantum Physics, Essential Oils, and the Mind-Body Connection.* Sound Concepts, American Fork, Utah. 20 pages. (Explains how your thoughts, feelings, and intentions determine which of the many possibilities possessed by an oil defined by its chemistry will actually manifest when applied. Offers a scientific explanation of why prayer and faith cause oils to work better. HIghly recommended.)   No ISBN

Thibodeau, Gary A., and Patton, Kevin T. (2000) *Structure and Function of the Body.* 11th edition. Mosby, St. Louis, Missouri. 528 pages. (Excellent and easy-to-understand reference on human physiology and bodily functions, including the biochemistry of bodily processes. Used in many medical schools as a required text for medical students. Beautifully and profusely illustrated. Very user friendly. Presented in a manner that even medical students can understand. Comes with a CD. Contains a short chapter on biochemistry in the back. Highly recommended.)   ISBN 0-323-01081-4

Thomas the Disciple (2004) *The Gospel of Thomas.* 4th prtg. (Translated and annotated by Stevan Davies) Skylight Paths Publishing, Woodstock, Vermont. 141 pages. (This is considered by most theological scholars as an authentic gospel by the Biblical Thomas (Didymas), one of the twelve principle disciples of Jesus. It's existence has been known for centuries inasmuch as it is referred to by several other works. A complete manuscript of the book was not found until 1945 when a copy was found in a large jar in a cave near Dag Hammadi, Egypt. However, it was not available in English until 1955. The book appears to have been written during the lifetime of Jesus, before his death. It catalogues many of the same sayings (slightly reworded) found in the synoptic gospels, but includes many quotes attributed to Jesus not found in the *New Testament*. Some theologians want to include it as a canonical book and legitimate scripture—a fifth gospel to be ranked as equal in authority to Matthew, Mark, Luke, and John. Highly recommended for those who want to gain deeper insight into the teachings of Christ and into his plan for the personal salvation of us all.)   ISBN 1-893361-45-4

Tiran, Denise. (2000) **Clinical Aromatherapy for Pregnancy and Childbirth.** 2nd edition. Churchill Livingstone, London. 196 pages. (This British author writes from the British school of aromatherapy which is incompatible with the principles and practice of aromatherapy as a true healing modality. Does not recognize difference between perfume/cosmetic/food grade oils and therapeutic healing grade oils. Book contains false and erroneous information. For example, on p. 46 she considers the following oils to have no use in aromatherapy whatsoever: basil, birch, calamus, cassia, cinnamon bark, clove, fennel, oregano, pine, savory, tansy, thuja, and wintergreen. While she may be correct when referring to fragrance grade oils, she is incorrect when referring to therapeutic grade oils in which case all of these oils are beneficial and pose no real risks with common sense application. The safety restrictions stated by Tiran are so great that an uninformed person would probably be afraid to use essential oils. Not Recommended.)   ISBN 0-443-06427-X

Tisserand, Robert, and Balacs, Tony. (1995) **Essential Oil Safety.** Churchill Livingstone, London. 277 pages. (Tisserand is considered the foremost aromatherapist in England. He also owns his own oil company. This book epitomizes the British point of view on using essential oils, a perspective that is so concerned about minimizing risk, that there is little possibility of real therapy taking place. In the British school, essential oils should never be taken orally or applied undiluted) to the skin. To the British, aromatherapy is massage with neutral carrier oils containing no more than 1-5% essential oils. In the preface, on p. x, the authors state, "This text was largely an extrapolation of toxicological reports from the Research Institute for Fragrant Materials (RIFM)." In other words, this book is based on data that apply only to perfume grade oils which are customarily refined, denatured, and laced with synthetics. The perfume industry cares only for fragrance and places no value on the hundreds of components of a natural oil that contribute to its healing powers but which do not contribute to its smell. Furthermore, as the authors further state, the research upon which this book is based is on animals, not humans. In addition, much of the research cited is on the toxic effects of single components of an oil, which, when extrapolated to the whole oil, is an invalid application of science. There is not one study cited in this book that applies to genuine therapeutic grade essential oil. However, without a critical understanding of the research upon which this book is based, one could be misled into believing that many oils, which are perfectly safe as therapeutic grade oils, are actually dangerous, which they are not. The chemistry in this book is well presented, but the safety recommendations are inappropriately conservative and would cause unwarranted fears against using essential oils, thus depriving many of the healing they could receive. These authors state on p. ix, "the majority of essential oils we recommend should not be available to the general public." In their opinion, the administration of essential oils should be restricted only to what they would regard as "qualified aromatherapists." Therefore, this book (Tisserand & Balacs) is incompatible with this book (*Chemistry of Essential Oils Made Simple*). This book could be useful in studying to take the ARC Exam, which is biased toward the British school of aromatherapy, however for that purpose, you are better off studying the book by Jane Buckle cited earlier in this bibliography. This book is recommended only if you are in the perfume industry or are interested in inexpensive, non-therapeutic oils for recreational aromatherapy such as scented candles and potpourri. Not recommended for those who apply oils for healing purposes.)   ISBN 0-443-05260-3

Tompkins, Peter, and Bird, Christopher (1989) *The Secret Life of Plants.* Harper & Row, New York. 402 pp. (This fascinating book concerns the astonishing abilities of plants to communicate among themselves as well as between animals, and people. The inspiring biographies of the great researchers, such as Burbank, Bose, and Carver, who discovered so much about plant behavior is woven into the text of scientific information presented in the book. This book contains nothing directly about oils, but by understanding the personalities of the plants from which they come, much insight is gained into how and why oils are what they are. Highly recommended.)   ISBN 0-06-091587-0

Valnet, Jean, (1990) *The Practice of Aromatherapy*. Healing Arts Press, Rochester, Vermont. 279 pp. (This is the first modern book written on aromatherapy. Its author, a French medical doctor, is considered by many to be "The Father of Modern Aromatherapy," because he did so much to develop and promote its practice. First published in the 1950s in France, the first English translation appeared in 1982. We can thank Robert Tisserand, British aromatherapist, for making this happen and ushering the world of aromatherapy to English speaking lands.   The decades of experience and research catalogued in his classic book are still valid today. While there is little chemistry in this book, it is a must read for everyone who wants to understand aromatherapy practice and its roots. Even though it was edited and made available in English by an aromatherapist of the British school (Tisserand), this book is definitely of the French school of aromatherapy. In fact, it is a defining text of that school. Highly recommended.)   ISBN 0-89281-398-9

Watt, Martin. (1995) ***Plant Aromatics: Oral and Dermal Toxicity of Essential Oils and Absolutes.*** Atlantic Institute of Aromatherapy (AIA), Tampa, Florida. 225 pp. (This is a revised American edition of a 1994 British publication and has the same limitations and biases as Tisserand and Balacs cited earlier. As a complication of research on perfume grade oils, it is excellent and very thorough, but has little or no information that applies to therapeutic grade oils. Therefore for those who are interested in aromatherapy for healing purposes, this publication would not be helpful and is not recommended. This publication could serve as a resource for preparation to take the ARC Exam, mentioned in the commentary under the books by Buckle and Tisserand. However, one would be better served to study for the ARC exam using Buckle's book than this one.) No ISBN.

Watt, Martin (1998) ***Reference Guide to Precautions in the Use of Aromatic Extracts from Plants.*** M. Watt, Blackmore, United Kingdom. 44 pp. (This little booklet deals with skin irritation, skin sensitization, skin photosensitization, and systemic toxicity resulting from essential oils. It is typically British and applicable only to perfume grade oils where fragrance is everything and therapy counts for nothing. A person newly acquainted with aromatherapy would, upon reading this booklet, be afraid to use any oil without the expertise of a professional aromatherapist or health care provider. This attitude is unjustifiably restrictive to the beneficial use of essential oils. Not recommended.) No ISBN

Whitaker, Julian. (1995) ***Dr. Whitaker's Guide to Natural Healing.*** Prima Publishing, Rocklin, California. 418 pp. (This is an encyclopedic treatment on dealing with disease and maintaining health by natural means. It does not contain anything about essential oils, however, but is a valuable research to have in your library for family and personal health care as an adjunct to essential oils. Recommended.)   ISBN 1-55958-495-5

Williams, David G. (1997) ***Chemistry of Essential Oils: Introduction for Aromatherapists, Beauticians, Retailers and Students.*** Michelle Press, Weymouth, England. Distributed by Scholium International, Port Washington, NY 11050. (Written for the perfume industry in the United Kingdom, this is not a book on therapeutic grade essential oils and their healing application, and the author makes that clear. Well written, the book has excellent info on the basic chemistry of oils. David Williams is an excellent teacher and presents the esoteric concepts of chemistry in very graphic and down-to-earth terms. An excellent book, but recommended only if you are very serious about the chemistry of essential oils or have a particularly strong interest in perfumes and their constituents.)   ISBN 1-870228-12-X

Worwood,Valerie Ann (1991) *Complete Book of Essential Oils & Aromatherapy*. New World Library, Novato, California. 423 pp. (While there is virtually no chemistry in this book, it is a fascinating and well-written source of historical, practical, and healing information with hundreds of formulas and applications from pregnancy, home care, and working environments, to beauty, sports and many diseases or conditions known to man. Well indexed and easy to use. It is British in its point of view, however, so disregard some of the extreme warnings such as her statement on p. xix that "calamus, tansy, and wintergreen oils should NOT be used under any circumstances." She's wrong. Calamus is a Biblical oil given in Exodus 30:22-25 as part of the holy anointing oil of Moses. Tansy is an excellent healing oil with estrogenic properties and can even be taken internally, Wintergreen applied neat is particularly good for arthritis and is a principle oil applied in raindrop therapy, which has healed thousands of many conditions. While she distinguishes perfume oils (that are largely synthetic and manipulated) from therapeutic grade oils (which are pure, natural and untampered with), she also includes oils extracted by solvents as being therapeutic grade, which we do not. She is also against all neat applications (p. 15). We recommend the book for its useful, unique and vast content not found elsewhere, but if you are looking for chemistry, you won't find it here.)   ISBN 0-931432-82-0

Wright, Henry. (2009) *A More Excellent Way*, Pleasant Valley Church, Thomaston, Georgia. 526 pp. (Based on Bible scripture and the insights of medical research, this one of the best books I know on the spiritual roots of disease. Henry Wright is not only a pastor, but has spent considerable time studying medicine as well as the physiology and microbiology of the human body. The book inclludes numerous testimonials and comes with a DVD. While there is nothing about essential oils in this book, it is highly recommended.)   ISBN 978-1-60374-101-9

Wright, Henry. (2002) *New Insights into Cancer*, Pleasant Valley Church, Thomaston, Georgia. 32 pp. (This brief booklet contains both spiritual and medical insights into the causes and cures of cancer. Discusses the physiological/spiritual/emotional connections to the body's cancer defense mechanisms in terms of hormones and cytokines, viz interleukin 2. Highly recommended.)   No ISBN

Young, D. Gary. (2000) *Science and Application of Essential Oils, Level I*. Young Living Essential Oils (YLEO), Payson, Utah. 100 pp. (This set of notes was published and distributed for participants in introductory YLEO-sponsored training programs taught by Dr. Young and his trained instructors. It contains a lot of easy-to-understand chemistry with a large number of structural formulas of the main ingredients of oils. Also contains excellent color illustrations of the biochemistry of oils and how they work at a cellular level. The only way to obtain these notes is to take the YLEO Level I Seminar which is also entitled a seminar on the "Science and Application of Essential Oils." Highly recommended.) No ISBN.

Young, D. Gary (2000) *Science and Application of Essential Oils, Level II*. Young Living Essential Oils (YLEO), Payson, Utah. 200 pp. (This set of notes was published and distributed for participants in advanced YLEO-sponsored training programs taught exclusively by Dr. Young. Contains a lot of essential oil chemistry as well as abstracts of research publications on essential oils.The only way to obtain these notes is to take the YLEO Level II Seminar. Highly recommended.) No ISBN.

Young, D. Gary. (2003) *Essential Oils Integrative Medical Guide,* Essential Science Publishing (ESP), Orem, Utah. 608 pages. (This is one of the best general references on the science and application of essential oils in print and espouses the French school of aromatherapy including all routes of administration—orally, rectally, by massage, and by inhalation. It is totally compatible with the point of view of this book (*Chemistry of Essential Oils Made Simple*). Includes listings of principal constituents of more than 90 different species of aromatic oils. This is a professional version of the book, *Essential Oils Desk Reference* (EODR), (2002) edited by Brian Manwaring listed earlier in this bibliography. All mentions of oils and oil blends are generic and not associated with any brand name as they are in the EODR. Highly recommended for serious students of essential oils interested in their healing attributes.) ISBN 0-943685-34-6

Yukteswar Giri, Sri. (1977) *The Holy Science.* SRF Publications, Los Angeles, California. 78 pp. (Originally published in 1894, this work quotes from *The Bible*—the books of Genesis, Psalms, John, I Corinthians, Hebrews and Revelation—as supporting scripture for certain scientific principles discovered by scientists and accepted by the public in general only in the the last one or two centuries. Also compares ancient scriptures from the *Hindu Vedas* that stand in harmony with those of the *Judo-Christian Scriptures*. HIghly recommended.) ISBN 0-87612-015-6

♥ Index

804   Index

808

Index

Index

Index

♥ About the Author

D avid Stewart, PhD, DNM, IASP, BCRS, LSH, studied theology, philosophy, and English literature at Central Methodist College in Fayette, Missouri (1955–58) and studied chemistry, biology, and social sciences at Central Missouri State University in Warrensburg (1962–63). He also studied commercial photography at Los Angeles Trade Technical College (1959-60). He completed a BS degree in Mathematics and Physics at Missouri School of Mines and Metallurgy in 1965 and was salutatorian of his graduating class. His MS and PhD degrees are in geophysics (theoretical seismology) and were earned from the University of Missouri at Rolla in 1969 and 1971 respectively.

He spent a semester in medical school at the University of North Carolina (1973) and has been a Certified Childbirth Educator (CCE) with the American Academy of Husband-Coached Childbirth (AAHCC) since 1975. He has spent more than 400 hours in training with D. Gary Young — internationally recognized authority on aromatherapy, essential oils, and the originator of Raindrop Technique.

Dr. Stewart became a Registered Aromatherapist (RA) in 2001. He is also an Integrated Aromatic Science Practitioner (IASP) recognized by the Canadian Government, a Board Certified Raindrop Specialist (BCRS), and a Licensed Spiritual Healer (LSH).

David Stewart is also a Doctor of Natural Medicine (DNM), His DNM degree was awarded in 2004 by the World Organization of Natural Medicine Practitioners (WONMP). He is a former faculty member of the Institute for Energy Wellness Studies (IEWS) in Brampton, Ontario, Canada.

He has held positions as a hydraulic engineer and hydrologist with the U.S. Geological Survey in Southern California (1965-67). He was a professor on the faculty of the University of North Carolina, Chapel Hill (1971–1978) where he was director of the MacCarthy Geophysics Laboratory. He also held a professorship at Southeast Missouri State University, Cape Girardeau (1988–1993) where he was founder and director of the Center for Earthquake Studies. He was a part-time United Methodist Pastor (1993–94, 1997–99) in rural Missouri. He has been the Executive Director of the InterNational Association of Parents and Professionals for Safe Alternatives in Childbirth (NAPSAC International) since its founding in 1975 until 1990.

For most of his life he has been self-employed as an author and lecturer, mainly in the area of alternative health care. He has served on advisory committees to the American Public Health Association

(APHA) and the American College of Nurse-Midwives (ACNM). He has testified as an expert on health matters before state legislative committees, U.S. congressional committees, medical licensing boards, and courts of law throughout the U.S. and Canada.

He has authored or co-authored over 300 published works, including seventeen books. Two of his publications won the "Books of the Year" Award from the *American Journal of Nursing*. One of his flyers on breastfeeding (published by La Leche League International, LLLI) sold over two million copies in ten languages. Besides this book, he is author of three other books featuring essential oils: *Healing Oils of the Bible* (available in four languages), *Statistical Validation of Raindrop Technique*, and a Bible study series entitled: *Healing: God's Forgotten Gift* (with Don Clair and Sandy Sutter). He has published numerous bookets and brochure on aromatherapy..

He has taught seminars throughout the U.S., Canada, Japan, and Australia, as well as Austria, Great Britain, Iceland, Malaysia, Romania, and Singapore. He has lectured in Lima, Peru, for the Pan American Health Organization (PAHO) and in Bogota, Colombia, for the United Nations Disaster Relief Organization (UNDRO). He has been quoted in newspapers and magazines throughout the world and has made numerous radio interviews. He has appeared on television in more than 40 countries.

As president and co-founder (with his wife, Lee) of the Center for Aromatherapy Research and Education (CARE International), he conducts training seminars leading to status as a Certified CARE Instructor (CCI), a Certified Raindrop Technique Specialist (CRTS), a Licensed Spiritual Healer (LSH), and Board Certified Raindrop Specialist (BCRS). His courses include: Healing Oils of the *Bible*, Raindrop Technique, Applied Vitaflex, Essential Oil Chemistry, and Emotional Release. If you would like to learn more about CARE's programs or attend one of Dr. Stewart's seminars, visit the website below or contact CARE and express your interest:

CARE International, RR 4, Box 646, Marble Hill, MO 63764 USA
(800) 758-8629 • careclasses@raindroptraining.com
• www.RaindropTraining.com •

Dr. Stewart lives on a 105 acre farm in Southeast Missouri with his wife, Lee. They have been married since September 1962 and have five children. They also have 12 grandchildren and two great-grandchidren (as of 2013). They attend the Marble Hill United Methodist Church where Lee is a former church treasurer, plays the piano, and directs the choir, and where David sings tenor, plays the organ, and teaches Sunday School from time to time when he is not traveling. He relaxes while beautifying his farm with his favorite toys: a tractor, brush hog, bulldozer, dump truck, and a chain saw.

♥ RESOURCES FOR TRAINING, BOOKS, DVDs, & ESSENTIAL OILS

AH   **BOOKS, VIDEOS, AROMATHERAPY SUPPLIES**
Abundant Health
222 West 3560 North
Spanish Fork, UT 84660
(888) 718-3068, (801) 798-0642, Fax: (877) 568-1988
orders@abundanthealth4u.com • www.abundanthealth4u.com

Excellent source for books, videos, DVDs, audio tapes, and a variety of useful aromatherapy supplies including essential oil carrying/storage cases, diffusers, amber glass bottles, and massage tables. Abundant Health is publisher of the *Reference Guide for Essential Oils*, by Connie & Alan Higley, a classic and essential reference for the optimal use of essential oils and which is one of the sources for the chemical compositions of essential oils cited in this book. For more info visit their website given above.

AIA   **TRAINING, BOOKS**
Atlantic Institute of Aromatherapy
16018 Saddlestring Drive
Tampa, FL 33618
(813) 265-2222
sylla@atlanticinstitute.com • www.Atlantic Institute.com

AIA offers educational opportunities through courses and books. They offer seminars on a variety of aromatherapy topics including essential oil chemistry. The AIA reflects the British viewpoint of aromatherapy. For more information visit their website given above.

CARE   **TRAINING, BOOKS, DVDS, FREE NEWSLETTER**
CARE International
Center for Aromatherapy Research & Education
RR 4, Box 646
Marble Hill, MO 63764
(800) 758-8629
careclasses@raindroptraining.com • www.RaindropTraining.com

CARE International publishes books, CDs and DVDs on the art and science of therapeutic applications of essential oils. CARE offers a 164 hour program toward becoming a Certified CARE Instructor (CCI). Included are 25 hours of formal course work in Applied Vitaflex, Raindrop Technique, Essential Oil Chemistry, Emotional Release with Oils, and Healing Oils of the Bible. Seminars offering one or more of these courses are taught by CCIs throughout Canada and the United States, more than 150 seminars each year, and sometimes in other countries. CARE also sponsors trainings in Vibrational Raindrop Technique and Animal Raindrop Technique.

The Center for Aromatherapy Research and Education is approved by the National Certification Board for Therapeutic Massage and Bodywork (NCBTMB) and the International Association of Continuing Education Training (IACET) as a continuing education Approved Provider. (Provider numbers are 408294-00 & 1307732 respectively). CARE's courses and credits are also recognied by the Natural Therapies Certification Board (NTCB).

CARE offers professional credits for Vitaflex, Raindrop, Chemistry, Emotional Release, Oils of Scripture, and Vibrational Raindrop Technique at both basic and advanced levels.

Visit www.RaindropTraining.com for more details as well as a calendar of courses and seminars. Subscribe to the FREE e-line newsletter (*The Raindrop Messenger*) by visiting the CARE website. For information on becoming a CCI, you need a *CCI Handbook* ($9.95, 128 pp.) available on the website or by calling the toll-free number.

HTSM   **TRAINING, BOOKS, DVDS**
Healing Touch Spiritual Ministry
P.O. Box 741239
Arvada, CO 80006
(303) 467-7829, Fax (303) 467-2328
staff@HTSpiritualMinistry.com • www.HTSpiritualMinistry.com
And also, www.ISHAaromatherapy.com

HTSM offers classes throughout North America leading to several types of certificates, one of which entitles you to use the title "Certified Clinical Aromatherapist" or CCA. Approved by the National Association of Holistic Aromatherapists (NAHA), completing requirements to be an HTSM-CCA prepares you and makes you eligible to sit for the Aromatherapy Registration Council (ARC) exam and become a "Registered Aromatherapist" or RA. One may also become an HTSM Instructor. Visit their website for details. HTSM uses this and other books by Dr. Stewart, in their courses. HTSM President and Founder, Linda L. Smith, is author of the book, *Healing Hands Healing Oils* which is subtitled, "Discovering the Power of Prayer, Hands On Healing, and Anointing." It is available from CARE at www.RaindropTraining.com.

IEWS   TRAINING, BOOKS, DVDS
Institute for Energy Wellness Studies
7700 Hurontario St. S., Suite 408
Brampton, Ontario, Canada L6Y 4M3
(905) 451-4475, Fax (905) 451-5036
sabinadevita@idirect.com • www.energywellnessstudies.com

    IEWS classes are taught on campus in Brampton, near Toronto. They train people to be practitioners in a variety of modalities offering certificates, degrees, and diplomas recognized throughout Canada and the 16 other countries of the British Commonwealth. One may earn the title of Integrated Aromatic Science Practitioner (IASP) or Certified Natural Medicine Practitioner, which are recognized by the Canadian Examining Board. IASP entitles you to legally practice vitaflex, raindrop and other hands on techniques without any other license. IEWS training requires all three of Dr. Stewart's aromatherapy books, including this one. Dr. Stewart, who is a former IEWS faculty member.

LSP   BOOKS, DVDS
Life Science Publications
1216 South 1580 West, Suite A
Orem, UT 84058
(800) 336-6308, (801) 224-6228, Fax: (801) 224-6229
www.LifeSciencePublishers.com

    LSP offers a wide selection of aromatherapy related books, videos, DVDs, audiotapes, training CDs and other items for sale. They are publishers of the *Essential Oils Desk Reference*, an essential reference on therapeutic applications of aromatic oils and which is one of the sources for the chemical composition of essential oils cited in this book. For more info visit their website given above. LSP sells all of Dr. Stewart's aromatherapy books and packages his book, *A Statistical Validation of Raindrop*, with Dr. Gary Young's booklet on raindrop technique.

PIA   TRAINING, AV PRODUCTS, BOOKS
Pacific Institute of Aromatherapy
P.O. Box 6723
San Rafael, CA 94903
(415) 479-9121, Fax: (415) 479-0119
www.pacificinstituteofaromatherapy.com

    PIA offers educational opportunities through courses, seminars, conferences, powerpoint presentations, videos, DVDs, and books. PIA offers two levels of aromatherapy education. The Aromatherapy Course is a Level One, three-day certification seminar; and Level Two is the PIA

<u>Masters Program</u>, available as home study or on location over six weekends in San Rafael. Kurt Schnaubelt, Ph.D., author of several books we recommend, is a German aromatherapist trained in France by Daniel Penoel, MD. Dr. Schnaubelt is the founder and executive director of this school. On the PIA website you may choose either English or German.

SC   BOOKS, BOOKLETS, PAMPHLETS, DVDs, CDs, TABLOIDS
Sound Concepts
782 South Auto Mall Drive
American Fork, UT 84003
(800) 524-4195 or (801) 225-9520
www.EssentialProductInfo.com or www.crowndiamondtools.com

   Sound Concepts publishes a large variety of excellent top quality informational and promotional materials specifically made for Young Living products. Several of their books, booklets, brochures, newspapers, and CDs are written or narrated by Dr. David Stewart and can help you build your YL Business. Visit their two websites and browse. You will also want to visit the Sound Concepts booth at the Young Living Grand Convention each year to see and experience samples of the great resources they can provide for you.

YLEO   TRAINING, THERAPEUTIC OILS
Young Living Essential Oils
Thanksgiving Point Business Park
3125 West Executive Parkway
Lehi, UT 84043
(800) 371-3515, Fax: (866) 203-5666
www.YoungLiving.com

   YLEO sells a wide variety of top grade therapeutic essential oils and offers training on a variety of aspects of aromatherapy. The American Botanical Council (ABC) data bank with comprehensive information on herbs and their medicinal properties is available via the YLEO website. YLEO recommended Dr. Stewart's Chemistry book in their June 2005 issue of *The Essential Edge.*.
   Young Living markets their oils by a network of distributors. One can enroll with the company to purchase these oils as a customer or as a distributor via the website or phone number given above or by contacting any YLEO distributor.
   If you do not know a YLEO distributor and cannot find one, you may also purchase YLEO therapeutic oils on the internet at this website: http://BibleOils.YoungLivingWorld.com. Any oil blends mentioned in this book by a brand name and designated with TM or ® are registered with YLEO.